Harries' Paediatric Gastroenterology

Harries' Paediatric Gastroenterology

EDITED BY

Peter J. Milla MSc, MB BS, FRCP

Senior Lecturer in Child Health, Department of Child Health, Institute of Child Health, London; Honorary Consultant Paediatric Gastroenterologist, The Hospital for Sick Children, Great Ormond Street, London

D. P. R. Muller BSc, PhD

Senior Lecturer in Biochemistry, Department of Child Health, Institute of Child Health, London

SECOND EDITION

CHURCHILL LIVINGSTONE
EDINBURGH LONDON MELBOURNE AND NEW YORK 1988

CHURCHILL LIVINGSTONE
Medical Division of Longman Group UK Limited

Distributed in the United States of America by
Churchill Livingstone Inc., 1560 Broadway, New
York, N.Y. 10036, and by associated companies,
branches and representatives throughout the world.

First edition 1977
Second edition 1988

ISBN 0-443-03058-8

British Library Cataloguing in Publication Data
Harries' Paediatric gastroenterology.
— 2nd ed.
1. Pediatric gastroenterology
I. Harries, J. T. II. Milla, Peter J.
III. Essentials of paediatric
gastroenterology
618.92'3   RJ446

Library of Congress Cataloging in Publication Data
Essentials of paediatric gastroenterology.
Harries' paediatric gastroenterology.

Rev. ed. of: Essentials of paediatric gastro-
enterology/edited by J. T. Harries. 1977.
Includes index.
1. Pediatric gastroenterology. I. Harries,
J. T. (John Thomas) II. Milla, Peter J. III. Title.
[DNLM: 1. Gastrointestinal Diseases — in infancy &
childhood. WS 310 E78]
RJ446.E87   1987   618.92'33   87–8077

Produced by Longman Singapore
Publishers (Pte) Ltd
Printed in Singapore

In memory of 'J. T. H.'

Preface to the Second Edition

In the months prior to his untimely death John Harries had been planning the second edition of *Essentials of Paediatric Gastroenterology* — a task that he undertook with great enthusiasm. Since the first edition, paediatric gastroenterology has come of age and there has been an explosion of new knowledge. Thus the second edition was to be bigger in order to take account of all the exciting advances that had been made and to include many contributors from overseas, yet, it was to retain the style of the original edition. The death of John Harries was a great blow not only to his family, colleagues and friends but also to paediatric gastroenterology to which he brought a unique blend of clinical and scientific skills. We, his closest colleagues, had no hesitation in deciding that the second edition should go ahead and were delighted to accept the task of coediting this volume. The book is therefore dedicated to a remarkable man who awoke our interest in paediatric gastroenterology and showed us that clinical practice combined with laboratory research could be stimulating, rewarding and above all, fun.

The purpose of this book is to cover in a moderate sized volume the important areas of paediatric gastroenterology. Although it is written primarily for the general paediatrician we hope that paediatric surgeons, undergraduate and postgraduate students and those with a special interest in paediatric gastroenterology will find the book a source of useful information.

The book is arranged in four sections. The first which is essential for a proper understanding of the subject considers the development, organization, physiology and biochemistry of the gastrointestinal tract and associated organs, together with the relevant investigatory techniques. The second and third parts deal with clinical questions relating principally to the alimentary tract and the liver respectively. The last section is concerned with a major raison d'être for the gastrointestinal tract, namely the provision of nutrition. An extended and up-to-date bibliography is included at the end of each chapter.

This book would not have been possible without the support of our families, colleagues and friends and we are particularly indebted to Professors Otto Wolff and June Lloyd for their constant support and encouragement. We would like to thank our contributors for their cooperation, our publishers for their guidance and forbearance and Miss Elisabeth Moore for secretarial help.

1988   P. J. Milla and D. P. R. Muller

Preface to the First Edition

The purpose of this book is to present a volume of moderate size which attempts to cover the important areas of a rapidly growing specialty, paediatric gastroenterology. It is written primarily for the practising general paediatrician, but hopefully it will also be a useful source of information to the paediatric surgeon, the undergraduate and postgraduate student, as well as to those with a special interest in paediatric gastroenterology. To this end moderately extensive bibliographies have been included in selected parts of the book, providing an opportunity for readers to pursue certain subjects in greater depth.

The book is arranged in three parts. The first deals with the prenatal development of structure and function, the interrelationships between structure and function with particular emphasis on the small gut, and an account of the currently available investigatory techniques. The pre- and postnatal development of hepatic, pancreatic and alimentary tract structure and function represents a relatively neglected, albeit extremely important, area of paediatric gastroenterology which has major implications with regard to nutritional practices in the newborn as well as in the older infant. In recent years major advances have been made in our understanding of the intricate and subtle relationships which exist between the structure and function of biological tissues involved in the digestion, transport and metabolism of nutrients, and an understanding of these interrelationships can only lead to the enhanced clinical care of patients. A wide range of techniques are now available for investigating children with gastroenterological problems, and these are described in Chapter 3.

The second part of the book considers a variety of conditions but, in the main, is orientated towards the alimentary tract. It begins with an account of the surgical conditions which can affect the newborn and older child, and of chronic inflammatory bowel disease. It continues with chapters on the long-term effects and management of children following intestinal resections, and on the effects of malnutrition on the structure and function of the alimentary tract, liver and pancreas. The important area of small intestinal enteropathies is covered in detail, as is infective diarrhoea and vomiting; both represent major world problems. The selective inborn errors of absorption are 'accidents of nature' and represent a unique group of disorders which are only rarely encountered in paediatric practice. Nevertheless they are important, since early diagnosis and treatment may be life-saving as, for example, in congenital glucose-galactose malabsorption; diagnosis is also important in terms of genetic counselling. Moreover, there is much to be learnt about 'alternative' transport systems from these genetically determined disorders of absorption, since the clinical manifestations invariably improve with age. For these reasons, a brief account is included. Parasitic infestations, protein-losing enteropathies and gastrointestinal disturbances related to psychological disturbances conclude this section of the book.

The third and final part of the book is devoted to disorders of the liver and pancreas in childhood. The inborn errors of hepatic metabolism, persistent neonatal jaundice, infections of the liver and chronic liver disease are considered in some detail; tumours of the liver and disorders of the pancreas are discussed in the two concluding chapters.

The role of gastrointestinal hormones and disturbed immune function in the pathogenesis of gastrointestinal disturbances have been integrated into the appropriate sections of the book, rather than given individual attention.

The clinical conditions encountered in paediatric gastroenterology pose fundamentally different problems to those encountered in adult patients, and this is particularly the case during the first few years of life. For example, during the first year of life a variety of biological processes are immature, and disease may have irreversible and permanent effects. Malnutrition secondary to malabsorption can interfere with brain cell replication and result in permanent intellectual defects. Acute infectious diarrhoea and/or vomiting, and its complications, may be a devastating event in the life of a young child and his family. Similarly, surgical procedures in the newborn and older infant present problems which are different to those encountered in the adult patient. The relationship between gastrointestinal symptoms and psychological disturbances in the child and its family, and the diseases which affect the liver in childhood, are other examples which emphasise some of the differences between paediatric and adult gastroenterology. These are some of the reasons why I accepted an invitation to edit a book which I thought should be concerned with the 'essentials' of paediatric gastroenterology, and why the above areas of paediatrics were selected as prominent items in the genesis of this volume. They delineate but do not separate the concept of adult from paediatric gastroenterology. Collaboration between paediatric and adult physicians and surgeons concerned with gastroenterological problems is critical to our understanding and to the clinical care of gastrointestinal disease at any age.

This book would not have been possible without the generous advice and support of my colleagues and family, to whom I am deeply grateful and to whom the book is dedicated. My interest in paediatric gastroenterology was born within myself, but was catalysed by Sir Wilfrid Sheldon and Dr Tony Dawson. The opportunity to establish a clinical and research team in paediatric gastroenterology resulted from the efforts, encouragement and support of Professor Otto Wolff and Professor June Lloyd. David Muller has been a constant source of intellectual and friendly inspiration. I am indebted to John Tripp, John McCollum and Peter Milla for many helpful discussions. I have been fortunate to be associated with the above mentioned people and have learnt much from them.

I wish to record my thanks to all the contributors for their tolerance and co-operation in my editorial duties, and I am indebted to my publishers for their patience and guidance. Last, but not least, I extend my gratitude to Miss Anna Curtis for an enormous amount of secretarial help.

1977   J. T. Harries

Contributors

I. W. Booth, MSc, BSc, MB, MRCP, DObstRCOG, DCH
Senior Lecturer in Paediatrics and Child Health, Institute of Child Health, University of Birmingham; Honorary Consultant Physician, The Children's Hospital, Birmingham

David C. A. Candy, MB BS, MSc, MRCP, MD
Wellcome Senior Lecturer, Department of Paediatrics and Child Health, University of Birmingham; Honorary Consultant Paediatrician, The Children's Hospital, Birmingham

R. K. Chandra, MD, FRCP(C)
Professor, Departments of Paediatrics, Medicine and Biochemistry, Memorial University of Newfoundland, St. John's, Newfoundland, Canada

James A. S. Dickson, MB ChB, FRCS(Edin), FRCS
Consultant Paediatric Surgeon, Children's Hospital, Sheffield

T. R. Fenton, MB BS, MRCP, MSc
Research Fellow, Institute of Child Health, London; Honorary Senior Registrar, The Hospital for Sick Children, London

Dorothy E. M. Francis, SRD
Group Chief Dietitian, The Hospital for Sick Children, London

Richard J. Grand, MB
Chief, Division of Pediatric Gastroenterology and Nutrition, The Floating Hospital, New England Medical Centre; Professor of Pediatrics, Tufts University School of Medicine, Boston, USA

Leo A. Heitlinger, MD
Research Assistant Professor, Department of Pediatrics, State University of New York at Buffalo; Attending Physician for Gastroenterology and Nutrition, Children's Hospital at Buffalo, USA

Vinay K. Jain, MD
Associate Professor, Department of Paediatrics, Memorial University of Newfoundland, St. John's, Newfoundland, Canada

Jean W. Keeling, MB BS, FRCPath
Consultant Paediatric Pathologist, John Radcliffe Maternity Hospital, Oxford

Bryan Lask, MB BS, MPhil, MRCPsych
Consultant Psychiatrist, The Hospital for Sick Children, London

Emanuel Lebenthal, MD
Professor of Pediatrics, State University of New York at Buffalo, Medical School; Director, International Institute for Infant Nutrition and Gastrointestinal Disease, and Chief, Division of Gastroenterology and Nutrition, Children's Hospital at Buffalo, USA

J. V. Leonard, PhD, FRCP
Reader in Child Health, Institute of Child Health, London; Honorary Consultant Physician, The Hospital for Sick Children, London

Fima Lifshitz, MD
Associate Director of Pediatrics, Chief of Pediatric Endocrinology, Metabolism and Nutrition, and Chief of Pediatric Research, North Shore University Hospital, New York; Professor of Pediatrics, Cornell University Medical College, New York, USA

June K. Lloyd, MD, FRCP
Nuffield Professor of Child Health, Institute of Child Health, University of London

Alan Lucas, MA, MB BChir, MRCP
Medical Research Council Dunn Nutrition Unit and University Department of Paediatrics Cambridge

A. S. McNeish, MSc, MB ChB(Glas), FRCP, FRCP(Glas)
Professor of Paediatrics and Child Health, and Director of the Institute of Child Health, London

Giorgina Mieli-Vergani, MD(Milan), PhD
Senior Lecturer in Paediatric Hepatology, King's College Hospital, London

Peter J. Milla, MSc, MB BS, FRCP
Senior Lecturer in Child Health, Department of Child Health, Institute of Child Health, London; Honorary Consultant Paediatric Gastroenterologist, The Hospital for Sick Children, Great Ormond Street, London

Alex P. Mowat, MB ChB, FRCP, DCH, DObstRCOG
Consultant Paediatrician and Paediatric Hepatologist, Department of Child Health, King's College School of Medicine and Dentistry, London

D. P. R. Muller, BSc, PhD
Senior Lecturer in Biochemistry, Department of Child Health, Institute of Child Health, London

Alan D. Phillips, BA(Hons)
Principal Electron Microscopist, Queen Elizabeth Hospital for Children, London

Ross Pinkerton, MD, MRCP, DCH
Clinical Research Fellow, Department of Haematology and Oncology, The Hospital for Sick Children, London

Jon Pritchard, FRCP
Consultant Paediatric Oncologist, The Hospital for Sick Children and (Hon) St Bartholomew's Hospital, London; Senior Lecturer in Paediatric Oncology, Institute of Child Health, London

Jacques Schmitz, MD
Associate Professor of Paediatrics, Département de Pédiatrie, Hôpital des Enfants-Malades, Paris, France

Val Shaw, BPharm
Staff Pharmacist, The Hospital for Sick Children, London

Lewis Spitz, PhD, FRCS
Nuffield Professor of Paediatric Surgery, Institute of Child Health, University of London;
Consultant Paediatric Surgeon, The Hospital for Sick Children, London

R. J. Stafford, MD
Clinical Instructor, Department of Pediatrics, University of Minnesota, Minneapolis, USA

Saul Teichberg, PhD
Associate Professor of Cell Biology in Pediatrics, Cornell University Medical College, New
York; Head, Electron Microscopy Laboratory, North Shore University Hospital, New
York, USA

J. A. Walker-Smith, MD(Sydney), FRCP, FRCP(Edin), FRACP
Professor of Paediatric Gastroenterology, Medical College of St Bartholomew's Hospital at
Queen Elizabeth Hospital for Children, London

Raul A. Wapnir, PhD, MPH
Professor of Biochemistry in Pediatrics, Cornell University Medical College, New York;
Head, Special Studies Laboratory, Division of Pediatric Endocrinology, Metabolism and
Nutrition, Department of Pediatrics, North Shore University Hospital, New York, USA

Edward R. Wozniak, BSc, MB BS, MRCP, DCH
Consultant Paediatrician, St Mary's Hospital, Portsmouth

S. G. Wright, MB, MRCP
Associate Professor, Department of Medicine, College of Medicine, King Saud University,
Riyadh, Saudi Arabia

Contents

PART 1

Prenatal and perinatal development of the gastrointestinal tract

INTRODUCTION

The improved care of respiratory disease in the preterm infant has resulted in nutrition becoming the critical factor for their survival. Thus the state of maturation of the gastrointestinal tract will largely determine whether the transition from intrauterine to extrauterine life will be successful or not. In the preterm and to a much lesser extent the full term infant, gastrointestinal function may be insufficiently developed to allow adequate nutrition and to regulate hydration.

The morphological and functional maturation of the digestive system begins during gestation and continues postnatally. The anatomical differentiation of the fetal gut resembles that of the newborn infant by 28 weeks of gestation, but the segmental rates of maturation are distinctly different from one region to another, and follow a predictable species-specific pattern (Lebenthal & Lee 1981). Therefore, in order to define morphological and functional maturity, each component of the digestive system must be reviewed separately.

A sound understanding of pre- and perinatal gastrointestinal tract development is crucial to the successful nutritional care of the premature and compromised infant. In this chapter developmental patterns in the human fetus, neonate and infant will be discussed and the physiological basis of neonatal and infant nutrition reviewed.

EARLY DEVELOPMENT OF THE FERTILIZED OVUM

The spherical fertilized ovum, within its trophoblastic covering embedded in the uterine wall, divides into numerous cells from which the different systems and organs of the body will develop. The germ layers are the inner

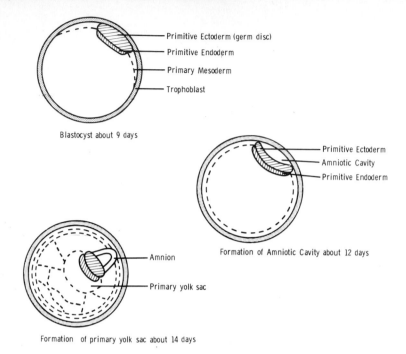

Fig. 1.1 Formation of amniotic cavity and primary yolk sac from the fertilized ovum.

endoderm, the outer ectoderm and between them the mesoderm. These layers are laid down in the first three weeks of prenatal life, and between three and eight weeks rapid growth and differentiation takes place during which time all the major systems and organs of the body are established. During the first seven days the fertilized ovum or blastocyst is embedding itself in the uterine wall. The primitive ectoderm separates from the trophoblast by the formation of a cavity, the amniotic cavity. On the opposite surface a single layer of primitive endoderm forms between the ectoderm and the blastocyst cavity. In the succeeding stages the blastocyst cavity becomes lined with mesodermal cells which are in continuity with the endoderm around its margins. These stages are shown in Figure 1.1. The cells of the primitive germ layers now become arranged in a more regular manner and the primary yolk sac undergoes a marked reduction in size, during which time a cavity appears within the endoderm, the secondary yolk sac. In the roof of the sac the endoderm is in contact with the ectoderm and forms a bilaminar embryonic disc, which is roughly circular in shape. This stage occurs towards the end of the second week and is show in Figure 1.2. Only the tissue of the embryonic disc contributes to the formation of the embryo.

The alimentary tract and its derivatives originate from the splanchnopleure of the embryonic disc. As shown in Figure 1.2, the splanchnopleure is composed of two layers, a mesodermal layer which gives rise to muscle

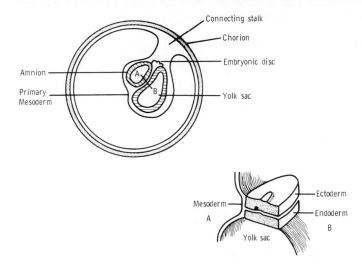

Fig. 1.2 Development of the splanchnopleure of the embryonic disc.

and connective tissue elements, and an endodermal layer which forms the epithelium of the intestinal tract and the parenchyma of the liver and pancreas.

From Figure 1.2 it will be seen that the yolk sac is an ovoid cavity with a roof of endoderm. With development of the cranial and caudal extensions of the embryonic disc the yolk sac becomes differentiated into fore-, mid-, and hindgut, as shown in Figure 1.3. The foregut gives rise to the pharynx, thyroid, thymus, parathyroid glands, respiratory tract, oesophagus, stomach, upper duodenum, liver and pancreas. The lower duodenum, small and large intestine, as far as the distal third of the transverse colon, are formed from the midgut. The remainder of the large bowel arises from the hindgut.

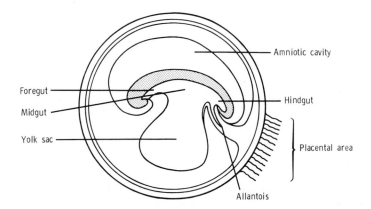

Fig. 1.3 Differentiation of yolk sac into fore-, mid- and hindgut.

MORPHOLOGICAL DEVELOPMENT

Gross structural development

By four weeks the primitive gut is identifiable as a tubular structure extending from mouth to cloaca. It is suspended dorsally by the dorsal mesentery which extends along the whole length of the intra-abdominal gut, and ventrally by a thick mesentery which extends from the septum transversum to the intra-abdominal portion of the foregut. Between four and six weeks the cranial part of the foregut changes from a flattened tube into a complicated series of structures, the branchial arch system; in man this system is transitory and is almost entirely obliterated by seven weeks. Occasionally, however, epithelial-lined cysts, sinuses or fistulae may result from incomplete obliteration of the branchial arch system.

The pharynx and oesophagus

Concurrent with the development of the pharynx the cranial ends of the oesophagus and trachea become demarcated, growth of the former occurring at a later stage when the embryo grows cranially. Two events may result in congenital malformation. Partitioning of the foregut into oesophagus and trachea can result in one of the various types of tracheo-oesophageal fistulae, with or without oesophageal atresia. The formation of the cardia results from the coordinated development of the oesophagus, stomach, diaphragm and their autonomic innervation; failure of coordination may result in either a structural abnormality, such as an oesophageal web, or in a functional defect, such as achalasia.

The stomach

The rudimentary stomach appears at the caudal end of the foregut as a fusiform dilatation, and beyond this the gut opens into the yolk sac (see Fig. 1.3). At first the opening is wide but by the fifth week it has become narrowed into a tubular stalk, the vitellointestinal duct, following which the stomach soon loses its connection with the duct. Growth alterations lead to the final shape and position of the stomach. The dorsal mesentery increases in depth and folds upon itself to form the greater omentum, and the ventral mesentery forms the lesser omentum. During its development there is little alteration in the form of the stomach, and malformations are consequently very rare.

The small and large intestine

The terminal portion of the foregut and the cranial end of the midgut grow rapidly to form a loop which becomes the duodenum, the apex of the loop representing the junction between the fore- and midgut. During gastric

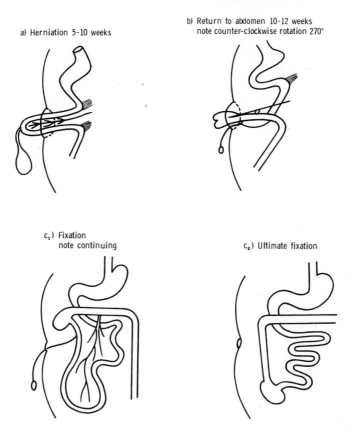

a) Herniation 5-10 weeks

b) Return to abdomen 10-12 weeks
note counter-clockwise rotation 270°

c₁) Fixation
note continuing

c₂) Ultimate fixation

Fig. 1.4 Sequential events leading to the ultimate fixation and position of the gut within the abdomen.

growth the duodenum is carried dorsally and to the right, and the mesentery is ultimately approximated to and absorbed by the dorsal peritoneum, rendering the duodenum retroperitoneal. While the stomach is growing, the midgut is increasing its length more rapidly than the embryo and forms a U-shaped loop which acquires a dorsal mesentery. At the apex of the loop is the vitellointestinal duct demarcating a cranial and caudal limb. As a result of this growth discrepancy, a series of manoeuvres occur which culminate in the final position of the gut within the abdomen, and these are depicted in Figure 1.4. From a simple straight tube the gut has undergone a counter-clockwise rotation of 270°.

The dorsal mesentery from the duodenojejunal flexure to the ileocaecal junction remains as the mesentery of the small intestine, and the mesenteries of the ascending and descending colon become fused with the parietal peritoneum. The transverse colon retains its mesentery which later fuses with the greater omentum.

The majority of small intestinal and proximal large intestinal malformations are related to three events: (1) failure of the endoderm of the yolk sac to separate from the notochord during the third week, which results in a variety of reduplications of the intestine, (2) failure of the vitellointestinal duct to regress during the fifth week, which results in a Meckel's diverticulum and other vestigial abnormalities, and (3) failures in herniation, return and fixation of the intestine between the fifth and twelfth weeks; failure at any stage may result in anomalies such as malrotation, exomphalos or an undescended caecum.

The hindgut becomes established early and a ventral diverticulum, the allantois, arises from it (see Fig. 1.3). Just caudal to the junction of the allantois and hindgut the cloaca develops, and the junction between the allantois and hindgut becomes the cloacal membrane. During the sixth week the cloaca becomes flattened from side to side and elongates in the sagittal plane. A septum forms to divide the cloaca dorsally into rectum and ventrally into the urogenital sinus. The part of the cloacal membrane sealing the rectum usually ruptures between the eighth and ninth weeks. Congenital defects of the anus and rectum resemble those of the oesophagus and are associated one with another more frequently than by chance; anal and rectal anomalies may arise from abnormalities occurring at several different stages of development. Duhamel (1961) has proposed a syndrome of caudal regression, with anorectal malformations as the milder expression, and sirenoid monsters as the most extreme form.

The liver and biliary system

The liver and biliary system arise from that region of the gut endoderm which also gives rise to the duodenum. At four weeks an hepatic diverticulum can be seen at the ventral aspect of the duodenum which has two portions, a cranial bud which differentiates into hepatic cells and bile ducts, and a caudal bud which becomes the gall bladder and cystic duct. The developmental events are depicted in Figure 1.5. The cranial bud divides into two main branches which form the right and left lobes of the liver. Initially these are of equal size, but after the third month the right lobe becomes larger and parts of this lobe then form the subordinate lobes. The hepatic cells divide rapidly so that the liver increases rapidly in size, and at 10 weeks it occupies most of the abdominal cavity. At the same time the original diverticulum elongates and differentiates into the hepatic duct and common bile duct. At birth the liver is relatively large in size but it is unusual for any anomalies to occur in its development. Occasionally an accessory lobe (Riedel's lobe) grows from the right lobe and can be easily palpated below the right costal margin.

Whilst the cranial bud of the hepatic diverticulum is developing into the liver and common bile duct, the caudal region of the diverticulum elongates to form the cystic duct during the fifth week of embryonic life. This

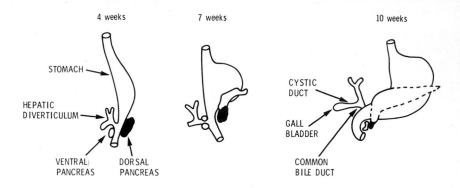

4 weeks   7 weeks   10 weeks

STOMACH

HEPATIC
DIVERTICULUM

VENTRAL   DORSAL
PANCREAS   PANCREAS

CYSTIC
DUCT

GALL
BLADDER

COMMON
BILE DUCT

Fig. 1.5 Origin and development of the hepatic diverticulum and pancreas.

expands at its distal end to form the gall bladder. Initially the gall bladder and hepatic ducts are hollow; proliferation of the epithelial lining temporarily converts them into solid cords and recanalization takes place by seven weeks. The gall bladder usually lies in a shallow bed on the undersurface of the liver, but congenital anomalies involving the biliary tract are relatively common with a frequency of 10%. The gall bladder may be absent, as in certain animals (e.g. the rat and the horse), a double gall bladder may be present and occasionally it may develop a mesentery of its own and hence be liable to torsion. Rarely a cystic dilation of the common bile duct (choledochal cyst) may develop. The commonest congenital anomaly is atresia of the bile ducts, which was considered to be due to failure of recanalization of the ducts, but this is almost certainly not the sole explanation; for example, atresia may represent the end result of an inflammatory process during fetal development.

As soon as the cranial portion of the hepatic diverticulum is formed it rapidly proliferates to form cords of epithelial cells. These grow rapidly to develop into a network of branching epithelial strands. The intrahepatic bile ducts arise as tributaries of the hepatic duct at eight weeks, differentiating into interlobular ducts at points of contact with connective tissue. The bile canaliculi extend between the hepatic cells and are continuous with the interlobular bile ducts. The canaliculi and intrahepatic ducts are probably formed from the liver cells.

The pancreas

Like the hepatobiliary system the pancreas also develops from the gut endoderm. Between three and four weeks two outpocketings arise from opposite sides of the duodenum, representing the earliest signs of pancreatic development. The dorsal pancreas extends out from the duodenum just cranial to the level of the hepatic diverticulum, and the ventral pancreas appears in the caudal angle between the gut and hepatic diverticulum (see

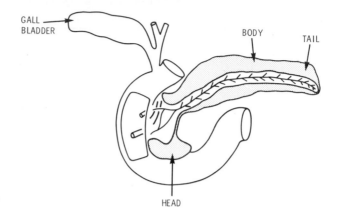

Fig. 1.6 Fusion of dorsal and ventral pancreas to form the head, body and tail of the pancreas.

Fig. 1.5). The dorsal pancreas grows rapidly into the dorsal mesentery, and by six weeks it is an elongated nodular structure. The ventral pancreas grows more slowly and remains closely associated with the developing hepatic diverticulum. The hepatic diverticulum forms the common bile duct and, as a result of this close relationship, a common exit into the duodenum develops for the biliary system and the pancreas.

As the duodenum grows the ventral pancreas and bile ducts are swept behind the duodenum to meet the dorsal pancreas, and at eight weeks the dorsal and ventral primordia fuse, the dorsal pancreas forms the tail, body and part of the head, whilst the majority of the head and the uncinate process arise from the ventral pancreas (Fig. 1.6). Failure of migration of the ventral pancreas may result in the formation of an annular pancreas, which in one study was found in 13.7% of 410 autopsies (Feldman & Weinberg 1952).

Both the dorsal and ventral pancreas have an axial duct. The dorsal duct arises directly from the duodenal wall, and the ventral duct unites with the common bile duct as it arises from the duodenum. At eight weeks, when the pancreas is relatively mature, the dorsal duct drains the body and tail and unites with the ventral duct to form the main pancreatic duct of Wirsung. Thus, bile and pancreatic juice have a common outlet into the duodenum at the ampulla of Vater. A circular layer of muscle develops around this outlet to form the sphincter of Oddi. The proximal end of the dorsal duct may either become a tributary of the main pancreatic duct or retain its opening into the duodenum, when it is known as the accessory duct of Santorini. This accessory duct is patent in up to 70% of adult subjects (Kleitsch 1955), but in only 10% is it the only exit into the duodenum; in the remainder pancreatic juice reaches the duodenum through both openings.

The mature pancreas is an elongated lobular gland, the head lying in close proximity to the duodenal loop. It is covered by a thin layer of connective tissue derived from the dorsal mesenchyme; the dorsal mesenchyme also grows into the developing gland, giving the mature pancreas its characteristic lobular appearance.

Differentiation

The various tissues of the gastrointestinal tract differentiate in an inherent species-dependent pattern upon which some individual variation occurs. The pattern is ill-understood but includes genetic, species-specific endogenous regulatory mechanisms, and environmental factors. The pattern of development follows a fairly well established sequence of primordial differentiation into ecto-, meso-, and endoderm, followed by anatomical specialization involving interactions of these three germ layers. Specific organs of the alimentary tract develop at different rates. Active transport occurs in the small intestine by 14 weeks gestation (Koldovsky et al 1965), yet in the neonate the pancreas can hardly be stimulated to secrete (Lebenthal & Lee 1980).

The oesophagus, stomach and intestine

Although the epithelium of most of the alimentary tract is of endodermal origin, differentiation varies according to the region of the tract. Thus in the oesophagus it differentiates to stratified squamous epithelium, in the stomach it forms gastric glands which contain a variety of secretory cells and in the small and large intestine both absorptive and secretory cells develop. Epithelial differentiation is initiated by exuberant proliferation of cells which may completely occlude the lumen, particularly in the oesophagus and small intestine. Failure of recanalization of the lumen may account for some congenital small gut atresias.

In the oesophagus a single lumen is restored by the ninth to tenth weeks and is lined by ciliated cells, which are replaced by stratified squamous cells during the fifth month.

The first glandular pits of the stomach appear at six weeks, and by 12 weeks parietal, chief and mucous cells have differentiated.

The differentiation and development of the small intestine has been more extensively studied than any other region of the gastrointestinal tract. Differentiation of the intestinal tract of the human occurs relatively much earlier in gestation than in the rat and thus extreme caution should be employed in extrapolating from such data.

Initially a single layer of cells is arranged radially towards the lumen; they contain large nuclei occupying most of the cytoplasm, the mitochondria are elongated and rough endoplasmic reticulum is present. Between eight and ten weeks a transition takes place in a craniocaudal direction from stratified to columnar cells; during this transition specialized junctional complexes and secondary lumina develop (Moxey & Trier 1978). The secondary lumina play a crucial role in the remodelling of the mucosa and eventual villus formation by a processs of fusion of the secondary lumina with the main lumen. Well defined villi are present by 10–11 weeks and crypts by 12 weeks. (Johnson 1910; Patzelt 1931; Moxey & Trier 1978).

The absorptive cells which line the villi resemble mature enteroytes with a well developed apical microvillus, and 'tight' junctions or desmosomes, but have an abundant apical tubular system. The Golgi apparatus has expanded and there are many lysosome-like meconium corpuscles (Bierring et al 1964, Anderson et al 1964). Goblet endocrine and Paneth cells are all present. (Moxey & Trier 1977). The presence of these cells suggests that they may play an important role in creating the correct microenvironment for morphogenesis and differentiation.

In the large intestine, villi and glandular cells appear in the colon during the third month. The villi reach their maximum development during the fourth month and thereafter gradually shorten and disappear; goblet and simple columnar cells appear by the eleventh week (Lacroix et al 1984).

The musculature of the bowel arises from mesoderm and develops in a craniocaudal direction, differentiation of the inner circular layer preceding that of the outer longitudinal layer.

Innervation of the bowel also proceeds in a craniocaudal direction. The neuroblasts of the myenteric plexus migrate down the alimentary tract with the vagus nerve preceding formation of the longitudinal muscle layer. The neuroblasts reach the oesophagus at six weeks, the cranial loop of the midgut by seven to eight weeks and innervation is complete by 12 weeks. Arrest in the migration of ganglion cells down the developing gut results in aganglionosis distal to the level of arrest, and leads classically to Hirschsprung's disease.

The liver

The anatomy of the hepatic architecture is complex and includes the portal venous system, which accounts for 60–80% of the total influx, the remainder being supplied by the hepatic artery. The vascular sinusoid spaces develop in the early weeks of embryonic life and serve to link the portal and hepatic venous systems. This venous network branches in a regular and uniform way, forming the hepatic lobules.

Layers of mesenchyme intervene between the endothelium of the sinusoids and the epithelial cells, and they give rise to blood-forming cells, haemocytoblasts, which rapidly proliferate to outnumber the hepatocytes and produce erythrocytes, which pass through the sinusoid walls to enter the general circulation. This source of haemopoietic activity subsides towards the end of gestation, and only small foci are present in the liver of the newborn.

The cells of the exocrine and endocrine pancreas develop from the cells which line the primitive pancreatic ducts, and at eight weeks the developing pancreas consists largely of a network of anastomosing ducts and ductules which are lined by a single layer of cells. Endocrine cells precede the development of exocrine cells, and there appear to be two generations of islet cells during embryonic life (Liv & Potter 1962). The first generation arises during the eighth week from cells lining the primitive pancreatic ducts. The second arises after the third month from the cells of the terminal ductules when the exocrine acinar cells have been formed. The islet cells disengage from the ductular system and appear as irregular structures scattered throughout the gland being separated from the acinar cells by a thin reticular membrane. They are particularly prominent in the tail of the pancreas.

Acinar cells also develop from cells lining the embryonic pancreatic ducts and first appear in both the dorsal and ventral pancreas during the third month of intrauterine life. The acinar cells are pyramidal in shape and rest on a reticular membrane, arranged in a circular or tubular fashion around a central lumen, and forming the intralobular ducts. These ducts drain into the interlobular ducts, which in turn drain into the main pancreatic duct.

FUNCTIONAL DEVELOPMENT

The gastrointestinal tract develops in an integrated fashion and in this section the various aspects are reviewed.

Motor activity

The motor activity of the gut moves the intraluminal contents from one specialized region of the gut to another and the pattern of motility is integrated with and related to the physiological function of particular regions of the gut. The oesophagus acts as a propulsive conduit conveying ingested food to the stomach which acts both as a mixing organ and a reservoir. In the stomach, food is processed for further digestion by intraluminal and brush border enzymes, and diluted to render its contents more isotonic. Gastric contents are discharged into the small intestine which is primarily a digestive and absorptive organ. Clear-cut patterns of motility are closely related to the functions of the small intestine, as are the segmenting and peristaltic en masse movements of the colon. Luminal contents are moved slowly in the colon to allow reabsorption of electrolytes against steep concentration gradients.

Sucking and swallowing

The fetus is able to swallow by 11 weeks in utero and an effective sucking mechanism develops by about 35 weeks gestation (Herbst 1981). Within a few days after birth, full term infants have a very effective suck and swallow mechanism. (Gryboski 1969). As the change is gradually made to ingestion of a more varied diet, sucking reflexes are repressed but may reappear in senility or fail to regress in patients with central nervous system damage (Herbst 1983).

The development of oesophageal peristalsis starts in utero at 11 weeks, long before the development of the oral phase of swallowing, and represents an exception to the usual cranio-caudal development. This may be related to the presence of amniotic fluid which has to be swallowed, but also ensures that the transport of food along the gut is developed before large amounts of food are presented to it.

Non-nutritive as well as nutritive sucking occurs in infants. Non-nutritive sucking develops first and is characterized by its rapidity usually exceeding two sucks per second, which is approximately twice that seen in nutritive sucking (Wolff 1968). In its most immature form, non-nutritive sucking consists of mouthing movements only, and this is usually first seen at approximately 24 weeks (Golubera et al 1959).

In its most immature form, nutritive sucking occurs in short bursts followed by a brief cessation of respiration and a swallow which is followed by uncoordinated oesophageal peristalsis. In the normal full term infant, a mature pattern develops within a few days of birth with prolonged bursts of rhythmical sucking. Nutrients are transported across the pharynx, swallowed and propelled to the stomach with a coordinated peristaltic wave. Normal movement of air across the pharynx into the lung also occurs simultaneously without interruption of the rhythmicity of either function. In premature infants the development of this mature pattern of swallowing may not develop for many weeks (Gryboski 1969). Neurological damage may also cause delayed development of mature sucking and swallowing patterns (Gryboski 1975).

Both nutritive and non-nutritive sucking can be altered by a number of factors. Even in the early neonatal period the presence of a nipple (Peiper 1963), visual stimuli (Milewski and Siqueland 1975) and the taste of the fluid, as well as nutrient content, can affect the efficiency of nutritive sucking. In general, there is more sucking activity with milk than with 5% dextrose (Dubignon & Campbell 1968) and with dextrose or sucrose than water (Ashmead 1980).

Awareness of the fact that the nonnutritive sucking of a premature infant of approximately 34 weeks gestational age does not suggest an effective nutritive suck should prompt the quick initiation of gavage feeding because oesophageal motility and intestinal motility will be inadequate.

The change from sucking of liquid nutrients to the mastication and swallowing of solid foods occurs later in life. Although solids deposited on the back of the tongue will be swallowed by most full term infants, the usual mechanisms whereby solid foods are transferred from the front of the tongue to the pharynx does not normally appear until about seven months. Illingworth & Lister (1964) have shown that if all solid foods are witheld because of illness or other reasons until approximately 15 months of age, infants accept solids poorly. This suggests that there is a critical period in developing the ability to handle solids.

Gastric emptying

Gastric emptying in both full term and premature infants appears to be relatively delayed in the first 12 hours of life when compared to that in the same infant at 24 or 48 hours (Gupta & Brans 1978). It is not clear whether overall there is any effect of gestational age on emptying (Siegel et al 1984a).

Studies of gastric emptying in infancy indicate that a receptor system in the duodenum regulates emptying and operates in a manner qualitatively similar to that of the adult. Modulation of gastric emptying is produced by food in the duodenum and, as in adults, digestion and caloric density seem important (Husband & Husband 1969, Siegal et al 1984b).

It may not be possible to explain all regulatory phenomena of gastric emptying in infancy on the basis of caloric density and digestibility. In healthy premature infants, human milk emptied faster than an adapted infant feeding contaning 20 cal/oz and having the same casein to whey ratio as human milk (Cavell 1979). This suggests that the macronutrient composition may also play a role in the regulation of gastric emptying. In a recent study, Siegel et al (1984b) observed the effects of altering the carbohydrate source (glucose, lactose, polycose) and fat source (long chain and medium chain triglyceride — LCT and MCT) on the gastric emptying profile in premature infants. The inhibition produced by LCT was much greater than that of MCT; alterations in carbohydrate source, in contrast, had minimal effects on gastric emptying rate. Thus, for infants with impaired gastric emptying a change from an LCT to MCT predominant formula might be logical.

Whilst posture, volume, and feeding temperature (Blumenthal et al 1979, 1980) appear to have little effect on gastric emptying, a number of pathological conditions are clearly associated with delayed gastric emptying and include cardiovascular disease (Cavell 1981a and b), respiratory distress syndrome (Yu 1975) and gastro-oesophageal reflux (Hillemeier et al 1981).

Small intestinal and colonic motor activity

The development of small intestinal motor function has been little studied. Amniography suggests that transit of contrast medium through the small intestine only occurs after 30 weeks gestation (McLain 1963). Recent studies in both the experimental animal and human preterm infants show a clear picture of fetal and neonatal development of fasting small intestinal motility.

Using chronically implanted electrodes, recordings have been made following surgery in utero and after birth in the dog and sheep (Bueno &

Ruckebusch 1979). Three stages of activity were seen: (1) disorganised; (2) groups of regular spike activity, the fetal pattern; and (3) a cyclical pattern with propagated migrating motor complexes (MMC). The first stage was not associated with luminal transit in contrast to the second and third stages. Birth was not accompanied by acute changes in the motility pattern but species variations became clear. In the sheep the MMC pattern starts 5 to 10 days before birth but in the dog the fetal pattern persists for up to 15 days after birth.

Studies in preterm human infants using nasojejunal feeding catheters have shown developmental patterns comparable to the above animal studies: between 27 and 30 weeks gestation, disorganised activity; 30 to 33 weeks repetitive groups of contractions, 'the fetal complex'; and from about 34 weeks the MMC pattern (Wozniak et al 1983). In full term infants a well established MMC pattern is seen. Acquisition of the MMC pattern seems to be closely associated with neurological development and coincides with the establishment of nutritive sucking. Extension of these studies should provide a rational basis for premature infant feeding practices.

Little is known regarding the development of colonic motor activity and studies are required in this area.

Secretion, digestion and absorption

The digestion and absorption of nutrients consists of an integrated series of intraluminal, brush border and cellular events. The amount of information derived from the human fetus is limited, most of the data referred to has been obtained from studies in the experimental animal.

Gastric secretory function

The stomach is both an exocrine and endocrine secretory organ. It secretes four major compounds from exocrine cells: hydrochloric acid, intrinsic factor, pepsinogen and mucoproteins. Several groups of investigators have shown that full term newborns (Agunod et al 1969; Ebers et al 1956; Avery et al 1966) and probably some preterm (Ames 1960) infants secrete hydrochloric acid within hours or minutes of birth. Each of these studies has shown that basal acid outputs are detectable within minutes and increase over the first hours of postnatal life. During this period, basal secretion is below that of older children, but is easily detectable particularly if the stomach is lavaged of amniotic fluid or swallowed maternal blood.

Development of gastric acid secretion after the first postnatal day is more controversial. Miller (1941) in a study of term infants showed that after a peak in basal acid output on the first or second postnatal day, a steady decline in basal acid output occurred over the subsequent ten days. Even by 30 days he observed no significant change in basal acid output. In contrast Ames (1960) found that two-thirds of the preterm infants at birthweights from 1000 to 2200 g secreted acid, and had maximum basal acid output on the fourth postnatal day, but no decrease in acid output was subsequently observed through the tenth postnatal day. The duration of the postnatal hyposecretory phase is not clear but most investigators have shown the period to be at least one month, although some have suggested several months or years (Agunod et al 1969; Deren 1971; Rodbro et al 1967; Euler et al 1979). In addition to depressed basal acid outputs during the first month of life, infants do not respond to the usual stimuli of acid secretion (Agunod et al 1969; Euler et al 1979). The undeveloped gastric secretory state during the neonatal period may be due to a decreased parietal cell mass, decreased secretogogue receptor density or affinity, or a decreased ability to respond due to postreceptor defects (Lichtenberger 1984). Elegant in vitro studies in the rat suggest that the ability to secrete acid was associated with the rate of acquisition of active proton secretion mechanisms (Ducroc et al 1981).

Pepsin has been detected in the term and preterm human infant and fetus and in the fetus, as early as the sixteenth week of gestation (Deren 1971). Werner (1948) found few if any zymogen granules in the 2300 g fetus, but substantially more granules nearer to term. Agunod et al (1969) found peptic activity to be about 2% of the adult at term; by the second week substantial increases in activity were found and by 2 to 3 months the protease activity was about 50% of the adult reference population.

Intrinsic factor can be detected in the human fetal gastric mucosa and gastric drainage of full term infants. It is first detected at about 14 weeks and increases approximately sevenfold by the third trimester (Christie 1981) and postnatally its secretion parallels that of acid. By day 10 to 14, levels are about 50% that of the adult (Agunod 1969) and appear similar in term and preterm infants (Marino et al 1984). Mucus production by the human neonatal stomach has to our knowledge not been studied.

Gastrin is detectable in cord blood at levels substantially greater than those of adults. The duration, magnitude and probable mechanisms of neonatal hypergastrinaemia have been recently reviewed by Lichtenberger (1984). Cord and neonatal blood gastrin levels greatly exceed maternal concentrations (Rodgers et al 1974; Lucas et al 1980) and this may persist for months (Euler et al 1977; Lucas et al 1980) or years (Sann et al 1975; Janik et al 1977). Whilst the precise origin and mechanism of neonatal hypergastrinaemia is unknown, an attractive and currently favoured hypothesis is that the hypergastrinaemia and hypochlorhydria are directly related to one another (Johnson 1984).

Since protein and amino acids are potent stimuli of gastrin release, changes in the infant diet may also be important in the regulation of neonatal hypergastrinaemia. Both term and preterm infants have been shown to have gastrin responses to milk feeds (Sann et al 1975; Aynsley-Green et al 1977). Patients of similar age receiving parenteral nutrition have substantially lower serum gastrin concentrations (Lucas et al 1980; Sann et al 1975; Janik et al 1977).

Exocrine pancreatic development

In man, zymogen granules and the several pancreatic enzymes are detectable in acinar cells and pancreatic homogenates respectively from mid-gestation; each of the enzymes displays a characteristic pattern of maturation which is discontinuous and continues until late infancy. Adult concentrations of the pancreatic enzymes are achieved by late infancy, but due to alternate pathways of digestion and the fact that significantly diminished enzyme concentrations correlate with partial digestion of dietary components, most term infants do not have significant malabsorptive problems. Preterm infants, however, and those with increased caloric demands, may have insufficient reserve to thrive on enteral feeds alone. In the perinatal period a transient physiological pancreatic insufficiency, characterized by depressed lipase and nearly absent amylase concentrations, contributes to incomplete digestion of fats and carbohydrate.

Normal exocrine pancreatic function requires normal morphology, patency of the ductular system, adequate stores of enzymes to be secreted, appropriate stimuli for secretion, response to the stimulus, and the ability to replenish enzyme stores following secretion. Each of these points will be addressed below.

As has been reviewed earlier in this chapter, the pancreatic morphology of newborns is similar to that of an adult (Lebenthal, Lev & Lee 1981). By mid-gestation the histological and ultrastructural appearance of the exocrine tissue becomes progressively more mature with the acquisition of the features of the mature acinar cell (Laito, Lev & Orlic 1974). Several of the pancreatic enzymes have been shown to be present in fetal pancreatic homogenates from fetuses between 16 and 40 weeks gestation.

Track et al (1975) conducted extensive studies, measuring trypsin, chymotrypsin, lipase, phospholipase and amylase activities in fetal tissues from 15 weeks until term. Activities of trypsin, chymotrypsin, lipase and phospholipase were detectable from mid-gestation but were substantially below (about 10%) adult values. Amylase was undetectable in mature concentrations during the perinatal period.

Exocrine pancreatic secretion in man is under hormonal and central nervous system control, and four phases have been described: cephalic, gastric, intestinal and postabsorptive. Hormonal responses have been shown to be qualitatively similar to those seen later in life and are reviewed in Chapter 14. The key hormones for pancreatic secretion, cholecystokinin and secretin, have not been studied in patients of this age. In view of the qualitative similarity between the hormone profiles of neonates and adults, it seems unlikely that lack of stimulus for secretion is the mechanism of the partial pancreatic insufficiency seen in infancy.

Response of the neonatal pancreas to cholecystokinin secretion in vivo (Delachaume-Salem & Sarles 1970; Zoppi et al 1972; Lebenthal & Lee 1980) is diminished compared to older children, with low intraduodenal enzyme concentrations which do not increase after secretogogue administration.

The mechanism of the lack of response of the neonatal pancreas to secretogogues is not clear. Experimental studies in the rat would suggest that in the neonatal pancreas post-receptor mechanisms are intact (Werlin & Stefaniak 1982).

Liver and biliary system

The metabolic development of the fetus is intimately associated with that of the liver.

Carbohydrate metabolism.   Glucose is the major source of energy during fetal life and anaerobic metabolism the most important component of glucose metabolism (Stembera & Hodr 1966; Villee et al 1958). Glycogen is stored solely in the liver, and rapid accumulation is initiated between 13 and 14 weeks' gestation (Capkova & Jirasek 1968) continuing until term. Small for dates neonates have a disproportionately reduced liver mass and glycogen reserve, and this is a major factor in the aetiology of the hypoglycaemia which they may experience (Shelley & Neligan 1966). Gluconeogenic and lipogenic pathways function from as early as the eleventh week of gestation (Villee et al 1958). In the fetus the glucose–fatty acid pathway is especially active, some 70% of fetal glucose uptake being converted to fat. This conversion, unlike other interconversions, releases energy which can fully cover the energy required for maintenance of metabolism. Thus the developing fetus has a highly economic energy balance.

Protein metabolism.   The fetal liver is a very active site of protein synthesis, though some of this undoubtedly represents haematopoietic activity. Albumin synthesis commences at about 12 weeks and gradually increases throughout gestation. In contrast coagulation proteins and caeruloplasmin concentrations are frequently low at term.

Cystine is not formed by the fetal liver because the transsulphuration pathway is incomplete due to the absence of cystathionase which does not appear until after birth (Sturman et al 1970). Cystine should therefore be regarded as an essential amino acid in the newborn, in contrast to older children and adults. The pathways involved in methionine, phenylalanine and tyrosine metabolism are also immature at birth despite the fact that phenylalanine hydroxylase activity can be detected as early as eight weeks (Raiha 1973) and the tyrosine oxidation system as early as the fourteenth week of gestation (Raiha et al 1971). Premature infants may have an impaired dietary tolerance to these amino acids due to defective cofactor metabolism (Light et al 1966).

Detoxication and excretion.   The nitrogen-excreting mechanism, the urea cycle, is closely coupled to kidney development. Thus the human fetal liver is capable of synthesizing urea at the same time as the mesonephric glomeruli are formed (Raiha & Suihkonen 1968). In general, however, the fetus relies on maternal tissues for the detoxication of noxious substances, and the term infant has a limited capacity for detoxication.

Bile secretion is also impaired as shown by decreased bile acid pool size, due to decreased bile acid synthesis and secretion and to impaired ileal uptake (Balistreri 1983). In addition to these quantitative changes there are qualitative differences in early life with the formation of atypical bile acids via fetal biosynthetic pathways. These atypical bile acids are not choleretic and do not mediate bile flow and some (monohydroxy bile acids) may be cholestatic. These qualitative differences indirectly contribute to decreased hepatic secretory function (Back & Walter 1980).

Small intestine

The small bowel is primarily an organ of digestion and absorption. In this section, membrane hydrolysis and the transport of nutrients across the brush border membrane from lumen to cytosol will be reviewed. The intracellular processing of nutrients, micronutrient, water, electrolytes and minerals is discussed in Chapter 9.

Carbohydrate digestion and absorption. Dietary di- and polysaccharides require hydrolysis to their component monosaccharides prior to absorption and utilization. The development of the capacity to hydrolyse dietary polysaccharides has been reviewed earlier in this chapter. In this section, the ontogeny of disaccharide hydrolysis and monosaccharide absorption will be discussed.

Dietary disaccharides are unaltered prior to contact with the enterocyte membrane where they are hydrolysed to their component monosaccharides by specific brush border enzymes located primarily on the villus.

The development of the intestinal disaccharidases, like many other brush border enzymes, is closely related to the maturation of the enterocyte. In the human fetus and newborn, the processes of maturation and epithelial cell renewal have not been fully explored. The first appearance of fetal disaccharidase activity correlates with the development of villous structure; similarly, epithelial renewal probably also occurs since disaccharidases are detectable in amniotic fluid and meconium (Antonowicz et al 1977). Information on mitotic rates, crypt cell populations and migration is not readily available in either the human fetus or infant.

The disaccharidases have a distinct topographical distribution along the small intestine. Initially, they appear throughout the intestine, but by term lactase, sucrase, isomaltase and maltase activities are highest in the proximal jejunum and decrease in both the orad and aborad directions (Newcomer & McGill 1966). The proximal distal gradient in disaccharidase activities thus established persists into adult life (Antonowicz et al 1974).

Compared to a number of laboratory animals, man is characterized by a unique pattern of disaccharidase development. In the mouse and rat, lactase is present during suckling, but sucrose-isomaltase and maltase are

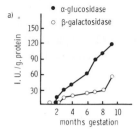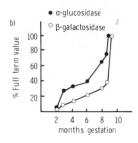

Fig. 1.7 Development of the brush border disaccharidases of the small intestine.

absent, and appear at or near weaning. In man, both lactase and the alpha-glucosidases (maltase and sucrase-isomaltase) are present in fetal mucosa prior to term. The relative activities of the brush border disaccharidases at different stages of gestation are shown in Figure 1.7. Sucrose-isomaltase activities can be identified from the first trimester (Sheehy & Anderson 1971), whereas lactase activity develops mainly during the latter portions of fetal life. Lactase, therefore, develops late in comparison to sucrase and maltase, but mature levels are present in term infants (Antonowicz and Lebenthal 1977).

Absorption of monosaccharides   Glucose, galactose and fructose are the products of oligosaccharide digestion in the small bowel. Glucose and galactose are primarily absorbed by a sodium-dependent active transport mechanism (see Chapter 9). Fructose, in contrast, is absorbed by sodium-independent facilitated diffusion.

Acquisition of active Na^+-dependent co-transport of glucose and galactose is associated with the development of an apical microvillus and junctional complexes by villous enterocytes. Studies in fetal jejunal and ileal everted sacs have shown that active transport occurs as early as the 10th week and a threefold increase occurs by 18 weeks (Koldovsky et al 1965).

There is little data available following birth but studies of potential difference evoked by glucose in preterm and full term infants have shown decreased numbers of transport sites with premature birth or compromised nutrition (McNeish et al 1983). The capacity for glucose absorption increases as gestation progresses and continues after birth (Milla 1983). There is thus not only increasing ability to absorb glucose but also Na^+ and hence water.

Protein digestion and absorption.   Digestion and absorption of dietary protein requires a series of events that is reasonably well defined in adults and older children (see Chapter 9) but much less well understood in the developing human. Since pancreatic protease concentrations within the duodenal lumen seem to be adequate (Borgstrom et al 1960; Lebenthal & Lee 1980), the diminished absorption of dietary protein in infants (Hirata et al 1965) may result from a diminished capacity to either hydrolyse oligopeptides or absorb amino acids, di- and tripeptides.

Studies in everted intestinal sacs from fetuses between 10 and 18 weeks' gestation have shown active absorption of L-alanine and L-leucine (Koldovsky et al 1965). There are no studies of peptide transport. It is likely, however, that perinatal and postnatal development of peptide transport is similar to that of glucose.

Brush border digestion has been studied to a limited extent in human fetuses. Gammaglutamyltranspeptidase, dipeptidyl aminopeptidase IV, folate conjugase and amino oligopeptidase are all present with similar activities to those found in the adult by the early part of the second trimester (Auricchio et al 1981). Aminopeptidase A is the only brush border peptidase which is markedly reduced during intrauterine gestation with less than one-third of adult values found in one study (Auricchio et al 1981). It would therefore appear that impaired oligopeptide hydrolysis is not the cause of the reduced absorption of dietary protein seen in the newborn.

Electrolyte transport   Little is known of the development of electrolyte transport processes other than that of the Na^+ coupled to the absorption of organic solutes. However, the presence of intrauterine diarrhoea in congenital chloridorrhoea (see Chapter 9) suggests the presence of specific electrolyte transport processes by the second trimester.

Similarly, basolateral enzymes which are intimately associated with transport processes such as adenylate cyclose and Na^+K^+ ATPase develop concomitantly with brush border translocation mechanisms and at a similar rate (Grand et al 1973).

Lipid digestion and absorption.   Triglyceride is the major dietary lipid and is hydrolysed by lipases to form more polar products prior to solubilization and absorption.

Three major lipases are active in the gastrointestinal tract in man: lingual lipase, bile salt stimulated lipase of human breast milk, and pancreatic lipase. The latter has been discussed earlier in this chapter.

Lingual lipase is secreted from Von Ebner's glands at the base of the tongue. Activity develops late in gestation and persists throughout life (Jensen et al 1982); it increases by 80% from 25 to 34 weeks and premature infants of 30 to 34 weeks gestation have sufficient intragastric activity to hydrolyse 15% of dietary fat in a formula within seven minutes of feeding (Hamosh et al 1978, 1981). Human milk contains two lipases, lipoprotein lipase and bile salt stimulated lipase which is active in the small intestine of the newborn. It is present in colostrum and its activity is similar in preterm and term milks, and does not vary significantly with length of lactation (Mehta et al 1982). Thus, lingual lipase and the bile salt stimulated lipase of human milk are able to hydrolyse dietary triglyceride and compensate for the low activity of pancreatic lipase in the newborn.

Intraluminal bile salts are important for the solubilization of the lipolytic products and other lipids such as cholesterol and for the fat soluble vitamins. In premature infants, however, intraluminal bile salt concentrations are commonly below the critical micellar concentration (2 mM) (Katz &

Hamilton 1974) due to a decreased bile salt pool size (Watkins et al 1973, 1975), which is thought to be secondary to inadequately developed hepatic and ileal function (Lester 1977).

Transport through the cell membrane seems to occur by simple diffusion. At the cell surface, the micellar aggregates are disassembled and mono-glycerides and fatty acids diffuse through the membrane. The phospholipid is hydrolysed by phospholipase A2, and the bile salts are utilized to generate new micelles further downstream as the products of lipase-mediated lipolysis are released from oil droplets (Roy 1981). The intra-cellular events of reesterification and chylomicron assembly have not been studied during development, and are beyond the scope of this review.

In summary, the intraluminal phase deficiency secondary to diminished lipase and bile acid concentrations impaired solubilization of the products of digestion so that they may pass through the unstirred layer, all contribute to the developmental steatorrhea seen in newborn and premature infants. Breast feeding, which supplies both lipases and more soluble lipids than cow's milk (Filer et al 1970), results in near normal lipid retention. Similarly, the use of MCT predominant formulae, which are not as dependent on lipases and bile salts for their digestion and absorption, may be helpful in premature and other infants with these deficiencies for whom breast milk is not available.

Immune systems.   During recent years a great deal of attention has been focused on the role of the gut in the body's overall immune competence in man, and it has become clear that it is of great importance. Perhaps this is not surprising since it is continually exposed to foreign antigenic material to which it must react to ensure the balanced survival of the host. The prenatal development of the immune systems of the gut is therefore a critical preparatory event to the newborn baby being suddenly exposed to its postnatal hostile environment. The development of the mucosal barrier against penetration by a variety of harmful agents from the intestinal lumen is critical. Knowledge on this aspect of paediatric gastroenterology is still fragmentary and continues to represent an important area for future investigation.

The density of the lymphoid Peyer's patches in the small intestine increases distally, and they are concentrated in the ileum; they are well developed by about the twentieth week of gestation. IgA-containing plasma cells are absent from the lamina propria of the fetal gut, and they first appear in the neonatal period preceding serum IgA. IgM-containing cells appear before birth during the third trimester. Of the specific immuno-globulin classes, only IgG can be transported across the placenta; this immunoglobulin represents an important source of passive immunity to the newborn against Gram-positive organisms but is relatively ineffective against Gram-negative species. There is no information on IgE or IgD immunoglobulins in the developing human fetus.

Bockman & Cooper (1975) have studied the fine structure of the human fetal appendix and found a relationship between the development of lymphoid follicles and the specialisation of the covering epithelium. They speculated that the follicle-associated epithelium provides a channel through which antigens can stimulate clonal proliferation and seeding of B lymphocytes in the lamina propria.

In the experimental animal, 'closure' to macromolecular uptake is a well established phenomenon (Walker 1979) but in the human it remains controversial. It is clear, however, that human milk contributes to gut defence not only with antibodies and viable leucocytes but also many other substances which interfere with bacterial colonization, prevent antigen penetration and enhance enterocyte maturation (Heird & Hansen 1977). Epidermal growth factor promises to be an important therapeutic tool in the future.

The large intestine

The large intestine is an organ of conservation particularly of water and electrolytes, but also of partially digested nutrients (see Chapter 2). Until recently there was no information regarding colonic transport in the neonate. Non-equilibrium rectal dialysis studies have shown that the pattern of movement of electrolytes was similar to that seen in later life, Na^+ absorption was electrogenic, and Cl^- absorption coupled to HCO_3^- secretion. HCO_3^- secretion was impaired, suggesting less well developed anion exchange (Milla 1983).

Enzymes During fetal life the colon possesses villi and an abundant brush border hydrolytic capacity with at least sucrase, amino-peptidase and alkaline phosphatase activities. The disaccharidases start to appear at about 11 weeks gestation and reach a peak at about 28 weeks then decline and disappear by term. In contrast peptidase and alkaline phosphatase activity persists in the adult colon. The significance of these changes is unknown but sucrase activity parallels villous formation and it is tempting to speculate that sucrase is in some way necessary for morphogenesis. Lactase is completely absent from the colon during the whole of fetal life (Lacroix et al 1984).

CONCLUSIONS

It is clear that the term infant is in a precarious state with regard to its ability to respond to increased nutritional demands (either increased losses or increased requirements). Relative inadequacy of primary mechanisms of nutrient acquisition render alternative pathways of nutrient retention more important than in later life.

Developing infants have diminished pancreatic amylase concentration in the duodenal lumen and several mechanisms of starch digestion may well be more important than later in life. Firstly, glucoamylase, a brush border alpha-glucosidase is present in nearly adult concentrations from the third trimester. Similarly, although salivary amylase is low at birth, it reaches adult values at a much earlier age than pancreatic amylase. Finally, human breast milk contains an amylase of salivary type which may also be important in the breastfed infant. These three alternate pathways of starch digestion can, therefore, act as compensatory factors to ameliorate the diminished capacities of neonates to digest, absorb and retain glucose derived from complex dietary carbohydrates.

In a similar fashion, human infants have physiological developmental steatorrhea which has been recognized for many years. The fat malabsorption is due to diminished intraduodenal pancreatic lipase concentrations in conjunction with bile salt concentrations below the critical micellar concentration. Alternative compensatory mechanisms for fat digestion include lingual lipase and bile salt stimulated lipase of human milk. Unlike the alternative pathways of starch digestion which appear only to be active distal to the pylorus, lingual lipase initiates lipolysis within the stomach.

Although the healthy term newborn is quite well adapted to a normal diet (i.e. breast milk) which is adequate for his needs, premature infants with inadequate stores of micronutrients and diminished capabilities to retain enteral nutrition are substantially less well adapted to extrauterine life. We hope that the data presented here will help those who care for premature infants and other nutritionally compromised neonates to make educated decisions regarding their nutritional support and also recognize areas of need for future research.

REFERENCES

Agunod M, Yamaguchi N, Lopez R, Lubby A L, Glass G B J 1969 Correlative study of hydrochloric acid, pepsin and intrinsic factor secretion in newborns and infants. American Journal of Digestive Disease 14: 400–414

Ames M D 1960 Gastric acidity in the first ten days of life in the prematurely born baby. American Journal of Diseases of Children 100: 252–256

Andersen H, Bierring F, Matthiessen M, Egeberg J, Bro-Rasnassen F 1964 On the nature of the meconium corpuscles in human foetal intestinal epithelium. II A cytochemical study. Acta Pathologica Microbiologica Scandinavica 61: 377–393

Antonowicz I, Lebenthal E 1977 Developmental pattern of small intestinal enterokinase and dissacharidase activities in the human fetus. Gastroenterology 72: 1299–1301

Antonowicz I, Chang S K, Grand R J 1974 Development and distribution of lysosomal enzymes and disaccharidases on human fetal intestine. Gastroenterology 67: 51–58

Antonowicz I, Milunsky A, Lebenthal E, Shwachman H 1977 Disaccharidase and lysosomal activities in amniotic fluid, intestinal mucosa and meconium. Biology of the Neonate 32: 280–289

Ashmead D H, Reilly B M, Lipsitt L P 1980 Neonates heart rate, sucking rhythm and sucking amplitude as a function of the sweet taste. Journal of Experimental Child Psychology 29: 264–281

Auricchio S, Stellato A, DeVizia B 1981 Development of brush border peptidases in human and rat small intestine during fetal and neonatal life. Paediatric Research 15: 991–995

Avery G B, Randolph J G, Weaver T 1966 Gastric acidity in the first day of life. Pediatrics 37: 1005–1007

Aynsley-Green A, Bloom S R, Williamson D H, Turner R C 1977 Endocrine and metabolic response in the human newborn to the first feed of breast milk. Archives of Disease in Childhood 52: 291–295

Back P, Walter K 1980 Developmental pattern of bile acid metabolism as revealed by bile acid analysis of meconium. Gastroenterology 78: 671–676

Balistreri W F 1983 Immaturity of hepatic excretory function and the ontogeny of bile acid metabolism. Journal of Pediatric Gastro-nutrition 2: S207–214

Bierring F, Andersen H F, Egeberg J, Bro-Rossmussen F, Matthieson M 1964 On the nature of the meconium corpuscles in human foetal intestinal epithelium. Acta Pathologica Microbiologica Scandinavica 61: 365–376

Blumenthal J, Ebel A, Pildes R S 1979 Effect of posture on the pattern of stomach emptying in the newborn. Pediatrics 63: 532–536

Blumenthal I, Lellman G T, Shoesmith D R 1980 Effect of feed temperature and phototheraphy on gastric emptying in the neonate. Archives of Disease in Childhood 55: 562–564

Bockman D E, Cooper M D 1975 Early lymphoepithelial relationships in human appendix. A combined light and electron-microscopic study. Gastroenterology 68: 1160–1168

Borgstrom B, Lindquist B, Lundh G 1960 Enzyme concentration and absorption of protein and glucose in the duodenum of premature infants. American Journal of Diseases of Children 99: 338–348

Bueno L, Ruckebusch Y 1979 Perinatal development of intestinal myoelectrical activity in dogs and sheep. American Journal of Physiology 237: E61–67

Capkova A, Jirasek J E 1968 Glycogen reserves in organs of human fetuses in the first half of pregnancy. Biologia Neonatorum 13: 129–142

Cavell B 1979 Gastric emptying in preterm infants. Acta Paediatrica Scandinavica 68: 725–730

Cavell B 1981a Effect of feeding an infant formula with high energy density on gastric emptying in infants with congenital heart disease. Acta Paediatrica Scandinavica 70: 513–516

Cavell B 1981b Gastric emptying in infants with congenital heart disease. Acta Paediatrica Scandinavica 70: 517–520

Christie D L 1981 Development of gastric function during the first month of life. In: Lebenthal E (ed) Textbook of gastroenterology and nutrition in infancy. Raven Press, New York, pp 109–120

Delachaume-Salem E, Sarles H 1970 Evolution en fonction de l'age de la secretion pancreatique humaine normale. Biologie et Gastroenterologie (Paris) 2: 135–146

Deren J S 1971 Development of structure and function in the fetal and newborn stomach. American Journal of Clinical Nutrition 24: 144–159

Dubignon J, Campbell D 1969 Sucking in the newborn in three conditions: non-nutritive, nutritive and a feed. Journal of Experimental Child Psychology 6: 335–350

Ducroc C R, Desjeux J F, Garyon B, Onoljo J P, Geloso J P 1981 Acid secretion in fetal rat stomach in vitro. American Journal of Physiology 240: G206–210

Duhamel B 1961 From the mermaid to anal imperforation; the syndrome of caudal regression. Archives of Disease in Childhood 36: 152–155

Ebers D W, Smith D T, Gibbs G E 1956 Gastric acidity on the first day of life. Pediatrics 18: 800–802

Euler A R, Byrne W J, Cousins L M, Ament M E, Leake R D, Walsh J H 1977 Increased serum gastrin concentrations and gastric acid hyposecretion in the immediate newborn period. Gastroenterology 72: 1271–1273

Euler A R, Byrne W J, Meis P J, Leake R D, Ament M E 1979 Basal and pentagastrin-stimulated acid secretion in newborn infants. Pediatric Research 13: 36–37

Feldman M, Weinberg T 1952 Aberrant pancreas: a cause of duodenal syndrome. Journal of the American Medical Association 148: 893–895

Filer L J, Mattson F H, Fomon S J 1970 Triglyceride configuration and fat absorption by the human infant. Journal of Nutrition 99: 293–298

Golubeva E L, Shuleikina K V, Vanshtein I I 1959 Development of reflex and spontaneous activity of the human fetus in the process of embryogenesis. Akusherstvo I Ginekologiia (USSR) 3: 59–62

Grand R J, Torti F, Jaksina S 1973 Development of adenylate cyclase and its response to cholera enterotoxin. Journal of Clinical Investigation 52: 2053–2059

Gryboski J 1969 Suck and swallow in the premature infant. Pediatrics 43: 96–101
Gryboski J 1975 Suck and swallow. In: Schaeffer A J, Markowitz M (eds) Gastrointestinal problems in the infant. W B Saunders, Philadelphia, pp 17–47
Gudmand-Hoyer E, Asp N G, Mollmann K M 1975 Disaccharidase activities in intestinal metaplasia — contribution of lysosomal and brush border enzymes. Scandinavian Journal of Gastroenterology 10: 653–656
Gupta M, Brans Y W 1978 Gastric retention in neonates. Pediatrics 62: 26–29
Hamosh M, Sivasurbramanian K N, Salzman-Mann C, Hamosh P 1978 Fat digestion in the stomach of premature infants. Journal of Pediatrics 93: 674–679
Hamosh M, Scanlon J W, Ganot D, Likel M, Scanlon K B, Hamosh P 1981 Fat digestion in the newborn: Characterisation of lipase in gastric aspirates of premature and term infants. Journal of Clinical Investigation 66: 838–846
Heird W C, Hansen J H 1977 The effect of colostrum on growth of intestinal mucosa. Pediatric Research 11: 406
Herbst J J 1981 Development of sucking and swallowing. In: Lebenthal E (ed) Textbook of gastroenterology and nutrition in infancy. Raven Press, New York, pp 97–108
Herbst J J 1983 Development of suck and swallow. Journal of Pediatric Gastroenterology and Nutrition 2: S131–135
Hillemeier A C, Lange R, McCallum R, Seashore J, Gryboski J 1981 Delayed gastric emptying in infants with gastroesophageal reflux. Journal of Pediatrics 98: 190–193
Hirata Y, Matsuo P, Kobuhu H 1965 Digestion and absorption of milk protein in infants' intestine. Kobe Journal of Medicine and Science 11: 103–106
Husband J, Husband P 1969 Gastric emptying of water and glucose solutions in the newborn. Lancet ii: 409–411
Husband J, Husband P 1970 Gastric emptying of starch meals in the newborn. Lancet ii: 290–292
Illingworth R S, Lister J J 1964 The critical or sensitive period, with special reference to certain feeding problems in infants and children. Journal of Pediatrics 65: 839–884
Janik J, Anbar A M, Burrington J D, Burke G 1977 Serum gastrin levels in infants and children. Pediatrics 60: 60–64
Jensen R G, Clark R M, de Jong F A, Hamosh M, Liao T H, Mehta N R 1982 The lipolytic triad: human lingual, breast milk and pancreatic lipases: Physiological implications of their characteristics in digestion of dietary fats. Journal of Pediatric Gastroenterology and Nutrition 1: 243–255
Johnson F P 1910 The development of the mucous membrane of the oesophagus, stomach and small intestine in the human embryo. American Journal of Anatomy 10: 521–561
Johnson L R 1984 Effects of somatostatin and acid inhibiting gastrin release in newborn rats. Endocrinology 114(3): 743–746
Katz L, Hamilton J R 1974 Fat absorption in infants of birthweight less than 1300 g. Journal of Pediatrics 85: 608–614
Kleitsch W P 1955 Anatomy of the pancreas. A study with special reference to the duct system. Archives of Surgery 71: 795–801
Koldovsky O, Heringova A, Jirsova V et al 1965 Transport of glucose against a concentration gradient in everted sacs of jejunum and ileum of human fetuses. Gastroenterology 48: 185–187
Lacroix B, Kedinger M, Simon-Assmann P, Roussel-M, Zeveibaum A, Haffen K 1984 Developmental pattern of brush border enzymes in the human fetal colon. Early Human Development 9: 95–103
Laito M, Lev R, Orlic D 1974 The developing human fetal pancreas: An ultrastructural and histochemical study with special reference to exocrine cells. Journal of Anatomy 117: 619–634
Lebenthal E, Lee P C 1980 Development of functional response in human exocrine pancreas. Pediatrics 66: 556–660
Lebenthal E, Lee P C 1981 Concepts in gastrointestinal development. In: Lebenthal E (ed) Textbook of gastroenterology and nutrition in infancy. Raven Press, New York, pp 3–6
Lebenthal E, Hatch T F, Lee P C 1981 Development of disaccharidase in premature, small for gestational age, and full-term infants. In: Lebenthal E (ed), Textbook of gastroenterology and nutrition in infancy. Raven Press, New York, pp 413–422
Lebenthal E, Lee P C, Heitlinger L A 1983 Impact of development of the gastrointestinal tract on infant feeding. Journal of Pediatrics 102: 1–9

Lebenthal E, Lev R, Lee P C 1981 Perinatal development of the exocrine pancreas. In: Lebenthal E (ed), Textbook of gastroenterology and nutrition in infancy. Raven Press, New York, pp 149–165

Lester R 1977 Diarrhoea and malabsorption in the newborn. New England Journal of Medicine 297: 505–506

Lichtenberger L 1984 A search for the origin of neonatal hypergastrinemia. Journal of Pediatric Gastroenterology and Nutrition 3: 161–166

Light I J, Berry H K, Sutherland J M 1966 Aminoacidaemia of prematurity. American Journal of Digestion in Children 112: 229–236

Liv H M, Potter E L 1962 Development of the human pancreas. Archives of Pathology 74: 439–450

Lucas A, Adrian T E, Christofides N, Blood S R, Aynsley-Green A 1980 Plasma motilin, gastrin, and enteroglucagon and feeding in the human newborn. Archives of Disease in Childhood 55: 673–677

Marino L R, Bacon B R, Hines J D, Halpin T C 1984 Parietal cell function of full-term and premature infants: Unstimulated gastric acid and intrinsic factor secretion. Journal of Pediatric Gastroenterology and Nutrition 3: 23–27

McLain C R 1963 Amniographic studies of gastrointestinal motility of the human foetus. American Journal of Obstetrics and Gynaecology 86: 1079–1087

McNeish A S, Mayne A, Ducker D A, Hughes C A 1983 Development of D-glucose absorption in the prenatal period. Journal of Pediatric Gastroenterology and Nutrition 2 (suppl 1): S222–226

Mehta N R, Jones J B, Hamosh M 1982 Lipases in preterm human milk: ontogeny and physiologic significance. Journal of Pediatric Gastroenterology and Nutrition 1: 317–326

Milewski A K, Siqueland E R 1975 Discrimination of color and pattern novelty in one month old infants. Journal of Experimental Child Psychology 19: 122–136

Milla P J 1983 Aspects of fluid and electrolyte absorption in the newborn. Journal of Pediatric Gastroenterology and Nutrition 2: S272–276

Miller R A 1941 Observations on the gastric acidity during the first month of life. Archives of Disease in Childhood 16: 22–30

Moran J R, Murell J, Ghishan F K 1984 Developmental maturation of glycine transport in the rat jejunum. Gastroenterology 86:1187 (abstract)

Moxey P C, Trier J S (1977) Endocrine cells in the human fetal small intestine. Cell Tissue Research 183: 33–50

Moxey P C, Trier J S (1978) Specialised cell types in the human fetal small intestine. Anatomical Record 191: 269–286

Newcomer A D, McGill D G 1966 Distribution of disaccharidase activity in the small bowel of normal and lactase deficient subjects. Gastroenterology 51: 481–488

Patzelt V 1931 Ausibildung des menschlichen Dames von der funften Woche bis zur Geburt. Zeitzchrift fur mikrosbopisch, anatomische Forschung (Leipzig) 27: 269–518

Peiper A (ed) 1963 Cerebral function in infancy and childhood. Consultants Bureau, New York

Raiha N C R 1973 Phenylalanine hydroxylase in human liver development. Pediatric Research 7: 1–4

Raiha N C R, Schwartz A L, Lindroos M C 1971 Induction of tyrosine and ketoglutarate transaminase in fetal rat and fetal human liver in organ culture. Pediatric Research 5: 70–76

Raiha N C, Suihkonen J 1968 Development of urea synthesizing enzymes in human liver. Acta Paediatrica Scandinavica 57: 121–124

Rodbro P, Krasilnikoff P A, Christiansen P M 1967 Parietal cell secretory function in early childhood. Scandinavian Journal of Gastroenterology 2: 209–213

Rodgers I M, Davidson D C, Lawrence J, Adrill J, Buchanan K D 1974 Neonatal secretion of gastrin and glucagon. Archives of Disease in Childhood 49: 796–801

Roy C C 1981 Unstirred water layer and epithelial brush border absorption of fatty acids and medium chain triglycerides in premature and term infants. In: Lebenthal E (ed) Textbook of gastroenterology and nutrition in infancy. Raven Press, New York pp 483–492

Sann L, Chayvialle J A P, Bremond A, Lambert R 1975 Serum gastrin level in early childhood. Archives of Disease in Childhood 50: 782–785

Sheehy T W, Anderson P R 1971 Fetal disaccharidases. American Journal of Diseases of Children 121: 464–468

Shelley H J, Neligan G A 1966 Neonatal hypoglycaemia. British Medical Bulletin 22: 34–39

Siegal M, Krantz B, Lebenthal E 1984a The effect of gastric emptying of isocaloric feedings in premature infants. Pediatric Research 18: (4) 212A

Siegal M, Lebenthal E, Krantz B 1984b Effect of caloric density on gastric emptying in premature infants. Journal of Pediatrics 104: 118–122

Stembera Z K, Hodr J 1966 Mutual relationships between the levels of glucose pyruvic acid lactic acid in the blood of the mother and of both umbilical vessels in hypoxic fetuses. Biologia Neonatorum 10: 303–315

Sturman J, Guall G, Raiha N C R 1970 Absence of cystathionase in human fetal liver: is cystine essential? Science 169:74

Track N S, Creutzfeldt C, Bockermann M 1975 Enzymatic, functional and ultrastructural development of the exocrine pancreas. Comparative Biochemistry and Physiology 51A: 95–100

Villee C A, Hagerman D D, Holmberg N, Lind J, Villee D B 1958 The effects of anoxia on the metabolism of human fetal tissues. Pediatrics 22: 953–971

Walker W A 1979 Gut closure and antigen uptake. In: Development of mammalian absorptive processes. Ciba, London, pp 201–216

Watkins J B, Ingall D, Szczepanik P, Klein P D, Lester R 1973 Bile salt metabolism in the newborn: measurement of pool size and synthesis by stable isotope technique. New England Journal of Medicine 288: 431–434

Watkins J B, Szczepanik P, Gould J Bk, Klein P D, Lester R 1975 Bile salt kinetics in premature infants: an explanation for inefficient lipid absorption. Gastroenterology 69: 706–713

Werlin S L, Stefaniak J 1982 Maturation of secretory function in rat pancreas. Pediatric Research 16: 123–125

Werner B 1948 Pepsin and pancreas proteinase in premature compared to full term infants. Annals of Paediatrics 170: 8–14

Wolff P H 1968 The serial organisation of sucking in the young infant. Pediatrics 42: 943–56

Wozniak E R, Fenton T R, Milla P J 1983 The development of fasting small intestinal motility in the human neonate. In Roman C (ed) Gastrointestinal motility. MTP Press, Lancaster, pp 265–270

Yu V Y H 1975 Effect of body position on gastric emptying in the neonate. Archives of Disease in Childhood 50: 500–504

Zoppi G, Andreotti G, Pajno-Ferrara F, Njail D M, Gaburra D 1972 Exocrine pancreas function in premature and full term neonates. Pediatric Research 6: 880–886

Structure and function

For practical purposes the digestive system may be thought of as a long muscular tube beginning at the lips and ending at the anus with certain large glands and organs such as the salivary glands, gallbladder, pancreas and liver situated outside this tube but emptying secretions into it. This chapter considers the relationships between the structure and the function of the mature alimentary canal, placing particular emphasis on the small intestine, and briefly reviews the associated digestive glands and organs; where appropriate, disturbances in the relationships between structure and function are described in the context of disease states.

The major function of the alimentary canal is the absorption of foodstuffs; it is, however, also a secretory and defensive organ and its structure will be considered in relation to these different aspects. The gross anatomical arrangement of the alimentary tract is similar throughout its length and consists of four layers, the serosa, the submucosa, the muscularis mucosa and the mucosa. These will be discussed in detail when describing the small intestine, the most important absorptive region of the tract. The alimentary tract is taken as extending from the oesophagus to the rectum, and other parts, such as the lips, tongue, teeth and pharynx, are not considered.

THE OESOPHAGUS

Anatomically the oesophagus begins at the inferior border of the cricopharyngeus and extends to the cardiac orifice of the stomach. Functionally, however, it extends from the lower border of the upper oesophageal sphincter to the upper edge of the lower oesophageal sphincter. These sphincters are operational terms rather than well-defined anatomical sites, and are identifiable in manometric studies as zones of high pressure (Goyal & Cobb 1981).

In achalasia (cardiospasm) the lower oesophageal sphincter fails to relax on swallowing, apparently as a result of a neuropathic disorder (Christensen 1983). In reflux oesophagitis, oesophageal motility and the tonic closure of the lower oesophageal sphincter is faulty (Christensen 1983).

As with all parts of the alimentary tract the oesophagus consists of four layers, but because of its specialized function structural differences exist compared with the small intestine. For example, because of the rapid luminal transit of food there is no requirement for an absorptive surface epithelial layer or for the secretion of digestive enzymes. Similarly there is not the same requirement for lymphoid tissue as a protection against invading microorganisms and, as it is well lubricated by saliva, mucus-secreting cells are not plentiful. However, because of the relatively undigested nature of the food which passes along its length, a stratified squamous epithelium is provided.

THE STOMACH

Structure

The mucosa is relatively thick and contains many mucus-producing cells and, when the stomach is partially empty, the mucosa is principally arranged in longitudinal folds or rugae. The only glands present in the submucosa are found in the pyloric region, adjacent to the duodenum. The muscularis mucosa consists of three rather than the usual two layers: an outer longitudinal, a middle circular and an inner oblique layer. The pyloric sphincter is a thickening predominantly of the middle circular layer.

The gastric mucosa contains three distinct types of glands. Firstly, the cardiac glands, which occupy the first few millimetres near the junction of the oesophagus, and are predominantly mucus-secreting glands, also contain undifferentiated and endocrine cells. Secondly, the pyloric glands, which occupy an area adjacent to the duodenum, produce mucus and

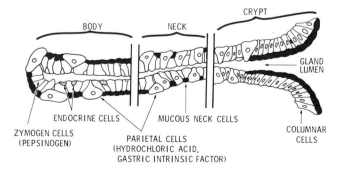

Fig. 2.1 The foveolae gastricae of the gastric mucosa showing the differrent regions and cell types.

contain type G endocrine cells which secrete gastrin. For a review of the physiology and pathology of gastrin see Walsh & Lam (1980). The remainder of the stomach (body and fundus) contains the third type of gland, i.e. the oxyntic or acid-secreting gland (Fig. 2.1) which contains chief or zymogen cells, parietal or oxyntic cells, mucosa neck cells and endocrine cells. The chief cell is a typical protein-secreting exocrine cell which synthesizes, stores and secretes pepsinogen. The parietal cell secretes hydrochloric acid and the gastric intrinsic factor which is necessary for the absorption of vitamin B_{12}. The mucous cells are located between the parietal cells in the neck region of the pits. The endocrine cells are scattered between the basement layer and chief cells and are important as a source of polypeptide hormones and biogenic amines. For a full review of the endocrine cells of the stomach see Ito (1981).

The surface epithelium of the stomach is made up of tall columnar cells which start abruptly at the cardiac region. They form a membrane which is one cell thick and secrete the mucus which coats and protects the lining of the stomach. The cells appear to originate at the pit openings and migrate upwards to replace those lost by desquamation, complete renewal of the surface cells taking place approximately every one to three days.

Function

The stomach has several important functions, which are listed in Table 2.1.

Table 2.1 Functions of the stomach

Storage, mixing and controlled emptying of food
Antibacterial properties of hydrochloric acid
Release of vitamin B_{12} from dietary protein
Synthesis of intrinsic factor
Initiation of protein digestion by pepsin
Initiation of fat digestion by lingual lipase
Synthesis of hormones
Facilitation of iron absorption

It receives and stores food, mixes it to form chyme and delivers the chyme in a controlled fashion to the small intestine. The function of the proximal stomach (fundus and body) as a reservoir is facilitated by the elasticity of its walls. The process of gastric filling is poorly understood, but it is probably not a completely passive process since gastric muscle appears to contract or relax to maintain the intragastric pressure constant over a wide range of volumes, implying that the process is regulated by a control mechanism. Immediately following the entry of food the gastric contents are composed of a liquid and solid phase which undergoes mixing and digestion to form a semisolid fluid or chyme which has an even consistency. This is achieved by the muscular movements of the stomach and by the digestive properties of gastric juice.

Gastric emptying is regulated by many factors all of which, with the exception of distension, are inhibitory (Hunt & Knox 1968, Cooke 1975, Heading 1983). Liquids are emptied faster than solids and probably by different mechanisms (Heading 1983). Delivery of the gastric contents to the duodenum is thought to depend on the force and frequency of antral peristaltic contractions. The osmolarity of the gastric contents is a sensitive and important mechanism regulating gastric emptying, isotonic contents leaving the stomach faster than hypo- or hypertonic ones. The effects of osmolarity on gastric emptying are mediated via sensitive osmoreceptors located in the proximal small intestinal mucosa. Acids, particularly hydrochloric acid, and fats (the longer the chain length of the fatty acids the greater the effect) both delay emptying. The mechanisms responsible for these inhibitory effects are likely to be both neural and humoral. Thus, pain or distension of the intestine inhibits gastric emptying by way of the sympathetic motor innervation to the stomach. Vagotomy has also been shown to abolish the inhibitory effect of hyperosmolar and fatty meals. The gastrointestinal hormones gastrin, secretin, cholecystokinin and gastric inhibitory polypeptide slow gastric emptying although the action of secretin is probably not physiological. Motilin increases gastric motility by inducing fasting propagative gastric motor activity. Despite the number and variety of the regulatory mechanisms the net result is that emptying occurs as a single exponential function, which implies a high degree of control between the various systems.

The acidity of gastric contents provides an important defence mechanism against ingested enteropathogenic bacteria, and patients with impaired gastric acid secretion are more susceptible to infective enteritis (Drasar et al 1969).

Vitamin B_{12} (cobalamin) does not exist in the free form but is attached to dietary protein, and a series of complex events is involved in its absorption (Seetharam & Alpers 1982). The first step is the release of the free vitamin from the dietary protein which is achieved by peptic digestion in the acid environment of the stomach. The free vitamin then complexes with R protein, a glycoprotein secreted by the stomach and salivary glands. This complex passes into the small intestine where it is degraded by trypsin and chymotrypsin and the free vitamin is again released. It is then complexed with gastric intrinsic factor, a glycoprotein of molecular weight 50 000 to 60 000 which is secreted by the gastric parietal cell. The cobalamin intrinsic factor complex stabilizes and protects the vitamin during intestinal transit and binds to specific receptors in the distal ileum prior to the release and absorption of the free vitamin. In general, intrinsic factor and acid are secreted in parallel and patients with achlorhydria usually have a reduced secretion of intrinsic factor. However, a continued secretion of small amounts of intrinsic factor may be sufficient to prevent the development of pernicious anaemia.

An ordinary meal remains in the stomach for about four hours and during this time it undergoes some digestion. The principal enzyme found in gastric juice is pepsin (Samloff 1971). This is formed from the inactive precursor pepsinogen, firstly by the action of hydrochloric acid and then by the autocatalytic action of free pepsin in the presence of hydrochloric acid. Pepsin is stable under acid conditions with a pH optimum at about 1.0–1.5. It initiates proteolysis in the stomach by hydrolysing peptide bonds at the amino groups of aromatic or acidic amino acids.

The first step in the hydrolysis of dietary triglyceride occurs in the stomach as a result of the action of lingual lipase which is secreted from the von-Ebner's glands on the proximal dorsal site of the tongue (Hamosh & Scow 1973) and possibly also by a gastric lipase secreted from glands within the gastric mucosa (De Nigris et al 1985). Lingual lipase differs from pancreatic lipase in that it has a low pH optimum (3.5–6.0), is relatively resistant to acid and does not require bile salts or colipase for activity (Hamosh et al 1981). In patients with cystic fibrosis and isolated pancreatic lipase deficiency, lingual lipase activity probably accounts for the major proportion of the hydrolysis of the triglyceride which is absorbed (Fredrikzon & Blackberg 1980, Muller et al 1975). Lingual lipase activity is also of major importance in the newborn and particularly the premature infant where it appears to compensate for both the low activity of pancreatic lipase and also the reduced bile salt concentration (Hamosh et al 1981).

Gastrin is synthesized and secreted by the 'G' cells of the antrum of the stomach, and the reader is referred to excellent reviews of this hormone by Walsh & Grossman 1975 and Walsh & Lam 1980. There are at least three human gastrins, 'big-', 'little-' and 'mini-' gastrin, with molecular weights of 3839, 2098 and 1647, respectively. The regulation of gastrin release from the 'G' cells is complex and is influenced by many factors. Stimulating factors include certain peptides and amino acids, gastric distension (acting via reflexes), vagal cholinergic stimulation (initiated from head or stomach), and blood-borne calcium or adrenaline (epinephrine). Inhibitory factors include acid and a variety of blood-borne peptide hormones such as secretin, gastric inhibitory peptide, vasoactive intestinal peptide and calcitonin. In addition to its stimulatory effect on gastric acidity, gastrin has a variety of other effects on gastric function and also on the function of other organs such as the small intestine, pancreas, colon and liver. Some of these effects require pharmacological doses and include secretion and inhibition of water and electrolyte transport, stimulation and inhibition of smooth muscle, enzyme secretion, release of hormones and trophic effects (see Walsh & Grossman 1975).

The acidity of the stomach facilitates the absorption of inorganic iron. At an acid pH precipitation of iron is prevented and chelation by ascorbate, dietary carbohydrates and amino acids is enhanced (Conrad & Schade 1968); these effects result in increased solubilization and absorption of iron.

THE SMALL INTESTINE

Basic structure and cell types (see Trier & Madara 1981)

Before discussing the function of the small intestine in some detail it is important to consider its basic structure and the cell types present.

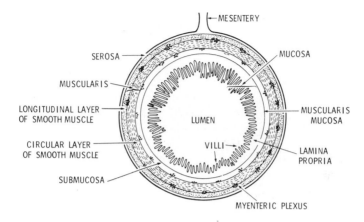

Fig. 2.2 Schematic cross-section of the small intestine showing its gross anatomical arrangement.

The wall of the small intestine consists of the four layers which are common to the whole alimentary tract (see Fig. 2.2). The outermost layer or serosa is an extension of the peritoneum and is made up of a single layer of flattened mesothelial cells which lie over some loose connective tissue. The muscularis comprises an outer longitudinal and an inner circular layer of smooth muscle, which together provide the primary mechanism for propelling the contents of the alimentary canal along its length. This is achieved by waves of constriction (peristalsis) which sweep downward, pushing the contents of the bowel ahead of them. Situated between the two muscle layers is a plexus of nerve fibres with numerous ganglia (myenteric plexus), which produces excitation above and inhibition below the stimulated area (Pescatori 1984).

The control of intestinal motility is a complicated and as yet poorly understood field, but it is clear that the autonomic nervous system and certain gastrointestinal peptides such as motilin and somatostatin play an important role (Wingate 1983).

The submucosa consists largely of dense connective tissue sparsely infiltrated by lymphocytes, macrophages, eosinophils, mast cells and plasma cells. It contains elaborate venous and lymphatic plexuses which drain the respective capillaries of the lamina propria of the mucosa. In addition it contains an extensive network of arterioles, ganglion cells and nerve fibres which form the autonomic submucosal plexus. Branched acinar glands

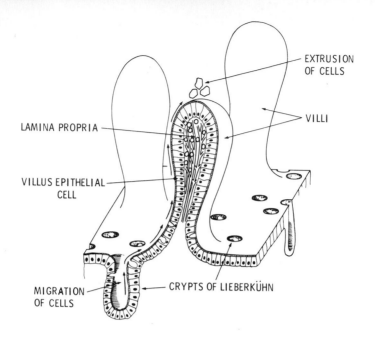

Fig. 2.3 The villi and crypts of the small intestinal mucosa.

(Brunner's glands) are found in the submucosa of the duodenum; their secretions are rich in mucus and bicarbonate and may provide protection against acid-peptic digestion of the proximal duodenum.

The innermost layer or mucosa can be subdivided into three further layers, the muscularis mucosa, the lamina propria and the epithelium. With the exception of the ileum the mucosa is thrown into a series of folds (folds of Kerckring) from which slender villi (0.2–1.0 mm in height) project into the lumen of the gut. As will be discussed later these folds and villi provide a mechanism to increase the absorptive surface area of the intestine. Between the villi are the crypts of Lieberkühn which dip down from the surface of the mucosa almost as far as the muscularis mucosa (Fig. 2.3). The villus: crypt length ratio is approximately 2:1, and there are about three times as many crypts as villi. The muscularis mucosa separates the mucosa from the submucosa and consists of a thin sheet of smooth muscle; one of the functions of the muscularis is to counteract stretching forces and so maintain the tall slender architecture of the villi.

The lamina propria

The lamina propria forms the connective tissue core of the villus, surrounds the crypts (Fig. 2.3) and has numerous functions. It provides structural support for the epithelium as well as for the many vascular and lymphatic channels that nourish the mucosa and transports absorbed material away to the systemic circulation. It contains numerous cell types, such as plasma cells, lymphocytes, mast cells, eosinophils and macrophages, and presents a defensive barrier to microorganisms and other foreign substances which may penetrate the surface epithelium. The lamina propria of the small intestine, particularly the distal part, contains isolated collections of lymphoid nodules. The larger ones may occupy the whole thickness of the mucosa, bulge onto its surface and even extend through the muscularis mucosa into the submucosal layer. When groups of nodules are massed together they form Peyer's patches which occur predominantly in the ileum. Immunoglobulins (IgA, IgM and IgG) are synthesized by the plasma cells and act as a first line of defence against invasion by microorganisms and other substances which may be involved in the production of local intestinal or systemic disease states (see Walker & Hong 1973). About 80 to 90% of the IgA in intestinal secretions (secretory IgA) is structurally and antigenically different to that found in serum. Secretory IgA consists of two molecules of IgA stabilized by a glycoprotein, secretory piece. It is likely that IgA molecules synthesized in the lamina propria pass into the epithelial cells where they complex with secretory piece and pass into the lumen as secretory IgA. The presence of secretory piece protects the IgA molecule from enzymatic digestion by the proteolytic enzymes normally present in the intestinal lumen. Immunoglobulins produced in the lamina propria probably also make an important contribution to the serum immunoglobulins. Indeed, the gut can be considered as an organ which makes an important contribution to the immune competence of the host as a whole.

Small unmyelinated nerve fibres are present in the lamina propria, and these may play a role in regulating mucosal blood flow and possibly also mucosal secretory activity. Smooth muscle fibres are present which may control villus motility. The activity (contraction and relaxation) of the villi is low during periods of fasting and increases during the absorption of a meal. By contracting and relaxing, the villi act as a 'micromixer' assuring optimal conditions for absorption, and may also be of importance in forcing lymph along the lymphatics.

The surface epithelium

The crypt epithelium is composed of at least four distinct cell types: Paneth, undifferentiated, goblet and endocrine cells, none of which have a brush border. The Paneth cells are located at the base of the crypts, are similar to salivary acinar glands and secrete large amounts of protein-rich materials. The observation that Paneth cells contain lysozyme (Peeters & Vantrappen 1975) and immunoglobulin (Rodning et al 1976) together with the demonstration of degenerating protozoa and bacteria within their lysosomes suggest that these cells are involved in the regulation of the microbiological flora of the small intestine, especially in the crypt region.

The most abundant cells in crypts are the undifferentiated or principal cells which form the lateral walls of the crypts and are also dispersed between the Paneth cells. Their cytoplasm contains many secretory granules. Goblet cells are found on the lateral wall of the crypts and are so named because of their shape. The thin basal half of the cell contains the nucleus and the apical half is distended by secretory material having the staining characteristics of sulphated mucoprotein. The function of intestinal mucus has not been completely defined, but it is believed to be important in protecting and lubricating the intestinal mucosa. The endocrine cells, also termed enterochromaffin, argentaffin, basal granular or more recently APUD (amine precursor uptake and decarboxylation) cells, are characterized by their inverted appearance compared to the order crypt cells. Their small secretory granules are distributed in the basal cytoplasm between the cell apex and the nucleus and are liberated into the lamina propria as opposed to the lumen of the gut. These cells synthesize and secrete the gastrointestinal hormones including gastrin, secretin and cholecystokinin as well as serotonin.

A major role of the crypt epithelium is that of cell proliferation and renewal of the intestinal epithelium (Creamer 1967). Within the crypts the undifferentiated cells divide and, as replication proceeds, new cells migrate up the wall of the crypt and on to the base of the villus where they begin to differentiate into mature cells. Differentiation continues as the cells migrate until the upper third of the villus is reached, where absorptive capacity is at a peak. At the extreme villus tip the cells degenerate, lose their absorptive capacity and are extruded into the intestinal lumen. The entire process of cell migration and maturation takes from four to five days in the ileum and five to seven days in the duodenum and jejunum. The epithelium covering the villus is composed of absorptive cells or enterocytes, goblet cells and a few endocrine cells. The latter types of cells closely resemble those found in the crypt epithelium. The enterocytes are the principal cells of the villus with the major role of digestion and absorption of the luminal contents.

The active absorptive and secretory processes in the small intestine appear to be spatially separated. There is an increasing body of evidence which suggests that undifferentiated crypt cells play an important role in the secretion of water and electrolytes into the lumen of the small intestine (Field 1981, Welsh et al 1982, Booth & Harries 1984).

Relationship between structure and function

Following the controlled emptying of chyme from the stomach, the duodenum is the area where neutralization, mixing, equilibration and the continuation of digestion takes place. By the time the intestinal contents reach the jejunum conditions are optimal for absorption. The ileum provides reserve capacity for absorption, as well as possessing specialized functions such as the absorption of vitamin B_{12}, and the sodium-dependent active absorption of bile salts.

Surface area and absorptive efficiency

The structure of the small intestine is so arranged as to provide the maximum available functional surface area, and this is achieved in three ways (Laster & Ingelfinger 1961, Trier 1968):

1. The luminal surface is thrown into a series of spiral or circular horizontal folds (i.e. folds of Kerckring) which increase the surface area by a factor of about three. They begin at the duodenum and end at the middle or distal third of the ileum, and are most abundant and highly developed in the distal duodenum and proximal jejunum where they may reach a length of 1 cm.

2. The numerous villi which extend from the mucosa amplify the surface area by a factor of 8 to 10 and they are approximately 0.5–1 mm in length. In the proximal duodenum they are normally broad and ridge-shaped, in the distal duodenum and proximal jejunum they are commonly leaf-shaped, whereas in the distal jejunum and ileum they are normally finger-like in shape. The villi are tallest in the distal duodenum and proximal jejunum and become progressively shorter as the ileocaecal valve is approached.

3. Finally, the brush border of the individual absorptive cells lining the villus is made up of slender microvilli which project into the lumen (Fig. 2.4). In man the microvilli average 1 μm in length with a width of

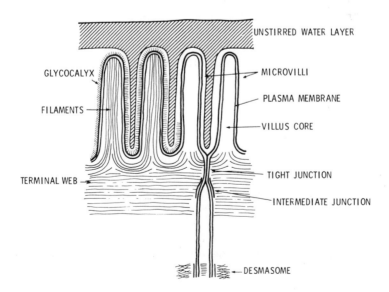

Fig. 2.4 The brush border of the absorptive cells of the small intestinal mucosa.

approximately 0.1 μm, and it has been estimated that they increase the absorptive surface of the cell by a further 15 to 40 times. Thus, the total surface area of the small intestine compared to a simple cylinder may be increased by a factor of up to 1200. Any reduction in villus size and/or number will result in a reduced surface area and impaired absorption. This mechanism partially explains the malabsorption in coeliac disease and intestinal resection.

The absorptive cell

The transport of dietary substances from the lumen to the bloodstream is regulated by the absorptive cell or enterocyte. Although the individual features of the enterocyte are not unique, its general appearance is distinctive and readily permits identification; the cells are tall columnar cells with a basally located oval-shaped nucleus. The arrangement of the enterocytes along the villus allows them to act as a transporting epithelium. They are polarized so that the apical brush border membrane faces the lumen of the intestine. The lateral borders of the enterocyte are joined at the tight junction with a potential space (lateral intercellular space) between adjoining cells.

The brush border. The brush border can be regarded as a subcellular organelle consisting of an apical plasma membrane surrounded by a surface coat or glycocalyx, a microvillous core and a terminal web (Fig. 2.4). The plasma membrane of the microvillus is both morphologically and biochemically different from the basal and lateral membranes of the absorptive cell; it is significantly wider (Palay & Karlin 1959) and has a different phospholipid composition (Lewis et al 1975). The glycocalyx is composed of a sulphated, weakly acidic mucopolysaccharide which differs structurally and histochemically from the mucus secreted by the goblet cell. It is an integral part of the cell, synthesized by the particular epithelial cell on which it is found and cannot be removed either by proteolytic or mucolytic agents (Holmes 1971). The microvillous core contains bundles of filaments which run parallel to the long axis of the microvillus and extend down into the cytoplasm of the cell where they interdigitate with the fibrils of the terminal web. The microvillous core and terminal web appear to provide important structural support for the brush border, thus ensuring that the maximum surface area is presented for absorption.

The microvilli together with the glycocalyx do much more than increase the available surface area. They actively participate in digestion and absorption in a number of ways. Firstly, intraluminal enzymes may be adsorbed on to the surface coat and thus some hydrolysis of substrates may take place at or in the glycocalyx with the theoretical advantage of releasing products near the microvillous plasma membrane (Ugolev 1972). The physiological importance of this digestive process compared to intraluminal digestion is probably minor. Secondly, a number of enzymes, particularly disaccharidases and peptidases, are located at or in the brush border membrane. The terminal digestion of carbohydrates and proteins occurs at the microvillous membrane prior to monosaccharide, amino acid or peptide transport into the cells. Thirdly, there appear to be specific receptors on the microvillous membrane–glycocalyx complex. For example, ileal absorptive cells have been shown to have specific receptors for the vitamin B_{12}-gastric intrinsic factor complex (Donaldson et al 1967). Fourthly, there is evidence that certain transport carriers are also located in the microvillous membrane. These are essential components of the overall transport process if the hydrophilic (water-loving) products of digestion, such as monosaccharides, amino acids and dipeptides, are to be transported across the lipid bilayer of the membrane. The close proximity of the hydrolytic enzymes and specific carriers of the brush border confers a 'kinetic advantage' for the transport of the terminal products of digestion across the plasma membrane into the cell (Crane 1968). For example, glucose is absorbed faster from sucrose than when presented to the mucosa as the free monosaccharide. Certain inborn errors of absorption are thought to result from a genetically determined defect or absence of protein carriers (see Ch. 9).

When considering the transport of substances from the lumen of the small intestine across the brush border there is a further barrier to take into account; the brush border is exposed to a predominantly aqueous environment, and a series of water lamellae extend outwards from the brush border becoming progressively more stirred until they blend imperceptibly with the bulk phase of the luminal contents. These relatively unstirred water layers immediately adjacent to the brush border present a barrier to uptake of substances by the mucosal cell and may be a rate-limiting factor in fat absorption (Wilson & Dietschy 1972).

The basolateral membranes. The basal and lateral membranes of the cell contain two enzymes which play a fundamental role in transport: sodium-potassium activated adenosine triphosphatase (Na^+–K^+)-ATPase and adenyl cyclase (Quigley & Gotterer 1969, Parkinson et al 1972). The former enzyme catalyses the hydrolysis of adenosine triphosphate (ATP) to adenosine diphosphate (ADP) and inorganic phosphate, which results in the liberation of energy; this energy is utilized by the 'sodium pump' to actively extrude sodium out of the cell across the basolateral membranes. This process generates and maintains a sodium concentration gradient between the intestinal lumen and the interior of the cell and allows for the active sodium-coupled transport of glucose and galactose and certain amino acids (Crane 1968); the resulting osmotic gradients result in water absorption. Thus the hydrolysis of ATP provides the cellular energy for the transport of electrolytes, certain sugars and amino acids against electrochemical gradients.

Adenyl cyclase catalyses the conversion of ATP to cyclic adenosine monophosphate (cAMP), and the role of this cyclic nucleotide in the regulation of water and electrolyte secretion is now well recognized (Field 1974).

Any factor which increases the intracellular concentration of cAMP also induces secretion of fluid and electrolytes, particularly monovalent anions, into the intestinal lumen. For example, the enterotoxin elaborated by *Vibrio cholerae* and the heat labile enterotoxin of *Escherichia coli* (Field 1974, 1976), prostaglandins (Kimberg et al 1971) and vasoactive inhibitory peptide (Schwartz et al 1974) all appear to exert their secretory effects via this system. Other intracellular mediators of intestinal secretion are cyclic guanosine monophosphate (cGMP) which is increased by the heat-stable enterotoxin of *E. coli* (Field et al 1978) and increased intracellular concentrations of calcium which appears to act by binding to and activating calmodulin, a calcium-dependent regulatory protein. For a review of secretion and the pathophysiology of diarrhoea see Dobbins & Binder (1981).

An important morphological specialization can be seen in the upper part of the lateral membrane where adjacent plasma membranes fuse for a short distance to form the so-called 'tight junction' (Fig. 2.4). It appears very likely that many small solutes, ions and water are able to traverse this junction (extracellular shunt pathway) during passive intestinal absorption or secretion. Other larger solutes, however, are unable to traverse this junction and must therefore cross the microvillous membrane, the cell cytoplasm and the lateral membrane before entering the intercellular spaces (Fordtran 1973). Immediately below the tight junction the lateral membranes diverge to form the intermediate junction which is approximately 200 Å wide. Below this is the third type of junctional complex, the desmosome, which serves to bind adjacent cells firmly together (Weinstein & McNutt 1972).

The basal membrane of the enterocyte is very close to the thin basement membrane on which the columnar cells lie and to the capillaries and lymphatics of the lamina propria. Absorbed material must always cross the basement membrane in order to reach these vascular and lymphatic channels. It has become increasingly clear that solute and water transport across the surface epithelium of the small intestine can occur via two routes, a transcellular route (i.e. the enterocyte) and an extracellular route (i.e. the paracellular shunt pathway), and the reader is referred to an excellent review by Schultz, Frizzell & Nellans (1974) for more detailed information.

Subcellular organelles. A variety of organelles, each with a specialized function, are distributed below the terminal web of the brush border; for example, mitochondria, lysosomes, the rough and smooth endoplasmic reticulum, and the Golgi apparatus. As in other cells the mitochondria provide metabolic energy and the lysosomes degrade waste and toxic substance. The endoplasmic reticulum has important roles in synthetic and transport processes. For example the smooth endoplasmic reticulum is the site of re-esterification of absorbed fatty acids and monoglycerides to triglyceride, and the rough endoplasmic reticulum synthesizes the protein moieties (apoproteins) which surround the packets of lipid (chylomicrons). The chylomicrons are then packaged within the Golgi apparatus, where it appears that the proteins also undergo glycosylation, prior to their secretion into the lymphatic system (Sabesin & Frase 1977). In abetalipoproteinaemia chylomicrons cannot be formed owing to a defect in the synthesis of an essential apoprotein designated apoprotein B (Gotto et al 1971).

THE LARGE INTESTINE

The wall of the part of the large intestine which lies within the peritoneal cavity consists of the four layers already discussed. The rectum, however, which lies outside the peritoneal cavity, has no serosa. The muscularis is composed of an inner circular and outer longitudinal muscle layer. The latter is distinctive because it is made up of three separate longitudinal strips (taeniae coli). The mucosa differs from that of the small intestine in that it has a flat absorptive surface with no villi; crypts are, however, present. The flat absorptive surface is lined by absorptive cells which have considerably less microvilli than the small intestine and which contain a moderate number of mucus-secreting goblet cells.

The main functions of the large intestine are the storage of intestinal contents prior to excretion, the absorption of water and electrolytes entering from the ileum and, in particular, the conservation of sodium ions and water (Cummings 1975). The colonic mucosa is able to absorb sodium from luminal concentrations as low as 15 mmol/l and against a potential difference of as much as 40 mV (lumen negative compared to the serosa), whereas the maximum potential difference generated by the ileum and jejunum is about 5 mV. Unlike the jejunum the absorption of sodium by the colon is not stimulated by glucose or amino acids. Patients with established ileostomies provide indirect evidence of the importance of the colon in sodium and water conservation, since they are susceptible to water and salt depletion especially in hot climates. The mineralocorticoid aldosterone influences colonic conservation of fluid, sodium and chloride. It promotes net absorption and increases the transmural potential difference, and in addition reduces the sodium : potassium ratio in the effluent of patients with an ileostomy (Sladen 1972). In patients with chronic inflammatory disease of the large bowel, transport of water and electrolytes may be impaired, which also emphasizes the importance of the large bowel in fluid conservation. The capacity of the large intestine to absorb declines progressively down the intestinal tract, with the rectum absorbing very little.

The factors which control the electrophysiology, the pharmacology and the motility of the large intestine and the act of defaecation are complex, and the reader is referred to the following reviews for detailed accounts of these processes: Duthie 1971, Bennett 1975, Edmonds 1975, Christensen 1981, 1984.

DIGESTIVE ORGANS AND GLANDS ASSOCIATED WITH THE ALIMENTARY TRACT

The salivary glands

There are three pairs of salivary glands, the parotid, mandibular and sublingual, all of which are of the compound tubuloalveolar type.

The parotid glands are the largest and are serous glands producing zymogen granules which are precursors of salivary amylase. The submandibular glands are predominantly serous but also contain mucous cells; the sublingual glands are also mixed but mainly secrete mucus. These three types of glands secrete saliva, which has several functions. It lubricates the buccal mucosa and lips, washes the mouth clear of cellular and food debris, moistens food and converts it to a semisolid or liquid mass prior to swallowing. Saliva is also involved in the initial stages of digestion with salivary amylase initiating starch digestion. Secretion of saliva is regulated by the autonomic nervous system and may be influenced by cephalic, mechanical or chemical factors.

The pancreas

The pancreas produces both exocrine and endocrine secretions, but in the context of intestinal function the exocrine secretion is of primary importance and its endocrine function will only be briefly mentioned. The endocrine and exocrine components are, however, functionally related and the former may effect the exocrine activity of the pancreas (Menderson et al 1981).

Structure (Gorelick & Jamieson 1981).

The pancreas is a compound acinous gland containing lobules which are bound together by loose connective tissue that is traversed by blood vessels, lymphatics, nerves and secretory ducts. The predominant acinar cells produce the exocrine secretion of the gland. Dispersed within these cells are isolated clumps of other species of cells (i.e. islets of Langerhans) which synthesize and secrete certain peptide hormones. The acinar cells consists of a single row of pyramidal epithelial cells which rest on a delicate reticular membrane and converge towards a central lumen, the size of which varies with the functional condition of the organ; it is small when at rest but becomes distended with secretory material during active secretion. The lumen of the acinus connects with small intercalated ducts; these are surrounded by centroacinar cells that drain into intralobular ducts which are covered by low columnar cells similar to centroacinar cells. These anastomose to form the interlobular ducts, which in turn communicate to become the main pancreatic duct of Wirsung. The interlobular ducts are lined with a columnar epithelium containing goblet cells, and the occasional argentaffin cell and mucous gland. The duct of Wirsung runs the whole length of the pancreas gradually increasing in size before opening into the duodenum at the ampulla of Vater. The islets of Langerhans, which produce the endocrine secretions, are separated from the surrounding acinar tissue by fine reticular fibres and do not connect with the pancreatic ducts. They contain three types of cells, designated alpha, beta and delta cells, which liberate glucagon, insulin and an unknown secretion, respectively.

Function (see Beck 1973, Brandborg 1973, Gorelick & Jamieson 1981).

The exocrine pancreas performs two important functions. Firstly the acinar cells synthesize and secrete a number of enzymes which take part in the luminal digestion of ingested protein, carbohydrate and fat.

The proteolytic enzymes are secreted as inactive precursors (zymogens) which, on entering the intestinal lumen, are activated by the action of a key enzyme, enterokinase. Enterokinase is a brush border enzyme which is released into the lumen and converts trypsinogen to trypsin, which in turn activates the other proteolytic zymogens. These enzymes convert proteins to amino acids and short-chain peptides, and these products are transported and further hydrolysed to enter the portal vein as amino acids. Salivary and pancreatic α-amylase hydrolyses starch to maltose, maltotriose and α-limit dextrins. Maltose and maltotriose are then split by brush border maltases to glucose, and α-limit dextrins are split by brush border sucrase-isomaltase to glucose; glucose then enters the cell by an active sodium-coupled transport system. The pancreas secretes three classes of enzymes which participate in the luminal digestion of lipids, phospholipases, lipase and esterase. The main function of the phospholipases is to convert leci-thin (phosphatidyl choline) to lysolecithin. Lipase converts triglyceride to monoglyceride and free fatty acids, and esterase hydrolyses molecules such as cholesterol esters to free cholesterol. The products of pancreatic lipolysis are solubilized by bile salt micelles and transported to the brush border for absorption.

The second important function of the pancreas is to secrete an alkaline aqueous fluid which is isosmotic with plasma; this neutralizes the acid chyme leaving the stomach and provides an optimal environment for luminal digestion. Sodium and potassium concentrations in pancreatic secretions are similar to those in plasma, and the chloride concentration is reciprocally related to that of bicarbonate and may reach 150 mmol/l. The intercalated ducts and centroacinar cells are the sites of water and electro-lyte secretion. Carbonic anhydrase, an enzyme involved in bicarbonate secretion, is found only in the ductular epithelium.

Exocrine pancreatic secretion is regulated by a complex series of neuro-humoral mechanisms (see Youngs 1972, Brooks 1973, Mayer 1981). The most important hormones involved in this regulatory process are gastrin, secretin and cholecystokinin-pancreozymin (CCK-PZ). Gastrin stimulates enzyme secretion and is under cholinergic control. A low intragastric pH is the principal inhibitory factor to gastrin release. Secretin-producing cells are located in the mucosa of the proximal small gut and its secretion results from the passage of acid from the stomach. Secretin stimulates pancreatic secretion of water and electrolytes, principally bicarbonate, and has relatively little effect on the secretion of enzymes. CCK-PZ is also synthesized and secreted by the proximal small intestinal mucosa in response to the arrival of chyme from the stomach. It stimulates the secretion of pancreatic enzymes and is approximately three times as potent as gastrin. The vagus appears to be involved in the release of secretin and CCK-PZ, but the presence of a local cholinergic mechanism is controversial. A cephalic phase of pancreatic secretion has also been demonstrated in man and results in stimulation of both bicarbonate and enzyme secretion.

Some implications of these control mechanisms are that hormonal stimulation of pancreatic secretion may be impaired because of (1) a reduction in the number of hormone-producing cells (i.e. APUD cells), as in coeliac disease or following gastric antrectomy; (2) a failure of hydrochloric acid and/or chyme to reach APUD cells, as is the case following gastrojejunostomy, or (3) a reduction in the number of pancreatic secretory cells, as may occur in cystic fibrosis, congenital pancreatic hypoplasia or pancreatitis.

The liver

The liver is the largest organ in the body and performs numerous functions, some of which are of fundamental importance in a consideration of intestinal function.

Structure

The liver is composed of lobules, the outlines of which are indistinct as a result of poorly developed connective tissue partitions between them. The central hepatic vein runs through the centre of the lobules, whereas the branches of the portal vein, hepatic artery, interlobular bile ducts and lymphatics run together in the connective tissue of the portal tracts at the periphery of the lobules. The lobules are made up of hepatocytes which extend radially from the central vein to the periphery. In order for the hepatocytes to perform both an exocrine and endocrine function they are arranged in such a way as to form anastomosing thin plates (Fig. 2.5). Each cell therefore abuts on to a blood vessel into which it delivers its endocrine secretions, and on to a canalicular lumen into which its exocrine secretion (i.e. bile) passes. Between the plates of cells are vascular sinusoids which receive blood from the portal vein and hepatic artery, and carry it to the centre of the lobule where it drains into the central vein. Lining the walls of the sinusoids are the Kupffer cells which have important phagocytic properties. The sinusoids and portal tracts also contain free round cells

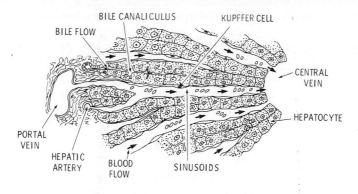

Fig. 2.5 The microstructure of the liver showing the arrangement of the hepatocytes, blood vessels and bile canaliculi.

which are precursors of both red and white blood cells. Within the plates but between adjacent rows of hepatocytes are the bile canaliculi into which the bile is secreted. The canaliculi anastomose with each other and drain the bile to the periphery of the lobule and into the canals of Herring, which are bordered in part by hepatocytes and also by duct-type cells. These canals are short and connect with small bile ducts in the portal tract.

Function

With respect to intestinal function the prime function of the liver is the secretion of bile. Bile is an iso-osmotic alkaline solution (pH 7.5 to 9.5) which contains an abundance of organic solutes such as conjugated bile salts, bilirubin, cholesterol and lecithin. Its main function is the solubiliz-ation of dietary lipids in the small intestine by bile salts prior to their absorption. Adequate intraluminal concentrations of bile salts are also important for other digestive events. For example, colipase and bile salts are necessary for optimum activity of pancreatic lipase (Borgstrom et al 1979). Similarly bile salts activate pancreatic esterase (Muller et al 1976), and may promote the activation of trypsinogen by trypsin (Hadorn et al 1974, Green & Nassett 1980). In addition, bile salts protect some of these enzymes against tryptic digestion and regulate the biosynthesis of choles-terol by the small gut mucosa.

There is a ductular and canalicular phase to the secretion of bile (Erlinger 1972). The ductular epithelium actively secretes sodium and bicarbonate into the lumen of the ducts by a coupled pump, which is under the influ-ence of gastrointestinal hormones such as secretin, CCK-PZ and gastrin, all of which increase bile flow and bicarbonate secretion. Vagal stimulation appears to enhance these humoral effects. The canalicular phase of secretion has two components, a bile acid-dependent and a bile acid-independent component. The active secretion of bile acids from the hepatocyte into the canaliculi establishes an osmotic gradient which results in the passive movement of water and cations to give an electrically neutral and isosmotic secretion. There is a linear relationship between bile flow and bile acid secretion rate, but if this is extrapolated to zero bile acid secretion, there is still significant bile flow. This and other evidence suggests that there is another mechanism for bile flow which is bile acid-independent. It is thought that the active transport of sodium ions may be responsible for this component, and this is supported by the fact that the bile acid-independent flow is suppressed or greatly decreased by inhibitors of the sodium pump. This component of bile flow can be stimulated by phenobarbitone, which produces no significant change either in the total bile acid secretion rate or in the relative output of individual bile acids.

In addition to synthesizing and transporting bile, the hepatocytes are ideally situated to perform their numerous metabolic functions as they come into intimate contact with the absorbed dietary constituents present in portal blood.

The gallbladder

The gallbladder is a distensible sac with a mucosa which is thrown into numerous folds, thereby increasing its surface area for absorption. The epithelium of the mucosa is columnar with microvilli and thus resembles the absorptive cells of the small intestine. Its wall also has submucosal, muscularis and serosal layers. In addition it has a well-developed layer of smooth muscle which is arranged in an interlocking pattern of longitudinal and spirally arranged fibres. The gallbladder is drained by the cystic duct, which enters the common hepatic duct to form the common bile duct. This terminates in the duodenum close to the point of entry of the pancreatic duct at the ampulla of Vater. The complex of smooth muscle fibres associated with the ampulla and the distal ends of the bile and pancreatic ducts form the sphincter of Oddi. The sphincter regulates the flow of bile into the intestine, inhibits the entry of bile into the pancreatic duct and prevents reflux of intestinal contents into the duct.

The function of the gallbladder is to concentrate and store bile, and to deliver it to the duodenum during meals (Banfield 1975). Hepatic bile is rapidly concentrated to the extent that about 90% of the fluid is removed as an isotonic solution composed principally of sodium, chloride and bicarbonate; sodium and chloride are absorbed by an electrogenically neutral coupled transport process. Fluid and electrolyte transport by the gallbladder has been recently reveiwed by Wood & Svanvick (1983). The flow of concentrated bile from the gallbladder is initiated by predominantly hormonal stimuli. Cholecystokinin-pancreozymin is released from the mucosa of the proximal small intestine following a meal, and the hormone simultaneously stimulates gallbladder contraction and relaxation of the sphincter of Oddi. Vagal stimulation may enhance the action of CCK-PZ on gallbladder contraction. As the products of digestion are absorbed so the hormonal stimuli diminish, sphincter tone returns, the gall bladder relaxes and thus bile is again retained and concentrated. The effects of CCK-PZ appear to be mediated by the cyclic nucleotide, cyclic guanosine monophosphate.

REFERENCES

Banfield W J 1975 Physiology of the gallbladder. Gastroenterology 69: 770–777
Beck I T 1973 The role of pancreatic enzymes in digestion. American Journal of Clinical Nutrition 26: 311–325
Bennett A 1975 Pharmacology of colonic muscle. Gut 16: 307–311
Booth I W, Harries J T 1984 Regulatory mechanisms of secretory diarrhoea and electrolyte imbalance in acute and chronic diarrhoea in infancy. In: Lebenthal E (ed). Chronic Diarrhoea in Children. Raven Press, New York, pp 307–317
Borgstrom B, Erlanson-Albertson C, Wieloch T 1979 Pancreatic colipase: chemistry and physiology. Journal of Lipid Research 20: 805–816
Brandborg L L 1973 Pancreatic physiology. In: Sleisenger M H, Fordtran J S (eds) Gastrointestinal Disease: Pathophysiology, Diagnosis, Management. Saunders, Philadelphia pp 359–364
Brooks F P 1973 The neurohumoral control of pancreatic exocrine secretion. American Journal of Clinical Nutrition 26: 291–310
Christensen J 1981 Motility of the colon. In: Johnson L R (ed) Physiology of the Gastrointestinal Tract. Raven Press, New York: pp 445–471
Christensen J 1983 Physiological characteristics of the gastro-oesophageal junction. The Italian Journal of Gastroenterology 15: 143–147
Christensen J 1984 Colonic motor activity. Italian Journal of Gastroenterology 16: 126–133
Conrad M E, Schade S G 1968 Ascorbic acid chelates in iron absorption: a role for hydrochloric acid and bile. Gastroenterology 55: 35–45
Cooke A R 1975 Control of gastric emptying and motility. Gastroenterology 68: 804–816
Crane R K 1968 Absorption of sugars. In: Code C F (ed) Handbook of Physiology, Section 6, Vol IV. American Physiological Society, Washington D C, pp 1323–1351
Creamer B 1967 The turnover of the epithelium of the small intestine. British Medical Bulletin 23: 226–230
Cummings J H 1975 Absorption and secretion by the colon. Gut 16: 323–329
Denigris S J, Hamosh M, Kasbekar D K, Fink C S, Lee T C, Hamosh P 1985 Secretion of human gastric lipase from dispersed gastric glands. Biochimica et Biophysica Acta 836: 67–72
Dobbins J W, Binder H J 1981 Pathophysiology of diarrhoea: alterations in fluid and electrolyte transport. Clinics in Gastroenterology 10 No 3: 605–625
Donaldson R M, MacKenzie I L, Trier J S 1967 Intrinsic factor-mediated attachment of vitamin B_{12} to brush borders and microvillous membranes of hamster intestine. Journal of Clinical Investigation 46: 1215–1228
Drasar B S, Shiner M, McLeod G M 1969 Studies on the intestinal flora. I. The bacterial flora of the gastrointestinal tract in healthy and achlorhydric persons. Gastroenterology 56: 71–79
Duthie H L 1971 Anal continence. Gut 12: 844–852
Edmonds C J 1975 Electrical potential difference of colonic mucosa. Gut 16: 315–323
Erlinger S 1972 Physiology of bile flow. Progress in Liver Disease 4: 63–82
Field M 1974 Intestinal secretion. Gastroenterology 66: 1063–1084
Field M 1976 Regulation of active ion transport in the small intestine. Ciba Foundation Symposium 42: 109–127
Field M 1981 Secretion of electrolytes and water by mammalian small intestine. In: Johnson L R (ed) Physiology of the Gastrointestinal Tract. Raven Press, New York, pp 963–982
Field M, Graf L H Jr, Laird W J, Smith P L 1978 Heat-stable enterotoxin of Escherichia coli: in vitro effect on guanylate cyclase activity, cyclic GMP concentration and ion

transport in the small intestine. Proceedings National Academy of Science USA
75: 2800–2804

Fordtran J S 1973 Diarrhea. In: Sleisenger M H, Fordtran J S (eds) Gastrointestinal
Disease: Pathophysiology, Diagnosis and Management. Saunders, Philadelphia,
pp 291–319

Fredrikzon B, Blackberg L 1980 Lingual lipase: an important lipase in the digestion of
dietary lipids in cystic fibrosis? Pediatric Research 14: 1387–1390

Gorelick F S, Jamieson J D 1981 Structure-function relationships of the pancreas. In:
Johnson L R (ed) Physiology of the Gastrointestinal Tract. Raven Press, New York,
pp 773–794

Gotto A M, Levy R I, John K, Fredrickson D S 1971 On the protein defect in
abetalipoproteinaemia. New England Journal of Medicine 284: 813–818

Goyal R J, Cobb B W 1981 Motility of the pharynx, esophagus and esophageal sphincters.
In: Johnson L R (ed) Physiology of the Gastrointestinal Tract. Raven Press, New York,
pp 359–391

Green G M, Nassett E S 1980 Importance of bile in regulation of intraluminal proteolytic
enzyme activities in the rat. Gastroenterology 79: 695–702

Hadorn B, Hess J, Troesch V, Verhaage W, Gotze H, Bender S W 1974 Role of bile acids
in the activation of trypsinogen by enterokinase: disturbance of trypsinogen activation in
patients with intrahepatic biliary atresia. Gastroenterology 66: 548–555

Hamosh M, Scow R O 1973 Lingual lipase and its role in the digestion of dietary fat.
Journal of Clinical Investigation 52: 88–95

Hamosh M, Scanlon J W, Ganot D, Likel M, Scanlon K B, Hamosh P 1981 Fat digestion
in the newborn. Characterization of lipase in gastric aspirates of premature and term
infants. Journal of Clinical Investigation 67: 838–846

Heading R C 1983 Control and measurement of gastric emptying. The Italian Journal of
Gastroenterology 15: 194–200

Henderson J R, Daniel P M, Fraser P A 1981 The pancreas as a single organ: the influence
of the endocrine upon the exocrine part of the gland. Gut 22: 158–167

Holmes R 1971 The intestinal brush border. Gut 12: 668–677

Hunt J N, Knox M T 1968 Regulation of gastric emptying. In: Code C F (ed) Handbook
of Physiology, Section 6, Vol. IV. American Physiological Society, Washington D C,
p 1917

Ito S 1981 Functional gastric morphology. In: Johnson L R (ed) Physiology of the
Gastrointestinal Tract. Raven Press, New York, pp 517–550

Kimberg D V, Field M, Johnson J, Henderson A, Gershon E 1971 Stimulation of intestinal
mucosal adenyl cyclase by cholera enterotoxin and prostaglandins. Journal of Clinical
Investigation 50: 1218–1230

Laster L, Ingelfinger F J 1961 Intestinal absorption — aspects of structure, function and
disease of the small intestinal mucosa. New England Journal of Medicine 264: 1138–1148

Lewis B A, Gray G M, Coleman R, Michell R H 1975. Differences in the enzymic,
polypeptide, glycopeptide, glycolipid and phospholipid compositions of plasma
membranes from the two surfaces of intestinal epithelial cells. Biochemical Society
Transactions 3: 752–753

Meyer J H 1981 Control of pancreatic exocrine secretion. In: Johnson L R (ed) Physiology
of the Gastrointestinal Tract. Raven Press, New York pp 821–829

Muller D P R, McCollum J P K, Trompeter R S, Harries J T 1975 Studies on the
mechanism of fat absorption in congenital isolated lipase deficiency. Gut 16:838

Muller D P R, Manning J A, Mathias P M, Harries J T 1976 Studies on the intestinal
hydrolysis of tocopherol esters. International Journal for Vitamin and Nutrition Research
46: 207–210

Palay S L, Karlin L J 1959 An electron microscopic study of the intestinal villus. I. The
fasting animal. Journal of Biophysical and Biochemical Cytology 5: 363–372

Parkinson D K, Ebel H, Dibona D, Sharp G W G 1972 Localisation of the action of
cholera toxin on adenyl cyclase in mucosal epithelial cells of rabbit intestine. Journal of
Clinical Investigation 51: 731–740

Peeters T, Vantrappen G 1975 The Paneth cell: a source of intestinal lysozyme. Gut
16: 553–558

Pescatori M 1984 The peristaltic reflex. Italian Journal of Gastroenterology 16: 48–53

Quigley J P, Gotterer G S 1969 Distribution of ($Na^+–K^+$)-stimulated ATPase activity in rat
intestinal mucosa. Biochimica et Biophysica Acta 173: 456–468

Rodning C B, Wilson I D, Erlandsen S L 1976 Immunoglobulins within human small intestinal Paneth cells. Lancet i: 984–987

Sabesin S M and Frase S 1977 Electron microscopic studies of the assembly, intracellular transport and secretion of chylomicrons by rat intestine. Journal of Lipid Research 18: 496–511

Samloff I M 1971 Pepsinogens, pepsins and pepsin inhibitors. Gastroenterology 60: 586–604

Schultz S G, Frizzell R A, Nellans H N 1974 Ion transport by mammalian small intestine. Annual Review of Physiology 36: 51–91

Schwartz C J, Kimberg D V, Sheerin H E, Field M, Said S I 1974 Vasoactive intestinal peptide stimulation of adenylate cyclase and active electrolyte secretion in intestinal mucosa. Journal of Clinical Investigation 54: 536–544

Seetharam B, Alpers D H 1982 Absorption and transport of cobalamin (vitamin B_{12}). Annual Reviews of Nutrition 2: 343–369

Sladen G E G 1972 A review of water and electrolyte transport. In: Burland W L, Samuel P D (eds) Churchill Livingstone, Edinburgh, pp 14–34

Trier J S 1968 Morphology of the epithelium of the small intestine. In: Code C F (ed) Handbook of Physiology, Section 6, Vol. III. American Physiological Society, Washington D C, pp 1125–1175

Trier J S, Madara J L 1981 Functional morphology of the mucosa of the small intestine. In: Johnson L R (ed) Physiology of the Gastrointestinal Tract. Raven Press, New York, pp 925–961

Ugolev A M 1972 Membrane digestion. Gut 13: 735–747

Walker W A, Hong R 1973 Immunology of the gastrointestinal tract. Journal of Pediatrics 83: 517–530

Walsh J H, Grossman M I 1975 Gastrin. New England Journal of Medicine 292: 1324–1334

Walsh J H, Lam S K 1980 Physiology and pathology of gastrin. Clinics in Gastroenterology 9: 567–591

Weinstein R S, McNutt N S 1972 Cell junctions. New England Journal of Medicine 286: 521–524

Welsh M J, Smith P L, Fromm M, Frizzell R A 1982 Crypts are the site of intestinal fluid and electrolyte secretion. Science 218: 1219–1221

Wilson F A, Dietschy J M 1972 Characterization of bile acid absorption across the unstirred water layer and brush border of the rat jejunum. Journal of Clinical Investigation 51: 3015–3025

Wingate D L 1983 The small intestine. In: Christensen J, Wingate D L (eds) A Guide to Gastrointestinal Motility. Wright, Bristol. pp. 128–156

Wood J R, Svanvick 1983 Gall-bladder water and electrolyte transport and its regulation. Gut 24: 579–593

Youngs G 1972 Hormonal control of pancreatic endocrine and exocrine secretion. Gut 13: 154–161

Investigatory techniques

Investigation of gastrointestinal disease in childhood usually requires relatively invasive techniques or exposure to radiation. Each technique examines only a small part of the structure or function of the gut and a careful clinical appraisal is necessary to enable the selection of a relevant and useful investigation. Even in expert hands, interpretation of the results of any investigation may be difficult, and close communication between clinical and laboratory staff is required to enable the sick child to reap the benefits of the recent advances in investigatory techniques.

The techniques described have been broadly divided into those which delineate structure and those which assess function; a degree of overlap is unavoidable but it is hoped that this subdivision will prove helpful in clinical practice.

STRUCTURAL STUDIES

Radiological techniques

Plain radiology

Plain abdominal films can provide important information for diagnosis and management in both acute and chronic gastroenterological disorders. These conditions are summarized in Table 3.1.

Contrast radiology

Alimentary tract. Barium sulphate is usually the contrast material of choice but may become inspissated by the absorption of water by the bowel and may cause bronchial obstruction if inhaled. Propyliodone (Dionosil) is preferable if a spillage into the trachea is likely.

Certain contrast agents can cause problems of fluid balance particularly

Table 3.1 Gastroenterological disorders found on plain radiology

Radiological sign	Condition	Comment
Fluid level	Intestinal obstruction Intestinal secretion	'Double Bubble' complete duodenal obstruction
Gut in chest	Diaphragmatic hernia	
Free gas	Intestinal perforation	Lateral decubitus film in the sick child
Pneumatosis	Necrotizing enterocolitis	Intramural gas and/or gas in the portal venous system
Gaseous distension	Toxic megacolon	Occurs in a variety of colonic inflammatory diseases, should be monitored 6 hourly
Calcification	Fetal or meconium peritonitis Chronic pancreatitis Liver disease and gallstones	Intrauterine infection or cystic fibrosis Gallstones seen uncommonly as most stones in childhood are pigment stones
	Renal calculi Neuroblastoma	
Foreign bodies		
Bony structures	Spina bifida Metastases Bony dysplasia	Histiocytosis Wilm's tumour Schwachmann's syndrome

in young infants, either because of high osmolarity (e.g. Gastrografin) or low osmolarity such as hypotonic barium enema suspensions (Gordon & Ross 1977). Recently, a number of alternative low ionic concentration contrast media such as metrizamide have become available. They are expensive but may have a place in sick infants or those in whom a perforation is suspected.

The indications for barium swallow are listed in Table 3.2. In certain circumstances, such as swallowing disorders in young infants, cine radiology may be useful.

A barium meal should always include the duodenal loop and the position of the duodenojejunal flexure should be assessed on an anterior and lateral film if malrotation is a possibility. The indications for a barium meal and follow through are listed in Table 3.3. In malabsorptive states this

Table 3.2 Indications for barium swallow

Dysphagia
Suspicion of oesophageal varices
Mediastinal masses
Vascular rings
Persistent respiratory stridor and aspiration
Foreign bodies
Assessment of oesophageal strictures

Table 3.3   Indications for barium meal and follow-through

Recurrent vomiting and failure to thrive
Congenital or postsurgical abnormalities
Hypertrophic pyloric stenosis when a tumour cannot be palpated
Suspected peptic ulcer
Gastrointestinal bleeding
Chronic inflammatory bowel disease
Intestinal malabsorption in association with a normal small intestinal biopsy

investigation should only be used if a peroral small intestinal biopsy is not diagnostic. Flocculation of contrast is seen in malabsorption but occurs in other conditions and is quite common in normal infants and may, therefore, be a nonspecific finding.

Table 3.4   Indications for barium enema

Neonatal intestinal obstruction
Intussusception
Chronic inflammatory bowel disease
Large bowel polyps
Chronic constipation

The indications for a barium enema are shown in Table 3.4. This procedure is of great importance in newborns with features of lower intestinal obstruction, as for example in Hirschsprung's disease or malrotation of the gut when a high caecum is found. We have, however, found a barium meal and follow-through of more help in the diagnosis of malrotation (Simpson et al 1972). In intussusception the procedure may be curative as well as diagnostic. Double contrast barium enemata are useful for demonstrating polyps or mucosal disease but in centres where skilled colonoscopy is available this is preferable. Chronic constipation with or without overflow is not usually associated with underlying organic disease but if Hirschsprung's disease is a possible cause a barium enema may be performed if rectal biopsies are not readily available.

Biliary tract.   For technical details of the procedures available for cholecystography and cholangiography the reader is referred to Harris & Caffey (1953) and Hodgson (1970). Oral cholecystography or intravenous cholangiography is contraindicated in patients with active hepatocellular disease or when the serum level of bilirubin is greater than 85 μmol/l (5 mg/100 ml).

Oral cholecystography and intravenous cholangiography provide information on the structure and function of the gall bladder, the presence of gallstones and the integrity of the extrahepatic biliary ducts. Both investigations have very limited application in childhood. Gallstones, except for pigment stones in patients with chronic haemolytic anaemia, are extremely rare before puberty. Neither investigation has a place in the diagnosis of persistent neonatal jaundice. Percutaneous and/or operative cholangiography in infants with persistent jaundice is useful in assessing how much of the extrahepatic biliary duct system is patent, and it is an important aid in the decision on the type of surgical approach to be adopted in patients with extrahepatic biliary atresia.

Splenoportography (see Melhem & Rizk 1970).   This procedure should only be used in the final assessment of portal hypertension when all preliminary investigations have been completed. It provides excellent visualization of the portal venous system, indicating the site of obstruction, the collateral circulation and its direction of flow, and it can be combined with splenic pulp pressure (i.e. portal vein pressure) measurements. It is not an emergency procedure and should be performed only when shunt surgery is being considered. In children under the age of 12 years it should be performed under general anaesthesia, and facilities for immediate surgery must be available if complications such as haemorrhage occur.

Selective angiography

Introduction of a catheter via a femoral artery enables selective angiography of the hepatic, coeliac, superior and inferior mesenteric arteries and may provide useful information in children with tumours, portal hypertension and circulatory abnormalities. The procedure is sometimes used to localize bleeding sites in massive continued gastrointestinal bleeding and embolization of vessels may be carried out (Irving & Northfield 1976).

Ultrasound

Ultrasound is non-invasive and does not involve exposure to ionizing radiation. It is extremely useful for assessing solid abdominal masses and has sometimes been used for the diagnosis of pyloric stenosis. Cystic lesions including duplication cysts and choledochal cysts may be identified. It is particularly useful for visualization of the liver, biliary tracts, spleen and varices, and in the child it is the method of choice for visualizing the pancreas (Caritz, Leopold & Wolf 1982).

Computerized tomography

Computerized tomography has not so far proved as useful in the investigation of gastroenterological disease as it has in neurology and neurosurgery. It may, however, be useful in those circumstances where ultrasonic visualization may be difficult, such as retroperitoneal pathology, mesenteric cysts and bowel lymphomas.

Radioisotopic scanning

The development of scintiscanning techniques following the administration of radioisotopes represents an important advance in the diagnosis of hepatic, pancreatic and gastrointestinal disease.

Liver

Scanning has proved most useful in the detection of space-occupying lesions such as abscesses, cysts and primary or secondary tumours. In addition, the technique can provide information on hepatocellular and reticuloendothelial function. The isotope most commonly used is [99]technetium sulphur colloid, which has a half-life of six hours. Following an intravenous injection the isotope is taken up by normally functioning hepatocytes and Kupffer cells. Cells which are diseased or compressed by space-occupying lesions have an impaired capacity to take up the isotope and appear as 'cold' areas on the photoscan. A large abscess or tumour is easily visualized as a distinct cold area, whereas more diffuse disease presents a patchy pattern. Liver scanning is a complementary diagnostic procedure and does not provide information for a definitive diagnosis (Rosenfield & Treves 1974).

[99]Technetium diethyliminodiacetic acid (DIDAD) is handled by biliary transport systems and hence is useful in biliary obstruction due to structural abnormalities such as choledochal cyst or extra-hepatic duct abnormalities. In biliary atresia when complete obstruction exists, no activity is detected in the intestine (Ryoji et al 1981).

Pancreas

Ultrasound and endoscopic retrograde choledochopancreatography have diminished the use of pancreatic isotope scans. [75]Se selenomethionine scan is useful in selected patients (McCarthy 1970). Liver uptake of the isotope can make interpretation difficult and by applying the radiosubtract principle (Agnew et al 1973) improved results may be obtained.

Gastrointestinal tract

In paediatric gastroenterological practice, radioisotopes are most commonly used to exclude a Meckel's diverticulum as a cause of gastrointestinal bleeding. Intravenously administered [99]technetium pertechnetate is excreted by gastric mucosa and if gastric mucosa is present in the diverticulum it may be identified. A negative result, however, does not exclude a Meckel's diverticulum.

Active gastrointestinal bleeding sites can sometimes be localized using [99]technetium-labelled red blood cells (Hattner & Engelstad 1982).

[99]Technetium sulphur colloid may be added to an infant's feed to perform a milk scan. This technique allows continuous monitoring of the stomach to assess gastro-oesophageal reflux and pulmonary aspiration of feed, and enables gastric emptying time to be measured (Jona & Glicklich 1981).

[111]Indium-labelled leucocytes are being investigated as a possible technique for assessing the site and extent of inflammatory bowel disease. In one study localization and extent of inflammatory disease was superior to contrast radiology and very nearly as good as endoscopy (Gordon & Vivian 1984). It is likely that it will prove most useful in small intestinal inflammatory bowel disease.

Biopsy

Peroral small intestinal biopsy

The development of this technique has undoubtedly been an important advance in the rational diagnosis and management of a variety of disorders affecting the small intestine (Rubin & Dobbins 1965, Trier 1971). It can provide information on both the morphology and the function of the small gut. For example, characteristic morphological abnormalities are found in children with coeliac disease, intestinal lymphangiectasia and abetalipoproteinaemia. Small intestinal biopsy is the diagnostic method of choice where an enteropathy is suspected. Despite the introduction of a variety of noninvasive screening tests (see pp 66–68) small intestinal biopsy has stood the test of time and has not been superseded. Assay of mucosal disaccharidase activities, coupled with morphological assessment, is important in differentiating primary from secondary sugar intolerance.

Instruments. A variety of instruments are available but we prefer the Crosby and Watson capsules (Crosby & Kugler 1957, Read et al 1962). Both capsules have a similar working mechanism, a spring-loaded knife block which fires by suction to cut off the mucosal biopsy specimen. Both are simple and straightforward to operate but their successful use is related to the experience of the operator. It is only by frequent practice that a reliable technique can be developed and maintained. Coupled with an experienced operator, a pathology department with the staff and facilities capable of utilizing the biopsy material correctly is essential for the provision of a good clinical service. For example, the misinterpretation of poorly prepared sections is still responsible for the incorrect diagnosis of coeliac disease. For these reasons biopsies are best performed in experienced centres. In addition to the conventional single porthole capsules, the Watson capsule may be obtained with two ports enabling two biopsy samples to be obtained simultaneously in the same patient (Kilby 1976). Instruments have also been developed to obtain multiple biopsy specimens from young infants (Carey 1964, Ament & Rubin 1973). We routinely use the Watson capsule mounted on a two lumen tube as described on page 72.

Recently, a steerable small bowel biopsy apparatus (MediTech Tube) has been introduced (Vanderhoof et al 1981). Although expensive, it has the advantage of reducing biopsy time while retaining the ability to obtain adequate biopsies safely with a low incidence of failure. It is also possible to obtain multiple biopsies with this instrument.

Preparation and technique. Platelet count, prothrombin and partial thromboplastin times, should precede biopsy. The prothrombin time is frequently prolonged in malabsorptive states and can be corrected within a few hours by intramuscular vitamin K_1. A period of fasting, allowing only fluids, is necessary since solid food particles can obstruct the capsule and interfere with firing. This period varies from four hours in an infant to an overnight fast in an older child.

The necessity for sedation depends on the age of the patient, and the extent to which the child understands what the procedure entails. Sedation should be avoided whenever possible since it tends to delay the passage of the capsule and is often unnecessary in young infants and children over the age of five years. In infants, the biopsy tubing can be passed through a dummy, allowing the baby to suck the dummy during the procedure. If sedation is necessary, chlorpromazine 2 mg/kg may be given intramuscularly 45 minutes before the procedure or diazepam 0.1 mg/kg intravenously during the procedure.

The passage of the capsule requires a quiet unflustered approach with frequent reassurance to the child. The patient should be seated at the edge of a chair or bed with an assistant steadying the forehead with one hand and holding both the child's hands with the other; infants and very young children can most conveniently be nursed in this position. The capsule is placed on the back of the tongue and then into the upper oesophagus with the first swallowing movement. The capsule tubing can be protected from teeth by a short length of firm outer tubing. Oesophageal passage of the capsule is encouraged by stiffening the tube with a cardiac catheter guide-wire and by gently pushing on the tubing. When the capsule is judged to be in the distal oesophagus the patient lies on his right side and the capsule is slowly advanced. By placing the patient in this position before the capsule enters the stomach, the capsule almost invariably drops towards and reaches the pylorus. The position of the instrument is checked by fluoroscopic screening, and its passage through the pylorus can be observed as a sudden downward turn into the first part of the duodenum. With the patient on his back the guide-wire is withdrawn to the pylorus, the capsule is then seen to travel round the duodenal curve to the duodenojejunal flexure. Throughout these manoeuvres the minimum of excess tubing should be advanced into the stomach so as to prevent looping. Looping can also be reduced by inserting a guide-wire into the proximal end of the tube. The assistance of a radiologist during the screening procedure is invaluable not only for recognizing the anatomy but also for techniques to encourage progression of the tube such as abdominal pressure to displace the pylorus.

Delay in the capsule leaving the stomach may be reduced by metaclopramide 0.3 mg/kg (to a maximum of 10 mg) given intravenously when the capsule is at the pylorus. When the capsule is in position just beyond the flexure it is flushed with a few millilitres of water and then with air in order to remove mucus or debris. It is then fired by suction using a 20 ml syringe; the movement of the knife block can usually be seen on fluoroscopy and confirms that the capsule has fired. The capsule is immediately withdrawn by steady traction; there may be a feeling of resistance initially, and then at the pylorus and cardia. The initial swallowing of the capsule and its subsequent withdrawal present the most distressing events of the whole procedure.

After completion of the investigation the patient's pulse rate and blood pressure are recorded at frequent intervals for 4–6 hours, but no dietary restrictions are imposed.

Handling of the biopsy specimen.   The laboratory requirements for each individual specimen should be determined beforehand and all the necessary equipment assembled. The tools for dismantling the capsule, a dissecting microscope and materials for fixing the specimen must be set out; dry ice should be available for snap-freezing a piece of the specimen if mucosal enzymes are to be assayed. The net weight of the specimen varies from 10 to 30 mg depending on the size of the porthole of the capsule. It should be promptly and carefully removed from the capsule, orientated mucosal side upwards in normal saline and examined under the dissecting microscope. Occasionally the dissecting microscopic appearances may be misleading and the parents should not be given a definitive diagnosis until stained sections of the biopsy have been carefully examined under the light microscope. A number of quantitative techniques have been developed and applied to biopsy sections in recent years; in clinical practice the most useful of these is that of Dunhill & Whitehead (1972) which determines the surface:volume ratio of the mucosa.

Complications.   In experienced centres serious complications arising from an intestinal biopsy are now extremely rare. We have not encountered any serious complications using the Watson capsule for the past 12 years, during which time over two thousand biopsies have been done.

Perforation and/or bleeding are most likely to occur in small marasmic infants weighing less than 4 kg, and biopsy should be avoided if at all possible in such patients. If coeliac disease is suspected in such patients it is probably wiser to institute a gluten-free diet without biopsy evidence and confirm the diagnosis at a later date by means of a formal gluten challenge. Occasionally the capsule can become firmly attached to the mucosa and cannot be withdrawn due to incomplete severing of the mucosa. Management is either to cut the tubing and await recovery of the capsule in the stools, or to leave the tubing loosely taped to the cheek allowing the child to eat, drink and move around normally. Attempts to dislodge the capsule by gentle traction should be made every 6–8 hours; epigastric discomfort indicates that the capsule is still attached. The capsule usually becomes detached within 24–48 hours. Premature firing or failure to fire is almost invariably related to poor maintenance of the capsule.

Liver biopsy

This investigation should always be carried out in an experienced centre which has all the available facilities. The procedure can provide extremely valuable diagnostic information following the application of a variety of laboratory techniques to the biopsy sample, e.g. light and electron microscopy, enzyme assays, histochemistry, determination of chemical contents, immunofluorescence, tissue culture and bacterial and viral culture. The clinical indications for liver biopsy in children are listed in Table 3.5.

Table 3.5   Indications for liver biopsy

Hepatomegaly of unknown cause
Glycogen and lipid storage diseases
Prolonged jaundice particularly neonatal jaundice
Evaluation of chronic liver diseases such as chronic active hepatitis and Wilson's disease
Suspected liver disease without jaundice
Toxic hepatitis
Portal hypertension

Contraindications. Liver biopsy is contraindicated in the presence of (1) clotting defects (prothrombin index less than 60% of control value; platelet count less than 50 000; prolonged bleeding time), (2) hydatid disease, because of the risk of dissemination and anaphylactoid shock, (3) vascular tumours of the liver, (4) infections of the pleura, lungs or peritoneum, and (5) suspected hepatic vein thrombosis. Moderate to severe ascites, a small impalpable liver and bile stasis (serum bilirubin greater than 425 μmol/l, i.e. 25 mg/100 ml) are relative contraindications depending on the experience of the operator and the urgency of diagnosis.

Biopsy instruments.   The two biopsy needles which are most suitable for use in children are the Menghini and Vim-Silverman needles, the former being almost invariably the instrument of choice (Menghini 1970).

The major concern in children is the increased risk of liver trauma with bleeding or biliary peritonitis resulting from movement during the biopsy. The extremely short intrahepatic phase using the Menghini needle minimizes this risk; its main disadvantage is the high failure rate in the presence of fibrosis. The needles are made with a variety of diameters (e.g. 1, 1.2, 1.4, 1.6, 1.9 and 2 mm), and generally speaking the larger the needle, the greater the risk of bleeding. In children the 1.2 or 1.4 mm needles are most frequently used, and the 1 mm needle is confined to high-risk patients. The needle has a specially bevelled tip which allows for the tissue to be removed by aspiration alone without rotation within the liver.

The chief advantage of the Vim-Silverman needle is the higher yield of tissue in patients with cirrhosis. The intrahepatic phase is much longer (5–15 seconds) than with the Menghini needle (one second), and consequently the risk of laceration is greater. The needle diameter is greater for an equivalent sized specimen. The apparatus consists of a cannula with an inner split cannula, the two sides of which tend to spring apart. The lumen is usually occluded with a trocar during insertion through the chest wall. After advancing to the liver and removing the trocar, the longer inner split cannula is advanced into the liver. The outer cannula is advanced to the lip of the split cannula, and the whole instrument is then rotated through 360° and withdrawn. Because of the necessary rotation the specimen is often distorted. This instrument should probably only be used in the investigation of cirrhosis when the Menghini technique may be unsuccessful.

Preparation and technique.   The success and safety of liver biopsy depends on meticulous attention to detail. Since the Menghini needle is almost invariably used in children, details concerning the preparation of the patient and the biopsy technique will be described for this instrument.

The patient is admitted to hospital, a full blood count and clotting studies are performed, and blood is cross-matched and available; the child should fast for at least four hours prior to the biopsy. Young children should be premedicated with sleep-inducing drugs (e.g. pentobarbitone 4 mg/kg) or receive general anaesthesia. In older children a detailed explanation of the procedure together with pentobarbitone (2–3 mg/kg) is usually sufficient. Full surgical aseptic techniques should be employed throughout the procedure. The upper border of liver dullness is percussed in the midaxillary line and the site of needle penetration is marked one intercostal space below. Two to three millilitres of local anaesthesia (e.g. 1% xylocaine) are injected to infiltrate the intercostal space down to the level of the pleura, and a 2–3 mm incision is made in the skin. Whilst an assistant presses firmly on the patient's chest the needle is inserted through the skin and continuous aspiration is applied to the attached syringe (10 ml Luer lock syringe containing 2–3 ml of saline); the needle is rapidly inserted into the liver and withdrawn in one movement, with no rotation or lateral movement. The placement of the index finger of the left hand on the needle should limit the depth of penetration, and the whole manoeuvre should take no longer than one second. The core of liver tissue is gently flushed from the needle into a sterile container, and a satisfactory specimen should be longer than 1 cm. It is reasonable to repeat the biopsy if tissue is not obtained at the first attempt.

Following the biopsy the child should lie on his right side and remain in bed for 24 hours. The pulse rate is recorded at 15 minute intervals for the first hour and at hourly intervals for the ensuing 4–6 hours, and a full blood count should be performed 24 hours after the biopsy.

Complications.   The incidence of complications is very variable and depends mainly on the general condition of the patient, the experience of the operator and the type and size of biopsy needle. The mortality rate varies from 0.02 to 0.1% in experienced hands.

The major complications are (1) haemorrhage requiring transfusion and occasionally surgery, (2) biliary peritonitis, (3) pneumothorax, and (4) puncture of other viscera such as the gall bladder or kidney. Failure to obtain a biopsy specimen may be related to cirrhosis, a blunt needle, or failure to maintain aspiration of the syringe during the passage of the needle through the chest cage into the liver. Local pain is not uncommon following biopsy and may require analgesia.

Rectal biopsy

Biopsy of the rectal mucosa and submucosa can provide diagnostic information. The main indication for suction rectal biopsy is Hirschsprung's disease but it is also useful in the diagnosis and management of chronic inflammatory bowel disease and for the diagnosis of neural lipidoses and amyloidosis.

The procedure may sometimes be worth considering in a wide variety of other disorders such as collagen diseases, pseudoxanthoma elasticum, Whipples disease and histiocytosis (Martin et al 1963). But here full thickness biopsies are necessary with their attendant risks.

Preparation and technique. The child should be sedated although occasionally general anaesthesia is required in uncooperative children.

Specimens can be obtained under direct vision through a proctoscope with angled cutting forceps and are usually taken from the posterior wall of the rectum just below the peritoneal reflection. In the very rare event of perforation of the rectum, specimens obtained from this site will not lead to peritonitis. Bleeding can usually be rapidly controlled with direct pressure.

A suction biopsy can be obtained without the aid of a proctoscope or sigmoidoscope and, if carefully performed, causes no discomfort to the child. The principle by which the available instruments operate is identical to that for peroral small gut biopsy instruments. Multiple biopsy specimens can be obtained at varying intervals from the anus and may be helpful in defining the length of the aganglionic segment in Hirschsprung's disease. Suction biopsy has the disadvantage of sometimes obtaining superficial specimens which contain little or no submucosa and therefore preclude any comments on the presence or absence of ganglion cells. However, the development of histochemical staining for cholinesterase activity in the mucosa allows for a presumptive diagnosis of Hirschsprung's disease on mucosal specimens in which ganglion cells are absent (Meier-Ruge 1974). This has become our diagnostic method of choice in Hirschsprung's disease (Lake et al 1978) but it is essential that biopsies are taken at carefully defined levels above the anal verge.

Endoscopy

The aims of endoscopy are to visualize diseased areas of the gastrointestinal tract, to obtain biopsy samples and to perform the procedures with the minimal discomfort to the patient. Endoscopy of the lower and upper parts of the alimentary tract is now established as an important diagnostic technique. The recent introduction of small diameter, second generation fibreoptic instruments, especially designed for children, represents a major advance in the field of endoscopy since it allows for a considerably more extensive examination of the alimentary tract than was previously possible. In addition, the technique may establish a diagnosis which was not apparent with conventional barium studies especially where the lesion is of the superficial mucosa only.

Proximal endoscopy

This enables the mucosa of the oesophagus, stomach and proximal duodenum to be visualized, as well as allowing biopsy samples to be obtained from apparently diseased areas. In the younger uncooperative child general anaesthesia is advisable to avoid the possible complication of perforation (Gleason et al 1974). In the older child premedicatory drugs, as used for adults, are usually adequate. The indications for proximal endoscopy include dysphagia, haematemesis (Cox & Ament 1979), gastro-oesophageal reflux, peptic ulceration, removal of foreign bodies and variceal sclerotherapy.

Endoscopic retrograde choledochopancreatography permits cannulation of the ampulla of Vater with injection of contrast into the common bile duct or pancreatic duct. Its use is limited to investigation of recurrent pancreatitis and some cases of obstructive jaundice, particularly if sclerosing lesions are suspected. Bile duct stones can sometimes be removed (Cotton & Williams 1980).

Distal endoscopy

Proctoscopy can be performed at the bedside and an auroscope can be used in very small infants. Rigid sigmoidoscopy is usually performed under general anaesthesia and allows examination of the rectum and sigmoid colon up to 12 cm in the infant and 25 cm in the older child. Fibreoptic endoscopy is superseding this technique.

The advent of small diameter floppy paediatric colonoscopes has enabled both sigmoidoscopy and total colonoscopy to be well tolerated by small infants and children without general anaesthesia. The mucosa can be closely examined and multiple biopsies taken for diagnostic purposes. It may also be used for therapeutic procedures such as snare polypectomy and electro-coagulation of bleeding sites. Careful preparation is required for the procedure. The child is put on clear fluids only from midday on the day preceding the examination. A large dose of a laxative such as senna syrup is given and if no response occurs, a phosphate enema is administered. On the day of the colonoscopy a further enema is given approximately one hour before the procedure and if the bowel is still not clear a saline washout may be required. Intramuscular chlorpromazine (2 mg/kg) is used as a pre-medication and intravenous diazepam and pethidine given to induce drowsiness.

Williams et al (1982) have reported a series of over one hundred total colonoscopies for the investigation of inflammatory bowel disease and rectal bleeding. Total colonoscopy was possible in 96% with examination of the terminal ileum in 50%, with no reported complications. In adults the incidence of perforation is less than 2 in 1000 and excessive bleeding from biopsy sites is uncommon.

FUNCTIONAL STUDIES

Before embarking on investigatory techniques designed to assess specific aspects of gastrointestinal function a careful clinical history and examination are essential in deciding which tests should be performed. As with all other investigations the critical and well informed physician can minimize the number of tests which are necessary to arrive at a diagnosis, thereby reducing patient discomfort and financial costs. For example, sequential documentation of height and weight and inspection of stools can provide important information with regard to the presence of underlying disease.

Oesophageal function

The use of contrast and radioisotope studies has been previously discussed. More detailed information of oesophageal motor activity can be obtained using perfused multilumen tubes connected to pressure trans-ducers to record intraluminal pressure changes at various points in the oesophagus. Using a sleeved catheter, lower oesophageal pressure, which is reduced in gastro-oesophageal reflux, can be measured as described by Dent (1976). The technique may be combined with simultaneous oeso-phageal pH recording (Werlin et al 1980).

Measurement of intraluminal oesophageal pH is carried out by passing a pH microelectrode into the lower oesophagus. Periods of fall in pH indicate acid reflux but these occur in normal children and the frequency and duration of the reflux is important. Several hours of study including a sleeping period are usually required for reliable interpretaton (Koch & Gass 1981, Sondheimer 1980).

Gastric acid secretion

The gastric parietal cells are functional and secrete acid within a few hours of birth (Avery et al 1966a). In children maximal stimulation of gastric acid secretion by pentagastrin results in the secretion of juice of comparable hydrochloric acid concentration to that in adults, but the volume and total acid output are only about a third of adult values in the first decade and less than a tenth of adult values during the first year of life (Agunod et al 1969).

The measurement of basal gastric acid and maximally stimulated acid outputs is a particularly useful investigation in children with intractable peptic ulcers and/or those suspected of having the Zollinger–Ellison syndrome; it may also be a useful test in patients following small gut resections.

Procedure

Following an overnight fast a nasogastric tube is passed under fluoroscopic control to the most dependent part of the stomach. The stomach contents are aspirated and discarded, and four 15 minute aspirate collections are performed to establish basal secretory volume, pH and titratable acidity (i.e. basal acid output = mEq of acid secreted per hour or per kg per hour). Maximal acid output is stimulated by intravenous pentagastrin (6 μg/kg), and gastric contents are collected at 15 minute intervals for two hours. Aliquots of each 15 minute collection pre- and post-stimulation are titrated to pH 7 with 0.2 N sodium hydroxide. Maximal acid output refers to the rate of acid secretion during the first hour after histamine or pentagastrin stimulation. Peak acid output refers to the two highest consecutive 15 minute acid secretory periods multiplied by two. Maximal and peak acid outputs are expessed as mEq of acid secreted per hour, or per kg per hour.

Results

Normal values and those found in peptic ulcer disease are shown in Table 3.6. In children with duodenal ulcers basal acid output is normal, whereas maximal and peak acid outputs are significantly increased (Christie & Ament 1976). In the Zollinger–Ellison syndrome basal and maximal outputs are markedly increased. There may be only a small and insignificant rise in peak output (Schwartz et al 1974); these findings constitute indications for a plasma gastrin assay. If the gastrin assay is equivocal

Table 3.6 Gastric acid output in control children and children with duodenal ulcer and Zollinger–Ellison syndrome

	Basal acid output	Peak acid output mEq/kg/h	Maximal acid output
[1]Controls (n = 14)	0.035 ± 0.01	0.332 ± 0.10	0.248 ± 0.09
Duodenal ulcer (n = 12)	0.064 ± 0.04	0.507 ± 0.14	0.486 ± 0.14
[2]Zollinger–Ellison syndrome (n = 3)	1.6–1.7	—	0.7–2.0

[1] Data from Christie & Ament (1976) as mean ± [1]SD
[2] Schwartz et al (1974), Roselund et al (1967), Burmester et al (1969)

(200–500 pg/ml), either a calcium infusion test (Schwartz et al 1974) or a secretin provocation test (McGuignan & Wolfe 1980) should be performed. Hypersecretion of gastric acid and hypergastrinaemia may also occur following resections of the small bowel (Avery et al 1966b; Strauss et al 1974). Reduced acid output occurs in conditions such as pernicious anaemia, the Verner–Morrison syndrome (Verner & Morrison 1958) and Menetrier's disease (Frank & Kern 1967)

Small intestinal function

Carbohydrate absorption

Tests of carbohydrate absorption are indicated in children with chronic diarrhoea and in those who fail to thrive or have persistent diarrhoea following an episode of acute gastroenteritis.

Examination of faeces. The characteristic stools of patients with carbohydrate malabsorption are frothy, liquid and acid, and the perianal region is often excoriated. The pH of the stool is generally less than 5.5 but this is an unreliable test and its routine use should be discouraged. The most useful screening procedure is to test for reducing substances. Five drops of a freshly collected aliquot of liquid stool are diluted with 10 drops of water, and a Clinitest tablet added (Kerry & Anderson 1964). The presence of more than 0.5 per cent reducing substances is taken as an indication of carbohydrate malabsorption. All carbohydrates consumed by children are reducing substances with the exception of sucrose. If sucrose intolerance is suspected an aliquot of stool should be boiled for a few minutes in the presence of hydrochloric acid (to hydrolyse the disaccharide to glucose and fructose) before testing for reducing substances. The application of thin layer chromatographic techniques enables the individual sugars to be identified and may be helpful in reaching a specific diagnosis (Soeparto et al 1972). Thus the presence of lactose, glucose and galactose in the absence of sucrose and fructose in a child consuming a diet which contains both lactose and sucrose strongly suggests lactase deficiency.

Oral load tests Oral loads of mono- or disaccharides can be performed in conjunction with the above tests. Following a fast, the duration of which will depend on the age and clinical state of the patient, the sugar under investigation is given in a dose of 1–2 g per kg body weight (maximum of 50 g) as a 10% solution together with a carmine marker. Body weight, stool frequency and volume are carefully recorded prior to and throughout the test, and the stools containing the marker are tested for reducing substances and individual sugars. Urine may be simultaneously collected and tested for sugars. As an adjunct serial determination of blood glucose can be performed, as for a glucose tolerance test. Normally blood glucose concentrations increase by at least 1.7 mmol/l (30 mg/100 ml) during the test, whereas this increment is less than 1.1 mmol/l (20 mg/100 ml) in patients with sugar intolerance. A flat glucose tolerance curve may also be secondary to delayed gastric emptying.

The presence of sugars in the stool and/or urine may be a normal finding in newborns, particularly if breastfed. Lactulose (a non-reducing disaccharide composed of fructose and galactose) is formed from lactose during the commercial preparation and storage of milk. It cannot be hydrolysed by the human small gut and may be detected in the urine of normal infants.

Oral loads of the relatively nonmetabolized pentose D-xylose have been widely used in the investigation of malabsorption, and the finding of a low one hour blood xylose has been recommended as a screening test for coeliac disease (Rolles et al 1973). Lamabadusuriya et al (1975), however, found the test unreliable and no substitute for the definitive investigation of intestinal biopsy. Recent refinements of this technique using other sugars (Menzies et al 1979) as a measure of intestinal permeability have not superseded intestinal biopsy as the means of excluding coeliac disease.

Breath tests. Unabsorbed carbohydrates are metabolized by colonic bacteria with the generation of hydrogen which is absorbed and then excreted by the lungs. There is a fairly good correlation between the amount of hydrogen produced and the amount excreted in breath. On this basis the quantification of hydrogen in breath following an oral load of sugar has been developed as a noninvasive test of sugar malabsorption in adults (Bond & Levitt 1972). False negative results, however, are not uncommon, and its application to young infants poses certain technical problems.

Initial enthusiasm for such noninvasive tests of mucosal function are now, however, waning as the sensitivity and specificity of these methods have become defined. At best they represent a noninvasive screening test but require expensive analytical apparatus.

Fat absorption

The most reliable clinical test for assessing fat absorption is the quantification of faecal fat over a period of at least 72 hours. An adequate dietary intake of fat before and during stool collections is essential; in infants this should be at least 5 g per kg per day, in young children about 40–50 g and in older children 70–80 g per day. A red or blue carmine marker is given and collections begun from the appearance of the first coloured stool. 72 hours (or five days) after administering the first marker the alternative coloured marker is given, and the collection of stools is completed by including the last stool before the appearance of the second marker. Infant stools may be collected using a polythene lining in the napkin, toddler stools using a potty or potty chair, and older children by careful cooperation with the child; if the stools are fluid a metabolic frame may be necessary. The stools are pooled and homogenized, and their fatty acid content analysed by the method of Van de Kamer et al (1949).

The results can be expressed either as absolute values of stool fat per day with an upper limit of normal of 5 g, or as a coefficient of absorption (i.e. per cent of fat absorbed). Fat excretion varies with age and the latter method is preferable in children. Normal values increase with age, being greater than 60% in premature infants, greater than 80% in full term infants, greater than 85% in children up to six months, and greater than 90% thereafter.

Lubrication of rectal thermometers or examining fingers, or the application of certain creams to the perianal region, may result in spuriously high faecal fat values. If the diet contains medium chain triglycerides the method for measuring faecal fat must be modified (Jeejeebhoy et al 1970).

The collection of stools and their subsequent analysis is unpleasant for the ward and the laboratory staff and the test should be reserved for those instances where there is a real indication for its use. We believe it to be overused in paediatric practice, such as in patients suspected of having coeliac disease when an early peroral jejunal biopsy can avoid the necessity for any further investigations.

A number of screening tests for fat malabsorption have been advocated but though no more reliable, stool microscopy for fat globules is probably the screening test of choice.

Protein absorption and loss

Total faecal nitrogen can be measured by the Kjeldahl method and can be combined with fat determinations. Coefficient of absorption for nitrogen provides information on net absorption but does not discriminate between nitrogen loss into the lumen and malabsorption. Generally speaking faecal nitrogen is a much less useful investigation in clinical practice compared with faecal fat. Moreover, since faecal nitrogen and fat correlate well with each other, nitrogen losses can be assumed to be excessive in the presence of steatorrhoea.

Excessive loss of serum proteins into the gastrointestinal tract may occur in a wide variety of diseases affecting the stomach, small and large intestine (see Chapter 13). The most widely used test to assess protein loss is the determination of radioactive chromium (^{51}Cr) in stools following the intravenous administration of ^{51}Cr-tagged albumin (Waldmann 1961). 25 microcuries of ^{51}Cr-tagged albumin (or ^{51}CrCl) are given intravenously, and all stools are collected for a period of four days; particular care must be taken to ensure that faeces are not contaminated by urine since this will result in spuriously high values of protein loss. The stools are pooled, homogenized and an aliquot counted for radioactivity. Normally, less than 1% of the dose is excreted in the stools, more than 4% being indicative of unequivocal protein loss. More recently faecal α^1-antitrypsin has been advocated as a marker of enteric protein loss, but this has not as yet found widespread favour (Hill et al 1981).

Albumin labelled with ^{131}I, ^{14}C or ^{75}Se has been used to study albumin synthesis and turnover in association with the ^{51}Cr test (Walker et al 1973).

Fluid and electrolyte absorption

Abnormalities of fluid and electrolyte absorption in the small and/or large bowel result in diarrhoea in a variety of disease states, but the available investigatory techniques are complex and, at present, unsuitable for routine clinical use.

Simple measurement of stool volume can, however, provide important information in assessing the course and response to therapy of children with severe and protracted diarrhoeal states. Determination of stool electrolytes may also be useful in such patients. There is only one condition where measurement of stool electrolytes is diagnostic and that is congenital chloridorrhoea (see Chapter 9). The finding of a stool concentration of chloride which exceeds the sum of the concentrations of sodium and potassium is pathognomonic of this rare disorder.

Absorption of haematinics

Tests which assess the capacity of the small intestine to absorb haematinic substances such as iron, folic acid and vitamin B_{12} can provide important information with regard to the presence of disease as well as its site in the small intestine. Defective iron and folate absorption occurs in proximal small intestinal diseases, whereas vitamin B_{12} malabsorption usually results from ileal disease but may also occur in proximal lesions which result in bacterial overgrowth, in pancreatic disease and in conditions in which gastric intrinsic factor secretion is impaired.

Iron and folate. The peripheral blood reticulocyte response to oral as compared to systemic treatment can be used as a test of absorption and utilization of iron and folate. The presence of iron deficiency as shown by a microcytic anaemia, low serum iron and high total iron binding capacity in the absence of blood loss may provide evidence of malabsorption. Similarly, if serum and red cell folate levels are low in the absence of malignancy, anticonvulsants or folic acid antagonists, folate malabsorption may be presumed. However, low blood levels and both macrocytic and microcytic anaemia may be due to deficient intake of these haematinics rather than malabsorption.

Vitamin B_{12}. Where there is apparent vitamin B_{12} deficiency and megaloblastosis, abnormalities of pancreatic (Allen et al 1978) and biliary function (Teo et al 1980), together with bacterial overgrowth of the small intestine, should be excluded before specific tests of gastric intrinsic factor secretion, ileal uptake and transport of vitamin B_{12} are undertaken. Malabsorption of vitamin B_{12} may be demonstrated either by whole body counting of ^{57}Cr vitamin B_{12} (Tait & Hesp 1976) or by the Schilling test. The former is preferred in girls who are not continent of urine due to the difficulty in ensuring that urine and stools are kept completely separate in these children. A modified Schilling test utilizing the 'Dicopac' dual isotope test kit, supplied by Amersham International Ltd, is preferred. In this test radiolabelled vitamin B_{12} as ^{58}Co-B_{12} and ^{57}Co-B_{12} bound to gastric intrinsic factor are given orally after a two hour fast. Following a further two hour fast, 1 mg of 'cold' vitamin B_{12} is given intramuscularly to saturate body stores and ensure a significant urinary secretion of the labelled vitamin B_{12}. Normally at least 10% of the labelled vitamin B_{12} will be excreted in the urine over the following 24 hours. Lower values indicate B_{12} malabsorption. Calculation of the ratio of ^{57}Co to ^{58}Co-B_{12} excreted will indicate whether the malabsorption is due to deficiency of active intrinsic factor. A ratio of ^{57}Co to ^{58}Co of more than two suggests intrinsic factor deficiency whereas a ratio around one suggests malabsorption due to other causes. Bacterial overgrowth may be associated with an abnormal test which is not corrected by the addition of intrinsic factor and hence a ratio of unity might be expected.

Small intestinal motility

Small intestinal motor activity in adults has been studied by gastroenterologists for many years but the technique has only recently been applied to paediatrics (Fenton et al 1983).

The available investigatory techniques are, however, complex, time-consuming and require considerable expertise in both their execution and interpretation. At present they are unsuitable for routine clinical use.

Pancreatic function

The assessment of pancreatic function involves the quantification of pancreatic enzymes, volume and bicarbonate in the proximal small intestine following stimulation of the gland. Enzyme activities reflect the function of the acinar cells, and volume and bicarbonate outputs are indicators of tubular function. The pancreas can be stimulated by the intravenous administration of cholecystokinin-pancreozymin and secretin, or by the administration of a test meal. The former method provides information on the maximal secretory capacity of the pancreas to a systemic stimulus, whereas the latter technique gives more physiological information on the response of the gland to intraluminal substrates. Variations in the stimulus applied, the collection of duodenal juice and in assay procedures and conditions result in differences in the observed enzyme activities. The test should therefore only be performed in experienced centres, and each centre must define its own reference data.

Intravenous cholecystokinin-pancreozymin (CCK-PZ) and secretin

Following an overnight fast, or for young infants a four-hour fast, the patient is sedated one hour before the tube is passed into the fourth part of the duodenum under fluoroscopic control. Contamination by gastric secretions can be minimized by means of continuous suction with a second tube positioned in the pyloric antrum, or by a proximal occlusive balloon in the first part of the duodenum. Duodenal secretions are collected on ice by siphonage. Prior to the administration of CCK-PZ and secretin, the patient should be tested against any hypersensitivity to the hormones. The hormones are given sequentially when it is necessary to quantitate HCO_3 secretion as, for example, in the diagnosis of cystic fibrosis. CCK-PZ (2 IU/kg) is administered by slow intravenous infusion and juice collected for 20 minutes; secretin (2 IU/kg) is then given and juice collected for a further 30 minutes. Alternatively, both hormones may be given together and juice collected for 30 minutes when a screening test of enzyme secretion is required.

Test meal

A test meal provides a more physiological stimulus to gall bladder contraction and pancreatic secretion and can also provide meaningful information on intraluminal digestion. McCollum et al (1977) have developed a modification of the Lundh test meal (Lundh 1962) containing 4 g% of glucose, comminuted chicken and corn oil which can be given to children with suspected cow's milk protein or gluten intolerance and to those with disaccharide intolerance without precipitating gastrointestinal symptoms.

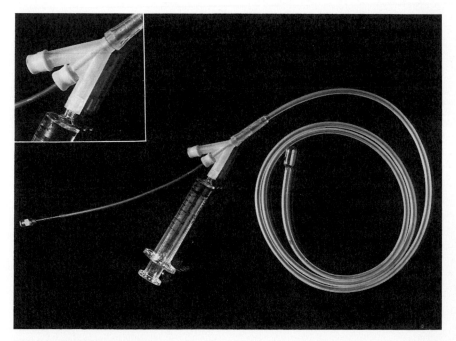

Fig. 3.1 Multipurpose biopsy tube

The meal is given via a nasogastric tube, and post-prandial juice is collected from the fourth part of the duodenum in aliquots for two hours.

Using either technique, samples of duodenal contents can be collected into appropriate transport media for culture of anaerobic and aerobic bacteria if bacterial overgrowth of the small intestine is suspected.

Over the past 10 years we have routinely used a combined two lumen investigation tube consisting of a Watson biopsy capsule on its tube (KIFA 17887-red)* over which a 12 FG nasoduodenal tube (Portex, Hythe, England) is placed. At the capsule end multiple holes are punched in the nasoduodenal tube for a distance of 5 cm. At the proximal end of the nasoduodenal tube an intravenous Y connector is inserted over the jejunal biopsy tube and sealed with a rubber bung as shown in Figure 3.1 (see p. 71). This leaves two outlets on the Y connector to which syringes may be attached or sealed with rubber bungs. This type of tube enables a number of different investigations involving duodenal intubation to be performed at the same intubation.

Indirect methods

Because of the problems encountered with duodenal intubation, proper specimen collection and accurate enzyme measurement, several alternative tests have been devised. These tests include measurement of pancreatic enzymes in blood and faeces and several so called 'tubeless' tests of intra-luminal hydrolysis.

Serum enzymes. Elevated serum amylase may be useful in suspected pancreatitis though 10% of children will maintain a normal level throughout the course of the illness (Jordan & Ament 1977). Isoelectric focusing allows the detection of three isoenzymes and greatly adds to the specificity of the abnormal serum amylase assay, but the assay is not readily available and this limits its usefulness.

Serum immunoreactive trypsin(ogen) (IRT) is a test which has great specificity as trypsin(ogen) cannot be detected in blood after pancreatectomy. The immunoreactive trypsin(ogen) level is almost invariably raised during acute pancreatitis and is of value in exocrine pancreatic insufficiency (Elias et al 1977, Masoero et al 1982). However, neonates with cystic fibrosis usually have elevated levels of IRT regardless of the presence or absence of pancreatic insufficiency. With advancing age, levels of IRT in cystic fibrosis correlate well with exocrine pancreatic insufficiency (Durie et al 1981).

Faecal Enzymes. Whilst testing faeces for pancreatic proteolytic enzymes seems an obvious way of detecting pancreatic insufficiency, in our opinion these are sufficiently unreliable tests as to be discouraged in clinical practice.

---

* KIFA S-17195 Solne-1-Sweden

'Tubeless' tests.   Several 'tubeless' tests have been devised which rely on a non-absorbable substance undergoing processing by pancreatic enzymes in the small intestine which then allows a product to be detected in urine, plasma or breath. The most popular of these tests employs N-benzoyl-L-tyrosyl-p-aminobenzoic acid which is taken by mouth. Following the action of chymotrypsin, para-aminobenzoic acid (PABA) is released which subsequently appears in the plasma or urine (Lang et al 1981, Toskes 1983).

Fluorescein dilaurate is another substance which can be used in a similar way and provides an estimate of lipolytic activity (Braganza 1982).

In both of these 'tubeless' tests the rate of false positive and false negative values limit their usefulness.

The simplest of all tubeless tests is breath analysis after labelled substrate administration. Whilst ^{14}C-labelled triolein provides complete separation of patients with exocrine pancreatic insufficiency (Goff 1982) ^{14}C substrates are not desirable in children. Use of the stable isotope ^{13}C provides encouraging results but availability of isotope and analysis limits its applicability.

Liver function

A variety of tests are available for the assessment of liver function, some reflecting hepatic damage and others providing information regarding the metabolic capacity of the organ.

Enzymes

Alteration in the activities of serum enzymes may reflect different processes. Elevated serum transaminases reflect tissue damage and hence hepatitis, whereas elevated hepatic alkaline phosphatase is seen in cholestatic liver disease. Alkaline phosphatase activities are normally higher in children than adults, particularly during periods of rapid growth due to alkaline phosphatase from bone. The isoenzyme arising from bone can be distinguished from that of the liver by electrophoretic techniques. Alternatively, 5-nucleotidase, which is a predominantly hepatic enzyme, can be measured if it is uncertain from which organ an elevated alkaline phosphatase arises.

Bile salts and bacteria

The qualitative and quantitative assessment of bile salts and aerobic and anaerobic bacteria in the lumen of the proximal small intestine can be made on duodenal juice after pancreatico-biliary stimulation, as discussed above. Total bile salt concentrations may be estimated following their extraction on Amberlite XAD resin (Ma Kino & Sjovall 1972) by an enzymatic method using 3α hydroxy steroid dehydrogenase (Iwata & Yamasaki 1964). Individual bile salts may be similarly quantified after separation by thin layer chromatography (McCollum et al 1977).

Decreased total bile salt concentration below the critical micellar concentration of approximately 2.2 mmol/l will result in impaired fat solubilization and absorption. This may occur from a variety of causes such as biliary obstruction due to various anatomical anomalies of the biliary tree, hepatitis, cholestasis and cholangitis or increased excretion as in ileal resection or pancreatic steatorrhoea and cystic fibrosis. Qualitative changes (i.e. increased glycine : taurine ratio, increased percentage of dihydroxy bile salts) may also occur where the enterohepatic circulation is broken and may cause impaired fat solubilization due to the lower solubility of glycine conjugates and higher critical micellar concentration of dihydroxy bile salts. The presence of deconjugated bile salts in significant quantity indicates the presence of bacterial overgrowth in the small intestine.

^{14}C-labelled glycocholic acid can be used to assess bile acid absorption and small intestinal bacterial overgrowth (Thaysen 1977). The labelled bile acid is given orally and the label measured in breath and in the stools. If increased amounts of glycine-l-^{14}C-labelled glycocholate reach the colon, bacterial deconjugation will result in increased amounts of radiolabelled glycine being absorbed and metabolized to radiolabelled carbon dioxide. Thus, impaired reabsorption and increased excretion of bile salts can be assessed by the measurement of ^{14}CO$_2$ in expired breath. The test can also be used as a measure of bacterial overgrowth of the small intestine, when a large peak of ^{14}CO$_2$ is seen within 2–8 hours after ingestion, while in controls the excretion is over a period of a few days without a large peak.

Evidence for bacterial overgrowth of the duodenum may be sought by culturing duodenal juice collected after pancreatic biliary stimulation. For the culture of anaerobic organisms a number of points are important. Anaerobic organisms are exquisitely sensitive to oxygen and it is therefore necessary to use pre-reduced transport medium, and in order for the juice to remain free of air it must be *expelled* under the transport medium. As with urinary infection quantitation is important, 0.5 ml of juice is cultured and colony counts greater than 10^5/ml are taken to be significant.

Bilirubin

Serum bilirubin is present in conjugated and unconjugated forms. Cholestasis causes a rise predominantly of conjugated bilirubin. In the neonate, unconjugated hyperbilirubinaemia frequently occurs but conjugated hyperbilirubinaemia implies neonatal hepatitis or biliary atresia. Bacterial flora convert conjugated bilirubin to urobilinogen. This appears in the urine when liver function is inadequate to clear absorbed bile pigment into bile or in conditions where there is increased bilirubin synthesis such as haemolytic states. In obstructive jaundice no bilirubin disappears from the urine but conjugated bilirubin is excreted in the urine.

Serum proteins

Separation of the different plasma protein fractions by electrophoresis can

Table 3.7   Serum protein patterns in different disease states

	Albumin	Serum concentrations in g/l				
		Total	Globulins α1	α2	β	γ
Normal	36–52	22–33	1–4	4–12	4–9	4–15
Cystic fibrosis	↓	↑	N	↑	N	↑↑
Biliary cirrhosis	↓	↑	↑	↑	↑↑↑	↑
Viral hepatitis	N or ↓	N or ↑	↓	↓	↑	N or ↑
Cirrhosis	↓↓	↑	N or ↑	N	↑	↑↑
Alpha₁-antitrypsin deficiency	N or ↑	N or ↑	absent	N	N	N or ↑

N = normal; ↑ and ↓ = increased and decreased concentrations, respectively

provide important information regarding the liver's capacity to synthesize proteins and in particular albumin. In addition, abnormalities in the globulin fractions may provide specific information on the aetiology of liver disease. Many disease entities alter serum protein patterns, and some examples are shown in Table 3.7.

Proteins involved in coagulation are also synthesized in the liver and factors II, VIII, IX, and X are dependent on vitamin K. These can be screened by estimating the prothrombin and partial thromboplastin times.

Alpha₁-antitrypsin deficiency has been associated with cirrhosis and emphysema. Caeruloplasmin or copper-binding globulin is deficient in Wilson's disease (hepatolenticular degeneration). Alpha-fetoprotein is synthesized by embryonic liver cells and disappears by the age of two months. It is found in the serum of patients with hepatoblastoma (Zeltzer et al 1974).

Bromosulphthalein (BSP) test

This is a sensitive test of the ability of the liver cells to excrete the anionic phthalein dye, bromosulpthalein. A 5% solution of BSP (5 mg/kg) is administered intravenously following an overnight fast, and a venous sample of blood is collected 45 minutes later from a site other than that where the dye was injected; the concentration of BSP is then determined. It is an extremely irritant dye and great care should be taken not to inject it subcutaneously. The test should not be performed in jaundiced patients or within a week of the administration of halogen-containing compounds or barbiturates. The results are expressed as a percentage of retention at 45 minutes: the normal values for neonates and older infants are less than 15 and 5%, respectively.

Rose Bengal ¹³¹I test

Rose Bengal is a red dye which is taken up by the liver and rapidly excreted in bile. The rate of hepatic uptake and/or excretion is impaired when liver cells are damaged or when biliary flow is impaired. It is a useful test in conjunction with others (e.g. liver biopsy) in differentiating extrahepatic biliary atresia from the neonatal hepatitis syndrome (Sharp et al 1967).

On the day before the test three drops of Lugol's iodine are given to block the uptake of ^{131}I by the thyroid. 1–10 mmol of ^{131}I rose bengal is given intravenously and urine free stools and urine are collected for three successive days. The excretion of radioactive rose bengal is determined in the stool and urine.

In normal infants 70 to 97% of the ^{131}I rose bengal is excreted in the faeces. In neonatal hepatitis 5 to 20%, and in extrahepatic biliary atresia less than 8% is present in the faeces. If the results are equivocal, the test can be repeated after two to four weeks treatment with cholestyramine. In this way about three quarters of patients studied can be divided into hepatitis or biliary atresia.

The separation of stool and urine is crucial since urine contamination will give falsely elevated results. This normally limits the technique to centres experienced in its use.

Examination of urine

The reducing sugars galactose and fructose are present in excessive amounts in the urine of patients with galactosaemia and hereditary fructose intolerance respectively, and paper chromatographic analysis of urine is an important investigation in patients suspected of either of these two diagnoses. The diagnosis is confirmed by specific enzyme assays. A generalized aminoaciduria occurs in Wilson's disease and galactosaemia. In tyrosinosis and fructosaemia, phenolic acids are excreted in excessive quantities.

Colonic function

Anorectal manometry

This technique is useful in the diagnosis of disorders of defaecation particularly when short segment Hirschsprung's disease is a possibility. The usual apparatus consists of three balloons. One is placed in the rectum and can be used to distend the rectum. The other two are placed in the anal canal at the internal and external sphincters respectively and pressure recordings are made at all three sites.

Normally, rectal distension causes relaxation of the internal sphincter with contraction of the external sphincter. In Hirschsprung's disease rectal distension causes contraction of the internal sphincter but external sphincter contraction is normal (Lawson & Nixon 1967, Aaronson & Nixon 1972).

Fluid and electrolyte absorption

The available investigatory techniques are complex and at present unsuitable for routine clinical use. Simple measurements of stool volume, osmolality and electrolyte concentration allowing separation of osmotic and secretory diarrhoea will not differentiate the contribution of colonic secretion from small intestinal secretion.

REFERENCES

Aaronson I, Nixon H H 1972 A clinical evaluation of anorectal pressure studies in the diagnosis of Hirschsprung's disease. Gut 13: 138–146

Agnew J E, Youngs G R, Bouchier A D 1973 Conventional subtraction scanning of the pancreas: an assessment based on blind reporting. British Journal of Radiology 46:83

Agunod M, Yamaguchi N, Lopez R, Lubey A L, Glass G B J 1969 Correlative study of hydrochloric acid, pepsin and intrinsic factor secretion in new borns and infants. American Journal of Digestive Diseases 14:400

Allen R H, Seetharam B, Podell E, Alpers D H 1978 Effect of proteolytic enzymes on the binding of cobalamin to R protein and intrinsic factor. Journal of Clinical Investigation 61: 47–54

Ament M E, Rubin C E 1973 An infant multipurpose biopsy tube. Gastroenterology 65:205

Avery G B, Randolph J G, Weaver T 1966a Gastric acidity on the first day of life. Pediatrics 37:1005

Avery G B, Randolph J G, Weaver T 1966b Gastric response to specific disease in infants. Pediatrics 38:874

Bond J H, Levitt M D 1972 Use of breath hydrogen (H_2) in the study of carbohydrate absorption. American Journal of Digestive Diseases 22: 379–382

Braganza, J M, 1982 Fluorescein dilaurate test. Lancet 2: 927–928

Burmester H B C, Hall R, Munawer N 1969 The Zollinger Ellison Syndrome in a child. Gut 10: 800–803

Carey J R 1964 A simplified gastrointestinal biopsy capsule. Gastroenterology 46:550

Caritz T G, Leopold G R, Wolf D A 1982 The spleen, liver, biliary tract, gastrointestinal tract and pancreas. In: Ultrasonography of Paediatric Surgical Disorders, New York, Grune & Stratton. pp 77–163.

Christie D L, Ament M E 1976 Gastric acid hypersection in children with duodenal ulcer. Gastroenterology 71: 242–246

Cotton P B, Williams C B 1980 Practical Gastrointestinal Endoscopy. Blackwell Scientific Publications, Oxford

Cox K, Ament M E 1979 Upper gastrointestinal bleeding in children and adolescents. Pediatrics 63: 408–413

Crosby W H, Kugler H W 1957 Intraluminal biopsy of the small intestine: the intestinal biopsy capsule. American Journal of Digestive Diseases 2:236

Dent J 1976 A new technique for continuous sphincter pressure measurement. Gastroenterology 80: 938–941

Dunhill M S, Whitehead R 1972 A method for the quantitation of small intestinal biopsy specimens. Journal of Clinical Pathology 25:243

Durie P R, Largman C, Brodrick J W, Johnson J H, Gaskin K J, Forstner G G, Geokas M C 1981 Plasma immunoreactive pancreatic cationic trypsinogen in cystic fibrosis: A sensitive indicator of exocrine pancreatic dysfunction. Pediatric Research, 15: 1351–1355

Elias E, Redshaw M, Wood T 1977 Diagnostic importance of changes in circulating concentrations of immunoreactive trypsin. Lancet, 2: 66–68

Fenton T R, Harries J T, Milla P J 1983 Disordered small intestinal motility: a rational basis for toddlers' diarrhoea. Gut 24: 897–903

Frank B F, Kern F 1967 Menetrier's disease. Gastroenterology 53:953

Gleason W A Jnr, Tedesco F J, Keating J P, Goldstein D P 1974 Fibreoptic gastrointestinal endoscopy in infants and children. Journal of Pediatrics 85: 810–813

Goff J S 1982 Two staged triolein breath test differentiates pancreatic insufficiency from other causes of malabsorption. Gastroenterology 83: 44–46

Gordon I R S, Rose F G M 1977 Diagnostic Radiology in Paediatrics. Postgraduate Paediatric Services, Butterworths, London

Gordon I, Vivian G 1984 Radiolabelled leucocytes: a new diagnostic tool in occult infection/inflammation. Archives of Disease in Childhood 59: 62–66

Harris R, Caffey J 1953 Cholecystography in infants. Journal of the American Medical Association 153:1333

Hattner R, Engelstad B L 1982 An advance in the identification and localisation of gastrointestinal haemorrhage. Gastroenterology 83: 484–485

Hill R E, Herez A, Corey M L, Gilday D L, Hamilton J R 1981 Faecal clearance of antitrypsin: a reliable measure of enteric protein loss in children. Journal of Paediatrics 99: 416–418

Hodgson J R 1970 The technical aspects of cholecystography. Radiology Clinics of North America 8:85

Irving J D, Northfield T C 1976 Emergency arteriography in acute gastrointestinal bleeding. British Medical Journal i: 929–931

Iwata T, Yamasaki K 1964 Enzymatic determination and thin layer chromatography of bile acids in blood. Journal of Biochemistry (Tokyo) 56: 429–431

Jeejeebhoy K N, Ahmad S, Kozak G 1970 Determination of faecal fats containing both medium and long chain triglycerides and fatty acids. Clinical Biochemistry 3: 157–162

Jona J Z, Glicklich M 1981 Simplified radioisotope technique for assessing gastroesophageal reflux in children. Journal of Pediatric Surgery 16: 114–117

Jordan S C, Ament M E 1977 Pancreatitis in children and adolescents. Journal of Pediatrics, 91: 211–216

Kerry K R, Anderson C M 1964 A ward test for sugar in faeces. Lancet i:981

Kilby A 1976 Paediatric small intestinal biopsy capsule with two ports. Gut 17:158

Koch A, Gass R 1981 Continuous 20–24 hour esophageal pH monitoring in infancy. Journal of Pediatric Surgery 16: 109–112

Lake B D, Puri P, Nixon H H, Claireaux A E 1978 Hirschsprung's Disease. An appraisal of histochemically demonstrated acetylcholinesterase activity in suction rectal biopsy specimens as an aid to diagnosis. Archives of Pathology and Laboratory Medicine 102: 244–247

Lamabadusuriya S P, Packer S, Harries J T 1975 Limitations of xylose tolerance test as a screening procedure in childhood coeliac disease. Archives of Disease in Childhood 50: 34–39

Lang C, Gyr K, Stalder G A, Gillessen D 1981 Assessment of exocrine pancreatic function by oral administration of B-benzoyl L-tyrosyl-p-aminobenzoic acid (Bentiromide): Five years clinical experience. British Journal of Surgery 68: 771–775

Lawson J O N, Nixon H H 1967 Anal canal pressure in the diagnosis of Hirschsprung's disease. Journal of Pediatric Surgery 2: 344–352

Lundh G 1962 Pancreatic exocrine function in neoplastic and inflammatory disease: a simple and reliable new test. Gastroenterology 42:275

Makino I, Sjovall J 1972 A versatile method for analysis of bile acids in plasma. Analytical Letters 5: 341–349

Martin L W, Landing B H, Nakai H 1963 Rectal biopsy as an aid in the diagnosis of diseases of infants and children. Journal of Pediatrics 62:197

Masoero G, Andriulli A, Bianco A, Benitti B, Marchetto M, De La Pierre M 1982 Diagnostic accuracy of serum cationic trypsinogen estimation for pancreatic diseases. Digestive Diseases and Sciences, 27: 1089–1094

McCarthy D M 1970 Pancreatic Scanning. A thesis on the clinical use of the amino acid Se[75]-I-selenomethionine in scintigraphic visualisation of the human pancreas in health and disease. Dublin, University College, National University of Ireland

McCollum J P K, Muller D P R, Harries J T 1977 A test meal for assessing the intraluminal phase of absorption in childhood. Archives of Disease in Childhood 52: 887–889

McGuignan J E, Wolfe M M 1980 Secretin injection test in the diagnosis of gastrinoma. Gastroenterology 79: 1324–1331

Meier-Ruge W 1974 Hirschsprung's disease: its aetiology, pathogenesis and differential diagnosis. In: Current Topics in Pathology, vol 59. Berlin: Springer-Verlag

Melham R E, Rizk G K 1970 Splenoportographic evaluation of portal hypertension in children. Journal of Pediatric Surgery 5: 522–526

Menghini G 1970 One second biopsy of liver — problems of its clinical application. New England Journal of Medicine 283: 582–585

Menzies L S, Laker M F, Pounder R et al 1979 Abnormal intestinal permeability to sugars in villous atrophy. Lancet ii: 1107–1109

Read A E, Gough K R, Bones J A, McCarthy C G 1962 An improvement to the Crosby peroral intestinal biopsy capsule. Lancet i: 894–895

Rolles C J, Kendall M J, Nutter S, Anderson C M 1973 One-hour blood xylose screening test for coeliac disease in infants and young children. Lancet ii: 1043–1045

Roselund M L, Crean G P, Johnson D G 1969 The Zollinger Ellison syndrome in a 10-year old boy. Journal of Pediatrics 75: 443–448

Rosenfield N, Treves S 1974 Liver-spleen scanning in pediatrics. Pediatrics 53: 692–701

Ryoji O, Klingensmith W C, Lilly J R 1981 Diagnosis of hepatobiliary disease in infants and children with Tc-99m-diethyl-IDA imaging. Clinical Nuclear Medicine 6: 297–302

Rubin C E, Dobbins W O 1965 Peroral biopsy of the small intestine. Gastroenterology 49: 676–699

Schwartz D L, White J J, Saulsbury F, Haller J R Jnr 1974 Gastrin response to calcium infusion: an aid to the improved diagnosis of Zollinger-Ellison syndrome in children. Pediatrics 54: 599–602

Sharp H L, Krivit W, Lowman J T 1967 The diagnosis of complete extra-hepatic obstruction by Rose Bengal ^{131}I. Journal of Pediatrics 70: 46–53

Simpson A J, Leonidas J C, Krasna I H, Becker J M, Schneider K M 1972 Roentgen diagnosis of midgut malrotation: value of upper gastrointestinal radiographic study. Journal of Pediatric Surgery 7: 243–252

Soeparto P, Stobo E A, Walker-Smith J A 1972 Role of chemical examination of the stool in the diagnosis of sugar malabsorption in children. Archives of Disease in Childhood 47: 56–61

Sondheimer J M 1980 Continuous monitoring of distal esophageal pH: A diagnostic test for gastroesophageal reflux in infants. Journal of Pediatrics 96: 804–807

Strauss E, Gerson C D, Yalow R S 1974 Hypersecretion of gastrin associated with short bowel syndrome. Gastroenterology 66: 175–180

Tait C E, Hesp R 1976 Measurement of ^{57}Co Vitamin B_{12} uptake using a static whole body counter. British Journal of Radiology 49: 948–950

Teo H N, Scott J M, Neale G, Weir D G 1980 Effect of bile on vitamin B_{12} absorption. British Medical Journal 2: 831–833

Thaysen E H 1977 Diagnostic value of the ^{14}C cholylglycine breath test. Clinical Gasroenterology 6(i): 227–244

Toskes P P 1983 Bentiromide as a test of exocrine pancreatic function in adult patients with pancreatic exocrine insufficiency: Determination of appropriate dose and urinary collection interval. Gastroenterology, 85: 565–569.

Trier J S 1971 Diagnostic value of peroral biopsy of the proximal small intestine. The New England Journal of Medicine 285: 1470–1473

Van de Kamer J H, Ten Bokkel Huinink, Weijers H A 1949 A rapid method for the determination of fat in faeces. Journal of Biological Chemistry 177: 347–352

Vanderhoof J A, Hunt L J, Antonson D L 1981 A rapid procedure for small intestinal biopsy in infants and children

Verner J V, Morrison A B 1958 Islet cell tumour and a syndrome of refractory watery diarrhoea and hypokalaemia. American Journal of Medicine 25: 374–386

Waldmann T A 1961 Gastrointestinal protein loss demonstrated by ^{51}Cr-labelled albumin. Lancet ii: 121–123

Walker W A, Lowman J T, Hong R A 1973 Measuring albumin turnover rates in patients with hypoproteinaemia. American Journal of Diseases in Children 125: 51–54

Werlin S C, Dodds W J, Hogan W J, Arndorfer R C 1980 Mechanisms of gastroesophageal reflux in children. Journal of Pediatrics 97: 244–249

Williams C B, Leage N J, Campbell C A, Douglas J R, Walker-Smith J A, Booth I W, Harries J T 1982 Total colonoscopy in children. Archives of Diseases in Childhood 57: 49–51

Zeltzer P M, Neerhout R C, Fonkalsrud E W, Steihm E R 1974 Differentiation between neonatal hepatitis and biliary atresia by measuring alpha fetoprotein. Lancet i: 373–375

PART 2

Surgical emergencies in the first few weeks of life

Surgery during the neonatal period is largely concentrated on the correction of congenital malformations. Ideally, such surgery should only be carried out in large centres by surgeons who are wholly committed to paediatrics or who have undergone specific training in paediatric surgical conditions. By concentrating the workload in major centres, the paediatric surgeons are able to acquire expertise in a wide variety of conditions and to assemble a group of dedicated anaesthetists, radiologists, pathologists and nurses who are essential to the successful outcome of major surgical interventions in this age group.

OESOPHAGUS

Oesophageal atresia and/or tracheo-oesophageal fistula

The incidence of oesophageal atresia in the United Kingdom is around one per 3000 live births. The anatomy of the various types of oesophageal anomalies is shown in Figure 4.1. The commonest variety (85%) consists of

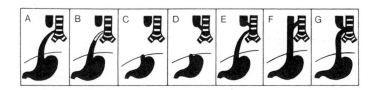

Fig. 4.1 The different varieties of oesophageal atresias and tracheo-oesophageal fistulae.

a proximal atresia with a distal tracheo-oesophageal fistula (Fig. 4.1A). In about 8% there is no fistula (Fig. 4.1C), and in 5% a fistula without atresia (Fig. 4.1F); the remainder covering a variety of defects are shown in Figure 4.1 B, D and G.

Clinical features

The presence of polyhydramnios in the mother during the last trimester of pregnancy should alert the clinician to the possibility of a high intestinal obstruction. This is a result of an interruption in the circulation of amniotic fluid due to the obstructive lesion. Polyhydramnios occurs in 20–25% of affected pregnancies. At birth, the infant is unable to swallow saliva and presents with froth at the mouth requiring repeated suctioning. Aspiration of saliva causes choking attacks and cyanotic episodes and may produce pneumonia which usually affects the right upper or middle lobe. In the common type this aspiration pneumonia may be aggravated by the reflux of highly acid gastric juice via the distal tracheo-oeosophageal fistula. It should be possible to establish the diagnosis before the first feed is offered.

Diagnosis

The diagnosis is confirmed by passing a large calibre (No. 10–12 French gauge) radio-opaque catheter into the oesophagus. In oesophageal atresia, progress of the catheter is arrested approximately 8–10 cm from the gum margin. A straight X-ray of the chest and abdomen will determine the level of the atresia. The presence of gas in the stomach is indicative of a distal tracheo-oesophageal fistula. The use of radio-opaque contrast material is both unnecessary and potentially dangerous since spill-over into the tracheo-bronchial tree may occur.

Associated anomalies

Associated anomalies are common, and in a survey of 1058 patients, Holder et al (1964) determined an incidence of 48% of additional malformations. The most frequent combination of anomalies may be conveniently grouped together as the VACTER association (V-vertebral, A-anorectal, C-cardiac, T-tracheal, E-(o)esophageal, R-renal, radial). In Table 4.1, the incidence

Table 4.1 The incidence of associated anomalies with oesophageal atresia (Holder et al 1964). Total number of cases = 1058

Congenital cardiac anomalies	201 (18.9%)
Gastrointestinal	134 (12.6%)
Genitourinary	109 (10.3%)
Anorectal anomalies	99 (9.3%)
Musculoskeletal	91 (8.6%)

of other congenital anomalies in association with oesophageal atresia is shown.

Management

Transfer of the infant to a recognized neonatal surgical centre for surgical treatment is recommended. During transfer it is essential to keep the upper oesophageal pouch empty to prevent aspiration of saliva. This is best achieved by continuous or frequent intermittent suction to an indwelling naso-oesophageal tube (the double lumen Repogle tube — size 10 French — is best suited for this purpose). Reflux of gastric content is restricted by placing the infant in the prone position.

Prior to surgery, chest physiotherapy and antibiotics may be required to resolve an aspiration pneumonia which may have developed. The aim of the operation is to disconnect the tracheo-oesophageal fistula, close the defect in the trachea and achieve a primary anastomosis of the oesophagus. This is possible in well over three-quarters of the cases. The procedure is best carried out via the extrapleural approach and at surgery either a fine transanastomotic Silastic® tube is passed, or a gastrostomy is fashioned, to permit early postoperative feeding with milk. Early postoperative complications include anastomotic leaks, pneumothorax, pneumonia, anastomotic strictures and recurrent fistulae. Late complications consist of oesophageal peristaltic incoordination resulting in swallowing difficulties, gastro-oesophageal reflux, tracheomalacia and an increased tendency to develop respiratory tract infections.

When primary oesophageal anastomosis is technically impossible, a situation found especially in atresia without fistula, the alternatives are either delayed primary anastomosis or oesophageal replacement. Delayed primary anastomosis involves continuous suction to the upper oesophageal pouch while awaiting selective growth of the proximal and distal oesophageal segments towards each other. This process may take 3–6 months, during which time the infant is fed by gastrostomy. Bouginage of the oesophageal pouches has been recommended (Rehbein & Schweder 1971) but its value is uncertain. The alternative approach, which is probably safer, is to abandon the oesophagus by performing an end-oesophagostomy in the neck and replacing the oesophagus at the age of 9–12 months by means of a colon interposition (Waterston 1969), a gastric tube (Anderson & Randolph 1978) or by the stomach itself (Spitz 1984).

Prognosis

The overall survival rate for oesophageal atresia should approach 90% (Rickham et al 1977, Myers 1979). With advances in neonatal care deaths should be restricted to those infants with multiple severe associated anomalies and chromosomal defects, and infants who are extremely premature (< 1000 g).

Tracheo-oesophageal fistula without atresia (H-type)

The clinical features of this lesion are due to the escape of food into the trachea and air into the oesophagus. The infant may present with choking and cyanosis with each feed, recurrent bouts of pneumonia or persistent abdominal distension.

The diagnosis is established by means of a cine-swallowing using Dionosil® as a contrast medium. The infant is placed in the prone position while contrast is introduced into the oesophagus via a nasogastric tube which is progressively withdrawn from the stomach until the site of the fistula is outlined. Identification of the fistula at endoscopy (oesophagoscopy and/or bronchoscopy) is important prior to surgical intervention. The fistula should be ligated and divided via either a cervical or thoracic route depending on its site.

STOMACH

Infantile hypertrophic pyloric stenosis

Infantile pyloric stenosis occurs in two to three infants per 1000 live births (Spicer 1982). The incidence is much lower among the black races of America and Africa (Klein & Cremin 1970). Males are affected four times as frequently as females and there is a preponderance among first-born infants.

Inheritance

A strong familial pattern of inheritance for pyloric stenosis is firmly established. The incidence among sons of male index patients is 5.5% and for daughters 2.4%, while for female index patients the incidence is 18.9% for sons and 7% for daughters. These proportions are 10, 25, 40 and 70 times the incidence for the same sex in the general population (Carter & Evans 1969).

Aetiology

The precise aetiology of the condition remains elusive — both hereditary and environmental factors have been implicated. A relatively low incidence in infants with blood Group A and an increased incidence in autumn and spring has been noted.

Numerous theories relating to the pathogenesis of pyloric stenosis have been postulated. These vary from muscular imbalances (Lehmann 1931), and mechanical trauma from ingested milk curds (Lynn 1960) to abnormalities of the myenteric nerve plexus (Alaroutu 1956, Belding & Kernohan 1953, Friesen et al 1956, Spitz & Kaufman 1975). The role of gastrin in the genesis of the condition remains speculative (Dodge 1970, 1974, Spitz & Zail 1976, Rodgers et al 1975).

Clinical features

Symptoms usually develop between the second and fourth weeks of life, although presentation soon after birth or as late as 4–6 months has been described. Classically, the vomiting is projectile in nature, occurs 10–20 minutes after a feed and never contains any bile. As a consequence of persistent vomiting the infant fails to thrive and bowel actions become infrequent and stools constipated. The presence of altered blood in the vomitus has been noted in 10–17% of the cases and is usually due to an ulcerated lower oesophageal mucosa (Spitz & Batcup 1979).

Most infants are referred before significant biochemical disturbances occur and initially are irritable and hungry. Only 10–15% of infants are clinically dehydrated on admission. When the stomach is full, visible peristalsis is easily seen and the palpation of a pyloric tumour, either during a test feed or shortly after a vomit establishes the diagnosis. The mass is characteristically olive-shaped, located deep in the right upper quadrant and is best felt soon after commencing a small 'test feed'. With care, over 90% of such tumours can be palpated.

Diagnosis

No further investigations are required once the pyloric 'tumour' has been palpated. In the absence of a palpable tumour, the diagnosis may be established on barium meal examination which characteristically demonstrates a narrow elongated pyloric canal with delayed gastric emptying and a 'mushroom' effect on the duodenal cap. Ultrasonography has recently been used to demonstrate the pyloric mass (see Ch. 3).

Management

The treatment of choice is Ramstedt's pyloromyotomy. The operative relief of the pyloric stenosis is *never* an emergency. Correction of dehydration, electrolyte and acid-base imbalance is essential prior to surgery. This may be achieved by oral rehydration with glucose saline solutions such as WHO oral rehydration solution or, where more severe deficits exist, by intravenous infusions of normal saline with added potassium chloride.

The operation is performed under a general endotracheal anaesthesia and basically consists of splitting the hypertrophied pyloric musculature down to, but not including, the mucosal layer. The incision in the pyloric canal should extend from the duodenogastric junction to the gastric antrum. A perforation of the duodenal mucosa occurs in approximately 5% of cases. This is not a disaster provided it is recognized and the defect closed.

Postoperatively, oral feeds are withheld for 18–24 hours. Earlier reintroduction of oral fluid substantially increases the incidence of vomiting (Spitz 1979).

Prognosis

Deaths as a consequence of pyloric stenosis are extremely rare. Complications which may occur include incomplete myotomy and wound sepsis and dehiscence.

DUODENUM

Duodenal atresia/stenosis

Congenital intrinsic duodenal obstruction may be caused by an atresia, stenosis or a diaphragm which may be complete or contain a small orifice. Extrinsic obstruction is most commonly associated with malrotation. Annular pancreas rarely causes obstruction to the duodenum unless accompanied by an underlying stenosis.

Aetiology

The frequent association with other congenital anomalies points to a developmental rather than an acquired origin for duodenal atresia. Tandler (1900) proposed a failure of recanalization following a temporary solid state as the embryological explanation for duodenal atresia. Boyden et al (1967) demonstrated that vacuoles develop in the duodenum as the occluding epithelium begins to disintegrate. Other investigators have shown that although the lumen of the duodenum may appear to be occluded, total obliteration of the lumen may not occur.

Clinical features

Persistent vomiting is the cardinal feature of duodenal atresia. In over three-quarters of cases, the vomitus is bile-tinged, while in the remainder i.e. those involving the supra-ampullary region of the duodenum, the vomitus is clear. Abdominal distension, if present at all, is confined to the upper abdomen. Small quantities of meconium may be passed in up to 50% of cases.

Diagnosis

The straight erect abdominal X-ray reveals the classical 'double-bubble' appearance. Contrast studies are necessary in cases with incomplete obstruction where it is important to differentiate duodenal stenosis from extrinsic compression due to malrotation with midgut volvulus.

Associated anomalies

Over 50% of the infants with duodenal atresia have additional congenital

Table 4.2 Anomalies associated with duodenal atresia and stenosis

	%
Down's syndrome	30
Malrotation	20
Congenital cardiac anomalies	20
Genitourinary anomalies	10
Oesophageal atresia	8
Anorectal malformations	7
Skeletal anomalies	6

anomalies. The frequency and type of anomalies are shown in Table 4.2 (Fonkalsrud et al 1969).

Management and Prognosis

Preoperative correction of fluid and electrolyte imbalances is required for infants in whom the diagnosis has been delayed beyond the first day of life.

The operative correction of duodenal atresia consists of fashioning a side-to-side duodenostomy. Duodenal diaphragms may be excised but particular attention must be directed to avoid damage to the biliary tract. A transanastomotic feeding tube is invaluable in providing a route for post-operative enteral nutrition without having to resort to parenteral nutrition.

The mortality in intrinsic duodenal obstructive lesions is directly related to the severity of the associated anomalies and to the degree of prematurity. The overall mortality rate is in the order of 25–30%.

Malrotation

Malrotation refers to an interference with the process of orderly fetal rotation of the midgut and the normal fixation of the mesenteries, which is described in detail in Chapter 1.

Malrotation is a constant feature of exomphalos and congenital diaphragmatic hernia and is frequently associated with intrinsic duodenal obstructions. It is also found in association with oesophageal atresia, anorectal anomalies, Hirschsprung's disease and biliary atresia.

Clinical features

The presentation of malrotation during the neonatal period is almost invariably with bile-stained vomiting which may be intermittent. The significance of bilious vomiting may not be appreciated until volvulus develops which is heralded by abdominal pain and the passage of dark blood per rectum. Ultimately, shock supervenes and unless urgent action is taken gangrene of the entire midgut loop develops. The risk of volvulus developing, which is of the order of 45–65% (Stewart et al 1976), makes an expectant approach to malrotation inadvisable. Operative correction of the malrotation should be carried out as soon as the diagnosis has been established. Recurrent abdominal pain with intermittent diarrhoea or obstructive jaundice are only rarely the presenting features in the neonatal period.

Diagnosis

A plain abdominal X-ray shows a dilated stomach and first part of the duodenum giving a 'double-bubble' appearance on the erect film. With the advent of volvulus, gas is forced out of the distal intestine producing the 'gasless abdomen' appearance. Confirmation of the diagnosis may be obtained by contrast studies of which a barium meal and follow-through is the examination of choice (see Ch. 3 pages 52–54). A barium enema may be helpful in showing the abnormal position of the caecum.

Management and prognosis

Because of the risk of strangulation the need for surgery is urgent. The volvulus is untwisted, all adhesions are divided, Ladd's bands are divided and the gut is freed until it is possible to lay the small bowel to the right and the large bowel to the left of the abdomen. No attempt should be made to restore the normal arrangement of the gut but the mesenteric isthmus must be widened to prevent recurrences. The gut may be sutured in its new position (Bill & Grauman 1966). Some surgeons perform an appendicectomy whereas others prefer not to open the gut lumen.

If strangulation has already occurred simple resection of the infarcted gut is performed when there is an adequate length of healthy gut remaining. When there is insufficient obviously viable bowel remaining a 'second look' policy is worth adopting. The bowel is arranged in its optimum position and the abdomen closed. 24 hours later the abdomen is re-explored in the hope that some of the previously non-viable gut may have recovered. This policy can sometimes offer the chance of survival in an otherwise hopeless situation.

In the absence of strangulation and infarction of the bowel, the results of surgery are excellent and recurrence of the volvulus is unusual. When resection is necessary, the prospects and quality of survival depend on the length of surviving gut.

Early management following resection

The average length of the small intestine in the newborn is 250 cm, and the minimum length compatible with survival is about 20–25 cm assuming that the ileocaecal valve is left intact (Wilmore 1972). Postoperative problems, however, should be anticipated even when there is a greater length of small gut remaining. The immediate problems are the body losses of fluid and electrolytes, and malabsorption; intravenous feeding is essential until an adequate oral intake has been achieved. Disaccharide and cow's milk protein intolerance not infrequently follows resection, and these two dietary constituents should be initially excluded from the feeding regime, particularly if a long length of gut has been removed. Feeds can be given by a continuous nasogastric drip at first, and later as small frequent feeds. Unabsorbed bile salts may exacerbate diarrhoea by their toxic effects on the colonic mucosa, and the oral administration of binding resins such as cholestyramine is sometimes helpful. When it has been necessary to remove the ileocaecal valve, bacterial overgrowth of the remaining small gut may contribute to the malabsorption and an appropriate antibiotic should be given. Even after an oral feeding regime has been established there is a tendency to recurrent episodes of diarrhoea, which may require fluid and electrolyte replacement. Adaptation of the remaining small bowel occurs gradually during the 2–3 months following surgery. The long-term effects of small intestinal resection are considered in Chapter 5.

SMALL INTESTINE

Intestinal atresia/stenosis

Atresias may occur at any level in the intestine but are most frequent in the small intestine. They vary from single occluding diaphragms to widely separated bowel ends with defects in the mesentery. They may be single or multiple.

Anatomy of the lesion

The classification of intestinal atresias has been only slightly modified since the early proposals of Bland-Sutton in 1889. The proximal segment is greatly hypertrophied and dilated while the distal intestine is narrow and collapsed ('unused').

Aetiology

Clinical and experimental evidence provide unequivocal support to the hypothesis that intestinal atresia results from an intrauterine vascular occlusion to the involved segment of intestine. The evidence may be summarized as follows:

1. bile pigments, squames and lanugo hairs are often found in the distal intestine.

2. careful pathological examination often reveals evidence of an intrauterine volvulus, intussusception, hernia or perforation (Tawes & Nixon 1971).

3. experimentally, atresias can be produced by interfering with the blood

supply to the fetal intestine (Barnard & Louw 1956, Courtois 1959, Santulli & Blanc 1961, Abrams 1968).

Clinical features

The most constant feature on clinical presentation is bilious vomiting. In low atresias, faeculent vomitus replaces the bilious vomit as the diagnosis is delayed.

Abdominal distension may be restricted to the upper abdomen in high jejunal atresias, but in the majority of cases abdominal distension is a prominent feature and may develop rapidly and become severe enough to cause respiratory embarrassment. The majority of infants fail to pass meconium and rectal washouts produce grey-white plugs of mucus. In 20% of infants, small amounts of normal-appearing meconium may be evacuated.

Diagnosis

Plain erect and supine abdominal X-rays will reveal air-fluid levels in the obstructed and dilated proximal bowel and an absence of gas beyond the level of the atresia. A rough estimation of the level of the obstruction may be gauged by the number of fluid levels present. Differentiation of low ileal and colonic obstruction is virtually impossible on plain abdominal radiography in the neonatal period. A diagnostic contrast enema under these circumstances is useful in distinguishing between a small intestinal atresia, meconium ileus and long-segment Hirschsprung's disease. Calcification, indicative of an antenatal perforation, is found in 10% of cases.

Management and Prognosis

Fluid and electrolyte replacement is generally not required in infants presenting in the first 24 hours of life, but where the diagnosis is delayed, replacement becomes an essential part of the preoperative preparation.

The operative treatment consists of resection of the grossly dilated proximal intestine and the fashioning of an end-to-end anastomosis to restore intestinal continuity. 'Tailoring' of the proximal bowel to permit an end-to-end anastomosis is required in high jejunal atresias and multiple anastomoses may be necessary in infants with multiple atresias involving long segments of the intestine. The minimum length of remaining small bowel compatible with long-term survival is 30–40 cm without an intact ileocaecal valve and 15–20 cm with an ileocaecal region (Wilmore 1972).

Results

The survival rate for intestinal atresia has steadily improved since the first successful correction in 1911. This improved prognosis is directly attributable to improved surgical and anaesthetic techniques and to refinements in postoperative management with particular emphasis on nursing care and the availability of parenteral nutrition. The overall survival rate should be in excess of 75–80% (Louw 1966, Tawes & Nixon 1971).

Meconium ileus

Meconium ileus occurs in 10–15% of infants with cystic fibrosis. The meconium, which in this condition, is thick, viscid, sticky and tenacious, forms an intraluminal bolus obstruction in the distal ileum. The deficiency of exocrine pancreatic secretions, the increase in albumin content of the meconium, and the associated abnormalities of intestinal secretion are all thought to be responsible for the abnormal consistency of the meconium.

In uncomplicated meconium ileus, the proximal ileum is enormously distended with the abnormal meconium. The distal bowel is narrow and contracted and contains greyish pellets of inspissated material. Approximately 50% of cases of meconium ileus are complicated by gangrene with or without perforation, volvulus, atresia or meconium peritonitis. The latter complication occurs as an antenatal event and causes an intense peritoneal inflammatory reaction. The extravasated meconium rapidly becomes calcified and is easily identifiable on a plain abdominal radiograph.

Clinical features

The outstanding feature of meconium ileus is the presence of abdominal distension at birth. Polyhydramnios occurs in about 20% of cases. A positive family history of cystic fibrosis is helpful in establishing a diagnosis. The distended meconium-filled loops of intestine may be visible and are often palpable on abdominal examination. Bilious vomiting occurs within the first 24 hours after birth. Generally, no meconium is passed and only small plugs of mucus are evacuated on rectal saline washouts.

Diagnosis

The plain abdominal X-ray classically reveals dilated loops of intestine of varying calibre with an absence or scarcity of air-fluid levels. Small bubbles of air within the meconium mass may give rise to the 'ground glass' appearance, a sign which is suggestive but not pathognomonic of meconium ileus. Calcification in the peritoneal cavity is indicative of meconium peritonitis, while air-fluid levels are suggestive of an associated atresia or volvulus.

Management

Nonoperative measures may be successful in treating the uncomplicated case. Any suspicion (clinical or radiological) of volvulus, gangrene, perforation, peritonitis or atresia, should be regarded as an absolute contraindication for this form of treatment. The procedure consists of an initial barium enema to exclude the possibility of a distal bowel lesion (Noblett 1969a) followed by the use of diatrizoate meglamine (Gastrografin®) to liquify the obstructing meconium mass. The Gastrografin® is hyperosmolar (osmolality 1900 mmol/l) and contains an emulsifying agent (Tween 80®). The former property causes fluid to be drawn into the lumen of the intestine while the latter property reduces the surface tension of the meconium, facilitating its expulsion. Massive fluid losses into the intestine are likely to occur during the procedure and it is essential to ensure that the infant is well hydrated prior to commencing the treatment. The procedure should be carried out under fluoroscopic control by an experienced paediatric radiologist. (Lillie & Chrispin 1972).

Surgical intervention is indicated for infants with 'complicated' meconium ileus and for those patients who fail to respond to nonoperative treatment. The aim of surgery is to relieve the obstruction by resecting any anatomical obstructive lesion e.g. atresia, and by evacuating the meconium mass from the distal intestine. Intestinal continuity may be restored by means of an end-to-side ileoileostomy with a distal (Bishop & Koop 1957) or proximal (Santulli & Blanc 1961) stoma. More recently, complete evacuation of the meconium from the intestine and end-to-end anastomosis has been preferred. Neonatal meconium obstruction has been reported in the absence of cystic fibrosis (Rickham & Boeckman 1965) and confirmation of the diagnosis by means of a sweat test is essential. Early survival rates of over 80% are now possible in uncomplicated cases.

Prognosis

It is rare for the infant with complicated meconium ileus to succumb to the intestinal lesion. There does not appear to be any evidence to suggest that the infant with meconium ileus is more severely affected than other infants with cystic fibrosis.

Duplications

Duplications can occur anywhere in the alimentary tract from the mouth to the anus. Characteristically, the wall of the duplication contains one or several layers of muscle and its mucosal lining is representative of some part of the gastrointestinal tract, however remote from the site of attachment. The lesion may be cystic or tubular and is invariably located on the mesenteric side of the bowel.

Aetiology

Three theories have been proposed:
1. persistence of transitory diverticuli (Lewis & Thyng 1907)
2. errors in recanalization of epithelial occlusion (Bremer 1944)
3. failure of separation of adhesions between the neural tube ectoderm and intestinal endoderm (Fallon et al 1954, Beardmore & Wiglesworth 1958).

Clinical features

Approximately half of all duplications are located in the small intestine, a quarter occur in the oesophagus while the remainder are roughly equally distributed in the stomach, duodenum, colon and rectum. Cystic duplications occur with far greater frequency than tubular duplications. The cystic lesions present with intestinal obstruction due to compression of the adjacent bowel. They are often palpable on clinical examination. The tubular duplications frequently contain ectopic gastric mucosa which is responsible for peptic ulceration of the adjacent intestinal mucosa and results in haemorrhage or perforation. Rarely, duplications are the cause of volvulus or intussusceptions.

Diagnosis

In addition to the features of intestinal obstruction, the plain abdominal X-ray in cystic duplications will reveal a radiolucent space-occupying lesion. Barium contrast studies may reveal a partial intestinal obstruction. Ultrasonography is undoubtedly the investigation of choice for unexplained abdominal masses in infancy and childhood. Cystic lesions are clearly differentiated from the solid tumours. Radioisotope scans with technetium (^{99}Tc) will assist in localizing ectopic gastric mucosa. The association of vertebral anomalies, particularly split vertebra or hemivertebra especially in the high thoracic region, should alert the clinician to the possibility of an intestinal duplication.

Treatment

Total excision which usually involves resection of the attached intestine is the treatment of choice. In certain situations, e.g. duodenal duplication, the risk of resection is so great that marsupialization into the adjacent intestine is recommended. Alternatively, the mucosal lining of the duplication may be stripped out. This method of treatment is particularly suitable for extensive tubular duplications, where resection would result in massive bowel loss.

Management

A brief period of intensive resuscitation is necessary to stabilize the clinically shocked infant prior to surgery. The period of resuscitation should not be prolonged lest irreversible gangrene supervenes.

The aim of surgery is to reduce the volvulus, to relieve any obstruction of the duodenum by the Ladd's bands and to widen the base of the small bowel mesentery in order to prevent a recurrence of the volvulus. Brennon & Bill (1974) advocate fixing the intestine in the nonrotated position, but most other surgeons are content to place the small bowel on the right of the peritoneal cavity and the colon on the left.

LARGE INTESTINE

Hirschsprung's disease

Hirschsprung first described a lethal condition of infancy characterized by intractable constipation, colonic dilatation and an empty rectum, in 1887. The disease is associated with a total absence of ganglion cells in the affected segment of intestine and an overgrowth of large nerve trunks in the intermuscular and submucosal zones. The defective innervation always affects the distal rectum and extends proximally for a variable distance. In 75% of cases the abnormal segment is restricted to the rectosigmoid region, while in 5% of cases there is total colonic involvement. The gross pathological changes consist of a narrow contracted aganglionic segment which extends proximally into a grossly dilated, thickened and hypertrophied normally innervated but functionally obstructed colon. The cone-shaped zone between the dilated and collapsed intestine is known as the 'transitional' area. The extent of this zone varies considerably.

Clinical features

Approximately 1 in 5000 infants are affected by Hirschsprung's disease. Overall, there is a 4:1 ratio in favour of male infants, but this discrepancy virtually disappears as the length of the involved segment increases. There is an increased risk of recurrence of the disease in subsequent siblings, ranging from 2% for short-segment disease to 12.5% in the case of long-segment involvement.

Presentation of Hirschsprung's disease is summarized in Figure 4.2 but commonly occurs as:

1. complete intestinal obstruction with bilious vomiting, complete obstipation and massive abdominal distension.

2. delayed passage of meconium, i.e. in excess of 24 hours after birth. This feature was present in 94% of patients in Swenson's series of 501 cases (1973). It is generally associated with bilious vomiting and abdominal distension. Temporary relief may be obtained following digital rectal examination or after a gentle rectal saline washout.

3. enterocolitis. This complication generally occurs during the second to

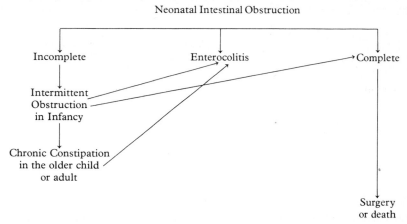

Fig. 4.2 The presentation of Hirschsprung's disease.

fourth weeks and results as a consequence of delayed diagnosis. The infant presents with profuse diarrhoea often containing blood and mucus, which is accompanied by abdominal distension and bilious vomiting. Fluid and electrolyte losses are rapid and the infant may present in hypovolaemic shock.

Diagnosis

Confirmation of the diagnosis may be achieved using one or more of the following investigations:

Radiology. The barium contrast enema is performed via a small soft rubber catheter inserted just within the anal canal in a previously *unprepared* colon. The barium solution is slowly introduced into the rectum with the infant in the lateral position, and is continued until an obviously dilated area becomes visible. This represents the classical 'cone' at the transition between aganglionic and ganglionic bowel. Where the diagnosis remains doubtful, delayed films taken 24 hours later characteristically show significant retention of contrast material (Berdon & Baker 1965).

Manometry. Failure of the internal anal sphincter to exhibit a relaxation wave in response to inflation of a balloon inserted into the rectum is diagnostic of Hirschsprung's disease (Aaronson & Nixon 1972). Holschneider (1982) has reported a diagnostic accuracy rate of 96% but this high success rate has not been universal experience, especially when the test is performed during the early neonatal period when the anal relaxation reflux may be physiologically absent.

Mucosal biopsy. The histopathological diagnosis of Hirschsprung's disease depends upon the demonstration of the absence of ganglion cells in the myenteric and submucosal plexus as well as the demonstration of increased nerve fibres and the presence of large trunks in these layers. The accuracy of diagnosis is facilitated by the advent of histochemical techniques (Meier-Ruge et al 1972) which specifically stain for acetyl-cholinesterase activity.

Until recently a full-thickness biopsy of the rectal wall was necessary, but this has been replaced by the suction biopsy technique introduced by Noblett (1969b). Suction biopsies from carefully defined levels in the rectum and staining for cholinesterase activity is our diagnostic method of choice (Lake et al 1978).

Treatment

The aim of treatment is to relieve the intestinal obstruction by either resecting or bypassing the aganglionic bowel. Temporary relief may be obtained by gentle washouts of the rectum using small quantities of a warm saline solution pending the results of the various investigations. The fashioning of a defunctioning colostomy sited in ganglionic bowel is generally recognized as the safest course of action until definitive surgery can be carried out. In some countries, regular rectal washouts are practised until the infant reaches the age of 3–6 months when the definitive operation is performed.

Infants presenting with established enterocolitis are often critically ill due to massive fluid and electrolyte losses in the diarrhoeae fluid as well as into the lumen of the bowel. Emergency colostomy under these circumstances is hazardous and could prove fatal. These infants require intensive resuscitative measures including urgent circulatory fluid volume expansion (20 ml/kg of plasma intravenously as rapidly as possible), correction of acid-base imbalance, and fluid and electrolyte deficiencies. Rectal washouts, using as much as 1–2 litres of warm normal saline may be required before adequate decompression of the intestine can be achieved. Antibiotic therapy is also invaluable in enterocolitis. A specific link between Hirschsprung's enterocolitis and toxin-producing *Clostridia difficile* has been established (Thomas et al 1982) and therapy with vancomycin, or Septrin® and metronidazole, is strongly indicated.

Definitive treatment may take the form of either of five recognized procedures:

1. Swenson's operation which consists of resection of the aganglionic intestine down to the internal anal sphincter i.e. rectosigmoidectomy (Swenson & Bill 1948).

2. Duhamel (1960) retrorectal pull-through procedure in which the proximal ganglionic bowel is pulled down to the anus behind the aganglionic rectum which is left in situ. A side-to-side anastomosis is achieved by one of a variety of methods, the most popular being by means of a stapling clamp.

3. Soave (1966) endorectal pull-through procedure in which the ganglionic bowel is pulled through the seromuscular cuff of the retained aganglionic rectum.

4. Rehbein's procedure (Rehbein 1958). This is in effect a low anterior

resection of the rectum and aganglionic bowel combined with forcible dilatation of the anal sphincter.

5. Rectal myomectomy.

Each of these procedures gives excellent results in experienced hands. There can be no place for the occasional operation performed by an inexperienced surgeon.

Prognosis

The majority of deaths in Hirschsprung's disease are due to enterocolitis which may occur even years after an apparently adequate and successful pull-through procedure. Other complications include anastomotic leaks and strictures, recurrent constipation, or incontinence and soiling.

Late onset Hirschsprung's disease

Although 80–90% of patients present in the neonatal period, some children present later with intractable constipation which may alternate with episodes of diarrhoea; the diagnosis may even be delayed to early adult life.

Clinical features and diagnosis

Once the condition has been suspected the diagnosis is much simpler than in the newborn and involves the same investigatory techniques. The disease is predominantly of the short-segment type. The only difficulty arises with very-short-segment disease, and this is considered separately.

Clinical differentiation from other causes of constipation is usually clear. Symptoms precede potty training, there may be failure to thrive and intermittent diarrhoea may be a feature. On rectal examination the anal canal and lower rectum are empty. This empty segment, with faecal loading in the proximal dilated gut which may be within reach of the examining finger, distinguishes Hirschsprung's disease from the loaded rectum and anal canal of 'rectal inertia'. Digital assessment of anal sphincter tone is too subjective to be generally useful. A barium enema must be performed without bowel preparation. The appearance of an empty, narrow and spastic rectum suddenly expanding into the dilated proximal bowel is extremely suggestive of this diagnosis. Histological diagnosis by suction biopsy is simple, but should be confirmed by examining frozen sections at the time of the pull-through surgical procedure. Anorectal pressure studies show the typical failure of relaxation of the internal sphincter.

Management

The same principles of treatment apply as in the newborn. If the bowel can be emptied by regular washouts and the child's general condition improves sufficiently, some surgeons prefer to proceed to a pull-through operation without a preliminary colostomy. Others consider that a preliminary colostomy, to rest and permit complete clearance of contents from the dilated colon and rectum, is safer. All the procedures described in the newborn are used in the older child and are technically easier to perform; postoperative problems with bowel training and control seem to be fewer in the older child.

Very-short- and ultra-short-segment Hirschsprung's disease

The term ultra-short-segment disease is applied to a group of patients in whom there is an abnormal sphincter response but in whom ganglion cells are present down to the level of the anal canal. As there is neither absence of ganglion cells nor any abnormality of the cholinesterase-staining reaction, 'internal sphincter spasm' is probably a better description of this entity.

Clinical features and diagnosis

The condition presents in a very similar fashion with severe chronic constipation; overflow faecal soiling is a common feature but failure to thrive is uncommon. On rectal examination the rectum is usually loaded with faeces down to the anal verge. This is due to a packing effect; the hypertrophied proximal bowel forcing the faecal bolus into the aganglionic segment, dilating it and moving the apparent cone distally. A barium enema will not differentiate this condition from 'rectal inertia' and the diagnosis can only be established by biopsy and anorectal manometry. A series of suction biopsies should be taken at 1 cm intervals so that a complete picture of the innervation of the anal canal and lower rectum can be obtained. Anorectal pressure studies will identify isolated internal sphincter spasm.

Management

Many patients can be managed along the lines established for 'rectal inertia', and the short length of affected bowel precludes any form of pull-through procedure. An extended internal sphincterotomy appears to be the logical operation, and good results have been reported (Lynn 1966); it is important, however, that the secondary rectal inertia be treated. A full anal sphincter stretch performed under general anaesthesia should probably precede an internal sphincterotomy since it is sometimes curative and avoids the permanent impairment of faecal control which may follow sphincterotomy.

Anorectal anomalies

The crucial factor in the management of infants affected by an anorectal anomaly is the distinction between the high or supralevator and the low or

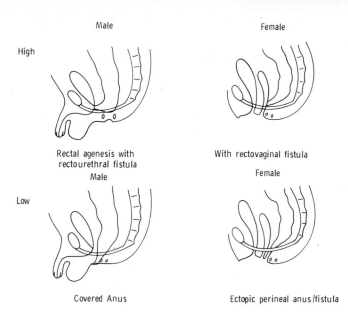

Fig. 4.3 Schematic representation of high and low anorectal anomalies.

translevator anomaly. The former requires an initial diverting colostomy followed by a pull-through procedure, while the latter is fully correctable by a local perineal procedure immediately after birth. The number and variety of abnormalities of this area is vast and complex. The international classification agreed in Melbourne in 1970 (Santulli et al 1970) attempted to standardize documentation of the anomalies. For practical purposes, a simple distinction between high and low anomalies of the most commonly encountered 9 abnormalities is presented in Figure 4.3.

Failure of complete separation of the primitive cloaca by the urorectal septum results in the formation of a high anomaly with a rectourinary or rectovaginal fistula. An error in posterior migration of the anal canal or excessive fusion of skin folds results in an ectopic or covered anus respectively (see also Chapter 1, p. 8).

Diagnosis

A careful clinical examination will elucidate the diagnosis in the majority of cases. The scheme of investigation for the male and female infant is shown in Figure 4.4 and is discussed below. Meticulous examination of the perineum is essential (Stephens & Smith 1971).

Special investigations. Invertogram: This depends on swallowed air outlining the blind rectal pouch. It generally takes 12–18 hours for swallowed air to reach the rectum, so that an X-ray taken before this time may be of no diagnostic value. The X-ray is taken as a true lateral with the

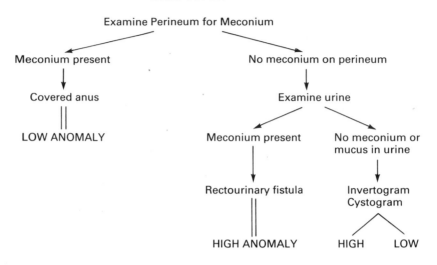

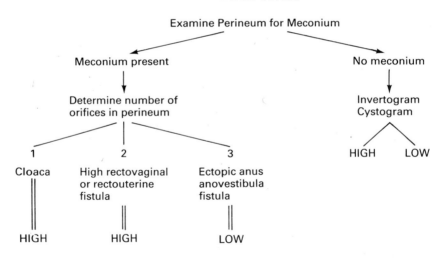

Fig. 4.4 Diagnostic algorithm for anorectal malformations in the male and female infant.

X-ray beam centred on the greater trochanter of the femur. The baby is held upside down for 3–5 minutes before the film is exposed. By measuring the level of the terminal gas shadow in relation to the bony landmarks of the pelvis (pubococcygeal line) the level of the obstruction can be determined (Wagensteen & Rice 1930).

Cystogram: The presence of a rectourinary fistula is diagnostic of a high anomaly.

Associated anomalies

A wide variety of anomalies occur in association with imperforate anus (see VACTER association under Oesophageal atresia, Associated anomalies). Hasse (1976) analysed the additional malformations in 1420 infants with anorectal anomalies and determined an overall incidence of 41.6%. The various systems affected were as follows:

Urogenital system	19.7%
Extremities and spine	13.1%
Cardiovascular system	7.9%
Gastrointestinal system	6.0%
Oesophageal atresia	5.6%
Abdominal wall defects	1.9%

Management

Low Lesions. An anoplasty (male) or cutback procedure (female) may be all that is required. Postoperatively, regular digital anal dilatations are carried out for approximately three months. This is to ensure that healing takes place without fibrosis and that the anal canal is of adequate size.

High lesions. A preliminary defunctioning colostomy is fashsioned. The definitive 'pull-through' procedure is postponed until the infant is of adequate size to withstand a major procedure. Various methods of fashioning an anus in the presence of a high anomaly have been advocated, but in all the aim is to utilize the puborectalis sling for reasons of continence (Stephens 1953), to fashion an anal orifice which is of normal calibre and to ensure that the distal 1–2 cm of the neoanus is lined with skin capable of transmitting sensory impulses (Stephens 1953, Rehbein 1959, Kiesewetter 1967, Mollard et al 1978, de Vries & Pena 1982).

Prognosis

Virtually all children with low imperforate anus acquire normal continence if the correct treatment and postoperative dilatations are carried out. For high lesions the prognosis is not so favourable. One-third are continent, one-third manage adequately but do not have normal control, and one-third are permanently incontinent. A terminal abdominal colostomy may be the best final solution for this latter group of patients.

Necrotizing enterocolitis (NEC)

Necrotizing enterocolitis is an acquired entity affecting predominantly premature infants who have experienced severe perinatal stress, e.g. anoxia, hypothermia, shock. It has emerged as the most common surgical emergency in the neonatal period, affecting 2–5% of all neonates admitted to special care nurseries.

The parts of the intestine most frequently affected are the terminal ileum and colon. The lesion varies from a mild inflammatory reaction to full-thickness gangrene of the bowel wall.

Aetiology and pathogenesis

The final common pathway in the pathogenesis of NEC is generally thought to be an ischaemic insult to the intestine. This causes mucosal damage which allows penetration of bacteria into the wall of the bowel. Lloyd (1969) proposed this aetiological sequence and likened the reaction to that of the diving response of certain mammals in which the cerebral circulation is protected at the expense of less vital organs e.g. the intestine. Touloukian et al (1972) and Barlow et al (1974) provided further experimental data to substantiate this theory. Predisposing factors which have been implicated in the aetiology of NEC include asphyxia, polycythaemia, umbilical arterial catheterization, respiratory distress syndrome, exchange transfusion and congenital cardiac disease (Kliegman et al 1982). Many bacteria have been isolated from the intestine of infants suffering from NEC but no specific organism has been linked with the onset of the disease (Thomas 1982).

Clinical features

The onset occurs most commonly between the second and tenth days of life. It may also occur in the early postoperative period following abdominal or cardiac surgery. The clinical features include reluctance to accept feeds, abdominal distension, passage of blood and mucus in the stools, vomiting which is generally bilious in character, hypothermia and apnoeic attacks.

Erythema and oedema of the anterior abdominal wall signifies imminent gangrene of the intestine. Thrombocytopenia, acidosis, and evidence of disseminated intravascular coagulation are commonly found on serological investigation.

Diagnosis

The demonstration on plain abdominal radiography of intramural gas (pneumatosis intestinalis) and gas in the portal venous system is diagnostic of NEC. Pneumoperitoneum signifies an intestinal perforation.

Treatment

Early diagnosis and prompt aggressive medical therapy has brought about an overall improvement in the survival rates of infants with NEC.

The medical management consists of complete cessation of oral intake for a minimum of 10–14 days during which nutrition is maintained by parenteral feeding. Nasogastric decompression is required during the period of paralytic ileus. Broad spectrum antibiotic therapy (penicillin, gentamicin, metronidazole) should be commenced immediately.

The indications for surgical intervention (Kosloske et al 1980) are intestinal perforation, mechanical intestinal obstruction and failure to improve on intensive medical therapy. The surgical treatment consists of the resection of all frankly gangrenous and perforated intestine and the establishment of proximal and distal enterostomies. Attempts at primary anastomosis may lead to anastomotic disruption, unless massive resections of potentially viable intestine are performed. Restoration of bowel continuity can be safely delayed until the infant is thriving and fully recovered from the episode of NEC, i.e. six weeks to six months later.

A long-term complication of conservative treatment is stricture formation. This develops in 10–15% of infants with moderate to severe NEC and manifests as either intermittent attacks of subacute incomplete intestinal obstruction, or as failure to thrive.

Prognosis

Early diagnosis treatment result in an overall 90% survival rate. Medical management is successful in avoiding surgery in 80–85% of cases.

Exomphalos and gastroschisis

This anomaly of the anterior abdominal wall varies from a relatively trivial hernia into the umbilical cord, to an intact major omphalocele containing most of the intraabdominal viscera or a gastroschisis. All these lesions result from a disturbance of the normal process of reduction of the physiological umbilical hernia as outlined in Figure 4.5.

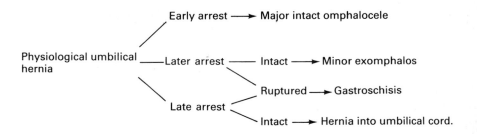

Fig. 4.5 Scheme for the development of the anterior abdominal wall.

Minor exomphalos and hernia into the umbilical cord

The defect at the base of the umbilicus measures less than 5 cm in diameter and the contents consist of small or large intestine. Reduction of the contents into the peritoneal cavity can be easily accomplished and repair of the abdominal wall defect is a safe and simple procedure.

Major exomphalos (omphalocele)

The defect in the anterior abdominal wall is greater than 5 cm and it may extend cranially to involve the sternum and anterior diaphragm (Cantrell et al 1958) or caudally with extrophy of the bladder or cloaca. The hernial contents invariably consist of liver and a major part of the intestine. These contents may be visible through the thin transparent covering membrane consisting of amnion on the outside and peritoneum on the inside. Treatment consists of primary surgical closure of a relatively small defect or of a staged repair which may either be accomplished conservatively by painting the sac with an antiseptic solution or by applying a prosthetic covering over the surface of the sac. Painting the sac causes cicatrization of the covering membrane and allows gradual epithelialization over a period of 3–4 months to occur. Repair of the hernia should not be delayed beyond 12–18 months. By applying prosthetic material (Silastic® or polypropylene mesh) over the dome of the omphalocele, staged reduction of the defect can be accomplished over a period of a few weeks with full repair of the abdominal wall.

Gastroschisis

This refers to an anomaly consisting of herniation of the intestine through a defect in the anterior abdominal wall, usually to the right of the umbilicus. There is no covering sac and the herniated intestine, which may extend from the stomach to the rectum, is grossly thickened, oedematous, matted together and appears to be shorter than normal. Associated anomalies are rare. In the majority of cases, reduction of the herniated contents into the peritoneal cavity may be affected following gradual forceful stretching of the abdominal musculature. If this cannot be accomplished without causing severe respiratory embarrassment, the application of a temporary prosthetic covering with gradual reduction of the contents over a period of a few weeks is the method of choice.

Associated anomalies

Malrotation is a constant associated anomaly in all major lesions. Meckel's diverticulum occurs in 10–20% of cases and intestinal atresias occur in approximately 5% of cases. Exomphalos is one of the features of the Beckwith syndrome (Irving 1967); the other features are macroglossia, gigantism, visceromegaly and neonatal hypoglycaemia.

OTHER LESIONS

Perforation of the stomach and rectum (Robarts 1968)

Perforation of the stomach may be due to trauma from overdistension of the stomach during resuscitation, or from rigid nasogastric tubes, congenital muscle defects or areas of vascular necrosis in the wall. Plain abdominal films reveal a gross pneumoperitoneum. Severe respiratory embarrassment can be temporarily relieved by peritoneal aspiration. The results of closure of the perforation are directly proportional to the speed with which this is achieved following the perforation.

The rectum may be perforated by clumsy insertion of a rectal thermometer or from saline washouts, particularly in babies with enterocolitis due to Hirschsprung's disease and in those with stercoral ulceration over a faecal plug. Intraperitoneal perforations result in abscess formation, and sometimes a lethal peritonitis. Closure of the defect and the treatment of any underlying cause are urgently required.

Meconium peritonitis (Rickham 1955)

Meconium peritonitis results from antenatal perforation of the bowel, usually due to one of the causes already discussed; meconium ileus should not be confused with meconium peritonitis. Minor degrees can sometimes be recognized on microscopic examination of a resected length of atretic small bowel. More severe leaks of meconium show up as speckled or diffuse intraperitoneal calcification on plain films of the abdomen. This appearance may occasionally be seen in the absence of any signs of intestinal obstruction or perforation. The most severe form, giant cystic meconium peritonitis, presents a major problem. The abdominal cavity is divided into two compartments: a meconium-filled anterior compartment into which air enters after birth; posterior to this lies the intestine, matted together by adhesions and covered by a thick inflammatory membrane and communicating with the cavity through a perforation.

The infant usually presents with gross abdominal distension and intestinal obstruction at birth. A plain film of the abdomen shows a large cavity containing fluid and air in the anterior abdomen, and intra-abdominal calcification. Surgery is mandatory for survival. The cavity should be emptied of its contents, the bowel freed and the perforation exteriorized; usually this procedure is technically difficult and often accompanied by severe bleeding.

Milk bolus obstruction (Cook & Rickham 1969)

The milk plug, inspissated milk curd, or milk bolus obstruction is a clearly defined entity, although certain features may overlap with those seen in necrotizing enterocolitis and functional intestinal obstruction. The condition appears to be related to feeding infants from birth with reconstituted full-cream powder preparations.

Typically, a previously normal baby develops signs of obstruction around the end of the first week of life. An unusual and confusing feature is that about half the affected infants have blood in their stools, or following rectal examination the finger is bloodstained. Plain films of the abdomen show small bowel obstruction with dilated loops and fluid levels; in the right iliac fossa bowel is replaced by an amorphous appearance suggesting a faecal bolus containing crescents of gas. The diagnosis is best confirmed by a Gastrografin® enema which may, in itself, relieve the obstruction. If the diagnosis is in doubt or the enema fails to relieve the obstruction, a laparotomy should be performed; the milk bolus can usually be broken up manually without opening the lumen and the fragments milked down into the colon.

Meconium plug syndrome (Clatworthy et al 1956, Ellis & Clatworthy 1966)

In this syndrome the bowel lumen becomes obstructed by a plug of normal meconium. The clinical features are those of an apparently low obstruction which are relieved by the passage of a bolus of meconium following a saline washout or a Gastrografin® enema. A similar appearance may be seen in short-segment Hirschsprung's disease, the functional intestinal obstruction associated with a premature or traumatic delivery, and in mild cases of meconium ileus. The long-term prognosis in uncomplicated cases is excellent. The diagnosis of Hirschsprung's disease *must* be positively excluded on suction rectal biopsy.

The small left colon syndrome

By providing a name for the apparent obstructions at the splenic flexure of the colon in neonatal period, Davis et al (1974) made an important contribution to paediatric surgery. Philippart et al (1975) further defined the condition in eight cases, all children of diabetic mothers.

The clinical presentation is identical to that of Hirschsprung's disease with failure to pass meconium and abdominal distension. The characteristic finding on a contrast enema is a narrow left colon which is less distensible than normal and relatively aperistaltic with an apparent 'cone' at the splenic flexure; this appearance has been confirmed at laparotomy. The distal colon is ganglionic, and in the majority of cases the obstruction recovers spontaneously with conservative management; rarely, caecal perforation has been recorded. The aetiology of the condition and its occurrence in infants of diabetic mothers is unexplained. The greater likelihood of a neonatal obstruction at the splenic flexure being of this nature rather than due to Hirschsprung's disease suggests that when facilities are available for the rapid exclusion of Hirschsprung's disease, the early management should be conservative.

Functional intestinal obstruction (Howat & Wilkinson, 1970)

Idiopathic and functional intestinal obstruction has been alluded to above. It occurs in premature infants, when it may be associated with immaturity of the ganglion cells and reflex arcs. It may also occur following traumatic deliveries in association with neonatal asphyxia, and occasionally for no obvious reason. The clinical features are those of subacute obstruction of the bowel. The baby fails to pass meconium in the first 24 hours of life. Plain films of the abdomen show uniform dilatation of the bowel with gas in the rectum and an absence of fluid levels. Complete recovery is the rule, and the only treatment required is withdrawal of feeds for a short period followed by their gradual resumption.

REFERENCES

Abrams J S 1968 Experimental intestinal atresia. Surgery 64: 185–191
Alaroutu H 1956 The histopathologic changes in the myenteric plexus of the pylorus in hypertrophic pyloric stenosis in infants. Acta Paediatrica 45: Supplement 107
Anderson K D, Randolph J G 1973 The gastric tube for esophageal replacement. Journal of Thoracic and Cardiovascular Surgery 66: 333–342
Barlow B, Santulli T V, Heird W C et al 1974 An experimental study of acute necrotizing enterocolitis; the importance of breast milk. Journal of Pediatric Surgery 9: 587–595
Barnard C N, Louw J H 1956 The genesis of intestinal atresia. Minnesota Medicine 39:745
Beardmore H E, Wiglesworth F W 1958 Vertebral anomalies and alimentary duplications. Pediatric Clinics of North America 5: 457–474
Belding H H, Kernohan J W 1953 A morphology study of the myenteric plexus and the musculature of the pylorus with special reference to changes in hypertrophic pyloric stenosis. Surgery, Gynecology and Obstetrics 97: 323–343
Berdon W E, Baker D H 1965 The roentgenographic diagnosis of Hirschsprung's disease in infancy. American Journal of Roentgenology 93: 432–446
Bill A M, Grauman D 1966 Rationale and technique for stabilization of the mesentery in cases of non rotation of the midgut. Journal of Pediatric Surgery 1: 127–132
Bishop H C, Koop C E 1957 Management of meconium ileus: Resection, Roux-en-Y anastomosis and ileostomy irrigation with pancreatic enzymes. Annals of Surgery 145: 410–414
Bland-Sutton J 1889 Imperforate ileum. American Journal of the Medical Sciences 98: 457–462
Boyden E A, Cope J G, Bill A H 1967 Anatomy and embryology of congenital intrinsic obstruction of the duodenum. American Journal of Surgery 114: 190–202
Bremer J L 1944 Diverticula and duplications of the intestinal tract. Archives of Pathology 38: 132–140
Brennon W S, Bill A H 1974 Prophylactic fixation of the intestine for midgut non-rotation. Surgery, Gynecology and Obstetrics 138: 181–184
Brereton R J, Zachary R B, Spitz L 1978 Preventable death in oesophageal atresia. Archives of Diseases in Childhood 53: 276–283
Cantrell J R, Haller J A and Ravitch M M 1958. A syndrome of congenital defects involving the abdominal wall, sternum, pericardium and heart. Surgery, Gynecology and Obstetrics. 107: 602–614
Carter C O, Evans K A 1969 Inheritance of congenital pyloric stenosis. Journal of Medical Genetics 6: 233–254

Clatworthy H W Jr et al 1956 The meconium plug syndrome. Surgery 39:131
Cook R M C, Rickham P P 1969 Neonatal intestinal obstruction due to milk curds. Journal of Pediatric Surgery 4: 599–605
Courtois B 1959 Les origines foetales des occlusions congénitales du grêle dites par atrésie. Journal de Chirurgie 78: 405–426
Davis W S, Allen R P, Favara B E 1974 Neonatal small left colon syndrome. American Journal of Roentgenology 120:322
de Vries P A, Pena A 1982 Posterior sagittal anorectoplasty. Journal of Pediatric Surgery 17: 638–634
Dodge J A 1970 Production of duodenal ulcers and hypertrophic pyloric stenosis by administration of pentogastrin to pregnant and newborn dogs. Nature 225: 284–285
Dodge J A 1974 A fresh-look at pyloric stenosis. In: Apley J (ed) Modern Trends in Paediatrics 4. Butterworth, London. pp 229–254
Duhamel B 1960 A new operation for the treatment of Hirschsprung's disease. Archives of Diseases in Childhood 35: 38–39
Ellis D G, Clatworthy H W Jr 1966 The meconium plug syndrome revisited. Journal of Pediatric Surgery 1: 54–61
Fallon M, Gordon A R G, Lendrum A C 1954 Mediastinal cysts of foregut origin associated with vertebral abnormalities. British Journal of Surgery 41: 520–533
Fonkalsrud E W, De Lorimier A A, Hays D M 1969 Congenital atresia and stenosis of the duodenum. Pediatrics 43: 79–83
Friesen S R, Boley J A, Miller D R 1956. The myenteric plexus of the pylorus. Its early normal development and its changes in hypertrophic pyloric stenosis. Surgery 39: 21–29
Hasse W 1976 Associated malformations with anal and rectal atresia. Progress in Pediatric Surgery 9: 99–103
Holder T M, Cloud D T, Lewis J E, Pilling G P 1964 Esophageal atresia and tracheoesophageal fistula. A survey of its members by the surgical section of the American Academy of Pediatrics. Pediatrics 34: 542–549
Holschneider A M (ed) 1982 Hirschsprung's Disease. Hippokrates Verlag, Stuttgart
Howat J M, Wilkinson A W 1970 Functional intestinal obstruction in the neonate. Archives of Disease in Childhood 45: 800–804
Irving I M 1967 Exomphalos with macroglossia: a study of eleven cases. Journal of Pediatric Surgery 2: 499–507
Kiesewetter W B 1967 Imperforate anus II. The rationale and technique of the sacro-abdomino-perineal operation. Journal of Pediatric Surgery 2: 106–117
Klein A, Cremin B S 1970 Racial significance in pyloric stenosis. South Africa Medical Journal 44:1131
Kliegman R M, Hack K, Zones P et al 1982 Epidemiologic study of necrotizing enterocolitis among low-birth-weight infants. Journal of Pediatrics 100: 440–444
Kosloske A M, Papile L A, Burnstein J 1980 Indications for operation in acute necrotizing enterocolitis of the neonate. Surgery 87: 502–508
Lake B D, Puri P, Nixon H H, Claireaux A E 1978 Hirshsprung's Disease. An appraisal of histochemically demonstrated acetyl cholinesterase activity in suction rectal biopsies as an aid to diagnosis. Archives of Pathology 102: 244–247
Lehmann W 1931 Nevere Anschauungen uber die sog. Kongenitale Pylorusstenose. Zeitschrift fur Kinderheilkunde 50: 691–704
Lewis F T, Thyng F W 1907 The regular occurrence of intestinal diverticula in embryos of the pig, rabbit and man. American Journal of Anatomy 7: 505–519
Lillie, J G, Chrispin A R 1972 Investigations and management of neonatal obstruction by gastrografin enema. Annals of Radiology 15:237
Lloyd J R 1969 The etiology of gastrointestinal perforations in the newborn. Journal of Pediatric Surgery 4: 77–84
Louw J H 1966 Jejunoileal atresia and stenosis. Journal of Pediatric Surgery 1: 8–23
Lynn H B 1960 The mechanism of pyloric stenosis and its relationship to preoperative preparation. Archives of Surgery 81: 453–459
Lynn H 1966 Rectal myectomy for aganglionic megacolon. Mayo Clinic Proceedings 41:289
Meier-Ruge W, Lutterbeck P M, Herzog B et al 1972 Acetylcholinesterase activity in suction biopsies of the rectum in the diagnosis of Hirschsprung's disease. Journal of Pediatric Surgery 7: 11–20

Mollard P, Marechal J M, Jaubert de Beaujeu et al 1978 Surgical treatment of high imperforate anus with definition of the puborectalis sling by an anterior perineal approach. Journal of Pediatric Surgery 13: 499–504

Myers N A 1979 Oesophageal atresia and/or tracheooesophageal fistula — A study of mortality. Progress in Pediatric Surgery 13: 141–165

Noblett H R 1969(a) Treatment of uncomplicated meconium ileus by Gastrografin enema: A preliminary report. Journal of Pediatric Surgery 4: 190–197

Noblett H R 1969(b) Rectal suction biopsy in the diagnosis of Hirschsprung's disease. Journal of Pediatric Surgery 4: 406–409

Philippart A I, Reed J O, Georgeson K E 1975 Neonatal small left colon syndrome: intramural not intraluminal obstruction. Journal of Pediatric Surgery 10: 733–740

Rehbein F 1958 Intraabdominelle Resektion oder Rektosigmoidektomie bei der Hirschsprung'schen Krankheit. Chirurg 29: 366–369

Rehbein F 1959 Operation for anal and rectal atresia with rectourethral fistula. Chirurg 30: 417–418

Rehbein F, Schweder N 1971 Reconstruction of esophagus without colon transplantation in cases of atresia. Journal of Pediatric Surgery 6: 746–752

Rickham P P 1955 Peritonitis in the neonatal period. Archives of Diseases In Childhood 30: 23–31

Rickham P P, Boeckman C R 1965 Neonatal meconium obstruction in the absence of mucoviscidosis. American Journal of Surgery 109:173

Rickham P P, Stauffer U G, Cheng S K 1977 Oesophageal atresia: triumph and tragedy. Australian and New Zealand Journal of Surgery 47: 138–143

Robarts F H 1968 Neonatal perforation of the stomach. Zeitschrift fur Kinderchirurgie, Suppl. Zu Bd, 5:62

Rodgers I M, Drainer I K, Moore M R, Buchanan K D 1975 Plasma gastrin in congenital hypertrophic pyloric stenosis. A hypothesis disproved. Archives of Diseases in Childhood 50: 467–471

Santulli T V, Blanc W A 1961 Congenital atresia of the intestine: Pathogenesis and treatment. Annals of Surgery 154: 939–948

Santulli T V, Kieswetter W B, Bill A H 1970 Anorectal anomalies; a suggested international classification. Journal of Pediatric Surgery 5: 281–287

Singleton E B 1963 Radiologic evaluation of intestinal obstruction in the newborn. Radiologic Clinics of North America 1: 571–580

Soave F 1966 Hirschsprung's disease: Technique and results of Soave's operation. British Journal of Surgery 53: 1023–1027

Spicer R D 1982 Infantile hypertrophic pyloric stenosis: a review. British Journal of Surgery 69: 128–135

Spitz L 1979 Vomiting after pyloromyotomy for infantile hypertrophic pyloric stenosis. Archives of Diseases in Childhood 54: 886–889

Spitz L 1984 Gastric transposition via the mediastinal route for infants with long-gap esophageal atresia. Journal of Pediatric Surgery 19: 149–154

Spitz L, Batcup G 1979 Haematemesis in infantile hypertrophic pyloric stenosis: the source of the bleeding. British Journal of Surgery 66: 827–828

Spitz L, Kaufman J C E 1975 The neuropathological changes in congenital hypertrophic pyloric stenosis. South Africa Journal of Surgery 13: 239–242

Spitz L, Zail S S 1976 Serum gastrin levels in congenital hypertrophic pyloric stenosis. Journal of Pediatric Surgery 11: 33–35

Stephens F D 1953 Imperforate rectum. A new surgical technique. Medical Journal of Australia 1: 202–203

Stephens F D, Smith E D 1971 Anorectal malformations in Children. Year Book Medical Publishers Chicago

Stewart D R, Colodny A L, Daggett W C 1976 Malrotation of the bowel in infants and children: a 15-year review. Surgery 79: 716–720

Swenson O, Bill A H 1948 Resection of rectum and rectosigmoid with preservation of sphincter for benign spastic lesions producing megacolon. Surgery 24: 212–220

Tandler J 1900 Zur Entwicklungsgeschichte des menschlichen Duodenum in fruhen Embryonalstadien. Morphologie Jahrb 29: 187–189

Tawes R, Nixon H H 1971 Etiology and treatment of small intestinal atresia: analysis of a series of 127 jejuno-ileal atresias and comparison with 62 duodenal atresias. Surgery 69: 41–51

Thomas D F M 1982 Pathogenesis of neonatal necrotizing enterocolitis. Journal of the Royal Society of Medicine 75: 838–840

Thomas D F M, Fernie D, Malone M, Bayston R, Spitz L 1982 Association between Clostridium Difficile and Enterocolitis in Hirschsprung's Disease. Lancet i: 78–79

Touloukian R J, Posch J N, Spencer R 1972 The pathogenesis in ischemic gastroenterocolitis of the neonate: Selective gut mucosal ischemia in asphyxiated neonatal piglets. Journal of Pediatric Surgery 7: 194–205

Wagensteen O H, Rice C O 1930 Imperforate Anus. A method of determining the surgical approach. Annals of Surgery 92: 77–81

Waterston D J 1969 Reconstruction of the esophagus. In: Mustard W T, Ravitch M M, Snyder W H, Welch K J, Benson C D (eds) Pediatric Surgery (ed 2) Year Book Medical Publishers, Chicago. 400–408

Wilmore D W 1972 Factors correlating with a successful outcome following extensive intestinal resection in newborn infants. Journal of Pediatrics 30:88

Surgical conditions in the infant and older child

The multiplicity and protean nature of the gastrointestinal disorders which require surgical treatment in infancy and later childhood prevent a clinically useful classification. Common problems will be considered in an order related to their frequency, followed by rarer associated conditions, concluding with a short discussion of causes of signs and symptoms. Many babies treated in the neonatal period may require further operations in infancy and childhood, e.g. late reconstructions of anorectal anomalies, repairs of pelvic floor musculature, and later surgery for Hirschsprung's disease: these are not discussed in this chapter.

Appendicitis

Acute appendicitis is the commonest surgical emergency affecting the abdomen and must always be considered in the differential diagnosis of any child presenting with sudden abdominal pain (Brown 1956). Although commonest in the older child and young adult, appendicitis occurs at all ages from the first few weeks of life to extreme old age: it is least common and most lethal at the extremes of life. Excluding the first few weeks of life when most reported cases were probably necrotizing enterocolitis, no child is too young to have appendicitis.

Aetiology and pathology

Studies in the experimental animal have demonstrated that obstruction with secondary infection results in acute inflammation of the appendix (Wagensteen & Bowers 1937). In man, obstruction appears to be the most important factor in the genesis of progressive disease. Obstruction, with the resultant increase in intraluminal pressure interferes with venous flow, leading to a mucosal breakdown, thrombosis, haemorrhage and oedema, and bacterial invasion of the wall of the appendix. Faecoliths, adhesions, lymphoid hyperplasia and strictures have all been implicated as causes of obstruction. Mucosal ulceration may be caused by viral infections and followed by secondary bacterial infection (Weiland 1977). The varying prevalence in different parts of the world suggests that both ethnic and dietary factors are important.

The pathological stages are the same at all ages. Acute inflammation progresses to a closed loop obstruction with transmural infection of the wall of the appendix, followed by necrosis and perforation. In the older child the omemtum envelops the appendix; in the younger child the omentum is short and tenuous, but the appendix is frequently in a retrocaecal, and therefore naturally walled-off, position. Even a free appendix may be sealed off from the general peritoneal cavity by the adherence of loops of bowel. An appendix abscess usually takes a few days to develop from the onset of symptoms. Only in their faster progression do the symptoms and signs in the younger child differ from those in the older.

Clinical features and diagnosis

The triad of abdominal pain, vomiting, and a low grade fever, with associated tenderness and guarding in the right iliac fossa are the typical clinical features of appendicitis in the older child. In the younger patient, particularly those under the age of 2 years, the presenting features of fever, vomiting, and crying are less specific and the correct diagnosis is often delayed.

In the early stages, body temperature is seldom raised above 38°C, but it increases rapidly with the onset of peritonitis; in younger children, especially the under fives, higher temperatures are seen in the early stages. The most helpful symptoms are central abdominal pain moving to the right iliac fossa, and pain on coughing and movement.

The most important signs are persistent tenderness and guarding over the appendix in the right iliac fossa. Rebound tenderness is unkind and not a helpful sign in childhood. Similarly, rectal examination is often unhelpful for children under the age of 5 years; in the older child, particularly when diarrhoea is a feature, rectal examination, looking for tenderness or bulging of the anterior rectal wall, is essential in the diagnosis of pelvic appendicitis. A tender mass in the right iliac fossa, or one arising from the pelvis, suggests an appendix abscess.

Differential diagnosis

In the early stages of the disease it can be difficult to distinguish appendicitis from simple colic but a short period of careful clinical observation usually resolves the dilemma.

A diagnosis of appendicitis should be suspected in any child with abdominal pain, but the list of differential diagnoses is formidable. Among the conditions which should be considered are simple colic, possibly related to dietary indiscretions or constipation, mesenteric adenitis, abdominal migraine, viral or bacterial infections of the bowel, urinary tract infections, intussusception, right sided basal pneumonia, torsion of an ovarian cyst or of a testis, occult abdominal trauma, primary peritonitis, infective hepatitis, deep iliac adenitis and, less frequently, discitis, diabetes mellitus, porphyria, and the Henoch–Schonlein syndrome. In children of ethnic groups among whom sickle-cell disease is prevalent (e.g. those of West African origin), abdominal pain may result from small infarcts in the bowel wall and is best treated conservatively. Appendicitis in these children may be complicated by progressive sickling and thrombosis in the mesentery of the terminal ileum and ascending colon.

Appendicitis is also seen in association with upper respiratory infections and with measles.

Management, complications and prognosis

In the early or uncomplicated case, appendicectomy is simple and satisfactory. After perforation, however, with local or generalized peritonitis, intravenous correction of fluid and electrolyte losses and control of the infection by antibiotics, should precede removal of the appendix. There is no clear evidence which antibiotics are best. Most frequently the organisms are those normally found in the large bowel, and antibiotics to which these are sensitive are generally used. These agents include ampicillin, second and third generation cephalosporins, and aminoglycosides — particularly gentamicin — in a variety of combinations. An appreciable proportion of intra-abdominal infections following perforation of the appendix are caused by nonsporing anaerobes, particularly by strains of bacteriodes. Metronidazole is effective in the prevention and treatment of bacteriodes infections; therapeutically effective serum levels are achieved when the drug is administered rectally as a suppository and its use is therefore logical (Othersen et al 1976, Willis et al 1976).

An appendix abscess should usually be drained surgically, and the appendix removed during the operation only if this can be achieved without disseminating the infection.

Conservative management is rarely indicated in children, in whom the infection progresses rapidly and unpredictably. However, a child with a history of longer than two days, who has a palpable, clearly defined mass, and who is definitely improving, should probably be treated conservatively with antibiotics and a fluid diet. Any child who requires intravenous fluids and gastric suction probably also requires an operation (Shipsey & O'Donnell 1985).

Whether an appendix abscess is treated conservatively or by surgical drainage, an appendicectomy should be performed after about six to eight weeks, since recurrent appendicitis is common.

Complications include abscess formation in the wound, the right and left iliac fossae, the pelvis, and in the subphrenic spaces. Intestinal obstruction secondary to sepsis may be an early complication or may develop later, secondary to adhesions. Incisional hernias are rare.

The overall mortality rate in appendicitis is less than 1%, and most deaths are secondary to infection or to problems in fluid management following delayed diagnosis (Pledger & Buchan 1969).

Carcinoid syndrome. Very rarely in children a carcinoid tumour will be found in an appendix removed for suspected appendicitis (Andersson & Bergdahl 1977). These tumours have the same low potential to metastasize as they do in adults, but the full caroinoid syndrome with diarrhoea, tachycardia, and flushing is very rare in children. The biochemical marker of metastatic carcinoids is the increased urinary output of 5-hydroxyindoleacetic acid (King et al 1985).

Intussusception

An intussusception is an invagination of a segment of bowel into an adjoining lower segment. This is usually followed by distal progression. It is an uncommon condition with an incidence of between one and two cases per 1000 live births. In the commonest form, the idiopathic intussusception of childhood, the apex and origin of the intussusception is usually in the terminal ileum or at the ileocaecal valve (Dennison & Shaker 1970, Raudkivi & Smith 1981)

Aetiology and pathology

Children between the ages of 3 months and 2 years are most frequently affected, with a peak incidence between 6 and 9 months. An obvious precipitating cause (e.g. Meckel's diverticulum, ileal polyp, or an enteric cyst) is present in only 2% of all affected patients. Although one of these lesions is more likely to be present in children over the age of 2 years, the idiopathic form is still the most common. Antenatal intussusceptions are among the causes of small bowel atresia. A seasonal incidence with peaks related to winter upper respiratory tract infections and summer enteritis, combined with a frequent association with mesenteric adenitis, suggests the possibility of a viral aetiology: there is some supportive evidence for this theory (Bell & Steyn 1962). The occurrence of intussusception in the Henoch-Schonlein syndrome, and following abdominal surgery, particularly after retroperitoneal dissection, suggests that disordered peristalsis may be important.

The intussuscepted bowel progresses round the colon, and if the diagnosis is delayed, it can reach and prolapse from the rectum. Strangulation of the gut and irreducibility of the intussusception are most likely when the apex is in the narrow small bowel. In tropical countries, particularly Africa, a form of intussusception in which the apex is in the anterior wall of the caecum is seen at all ages; strangulation and irreducibility are much less likely in this form (Olumide et al 1976).

Clinical features and diagnosis

The signs and symptoms are closely related to the progression of the disease. Initially these are colic and vomiting. The spasms of pain are associated with pallor which persists between them, and the child remains restless and irritable. After a normal stool the typical redcurrant jelly stool consisting of blood and mucus is passed in 30–50%. Later the abdomen becomes distended and the vomiting copious and bilestained. Dehydration and infection spreading through the bowel wall lead to fever and tachycardia. On examining the abdomen, the characteristic finding is a sausage-shaped mass with its curve and position following the line of the gut from the ascending colon round to the sigmoid colon. Any of the typical clinical features may be missing. The onset of vomiting may be delayed, colic is occasionally absent, and an abdominal mass may not be palpable because it lies behind the liver, muscle-guarding, or distended loops of small bowel.

Erect and supine plain films of the abdomen are very helpful in confirming the diagnosis. The caecal gas shadow is absent, and dilated loops of small bowel often lead to the site of the intussusception, which may appear as a soft tissue mass with a crescent of gas outlining its distal margin. If there is any clinical doubt a barium enema will outline the mass in the bowel lumen.

Management and prognosis

An intussusception is an acute surgical emergency: as in appendicitis most deaths are related to dehydration and infection, and when necessary these must be treated prior to any surgery.

The place of a therapeutic barium enema to reduce the intussusception, which can be successful in 50–75% of cases, is controversial. In many parts of the world this is the initial treatment of choice, whereas in the United Kingdom most centres prefer the speed and certainty of surgical reduction. When there is a history of less than 24 hours in a child who is in good condition, or when an enema is required for diagnosis, an attempt at reduction is safe and reasonable. Free reflux of barium into the terminal loop of the small bowel is the essential sign of successful reduction, and in its absence the abdomen should usually be explored. In the author's experience, if the criteria for safe barium enema reduction are met, performing the procedure under general anaesthesia makes it both simpler and more reliable. If the reduction fails, an immediate transfer to theatre under the same anaesthetic is necessary. Operative reduction is most easily performed through a transverse supraumbilical incision with most of the procedure under direct vision. There is often a sudden increase in pulse rate and a fall in blood pressure immediately following the reduction. If this happens, it is best treated by an infusion of blood or plasma. An irreducible intussusception should be resected through healthy gut and an end-to-end anastomosis performed. In uncomplicated cases with a healthy caecal wall, there is no contraindication to appendicectomy (Levick 1970).

Recurrences happen in about 5% of cases after both operative and barium enema reduction. The mortality rate is about 1%; deaths are usually associated with delay in diagnosis and treatment.

Remnants of the vitellointestinal duct

During early intrauterine development the vitellointestinal duct leads from the midpoint of the primitive gut through the umbilicus to the yolk sac. Normally it atrophies and disappears completely, but remnants persist in about 2% of individuals. Most commonly this is at the ileal end, as a Meckel's diverticulum. Persistence of the umbilical end produces a small everted umbilical polyp which is covered by mucosa; of the midportion an umbilical cyst; and of the whole tract a vitellointestinal fistula. Occasionally incomplete atrophy leaves a fibrous cord attaching the ileum to the umbilicus. This cord may form the apex for a volvulus or the trapping band for an internal hernia. An umbilical polyp can be distinguished from the more common umbilical granuloma by its velvety secreting surface which may cause excoriation of adjacent skin. Both lesions are treated by simple diathermy excision. A patent vitellointestinal duct allows bowel content to escape at the umbilicus; the duct is often associated with narrowing of the ileum at its base. Rarely, but dramatically, gut may intussuscept through the umbilicus. Excision of the duct and correction of any ileal narrowing is simple and effective. The rare cyst formed by persistence of the middle section of the duct presents either as an infected abscess or a symptomless mass behind the umbilicus. It should be excised.

Meckel's diverticulum

A Meckel's diverticulum arises from the antimesenteric border of the gut 40–60 cm from the ileal caecal valve, and is usually symptomless. It can contain pancreatic tissue or acid-secreting gastric mucosa; if the latter is present, there is a risk of peptic ulceration at the junction of the diverticulum with the normal ileum. The commonest presenting feature of this is painless bleeding, often exsanguinating, in the first two years of life. Perforation of the ulcer is uncommon. A Meckel's diverticulum must be suspected in any young child with severe rectal bleeding. The diagnosis is difficult to confirm using conventional contrast radiology, although it may be outlined by a small bowel barium enema. The acid-secreting mucosa takes up pertechnetate and this can be identified in about 70% of cases as a 'hot spot' on a technetium scan using Tc 99 as pertechnetate (Jewett et al 1970). The frequency of false negative results with this technique raises some doubts as to its value.

Surgical treatment involves excision of the diverticulum together with a segment of ileum, to include the ulcer. An inverted diverticulum may form the apex of an intussusception and must be excised following reduction.

Diverticulitis of these usually wide-necked diverticula is uncommon and clinically indistinguishable from appendicitis. The diverticulum is easily found and removed through a standard appendicectomy incision. It is usual to excise a Meckel's diverticulum found incidentally at laparotomy in order to prevent later complications, but in a wide-necked diverticulum with no thickening or other visible abnormality in the wall this is probably not essential, and the operation may carry more risks than leaving well alone.

Hiatus hernia and gastro-oesophageal reflux

The oesophagogastric junction, the lower oesophageal sphincter and oeso-phageal vestibule should all lie in the abdomen, with the lower oesophagus held to the right crus of the diaphragm by the phreno-oesophageal liga-ments. Two types of hernia occur at the hiatus. With the paraoesophageal or rolling hernia, which is rare in children, the fundus of the stomach rolls into the peritoneal sac protruding through an enlarged hiatus. The common hernia is the sliding hernia in which the oesophagogastric junction is displaced into the chest. Gastro-oesophageal reflux is usually associated with a sliding hernia but can occur without any demonstrable evidence of herniation, particularly in infants. Reflux and herniation are not synony-mous, but most frequently occur together (Carré 1959, Winter & Grand 1981).

In the newborn infant, the pressure developed in the lower oesophagus (sphincter zone) is lower relatively as well as absolutely than in adults. Maturation to the adult pattern should start around the third month of life. Gastric acid secretion is high at birth, then falls, and starts rising again also after the third month. Reflux occurs easily but, presumably because of the lower acidity of the stomach contents, it is less damaging to the oesophageal mucosa. This complex pattern of development explains the ease with which small babies can be 'burped', the frequency of posseting (regurgitation of small amounts of curdled feed), and the more severe persistent vomiting, which usually stops spontaneously towards the end of the first year of life. Reflux is least likely to occur when the baby lies prone. The sliding hernias associated with severe vomiting have been given several names; chalasia of the cardia, congenital short oesophagus, and partial thoracic stomach as well as hiatus hernia. The essential problem is the reflux, and most of the other features are secondary effects (Balistreri & Farrell 1983).

Clinical features, diagnosis and prognosis

The outstanding symptom is regurgitation and/or vomiting starting in the first week of life, occurring after and between feeds. The vomit does not contain bile but may be bloodstained. At this age the differential diagnosis rests between hiatus hernia, hypertrophic pyloric stenosis, simple feeding mismanagement, and infection. Minor degrees of reflux recover spontaneously, and in the majority of infants the vomiting resolves by 12 months of age. More severe reflux can be associated with failure to thrive, aspiration of gastric contents with chronic recurrent pulmonary infection, ulceration of the lower oesophagus leading to acute or chronic bleeding, dysphagia from spasm and finally stricture formation. It is also likely that excessive crying, irritability and sleep disturbance are caused by reflux (Carré 1984).

Associated lesions. There is a clear association between hiatus hernia and congenital hypertrophic pyloric stenosis. Following repair of an oesophageal atresia, the oesophagus may be short with reflux increasing the risk of stricture formation at the anastomosis, as well as in the usual position in the distal oesophagus. Reflux is common in severely mentally retarded children in whom it must be distinguished from rumination (Sondheimer & Morriss 1979). Occasionally reflux presents in the older child with symptoms similar to those seen in adults — heartburn and dysphagia, particularly on stooping or bending. More rarely abnormal postures and torsion dystonia of the neck will be the presenting symptom (Sutcliffe 1969).

Investigation. The available techniques are barium swallow and meal, ultrasound, oesophagoscopy and biopsy, pH testing short and long duration (18 or 24 hours), manometry, scintiscanning with a Tc^{99} sulphur colloid labelled meal, and 'string tests'. The tests used in any centre will depend on what is available. A barium swallow is essential to study the mechanism of swallowing, look for the presence of spasm or stricture in the lower oesophagus, and study the stomach, pylorus and duodenum. There is now agreement that the signs of herniation are different from those in adults. The most important features are the positions of the oesophageal vestibule and lower sphincter. It is debatable as to what lengths should be taken to provoke reflux. Ultrasound examination, which is noninvasive, can demonstrate fluid reflux in children even when a barium study has failed to show it. Oesophagoscopy — preferably with flexible fibre optic instrument — also allows examination of the stomach, pylorus and first part of the duodenum, differentiates stricture from spasm and reveals oesophagitis better than barium. Biopsy of the lower oesophagus should be routine. Of the pH studies, when these are available, the 18–24 hour study produces the most physiological assessment of what is happening in the lower oesophagus. Manometric studies have produced important evidence for the understanding of reflux. Scintiscanning, with a labelled milk feed, is also a physiological test, but requires prolonged access to a gamma camera, as pictures may need to be taken for up to 4 or 5 hours.

In the string tests, a thread protected by a feeding tube is passed and then methylene blue is instilled into the stomach through a nasogastric tube. The extent of dye-staining of the string gives an index of how far up the oesophagus the reflux extends. This is a cheap and simple test, but does not indicate the acidity, frequency, or duration of the reflux (Arasu et al 1980).

Management

The initial approach to a baby who is thriving, and has no evidence of oesophagitis or recurrent chest infection, should be reassurance. Investigations are reserved for those babies with severe vomiting, failure to thrive, recurrent chest infection, haematemesis, possibly severe sleep disturbance, and certainly dysphagia, suggesting early stricture formation. For those with minor symptoms, thickening the feeds and mild antacids are helpful. In babies under the age of 6 months alginate plus antacid (Gaviscon®) should not be used, because of its high sodium content.

Posture. It has been traditional to maintain babies with symptomatic reflux in an infant hernia seat with the back angled at 60° to the horizontal. Most clinicians have been satisfied that this is effective, but it has been shown that if the aim is to ensure that the oesophagus opens into the gastric air-bubble, this is more easily achieved by nursing the infant prone (Orenstein & Whitington 1983). Otherwise the infant must be kept bolt upright, a position which in small babies is neither practical nor safe. For the less severe degrees of reflux it seems reasonable to continue to recommend the sitting position at 60° from 1–1½ hours after feeds and that the child should sleep prone at night. In the more severe cases, nursing on a special frame prone at 60° may be helpful. H_2 antagonists (cimetidine and ranitidine) reduce the gastric acid output and may speed the healing of the oesophagitis.

Surgery is only indicated for those infants in whom medical measures fail to control the reflux and who fail to thrive, become anaemic, or develop a stricture (Fonkalsrud et al 1985). In infants under the age of 12 months, gastropexy, provided it produces an adequate length of oesophagus within the abdominal cavity combined with tightening of the hiatus, is a simple and effective procedure for reflux in the absence of stenosis. It is, however, more usual to treat all ages the same by using the Nissen fundoplication, or Belsey Mark IV operation, in which, after mobilization to ensure an adequate length of oesophagus within the abdomen, the body of the stomach is wrapped around and sutured in front of the oesophagus. For routine cases, the abdominal approach is satisfactory but where there is severe stricturing or shortening of the oesophagus, thoracotomy, which permits better mobilization, is preferable. At the time of operation the pylorus should be inspected, and, if it is narrowed, a pyloroplasty or pyloromyotomy should be performed. These procedures carry a risk of 'dumping', which has been reported following the Nissen operation, even without any procedure on the pylorus (Johnson et al 1977).

Caustic strictures of the oesophagus

The accidental ingestion of corrosives (most commonly liquid caustic soda preparations) causes ulceration of the mouth, and extensive destruction of the oesophagus, stomach and duodenum, frequently progressing to oesophageal stricture. Spillover into the upper respiratory tract may lead to scarring and strictures in and around the larynx. Emergency treatment includes systemic steroids and antibiotics to reduce scarring and infection. Early oesophagoscopy is essential to assess the damage, and the passage of a nasogastric tube, or stent, permits early feeding and should maintain a dilatable channel. If this fails, a feeding gastrostomy is required. Impenetrable strictures, after healing, must be excised and replaced by colon or stomach (Hawkins et al 1980).

Achalasia of the cardia

Achalasia of the cardia (cardiospasm) is due to failure of the lower end of the oesophagus to relax, and although primarily a disease of adult life, it does also occur in childhood. The typical clinical features are dysphagia, immediate regurgitation of food after eating, retrosternal discomfort relieved by the regurgitation, and weight loss.

The differential diagnosis is from oesophageal strictures and, in older children, anorexia nervosa. The appearances on a barium swallow are diagnostic; the oesophagus is dilated, terminating in a distal 'rat tail' through which barium passes slowly into the stomach. Oesophageal manometry will confirm the disorder of motility, and identify the length of oesophagus involved. Treatment is either by balloon dilatation or Heller's oesophageal myotomy. Immediate results are excellent but gastro-oesophageal reflux has led to later stricture formation. To prevent this, some surgeons include a Nissen fundoplication in the operation (Buick & Spitz 1985).

Apud (amine precursor uptake and decarboxylation) tumours

See Zollinger–Ellison syndrome on pages 124, 519–520.

Peptic ulcer

The incidence of peptic ulcer disease in childhood has not been clearly established. Fibreoptic endoscopy has increased the accuracy and certainty with which the diagnosis is made. (Curci et al 1976).

Clinical features and diagnosis

Acute ulcers. Acute gastric or duodenal ulcers occur in the neonatal period and infancy following acute stress in delivery, associated with neonatal asphyxia or severe respiratory distress. They can present with bleeding, perforation or obstruction.

In later childhood an acute peptic ulcer may also rarely occur following severe stress, as with severe burns (Curling's ulcer) or meningitis (Cushing's ulcer), or following the administration of corticosteroids. They are more likely to occur in children with previously proven ulcers or with conditions which are known to be associated with peptic ulceration (e.g. cirrhosis, chronic lung disease, and following small intestinal resection). These stress ulcers are equally distributed between the stomach and duodenum, and there is no sex predilection.

Severe bleeding with haematemesis or melaena is usually the presenting feature of acute stress ulcers irrespective of the age of the child. The bleeding does not often resolve with conservative measures and surgery may be necessary.

Where the risk of ulceration is high, prophylaxis with antacids or H_2 antagonists (cimetidine or ranitidine) is recommended. Surgical treatment is in a state of flux. Previously, emergency operation was often required: now a combination of suppression of acid secretion and endoscopic control of the bleeding point is a promising alternative.

Chronic ulcers. Chronic peptic ulcers are seen predominantly in children from school age upwards. The symptom of abdominal pain relieved by alkali, food or vomiting is similar to that seen in adults. There is frequently a strong family history of peptic ulcer disease. Males are affected more frequently than females (3:2), and duodenal ulcers are more common than gastric ulcers (8:1).

The diagnosis of acute or chronic peptic ulceration in childhood is based on the clinical features, radiology, and endoscopy. Barium studies should be interpreted by an experienced paediatric radiologist, since fear and anxiety may considerably influence the appearance of the duodenum. Gastric acid studies are of little help in diagnosis. Fibreoptic endoscopy, which is now simple to perform with the wide range of paediatric endoscopes available, is essential, and is the investigation of choice. Both the diagnosis of an ulcer and the rate of healing in response to treatment should be checked endoscopically (Tolia & Dubois 1983, Collins et al 1986).

Management. As in the adult type of peptic ulcer, medical treatment is aimed at neutralization of gastric acidity by food or antacid preparations. Frequent snacks are just as effective as antacids and easily become part of a child's routine. All the agents in use in adults can be given to children. H_2 antagonists (cimetidine, ranitidine and carbenoxolone) are the drugs of first choice. Other agents, pirenzepine and sucralfate, have still to be assessed. In very anxious patients a tranquilizer such as diazepam may be helpful. If the ulcer does not respond to medical treatment, surgery should be considered. Gastroenterostomy, partial gastrectomy and vagotomy with a drainage procedure have all been performed, but a highly selective vagotomy is probably the operation of choice.

The Zollinger–Ellison syndrome

The Zollinger–Ellison syndrome — a condition of intractable peptic ulceration due to gastric hypersecretion caused by a gastrinoma, has been described in children (Rosenlund 1967). The commonest, but not the only source for the gastrin is an adenoma (apudoma) of the pancreas, which may be benign (35%) or malignant. These tumours metastasize to lymph nodes and to the liver but only grow slowly. The condition should be suspected in older children who have multiple or post-bulbar ulcers, who develop recurrent ulcers after treatment, or who present with diarrhoea as well as peptic ulcer symptoms. Gastric secretion studies show an increased basal acid output close to maximal output (see Ch. 3 pages 64–66). The normal serum gastrin level range is 50–200 pg/ml fasting, and up to 600 pg/ml after a protein meal: in the Zollinger–Ellison syndrome levels range from 500–10 000 pg/ml. As the tumour may be one of the group seen in the Multiple Endocrine Adenomatosis syndrome, the rest of the endocrine system should be investigated. The primary tumours, though usually small, may be identified by computed tomography (CT) scanning; and liver metastases by CT scanning or ultrasound examination (Newsome 1974).

Management. An operation is required to look for the primary tumour and metastases and where possible the tumour and lymph nodes metastases are excised. The presence of hepatic metastases removes any prospect of a cure, but survival for many years can still be expected. If, following tumour resection, the serum gastrin level falls to normal, no further treatment is required, but the level should be kept under review as a further rise, indicating the presence of metastases, is common. The acid hypersecretion should be controlled by H_2 antagonists prior to operation. Total gastrectomy is only required for those patients who do not come under control, but can be undertaken with confidence as children of all ages thrive remarkably well after total gastrectomy (Wilson et al 1971).

Polyps

Gut polyps in children can be classified into three groups: a) the common benign juvenile polyps; b) the premalignant conditions of adenomatous polyp, familial adenomatous polyposis coli, and familial juvenile polyposis coli; and c) the eponymous syndromes with features in other systems, Peutz–Jeghers syndrome, Gardner's syndrome, Cronkhite Canada syndrome and Turcot syndrome.

Benign Juvenile Polyps. Juvenile polyps are benign hamartomatous smooth or lobulated lesions on a long stalk containing small mucus cysts, and are most frequently seen in the distal colon or rectum. They may be single or up to five may be scattered throughout the colon. They cause painless rectal bleeding separate from bowel action, prolapse from the anus, or much less often, lead to recurrent abdominal pain from intussusception. The flexible sigmoidoscope and paediatric colonoscope have revolutionized the management of these lesions. Flexible sigmoidoscopy can be safely performed without anaesthesia in nearly all children and the polyps removed by snare diathermy. Total colonoscopy is preferred. This, in the most skilled hands, can be performed under sedation: others prefer to have the children under a general anaesthetic. The polyp must be examined histologically to identify the rarer adenomatous polyps which require more careful obliteration of the base, and follow-up examination, as they are premalignant (Veale et al 1966).

Multiple juvenile polyps (more than five) suggest the familial juvenile polyposis syndrome in which the polyps are both juvenile and adenomatous, are more widely distributed in the gut, and are premalignant. For this condition, a colectomy, as for familial polyposis coli, is required (Sachatello et al 1970).

Familial polyposis coli. Familial polyposis coli is a rare disease with an incidence of about one in every 8 300 births; it is transmitted as an autosomal dominant. Multiple adenomatous polyps develop insidiously throughout the large intestine and, if left, invariably undergo malignant change. Symptoms rarely develop before the age of 10 years, although cases have been identified as early as 2 years of age and malignant changes have been reported by the age of 13 years (Calabro 1962).

The children of affected parents, who have a 50% chance of inheriting the disease, should be colonoscoped every six to 12 months from the age of 5 years into early adult life. The early lesions are small and may be missed, but progress eventually to the easily recognized colon carpeted with small adenomatous tumours. The symptons in new cases are diarrhoea with the passage of blood and mucus. In these, a barium enema is a reasonable first investigation, but the diagnosis should be confirmed by colonoscopy and biopsy.

It is now clear that this syndrome also includes children with polyps throughout the gastrointestinal tract. Because of the malignant potential of the polyps, a total colectomy is required. It is not yet clear whether an ileorectal anastomosis with 6-monthly clearing of the rectum, or the mucosal stripping operation with an endorectal anastomosis (possibly including an ileal pouch, triple (Parks), double or quadruple) is the best form of treatment (Parks et al 1980). There is much to commend the security of the complete mucosal strip.

The Peutz–Jeghers syndrome. The Peutz–Jeghers syndrome is less common than familial polyposis. The clinical features are characterized by mucocutaneous pigmentation of the lips, face and fingers, and the polyps are distributed throughout the gastrointestinal tract. The polyps are usually benign although malignant change has been recorded. The condition is inherited as an autosomal dominant. Treatment is chiefly supportive, surgery being reserved for the relief of complications, since excision of all the polyps is seldom possible (Dormandy 1957).

In Gardner's syndrome, adenomatous polyps are found in association with osteomas of the skull and mandible, epidermoid cysts, and skin tumours. The polyps are found throughout the gut.

In the Cronkhite–Canada syndrome polyps are found throughout the gut and there is an association with atrophy of the nails and skin pigmentation.

In Turcot's syndrome, colonic polyps are found in association with central nervous system (CNS) tumours.

Anal lesions

Anal fissure

Anal fissures are common lesions in childhood, particularly in infants and young children. In the infant fissures may be multiple and secondary to oedema and inflammation of the perianal skin, as well as to passage of hard stools. Treatment should be directed to the underlying cause (e.g. ammoniacal dermatitis or candidiasis).

In the older child fissures nearly always result from the passage of hard stools. The fissure is a mucosal split which may be associated with a sentinel pile from the tearing down of one of the anal valves. The lesion is initially very painful and accompanied by bleeding. This pain is usually of short duration, and problems chiefly arise from the pain of defaecation leading to a deliberate holding back of stool with further stretching of the fissure when it is passed. Crohn's disease should be considered in children with chronic recurrent fissures.

Most fissures heal spontaneously. Treatment is aimed at maintaining soft stools until the fissure has healed; topical anaesthetic creams, helpful in adults, are of little value, except in older children, since they must be applied immediately before the passage of a stool to be effective. Fissures which do not heal within a few weeks should be biopsied and examined histologically, and at the same time the anus should be dilated. Occasionally a subcutaneous internal sphincterotomy will be required for very resistant cases (Watts et al 1965). In unexplained or difficult cases the possibility of sexual abuse should be considered (Hobbs & Wynne 1986).

Perianal sepsis

Perianal abscess

Perianal abscesses are common and present with a painful swelling in the anal region. They arise from subcutaneous bleeding (the acute thrombotic pile), from cracks or fissures, or with no apparent precipitating cause. Early incision and unroofing of the abscess is essential to avoid extension and fistula formation. Abscesses also arise from infection in anal glands extending through the anal wall to form fistulae.

Ischiorectal abscesses are less common and require early incision and free drainage; occasionally these may be secondary to foreign bodies perforating the rectum or anal canal.

Fistula in ano

A fistula in ano can arise as described above or as a complication of Crohn's disease. Fistulae usually present as abscesses which recur after apparent healing following incision and drainage. Superficial fistulae are easily treated by excision and laying open of the track. Histological examination of the specimen for evidence of Crohn's disease is essential. High level fistulae with an internal opening above the puborectalis are more difficult to manage but are fortunately rare.

Rectal prolapse

Prolapse of the rectum may be due to herniation of the rectal wall in association with paralysis or defects of the pelvic floor muscles, as in children with spina bifida. The more usual prolapse is of the mucosal lining and is associated with chronic diarrhoea, as in cystic fibrosis, or with constipation. The first essential in treatment is correction of the underlying cause. Manual reduction of the prolapse is usually simple but recurrence with the next bowel action is common. Prolapses are most easily reduced immediately after they occur, and this is usually necessary with decreasing frequency. Occasionally, strapping together of the buttocks is necessary to maintain reduction of the prolapse. When these measures are unsuccessful, submucosal injection of phenol in almond oil, as for haemorrhoids in adults, is often effective. Only rarely should it be necessary to resort to a circumferential perianal stitch or a more complicated repair procedure.

Haemorrhoids

Internal haemorrhoids are rare in childhood and seldom require any treatment. They may not be apparent in patients examined under general anaesthesia, since they are best seen in the conscious child who is voluntarily straining during examination with an anal speculum.

Abdominal hernias

External abdominal hernias in children occur in the inguinal regions through a persistent processus vaginalis, at the umbilicus through an incompletely closed umbilical ring, through defects in the supraumbilical linea alba (i.e. supraumbilical and epigastric hernias), or down the femoral canal. Incisional hernias may be left following the repair of difficult diaphragmatic hernias and congenital umbilical defects, or may result from sepsis and faulty healing of abdominal wounds. Rare hernias, like gluteal and obturator hernias, are only diagnosed at laparotomy for intestinal obstruction. Direct inguinal hernias and false hernias secondary to muscle paralysis are rare and seldom seen apart from children with spina bifida. The importance of all hernias lies in the risk of irreducibility with obstruction and possible strangulation of loops of gut.

Inguinal hernia

Indirect inguinal hernias occur in 1% of children with a male to female ratio of 10:1. A swelling in the inguinal region and/or scrotum may be noticed at any age, and irreducible hernias are most likely at the time of their initial appearance or during the first six months of life. True strangulation with infarction of gut is rare, but pressure on the testicular vessels can result in thrombosis and infarction of the testis. There is usually no difficulty in identifying an inguinal hernia as the cause of an intestinal obstruction; small hernias may, however, be missed or the hernia may have spontaneously reduced before the child is seen, when the only clues will be thickening and oedema of the cord and oedema of the testis.

In the differential diagnosis, other inguinal swellings such as a communicating hydrocele, particularly when associated with ascites, a hydrocele of the cord, an undescended testis and enlarged lymph nodes, should be considered. When there is a history of recurrent inguinal swelling and there is no obvious hernia apparent at the time of examination, gentle rolling of the spermatic cord over the pubic bone will enable the experienced examiner to identify the presence of a sac. Girls with bilateral indirect inguinal hernias should have full chromosome studies to exclude the testicular feminization syndrome.

Management. Management depends on whether the hernia is irreducible or not. Strangulation rarely complicates a 'stuck' inguinal hernia, and surgery can be technically very difficult. Most hernias can be reduced following sedation of the child and nursing in a head down position; gentle manual pressure may be necessary to complete reduction. An elective herniotomy should be performed two days later. If these conservative measures fail to reduce the hernia, emergency surgery is necessary.

An elective herniotomy for children with reducible hernias is a simple procedure in all except very small babies. It should be performed as soon as possible following diagnosis to avoid the risks of irreducibility and strangulation.

Umbilical hernia

Umbilical hernias result from a circular defect at the umbilical cicatrix and are particularly common in negroid children. Strangulation and rupture of the sac can occur but is very rare. Most umbilical hernias remain asymptomatic and close spontaneously. Surgery is only very occasionally performed before the age of 5, and hardly ever before the age of 2 years. A short period of strapping, not exceeding six weeks, should be considered in infants less than 3 months of age who have repeated episodes of crying with swelling of the hernia. In the older child omentum may become trapped in an almost closed hernia causing obscure abdominal pain which is completely relieved by herniotomy.

Supraumbilical and epigastric hernias

These are usually merely protrusions of extraperitoneal fat through defects in the linea alba. A supraumbilical hernia is distinguished from a true umbilical hernia not by its relation to the umbilicus but by its elliptical or transverse slit shape. Both supraumbilical and epigastric hernias may cause pain as a result of trapping of their contents. Surgical repair is simple and relieves any symptoms.

Femoral hernia

Femoral hernias are occasionally seen in children. The swelling is below the inguinal ligament and lateral to the pubic tubercle.

Swallowed foreign bodies

Children have a notorious tendency to swallow foreign bodies of all types. Objects such as coins or pebbles may become lodged in the upper oesophagus, where they may cause dysphagia and, if left for any length of time, lead to ulceration and stricture formation; alternatively they may be held up at the site of an already existing stricture. A particular problem is the ring pull of aluminium drink cans, which in the upper oesophagus and may easily be missed on an X-ray (Levick & Spitz 1977). They must be removed as soon as possible under direct vision through an oesophagoscope. Most foreign bodies which reach the stomach will pass through the remaining gut spontaneously. With blunt objects, such as coins and marbles, considerable patience may be required. Sharp objects may arrest at any part of the gut and result in perforation; long objects may arrest in the tight bends of the duodenum and ulcerate through the bowel wall. If objects such as these have failed to progress over a period of 24 hours or the child develops abdominal pain and tenderness, surgical exploration and removal is indicated. A recently recognized problem is the mercury cell, which if not passed rapidly through the gut, opens to release metallic mercury and caustic potash. A mercury cell remaining in the stomach after 24 hours should be removed by endoscopy if possible (Litovitz 1985).

Most objects, even those not normally considered radio-opaque, are visible on a soft tissue X-ray of the abdomen and their progress can be easily followed. This is fortunate since seraching the stools for foreign bodies, though always recommended, is often unsuccessful.

Trichobezoar

This term refers to a collection of hair as a ball in the stomach and results from a child swallowing his own hair, and wool and fluff from garments and blankets. It is usually associated with underlying emotional upsets. The clinical features are abdominal pain, anorexia and a mobile mass in the epigastrium. A barium meal shows the barium to be trapped in the interstices of the hair ball. Laparotomy and gastrotomy are necessary to remove hair balls. The surgeon should beware of the tail which may extend a long way distally.

Abdominal trauma

This diagnosis is easy when there is a clear-cut history of a fall or a road traffic accident, but it may be more difficult in children who deny injuries incurred in forbidden activities or in young children with non-accidental injuries inflicted by adults. The most frequently affected organs are the spleen, kidneys, liver, gut and mesentery, and pancreas. Gut lesions include rupture and haematomata of the duodenum and tears of the mesentery. Rupture of a hollow viscus is rapidly followed by peritonitis, and rupture of solid organs is accompanied by the signs of acute blood loss.

Duodenal haematomas are caused by blunt trauma from falls, such as on to the back of a chair or over the handlebars of a bicycle. The clinical features are those of duodenal obstruction and barium studies show narrowing and obstruction usually in the second part of the duodenum. If the diagnosis is in doubt, a laparotomy should be performed and the haematoma evacuated. If the diagnosis is certain, most cases will recover spontaneously after a week to 10 days with conservative management.

Peritonitis

Peritonitis may be primary or secondary to another focus within the peritoneal cavity. Primary infections of the peritoneum, which are becoming increasingly less common, are due to the pneumococcus or streptococcus or occasionally viruses. Patients with the nephrotic syndrome, immune deficiency states, and pneumococcal pneumonia are particularly likely to develop primary peritonitis. Secondary peritonitis may complicate appendicitis, intussusception, Meckel's diverticulum, peptic ulcer and intra-abdominal surgery.

Clinically there is abdominal pain, distension, generalized tenderness and guarding, vomiting, and often diarrhoea; there is associated general malaise, a high fever and sometimes shock. The white cell count is strikingly increased from 20 to $50 \times 10^9/l$, and although the diagnosis can be confirmed by needle aspiration of the peritoneum, it is more usually made at laparotomy. In addition to gastric suction and intravenous fluids, appropriate intravenous antibiotics should be administered in large doses for at least 10 days.

Tuberculous peritonitis

Tuberculous peritonitis remains a relatively common disease in the developing parts of the world but it is very rare in industrialized countries. The peritoneum becomes infected secondary to small bowel and/or mesenteric lymph node involvement. The diagnosis is confirmed by histology and culture, and treatment is with the conventional antituberculous drugs (Singh et al 1969).

Gastrointestinal bleeding and haemangiomas

Gastrointestinal bleeding in infancy is common but rarely serious. The essential decision must be to distinguish minor bleeding, which seldom has a serious cause, from major bleeds which cause a fall in the haemoglobin level and require intensive investigation. The commoner causes of bleeding and suggested investigations are included in Table 5.1. Endoscopy, if available, is the investigation of choice and should be carried out early in the course of the haemorrhage. A haematemesis indicates upper gastrointestinal tract bleeding, but in children, because of the rapid transit, even bleeding from oesophageal varices can present as the passage of bright red blood per rectum. Haemangiomas of the gut are a cause of occult (sometimes overt) and painless bleeding. They vary from multiple telangiectases, diffuse vascular hamartomas, or simple large cavernous haemangiomas, to multiple small submucous capillary lesions. In many children there are cutaneous or subcutaneous haemangiomas which serve as markers, as in Osler's disease and the Blue Rubber Bleb naevus syndrome. Here fibreoptic endoscopy has revolutionized diagnosis and treatment, except for the small bowel which is still only accessible by either isotope scanning (Gordon 1980) or laparotomy. Most of the gastric, duodenal and colonic lesions are small enough to be treated by injection. For large lesions, resection remains the best treatment.

Intestinal obstruction

Duodenal obstruction

Malrotation and intermittent volvulus occasionally cause recurrent episodes of vomiting outside the neonatal period. The condition should be considered in children with recurrent episodes of bile-stained vomiting.

Table 5.1 Gastrointestinal haemorrhage

Haematemesis

Age	Bleed	Cause	Vomit	Investigation
Neonate	Minor	Swallowed blood Pyloric stenosis Reflux oesophagitis	Fresh blood Coffee grounds	Test feed. Barium meal Barium swallow
	Severe	'Stress' peptic ulcer	Fresh blood	Barium meal
Infant and child	Minor	Hiatus hernia with reflux oesophagitis	Coffee grounds	Barium swallow and endoscopy
	Severe	Acute gastric erosions Peptic ulcer Mallory–Weiss syndrome Oesophageal varices	Fresh blood	Barium meal and endoscopy Endoscopy Endoscopy Barium swallow and endoscopy

Rectal bleeding

Age	Bleed	General condition	Cause	Stool	Investigation
Neonate	Minor	Well	Anal fissure	Bloodstreaked	Local examination
		Well	Haemorrhagic disease of the newborn	Fresh blood	Prothrombin time
			Mucosal erosions	Bloodstreaked	None
	Major	Ill	Necrotizing enterocolitis	Blood and stool mixed	Plain X-ray
		Ill	Volvulus	Fresh blood	Plain X-ray Barium meal Laparotomy
Toddler	Minor	Well	Fissure in ano	Bloodstreaked	Local examination
	Mixed	Usually well	Haemangioma	Fresh blood	Endoscopy
			Colitis	Blood and mucus	Barium enema, colonoscopy
		Ill	Intussusception	Fresh blood and mucus	Clinical examination Barium enema
	Major	Usually well	Meckel's diverticulum	Fresh blood or melaena	Technetium scan
Older child	Minor	Well	Fissure in ano	Bloodstreaked	Local examination
			Polyps	Fresh blood	Sigmoidoscopy
			Infective diarrhoea	Blood and pus	Stool culture
	Mixed		Ulcerative colitis ⎫ Crohn's disease ⎬	Blood and mucus ⎫ ⎬	Barium enema Colonoscopy
			Peptic ulcer ⎫ Haemangioma ⎬	Melaena	Barium meal Endoscopy
	Major		Oesophageal varices	Mixed blood and melaena	Barium meal Oesophagoscopy

Investigation and treatment follow the same plan as in the newborn (see Ch. 4).

Duodenal ileus

Duodenal ileus, an obstruction of the third part of the duodenum by the superior mesenteric vessels, is seen in the 'cast syndrome' following application of a plaster jacket, in association with weight loss and lordoscoliosis. This latter combination is seen in Duchenne muscular dystrophy. Duodenal ileus may also be part of a pseudo-obstructive syndrome. The symptoms are increasing discomfort and upper abdominal distension associated with vomiting of bile-stained fluid and food. The diagnosis is confirmed by a barium meal examination, which outlines the dilated proximal duodenum, with hold-up of contrast in the third part. The treatment should, where possible, be aimed at removal of the cause. Where this fails, a side-to-side duodenojejunostomy will relieve the obstruction. Obvious radiological signs may be associated with little apparent abnormality at operation, and treatment should proceed on the radiological evidence alone.

Distal obstruction

Acute bowel obstruction distal to the duodenum is either mechanical or paralytic. Mechanical lesions include external and internal hernias, adhesion bands, volvulus related to adhesion bands or a Meckel's Diverticulum, or more rarely of a sigmoid colon, Hirschsprung's disease, inflammatory strictures, and neoplasms involving or compressing the gut. Intraluminal obstructions can be caused in the small bowel by vegetable matter which swells as it absorbs fluid, or in the tropics by a mass of ascaris worms, and in children with cystic fibrosis a meconium ileus equivalent occurs. Paralytic ileus may be generalized, as in general peritonitis, or localized related to an intraperitoneal abscess e.g. an appendix abscess, or retroperitoneal sepsis e.g. pyonephrosis. In sickle cell disease thrombosis in the mesenteric vessels may lead to infarction with a mixed picture. More complicated are the adynamic gut or pseudo-obstructive syndromes, the rare acute gut dilatation which is seen in air swallowing, and the acute presentations of coeliac disease. Laparotomy should be avoided if possible as the resulting adhesions only increase the very difficult problem of treatment.

The cardinal clinical signs and symptoms of obstruction are vomiting, which progresses from gastric contents, through bile-stained, to faeculent; abdominal distension; and absolute constipation. The additional signs and symptoms of peritonitis have been discussed above. In mechanical obstruction, severe colicky abdominal pain is common, and ladder patterning from distended loops of gut, possibly showing visible peristalsis, is seen. Bowel sounds are absent in generalized peritonitis and increased or tinkling in mechanical obstruction. Plain abdominal X-rays are very helpful in confirming the diagnosis and identifying the cause of the obstruction.

The first essential in treatment is to correct fluid and electrolyte imbalance, control infection, and decompress the gut by nasogastric aspiration. The underlying lesion should be treated as soon as the patient is fit. Many cases of adhesion obstruction will respond to 6–12 hours of conservative nonoperative treatment. Very severe colic, pyrexia, abdominal tenderness, or a leucocytosis suggest impending infarction and demand early operation.

REFERENCES

Andersson A, Bergdahl L 1977 Carcinoid tumours of the appendix in children. A Report of 25 Cases. Acta Chirurgica Scandinavica 143: 173–175

Arasu T S, Wyllie R, Fitzgerald J F et al 1980 Gastroesophageal reflux in infants and children — comparative accuracy of diagnostic methods. Journal of Pediatrics 96: 798–803

Balistreri W F, Farrell M K 1983 Gastroesophageal reflux in infants. The New England Journal of Medicine 309(13): 790–792

Bell T M, Steyn J H 1962 Viruses in lymph nodes of children with mesenteric adenitis and intussusception. British Medical Journal 2:700

Brown J J M 1956 Acute appendicitis in infancy and childhood. Journal of the Royal College of Surgeons of Edinburgh 1:268

Buick R G, Spitz L Achalasia of the cardia in children. British Journal of Surgery 1985 72(5): 341–343

Calabro J J 1962 Hereditable multiple polyposis syndromes of the gastrointestinal tract. American Journal of Medicine 33: 276–281

Carre I J 1959 The natural history of partial thoracic stomach (hiatus hernia) in children. Archives of Disease in Childhood 34: 344–353

Carre I J 1984 Clinical significance of gastro-oesophageal reflux. Annotations. Archives of Disease in Childhood 59: 911–912

Collins J S A, Glasgow J F T, Trauton T G, McFarland R J, 1986 Twenty year review of duodenal ulcer. Archives of Disease in Childhood 61: 407–408

Curci M R, Little K, Sieber W K, Kiesewetter W B 1976 Peptic ulcer disease in childhood reexamined. Journal of Pediatric Surgery 11(3): 329–335

Dennison W M, Shaker M 1970 Intussusception in infancy and childhood. The British Journal of Surgery 57:679

Dormandy T L 1957 Gastrointestinal polyposis with mucocutaneous pigmentation. Peutz-Jeghers syndrome. New England Journal of Medicine 256: 1093, 1141, 1186

Fonkalsrud E W, Ament M E, Berquist W 1985 Surgical management of the gastro esophageal reflux syndrome in childhood. Surgery 97(1): 42–47

Gordon I 1980 Gastro-intestinal haemorrhage unrelated to gastric mucosa diagnosed on 99 Tcm pertechnetate scans. British Journal of Radiology 53: 322–324

Hawkins D B, Demeter M J, Barnett T E 1980 Caustic ingestion: controversies in management. A review of 214 cases. The Laryngoscope 90: 98–109

Hobbs C J, Wynne J M 1986 Buggery in Childhood — a common syndrome of child abuse Lancet 4: 792–796

Jewett T C, Duszynski D O, Allen J E 1970 The visualisation of Meckel's diverticulum with 99 mTc-pertechnetate. Surgery 68:567

Johnson D G, Herbst J J, Oliveros M A, Stewart D R 1977 Evaluation of gastroesophageal reflux surgery in children. Pediatrics 59: 62–68

King M D, Young D G, Hann I M, Patrick W J A 1985 Carcinoid Syndrome: an unusual cause of diarrhoea. Archives of Disease in Childhood 60: 269–271

Levick R K 1970 Management of Intussusception. Barium Enema versus Surgery. Clinical Pediatrics 9(8): 457–462

Levick R K, Spitz L 1977 The 'invisible' can top. British Journal of Radiology 50: 594–596

Litovitz T L 1985 Battery Ingestions: Product Accessibility and Clinical Course. Pediatrics 75(3): 469–476

Newsome H H 1974 Multiple Endocrine Adenomatosis. Surgical Clinics of North America 54(2): 387–393

Nicholls R J, Moskowitz R L, Shepherd N A 1985 Restorative proctocolectomy with ileal reservoir. British Journal of Surgery 72: 76–79

Olumide F, Adedeji A, Adesola A O 1976 Intestinal obstruction in Nigerian children. Journal of Pediatric Surgery 11:195

Orenstein S R, Whitington P F 1983 Positioning for prevention of infant gastroesohageal reflux. Pediatrics 103: 534–537

Othersen H B, Truluck T B, Loadholt C B 1976 Ruptured Appendicitis in Children: Continuing Controversy Over Antibiotic Combinations. Journal of Pediatric Surgery 11: 405–409

Parks A G, Nicholls R J, Belliveau P 1980 Proctocolectomy with ileal reservoir and anal anastomosis. British Journal of Surgery 67: 533–538

Pledger H G, Buchan R 1969 Deaths in children with acute appendicitis. British Medical Journal 2:466

Raudkivi P J, Smith H L M 1981 Intussusception: analysis of 98 cases. British Journal of Surgery 68: 645–648

Rosenlund M L 1967 The Zollinger–Ellison syndrome in children: a review. American Journal of Medical Science 254:884

Sachatello C R, Pickren J W, Grace J T 1970 Generalized juvenile gastrointestinal polyposis. Gastroenterology 58:699

Shipsey M R, O'Donnell B 1985 Conservative management of appendix mass in children. Annals of the Royal College of Surgeons of England 67:23

Singh M, Bhargava A, Jain K 1969 Tuberculous peritonitis. New England Journal of Medicine 281:1091

Sondheimer J M, Morris A 1979 Gastro-esophageal reflux among severely retarded children. Journal of Pediatrics 94: 710–714

Sutcliffe J 1969 Torsion spasms and abnormal postures in children with hiatus hernia: Sandifer's syndrome. Progress in Pediatric Radiology 2: 190–197

Tolia V, Dubois R S 1983 Peptic ulcer disease in children and adolescents. Clinical Pediatrics 22: 665–669

Veale A M, McCole I, Bussey H J, Morson B C 1966 Juvenile polyposis coli. Journal of Medical Genetics 3:5

Wagensteen O H, Bowers W F 1937 Significance of the obstructive factor in the genesis of acute appendicitis. Archives of Surgery 34:496

Watts J M, Bennett R C, Goligher J C 1965 Stretching of anal sphincters in the treatment of fissure-in-ano. British Medical Journal 2:342

Weiland L H 1977 Afflictions of the pesky appendix. Postgraduate Medicine 61(3): 54–62

Willis A T, Ferguson I R, Jones P H 1976 Metronidazole in prevention and treatment of bacteroides infections after appendicectomy. British Medical Journal 1:318

Wilson S D, Schulte W J, Meade R C 1971 Longevity studies following total gastrectomy in children with the Zollinger–Ellison syndrome. Archives of Surgery 103:108

Winter H S, Grand R J 1981 Gastroesophageal reflux. Pediatrics 68: 134–136

Chronic inflammatory bowel disease

INFLAMMATORY BOWEL DISEASE

The term 'inflammatory bowel disease' will be used in this chapter to denote ulcerative colitis and Crohn's disease which are the commonest causes in delevoped countries, although schistosomiasis, amoebiasis and tuberculosis account for more inflammatory colonic disease world-wide. Once considered rare in paediatric pratice, inflammatory bowel disease is now diagnosed much more frequently.

Ulcerative colitis is a recurrent, inflammatory and ulcerative disease involving only the mucosa of the colon. Almost invariably, the entire large bowel is affected.

Crohn's disease however is a transmural, focal, subacute or chronic inflammatory disorder, affecting any part of the gastrointestinal tract from mouth to anus, but most commonly the distal ileum, colon and anorectal areas.

As there is no specific diagnostic test for either disease, the diagnosis is made on the basis of clinical, radiological, colonoscopic and pathologic findings, and by excluding infective causes of colonic inflammation.

Incidence

From the 1950's to the 1970's, there has been a well recognized and dramatic increase in the incidence of Crohn's disease ranging from 100–400% in all age groups (Mendeloff et al 1970). In Northern Europe and North America, where the incidence is currently about 4 per 100 000, this trend has probably levelled off, but the incidence may still be rising in less industrialized areas (Gilat 1983). There are two peaks of incidence, in early and late adult life, but between a quarter to a third of patients with Crohn's disease present before the age of 20.

In contrast to Crohn's disease, the incidence of ulcerative colitis has not changed, and the overall incidence of Crohn's disease and ulcerative colitis now appears to be similar. Only 15% of patients with ulcerative colitis present before the age of 20, and then usually in adolescence. Although ulcerative colitis may present in early life, it now seems likely that many cases of inflammatory disease of the colon presenting in the first year of life are related to food allergy (Jenkins et al 1984).

Pathogenesis

The aetiology of both diseases is unknown, despite a massive research input. The various aetiological theories have recently been reviewed by Sachar et al (1980) and Kirsner & Shorter (1982). To date, no clear concept has emerged to suggest whether these diseases are primarily immunological, environmental or infective; for example many of the observed immunological abnormalities may be secondary phenomena.

The recognition of cases in which Crohn's disease and ulcerative colitis occur in the same patient has led to the notion that these two forms of inflammatory bowel disease are different manifestations of the same disease and represent different ends of a single histopathological spectrum. Well documented cases of such an occurence are, however, rare and the reported incidence of dual occurence is below that expected on the basis of chance (Eyer et al 1980).

Risk factors

Certain populations and subpopulations have been identified as being at higher risk of developing inflammatory bowel disease (Mendeloff et al 1970). Thus, ulcerative colitis and Crohn's disease occur more commonly amongst North European, Anglo-Saxon races; urban rather than rural dwellers; and in Jews living in Europe and North America (but less commonly in Israelis). Males and females are equally affected. Although not classically genetic disorders, multiple familial occurrences occur in 15–40% of patients with ulcerative colitis and Crohn's disease (Farmer et al 1980), and in a quarter of such families, both forms of inflammatory bowel disease may occur. With the exception of the association between HLA-B27 and ankylosing spondylitis complicating inflammatory bowel disease, no evidence exists to suggest that inflammatory bowel disease occurs with greater frequency in subjects of any given histocompatibility type (Kirsner & Shorter 1982).

Immune mechanisms

At present, there is no convincing evidence that the multiple immunological abnormalities observed in patients with inflammatory bowel disease have a primary pathogenetic role.

Serum antibodies reacting with colonic epithelial cells and cross-reacting with lipopolysaccharide antigens extracted from *Escherichia coli* (*Esch. coli*) have been demonstrated in patients with ulcerative colitis and Crohn's disease (Bartnik & Shorter 1980), but epithelial specific cytotoxic antibodies have not as yet been demonstrated in colonic tissue.

Circulating immune complexes have been reported in patients with inflammatory bowel disease (Hodgson et al 1977), which may contribute to tissue damage by complement activation. However, immune complexes may occur secondarily to the disease process and may represent nonspecific markers of acute inflammation.

Evidence to support the primary involvment of an immunoglobulin E (IgE)-mediated immediate hypersensitivity reaction in the pathogenesis of inflammatory bowel disease, other than that occurring in infancy as a result of food allergy (Jenkins et al 1984), is currently lacking. IgE plasma cells in the plasma and mucosa of patients with inflammatory bowel disease are not consistently elevated (Sachar et al 1980).

The role of lymphocyte-mediated reactions remains confused. Circulating T (thymus-derived)-lymphocytes, sensitized to a wide variety of colonic and enterobacterial antigens are present in patients with inflammatory bowel disease (Strickland & Sachar 1977). A certain class of circulating lymphocytes (crystallizable fragment (Fc) receptor-bearing killer cells) in patients with inflammatory bowel disease do exert a specific cytotoxicity *in vitro* against colonic epithelial cells (Kirsner & Shorter 1982). More recently impaired K-cell (killer cell) activity has been reported in patients with inflammatory bowel disease (Ginsburg et al 1983), but the degree of cytotoxicity does not correlate with disease activity or extent, and the phenomenon is only demonstrable in patients with small intestinal Crohn's disease.

Infectious agents

The possibility that infectious agents may play a role in the pathogenesis of inflammatory bowel disease is an attractive one, but to date the evidence is inconclusive and no organism has remotely fulfilled Koch's postulates. Bacterial agents have been sought, and interest is currently centred on intestinal anaerobes, such as (Clostridium difficile (*C. difficile*); cell-wall deficient L-forms, mycobacteria and chlamydia. Similarly, several investigators have reported the presence of cytopathic, virus-like agents from inflammatory bowel disease tissue. A virus-like agent has also been implicated as an explanation for the observed ability of bacteria-free filtrates of Crohn's disease and ulcerative colitis homogenates to produce granulomatous lesions (Cave et al 1973, 1976).

Dietary factors

The recent, marked rise in the incidence of Crohn's disease, its prevalence in industrialized areas and higher incidence amongst members of a low risk group who subsequently move to urban centres, point to the involvement of an environmental factor in the pathogenesis.

With the exception of allergic colitis in infancy, there is no good evidence to support an aetiological role for cow's milk or any other dietary protein in inflammatory bowel disease. The finding of raised anti-dietary protein antibodies in some patients with inflammatory bowel disease may merely reflect increased macromolecular absorption through an already damaged mucosa. The role of food stabilizers, heavy metals, fibre and sucrose remains confused.

Psychosomatic factors

The role of psychosomatic factors in the pathogenesis of inflammatory bowel disease remains controversial. There is no evidence to support the concept that a 'colitis personality' precedes the onset of ulcerative colitis, nor that there is a close temporal relationship between disease onset and stressful life events (Daniels 1984, Mendeloff et al 1970). A similar aetiologic relationship has not been suggested for Crohn's disease, although adults with Crohn's disease are said to be more neurotic and introverted than controls (Gazzard et al 1978). Such personality traits are perhaps not surprising in patients with a chronically disabling gastrointestinal disorder. A recent study has reported a significantly higher incidence of psychiatric illness, particularly depression, in adults with Crohn's disease than in control subjects with other chronic medical illnesses (Helzer et al 1984).

Although good scientific evidence to support an aetiological role for psychosomatic factors is lacking, many patients and their families encounter emotional problems as a result of their disease and the importance of careful, considerate support from their attending paediatricians should not be underestimated.

CROHN'S DISEASE

Pathology

The affected intestine is thickened. Inflammation is transmural and the peri-intestinal fat and serosa may be involved, with consequent fibrosis, and as a result, adhesions betweeen affected intestinal loops are common. Perianal skin tags, fissures or fistulae are common, especially when the large bowel is involved (Buchmann & Alexander-Williams 1980). In children, ileocolitis is the most common (52%) and colitis the least common (9%) form of disease, with diffuse small bowel disease and ileal disease each accounting for about 20% (Gryboski & Spiro 1978). Mucosal ulceration is often present. Early in the disease the ulcers are characteristically apthoid (small shallow ulcers with a white base and surrounding mucosal inflammation), later they are serpiginous and discontinuous. Stricturing may be present in more advanced disease as may the classic 'cobblestone' appearance of the mucosa which results from intercommunicating fissures surrounding inflamed, oedematous islands of intact epithelium. Microscopically, transmural inflammation is present, together with mucosal ulceration and fissuring. The diagnostic hallmark is the presence of noncaseating epitheloid granulomata, which are found in 50% of cases.

Clinical features

Abdominal pain (often colicky, periumbilical, and worse after meals), diarrhoea and growth failure are the dominant presenting symptoms (Table 6.1). However, the disease is frequently insidious in onset, and extraintestinal symptoms such as intermittent fever, arthritis (Lindsley & Schaller 1974), iridocyclitis, lassitude, erythema nodosum or growth retardation may dominate the picture, with little or no clinical pointers towards gastrointestinal disease (Burbige et al 1975). Not surprisingly, the initial diagnosis in children subsequently shown to have Crohn's disease is often incorrect, and the correct diagnosis may be considerably delayed. Thus, Burbige et al (1975), demonstrated a mean delay of 13 months between onset of symptoms and diagnosis, whilst delayed referral raised this figure to nearly 3 years in another series (O'Donoghue & Dawson 1977). The site and extent of disease has a considerable effect upon the delay in diagnosis; left-sided colonic disease (1.8 months) is more rapidly diagnosed than diffuse small bowel disease (5.4 months) or disease confined to the terminal ileum and

Table 6.1 Presenting symptoms in children with Crohn's disease and ulcerative colitis (Gryboski & Spiro 1978, Gryboski & Hillemeier 1980)

	Crohn's disease				Ulcerative colitis
	Diffuse small bowel	Terminal ileum	Ileocolitis	Colitis	
Number of patients	17	16	45	8	41
	%	%	%	%	%
Abdominal pain	71	75	51	75	25
Periumbilical	59	50	40	62	—
Right lower quadrant	0	12	7	13	—
Epigastric	12	12	4	0	—
Diarrhoea	87	37	62	100	72
Rectal bleeding	12	0	33	100	45
Fever	19	29	22	50	68
Arthritis	0	6	9	12	10
Fistula	0	6	0	0	0
Short stature	29	6	40	50	18

right colon (16 months) (Burbige et al 1975). The cause of the diarrhoea in patients with small intestinal Crohn's disease is probably multifactorial; extensive mucosal dysfunction, bile acid malabsorption in terminal ileal disease, bacterial overgrowth resulting from strictures and disordered motility, and protein exudation from inflamed surfaces all play a part. Frank blood in the stools is uncommon in the absence of colitis.

Many patients with a short history of a few months have evidence of weight loss, with a low weight for height. Those who present during adolescence may suffer severe growth failure; wasting may be extreme and hypoalbuminaemia may be present. Those with a longer history of perhaps years may be short in stature, but with a weight appropriate for their height. The importance of seeking diagnostic clues outside the abdomen cannot be overemphasized. 50% of patients are anaemic but this may not always be clinically detectable. The presence of clubbing, perianal disease (skin tags, fissures, fistulae), oral ulceration, uveitis or arthritis may provide valuable information on which a clinical diagnosis may be based. Abdominal examination may reveal an area of localized tenderness, possibly with a palpable mass.

Diagnosis

Laboratory assessment

Haematological examination reveals an iron deficiency anaemia in 50% of patients, presumably as a result of malabsorption and blood loss. An elevated erythrocyte sedimentation rate and a polymorphonuclear leucocytosis may be present although a lymphopenia may result from malnutrition. The degree of thrombocytosis (Harries et al 1983) and hypoalbuminaemia (Lloyd-Still & Green 1979) or the plasma levels of acute phase protein (Campbell et al 1982) may all correlate with disease activity. Liver function tests should be performed, and in this context a raised serum alkaline phosphatase is probably the best index of disturbed liver function in inflammatory bowel disease. It should be remembered, however, that an elevated alkaline phosphatase may result from bone, secondary to steatorrhoea and abnormal vitamin D and calcium absorption.

Diagnostic imaging (Lee 1983)

Plain abdominal film. In patients with colicky pain and distension, erect and supine films of the abdomen may reveal the presence of incomplete small intestinal obstruction, with distended loops and fluid levels. Occasionally an intra-abdominal abscess may be revealed by the abdominal displacement of loops of small intestine.

Barium meal and follow through. Examination of the small intestine should be performed in all patients and this is best done in a centre experienced in this examination. A small bowel meal, in which barium is introduced directly into the duodenum by a transpyloric tube probably gives more accurate information (Nolan 1981) but is much less comfortable for the child. The column of barium should be followed to the caecum and its passage through the terminal ileum screened, preferably during palpation of the right iliac fossa in an attempt to separate overlying loops of ileum and also to localize areas of tenderness. A number of abnormalities should be sought: dilated intestine proximal to narrowed segments, which when severe produces a 'string sign'; fissuring ('rose thorn' ulcers); mucosal irregularities or a mucosa in which the normal feathery pattern is not seen; increased separation of adjacent loops by mural thickening and fistulae.

Barium enema. In order to show adequate mucosal detail, it is essental to perform a double contrast examination, although this is not always easily done in children. The changes (colonic narrowing, loss of haustrations, discrete apthoid or linear mucosal ulceration, cobblestoning, fissuring, thumbprinting) are discontinuous and may be eccentric and often confined to the ascending or the transverse colon. The rectum is normal in 50% of cases but the thickening and mucosal abnormality may sometimes be recognized in the terminal ileum.

The radiological features useful in differentiating Crohn's colitis from ulcerative colitis are shown in Table 6.2.

[111]Indium-labelled leucocyte scan. Gamma camera scanning following the intravenous injection of [111]Indium-labelled autologous leucocytes is a useful method of assessing inflammatory bowel disease in adults (Savery Muttu et al 1983) and has recently been used in children (Gordon & Vivian 1984). Although apparently accurate in the localization of active disease, the technique involves a relatively high radiation exposure to the liver and

Table 6.2 Radiological features useful in differentiating chronic ulcerative colitis from Crohn's colitis

	Crohn's colitis	Idiopathic ulcerative colitis
Pattern and sites of involvement	Asymmetric and eccentric involvement. Rectum involved in 50%. Terminal ileum abnormal in majority of patients. Right-sided colitis only, 35%	Symmetric and contiguous involvement. Rectum almost always abnormal. Terminal ileum normal
Mucosal pattern in acute stage	Focal aphthous ulcers surrounded by normal adjacent mucosa	Diffuse granular pattern produced by oedema and superficial ulceration involving entire mucosal surface
Mucosal pattern in chronic stage	Deep ulceration with cobble-stone pattern. Pseudosacculations. Skip areas	Coarse granularity secondary to deep ulcers superimposed on granular pattern. Loss of haustra. Foreshortening
Abdominal complications	Fistulae and abscesses. Stricture formation with or without obstruction	Toxic megacolon. Carcinoma. Strictures (benign and malignant)

spleen which means that [111]Indium scanning in children with inflammatory bowel disease is indicated only when other methods have proved unsatisfactory.

Colonoscopy

The recent development of floppy, small-diameter paediatric colonoscopes has provided a safe, accurate method of directly and microscopically examining the entire colon in children (Williams et al 1982). The examination may be adequatelly performed under sedation, and general anaesthesia is not usually required. Biopsies are routinely obtained, and although small and superficial, they are adequate for diagnosis. Based on gross endoscopic and histological findings, diagnosis can be confirmed in over 90% of children with inflammatory bowel disease. Because of its ability to detect mucosal-only lesions, its great accuracy, and the difficulty in obtaining good double-contrast films with a barium enema in children, it is likely that colonoscopy will be increasingly used in the diagnosis and management of children with inflammatory bowel disease.

Differential diagnosis

10% of children at some time during childhood experience recurrent abdominal pain and a common diagnostic problem is to decide when to investigate such children for possible inflammatory bowel disease. Fortunately, as discussed earlier under 'Clinical Features', children with Crohn's disease rarely present with abdominal pain in the absence of other symptoms. Gryboski & Spiro (1978) have pointed out that abdominal pain in children with Crohn's disease is often periumbilical (Table 6.1). Careful screening is, therefore, necessary to be certain of the cause of any abdominal pain syndrome in childhood.

Crohn's disease may be differentiated from ulcerative colitis by the site and discontinuous nature of the inflammatory process, and the histological features of affected tissue.

Intestinal tuberculosis and amoebic colitis may mimic Crohn's disease, and are most reliably differentiated by histological examination and culture of colonoscopic biopsies. Other granulomatous diseases such as chronic granulomatous disease, sarcoidosis and histoplasmosis are rare in childhood as are small intestinal malignancies. Immunoproliferative disease of the small intestine although uncommon in children may also present with diarrhoea, abdominal pain and weight loss (Khojaste et al 1983).

Complications

Intestinal

Adhesions, strictures with stagnant loop syndrome, fistulae and abscesses result from the transmural nature of the inflammation in Crohn's disease.

Toxic megacolon may complicate Crohn's colitis but is a less common cause of this disorder than ulcerative colitis. Perianal disease may precede the appearance of the intestinal manifestations of Crohn's disease by several years and is most commonly seen in patients with a colitis (Buchmann & Alexander-Williams 1980). Similarly cheilitis granulomatosa may precede the appearance of intestinal disease.

The risk of intestinal and extraintestinal carcinoma is increased in Crohn's disease. Thus, in patients diagnosed before the age of 21 the risk of developing carcinoma is twenty times greater than normal (Weedon et al 1973). However, the incidence of small intestinal carcinoma complicating Crohn's disease is still exceedingly low and the risk of developing colonic carcinoma too low to warrant prophylactic colectomy.

Extraintestinal

Arthritis and arthralgia (Lindsley & Schaller 1974). Arthritis is the most common extraintestinal manifestation of Crohn's disease and occurs in about 11% of children, usually those with an ileocolitis (Gryboski & Spiro 1978). Typically both arthritis and arthralgia affect the large joints in the lower limbs and may even occur when intestinal disease is in remission. Arthritis may be mono- or polyarticular and synovitis with an effusion is commonly present. Sacroileitis and ankylosing spondylitis, in which most patients are HLA-B27 positive, may occur but are rare in children.

Skin lesions. Erythema nodosum or pyoderma gangrenosum occur in about 5% of patients, often at times of exacerbation of intestinal disease or when on reduced doses of steroids.

Uveitis. Although acute symptomatic uveitis occurs in only 0.5–3% of patients, the incidence of asymptomatic transient uveitis in childhood may be as high as 30%. Uveitis occurs particularly in male patients with a colitis (Daum et al 1979).

Urinary tract. Renal calculi complicate Crohn's disease in about 5% of children (Gryboski & Spiro 1978). Hyperoxaluria, secondary to increased colonic oxalate reabsorption, and resulting from steatorrhoea following extensive small intestinal disease, is a common cause (Dobbins & Binder 1977). Noncalculous hydronephrosis and hydroureter may follow compression of the ureter by an inflammatory mass, fibrosis or abscesses. Enterovesical fistulae present with pneumaturia and recurrent urinary tract infections.

Liver Disease. On the basis of biochemical abnormalities, hepatic dysfunction is found in 8% of patients with Crohn's disease (Dew et al 1979), and in this context a raised serum alkaline phosphatase activity is the best index of hepatic disease (Kane et al 1980). Occasionally, children with inflammatory bowel disease may present with chronic liver disease and only minimal gastrointestinal symptoms (Kane et al 1980) and it is therefore important to consider this diagnosis in those patients presenting with chronic liver disease of unknown aetiology.

The most common lesions are pericholangitis and fatty change; cirrhosis, chronic active hepatitis, sclerosing cholangitis and biliary tract carcinoma are rare. Colectomy in patients with Crohn's colitis, or alternatively intensive medical treatment of the intestinal disease, may halt the pericholangitic process (Freese et al 1980).

Cholelithiasis. Symptomatic cholelithiasis in children with Crohn's disease is exceedingly rare. However, gallstones occur in one-third of adults with Crohn's disease involving the terminal ileum but are not age related. Asymptomatic gallstones may be commoner than supposed in children with long-standing disease.

Nutritional deficiencies

Protein-energy malnutrition. Weight loss is present in three quarters of children at presentation and in some may be severe (Burbige et al 1975). There are a number of possible reasons for this nutritional depletion.

The caloric intake of children with Crohn's disease is commonly reduced. Reduced intake, often by as much as 50% (Kirschner et al 1981), may be due to anorexia and nausea associated with a severe systemic illness, bolus colic following food, or in some cases, by zinc deficiency producing loss of taste sensation (McClain et al 1980).

Absorptive defects in children are well recognized (Beeken 1973) and presumably result from widespread mucosal abnormalities, disordered motility, stagnant loops, fistulae or resections.

Steatorrhoea occurs in up to a third of patients. In adults with 100 cm or more of ileal disease/resection, marked steatorrhoea appears to be related to fatty acid malabsorption consequent upon markedly reduced luminal bile salt concentrations. Patients respond to reduced dietary fat, rather than to cholestyramine. When less than 100 cm of ileum is involved, marked diarrhoea and mild steatorrhoea result from increased faecal bile acid loss. Jejunal luminal bile salt concentrations are normal and these patients usually respond to cholestyramine (Poley & Hoffman 1976).

Upper small intestinal bacterial overgrowth is often present particularly if jejunal disease or enteroenteric fistulae are present (Beeken & Kanich 1973); the consequent bacterial deconjugation of bile salts leads to further impairment of fat absorption and secretion of fluid and electrolytes.

Increased losses of intestinal protein and blood are common and result from extensive areas of intestinal ulceration and exudation (Beeken 1973, Morson & Dawson 1979). Thus, faecal nitrogen excretion in children with Crohn's disease is raised but is not increased following supplementation with a completely assimilated defined formula, suggesting that this abnormality results from mucosal loss rather than true protein malabsorption (Motil et al 1982a). During treatment with corticosteroids and during periods of catabolism, large amounts of nitrogen are lost in the urine (Foster & Karran 1980). However the relationship between chronic inflammation in Crohn's disease and protein metabolism is controversial. Studies performed in adolescents with growth failure have failed to show that chronic inflammation or corticosteroid treatment alter rates of protein turnover or retention (Motil et al 1982a), whereas in adults, rates of protein turnover but not retention rates appear to correlate with disease activity (Powell-Tuck et al 1984).

Specific deficiencies. Sodium depletion is uncommon except in patients with fulminating colitis or in those with a small intestinal stoma, when the intestine is in a secretory state. Under these circumstances potassium depletion tends to occur as a result of secondary hyperaldosteronism. Symptomatic magnesium deficiency in Crohn's disease is well recognized but uncommon (Grand & Colodny 1972) and results from abnormal gut losses, particularly when watery diarrhoea (Harris & Wilkinson 1971) and anorexia are present, and intravenous therapy contains inadequate magnesium. Plasma magnesium concentrations poorly reflect total body magnesium and therefore urinary levels should also be estimated. Calcium deficiency, although uncommon may present as metabolic bone disease (Krawitt et al 1976).

Iron deficiency occurs in 50% of patients. It should be distinguished from the normocytic anaemia of chronic inflammation, in which total iron binding capacity is normal or low and does not respond to iron therapy.

A macrocytic anaemia may be present as a result of vitamin B_{12} or folic acid malabsorption. An abnormality in vitamin B_{12} absorption is seen in over 50% of children with Crohn's disease as a result of disturbed terminal ileal function (Beeken 1973). Folate deficiency may occur because of dietary insufficiency, jejunal disease, or as a consequence of administered sulphasalazine which is a competitive inhibitor of intestinal folate transport and metabolism (Reisenauer & Halsted 1981). Folic acid (1–5 mg daily) should therefore be given to patients receiving sulphasalazine.

Zinc deficiency is common in Crohn's disease. McClain et al (1980) have reported low serum zinc concentrations in 40% of a series of Crohn's disease patients with impaired zinc absorption and depression in taste sensation. Plasma concentrations of zinc are however subject to acute variation and a single low value should not be interpreted as necessarily indicative of true zinc deficiency. The activity of a zinc-dependent enzyme, such as alkaline phosphatase or carbonic anhydrase, which is depressed in zinc deficiency, should be measured concurrently (Aggett & Harries 1979). Administration of zinc in malnourished zinc-deficient children, coincides with periods of rapid growth (Golden & Golden 1981), but the relationship between zinc deficiency and growth failure in Crohn's disease has not been clearly defined.

Growth failure and sexual immaturity (Fig. 6.1)

Growth retardation and delay of sexual development occur in up to 30%

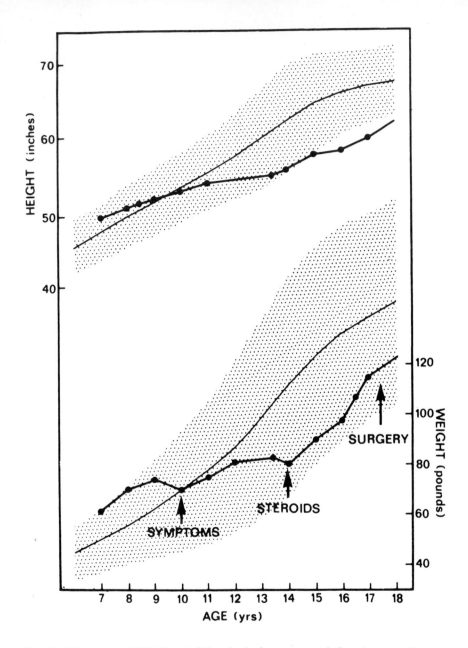

Fig. 6.1 (Homer et al 1977) Growth failure beginning two years before the onset of symptoms in a patient with Crohn's disease. Linear growth remained abnormal despite medical and surgical therapy and no recurrence. The patient had achieved puberty before surgery. The shaded area represents 97% confidence limits for height and weight, and the solid lines the 50th percentile.

of children and adolescents with Crohn's disease (O'Donoghue & Dawson 1977, Homer et al 1977). In addition to posing very difficult problems in management, growth failure may present difficult diagnostic problems, and may be the sole manifestation of disease in about 5% of patients (O'Donoghue & Dawson 1977, Burbige et al 1975). Despite its frequency, the pathogenesis of the growth failure has, until recently, remained unclear. It does not appear to be the result of a primary endocrine disturbance.

There is now accumulating evidence that nutritional deprivation is the most important single determinant of growth failure in Crohn's disease (Kelts et al 1979, Kirschner et al 1981, Motil et al 1982a). Body weight is generally appropriate for height (Homer et al 1977, Kelts et al 1979, Motil et al 1982b), which suggests that affected children are 'nutritional dwarfs'. In children with chronic renal insufficiency, reduced growth velocity occurs if caloric intake is reduced below 80% of that recommended for the child's age, and ceases altogether if intake falls below 40% (Betts & Magrath 1974). A similar situation seems to pertain in children with Crohn's disease, and estimated caloric intakes of 56% and 82% of recommended daily intake have been recorded in published series (Kirschner et al 1981, Kelts et al 1979). There is now also good evidence that calorie and protein supplementation will promote growth which continues beyond the period of supplementation in these growth retarded patients.

The results of the studies to date on the effect of enteral or parenteral nutrition on growth are summarized in Table 6.3. From these studies it is clear that chronic protein-calorie malnutrition consequent upon an impaired intake plays an important role in the growth failure in Crohn's disease. It has also become clear that nutritional supplementation is effective whether given by the oral or intravenous route (Morin et al 1980) and a recent study (Kirschner et al 1981) suggest that oral supplements need not be in an elemental form.

Medical management

The aims of treatment are to induce and maintain a remission of disease activity, to correct malnutriton and to restore growth. The importance of nutritional measures in trying to achieve all these aims cannot be overemphasized.

Drugs

There is no evidence that any drug alters the long-term natural history of Crohn's disease, yet a variety of agents are useful in the management of various manifestations of the disease.

Corticosteroids have been the mainstay of treatment in Crohn's disease, particularly of the small intestine. Remission may be achieved in about 70%

Table 6.3 Summary of nutritional supplementation studies in children and adolescents with inflammatory bowel disease and growth failure[1]

Author	Patients[2]	Age (yr)	Diagnosis	Duration of illness (yr)	Height (cm)	Average Weight (kg)	Bone age (years)	Drug therapy[3]	Mode/duration of nutrition[4]	Nutrient intakes protein (g/kg/d)	Nutrient intakes energy (kcal/kg/d)	Prior height velocity (cm/6 months)	Post height and weight (cm/6 months)	velocity (kg/months)
Kelts et al 1979	5 M 2 F	9–17	Crohn's	0.5–8	133	30	11	P,S	TPN + PO Food 6–8 weeks	2.1	75	0.9	3.2	1.2
Layden et al 1976	3 M 1 F	11–17	Crohn's	2–6	137	31	10	P,A	TPN, 4–6 weeks	1.7	80	0.6	4.1	3.1
Strobel et al 1979	6 M	11–16	Crohn's	—	—	—	—	P,S,N	HPN + PO Food, 0.5 years	—	70	0.5	4.3	—
Kirschner et al 1981	4 M 3 F	11–15	Crohn's	—	145	—	11	P,S	PO Food + Formula, 1 yr + TPN (P), 4 weeks	2.2	77	0.9	3.1	—
Morin et al 1980	3 M 1 F	12–13	Crohn's	2–5	134	28	(>2 SD)	P,S	PO Food, 16 weeks + IG Formula, 6 weeks	1.5	80	0.8	4.5	—
Motil et al 1982	6 M	13–16	Crohn's	2–5	145	38	12	P,S	IG Formula + PO Food 0.5 years	3.2	95	0.6	3.0	7.3

[1] Summary information estimated from available data listed in publications.
[2] M = Male, F = Female
[3] P = Prednisone, S = Sulphasalazine, A = Azathioprine
[4] TPN = Total Parenteral Nutrition, PO = Oral, HPN = Home Parenteral Nutrition, (P) = Peripheral, IG = Intragastric.

of patients, but is often short-term and 70% will have relapsed by 12 months (Jones & Lennard-Jones 1966). There is no evidence that these agents prevent relapse when given in relatively small doses to patients with quiescent disease (Summers et al 1979), and their use may not only be associated with an increased relapse rate following surgery (Cooke et al 1980), but also with growth retardation (Berger et al 1975). Correction of malnutrition, by either the enteral or parenteral routes (Strobel et al 1979, Morin et al 1980) is effective in inducing remission and, in some patients, may be at least as effective as corticosteroids (O'Morain et al 1984).

For induction of remission, prednisolone is begun in high dosage (2 mg/kg/24 h) and reduced following symptomatic improvement, usually by about 2–3 weeks. The dose is tailed off over 4–6 weeks and stopped if possible. Some patients experience a recurrence of their symptoms when the dose is reduced below about 0.3 mg/kg/24 h, and in these cases alternate day steroids may control symptoms without growth retardation (Whittington et al 1977). It seems likely that the problems of steroid-induced growth failure and steroid-dependent symptoms may now be overcome with nutritional support (see below).

Immunosuppressives (azathioprine, 6-mercaptopurine) have been widely used in Crohn's disease in adults, often as a means of maintaining remission. Although the results of clinical trials in adults are conflicting, these agents may have a useful role in maintaining remission (O'Donoghue et al 1978) or reducing steroid requirements (Present et al 1980) in patients with moderate or severe disease. It is noteworthy that the mean time to the recognition of improvement with 6-mercaptopurine in the study by Present et al (1980) was three months. Severe myelosuppression is an infrequent but serious complication of treatment and long-latency lymphoid malignancy a possible long-term hazard. Clearly, treatment must be monitored with frequent blood counts. It is difficult to know when to withdraw immunosuppressive agents, but this is usually done slowly after 12–24 months symptom-free remission.

Sulphasalazine (30–50 mg/kg/24 h) is useful in the management of patients with symptomatic Crohn's colitis, but in contrast to ulcerative colitis does not appear to have a prophylactic action (Summers et al 1979). Some patients experience nausea and vomiting soon after beginning treatment and occasionally have bloody diarrhoea (Werlin & Grand 1978); such symptoms can often be avoided by restarting with very small doses and increasing slowly (Holdsworth 1981). Oligospermia, a recently recognized side effect, appears to be reversible (Drife 1982) but is particularly worrying in children on long-term treatment.

Recently, metronidazole has been shown to be effective in the treatment of Crohn's disease, by a mechanism which may not just be related to a reduction in small intestinal overgrowth (Gilat 1982). It appears to be more effective in colonic than small intestinal disease and particularly in patients with perianal disease (Brandt et al 1982). At present it seems reasonable to use metronidazole in patients with colitis who fail to respond to sulpha-salazine, those with significant perianal disease, and in patients with demon-strable small intestinal bacterial overgrowth.

In patients with diarrhoea following extensive ileocolonic resection or dysfunction, an agent which increases transit time, such as loperamide, may provide useful symptomatic relief. The dose should be titrated carefully, so that the patient is free of diarrhoea at night and is able to sit through a school lesson without interruption.

Diarrhoea resulting from increased amounts of bile salts entering the colon, following the resection of less than 100 cm of ileum, usually responds to oral cholestyramine (Poley & Hoffman, 1976).

Nutritional therapy

The importance of nutritional therapy, not only in the correction of specific deficiencies, but also in the management of disease activity and of growth failure, is becoming increasingly recognized, and patients with Crohn's disease (and ulcerative colitis) demand considerable expertise in nutritional assessment and support. The nutritional status of all patients with inflam-matory bowel disease in relapse and/or those with growth failure should be regularly monitored. Those with a history of recent weight loss greater than 5% body weight, a decreased weight for height or a serum albumin below 35 g/l should have a complete nutritional assessment as outlined by Merrit & Blackburn (1981).

Patients with evidence of iron, folate or vitamin B_{12} deficiency should receive supplements, and those with terminal ileal disease and an abnormal Schilling test will require regular vitamin B_{12} supplements. Malnourished patients will also require multivitamin supplements. Zinc and magnesium deficiency should also be corrected by approriate supplementation. In the latter case this will probably be by the parenteral route as oral magnesium salts above a dose of 3 mmol/kg/24 h of magnesium usually result in diarrhoea.

The correction of malnutrition in Crohn's disease is commonly associated with symptomatic relief by a mechanism which is unknown. Experi-ence with parenteral nutrition in adults has been reviewed by Driscoll & Rosenberg (1978), and in 17 children on home parenteral nutrition by Strobel et al (1979). Relief of symptoms occurs in about 70% of patients and nutritional repletion in almost all, but remission is often short-lived and the number in remission after 3 months varies between 20 and 79%.

Enteral feeding, using an elemental diet has also been assessed as a means of inducing remission in Crohn's disease. To date, most studies have been uncontrolled, and the results should therefore be treated with caution. However, correction of protein-energy malnutrition, anaemia and hypoal-buminaemia may be achieved and remission induced (Goode et al 1976, Morin et al 1980, O'Morain et al 1984). The evidence to support the use of an amino acid (elemental) rather than a polymeric whole protein feed is lacking (Moriarty et al 1981) but preliminary evidence from a small controlled trial strongly suggests that an enteral elemental diet may be at least as effective as steroids in inducing remission in acute Crohn's disease (O'Morain et al 1984).

Currently the indications for parenteral/enteral nutrition as a means of inducing remission are severe malnutrition, failure of medical treatment, particularly in those patients in whom extensive or duodenal disease precludes surgery, and the improvement/maintainence of nutrition pre- and postoperatively. Where nutritional supplementation in growth failure is required, a 40% increase in calories and protein intake above that recommended for the patient's height–age is an appropriate point at which to start (Motil et al 1982a).

Oral foods may be introduced to replace tube feeds and maintain caloric intake, but in some patients overnight tube feeds may be required in order to maintain adequate growth.

Surgery

The indications for surgery are summarized in Table 6.4. Whether or not nutritional therapy (enteral or parenteral) will alter the natural history of Crohn's disease and lessen the frequency of surgical intervention is currently not clear. At present a trial of nutritional therapy is often indicated before surgery, for example in those patients requiring long-term continuous corticosteroids in whom an absolute indication for surgery does not exist.

Table 6.4 Indications for surgery in Crohn's disease

Intestinal obstruction
Intestinal fistula
Toxic megacolon
Haemorrhage
Perforation
Abscess
Failed medical treatment (including failed nutritional therapy)
Growth failure (some cases)

Perianal disease is rarely sufficiently severe to require proctectomy and can usually be managed conservatively, although drainage of abscesses is sometimes required.

Resection of ileocolonic disease is frequently complicated by fistulae and abscesses, and systemic complications such as arthritis or erythema nodosum (Korelitz et al 1968). However, the advent of nutritional therapy has provided a potent means of treating such disease and surgery will be required less often.

In intractable colonic disease a total proctocolectomy is the operation of choice, except in patients with relative sparing of the rectum, in whom an ileorectal anastomosis may be possible following medical treatment of the proctitis.

In children with small intestinal disease, the recurrence rate is less following local resection than in ileocolitis. Thus, children with only small intestinal disease have a reoperation rate of 3% at 1 year and 23% at 10 years compared to 10% and 65% respectively, when small bowel and colon are involved (Homer et al 1977).

The results of studies reporting the growth response to surgical resection in Crohn's disease are conflicting. At present, a relatively conservative approach to surgery is indicated when growth failure is the sole indication, particularly as nutritional therapy is likely to be more effective in inducing growth spurts. Growth following surgery is most likely to occur in the prepubertal child with a retarded bone age in whom all macroscopically abnormal bowel can be resected and when a sustained disease-free period follows surgery (Homer et al 1977).

Prognosis (Farmer 1981)

Comparison of published series outlining the prognosis in Crohn's disease is difficult because of differing treatment regimens, in particular the frequency of surgical intervention, and the extent to which steroids have been used. Furthermore, it is not yet known to what extent nutritional therapy will affect the long-term prognosis. In general, however, the long term prognosis of Crohn's disease beginning in childhood is fairly good. Most children go on to experience good general health and to lead productive lives, although morbidity during childhood and adolescence may be high (Puntis et al 1984). Despite a high morbidity, mortality is low; 2.4% of a large series of 522 patients died (Farmer & Michener 1979) and after 5 and 20 years of disease, the actuarial probability of survival was 98% and 89% respectively, of that expected.

The site of disease is an important determinant of morbidity and prognosis. Patients with colonic disease have more extraintestinal complications and operations, and fare worse in the long-term, than patients with small intestinal disease (Farmer & Michener 1979, Gryboski and Spiro 1978). This is in part related to a poorer response to drugs but also to a higher recurrence rate after surgery.

It has been suggested that the incidence of colorectal carcinoma in patients presenting with Crohn's disease under the age of 21 is greater than in a control population (Weedon et al 1973) but the exact risk requires further definition. Currently, the risk of developing colonic cancer does not justify prophylactic colectomy, although this view may need to be revised in the future as a larger number of patients are now surviving without colectomy as a result of successful medical therapy (Butt et al 1980).

ULCERATIVE COLITIS

Pathology

Ulcerative colitis is an inflammatory disease of the colonic mucosa. The rectum is almost invariably affected and although the entire colon may ultimately become involved, changes are usually most severe in the distal large bowel. The colon is usually reduced in length and there is loss of haustral pattern. In contrast to Crohn's disease, the inflammatory changes are always continuous and the mucosa has a granular haemorrhagic appearance and is extremely friable. Ulceration may be very superficial. It may be patchy, with intact, inflamed mucosa intervening, and adjacent to an area of ulcerated mucosa there may be vigorous proliferation of regenerating epithelium (pseudopolyps). Inflammation may also be present in the distal 5–25 cm of the terminal ileum ('back-wash' ileitis).

Microscopically, the inflammatory process is initially confined to the mucosa but may spread to the submucosa if the overlying epithelium is destroyed. Vascular congestion, crypt abscesses, loss of goblet cells, crypt branching and the appearance of Paneth cells within the crypts are all commonly seen, but none of these changes is diagnostic. Fibrosis is minimal, even in chronic disease. In fulminating disease, extensive mucosal ulceration is accompanied by severe destruction of submucosa to expose the colonic musculature, which may be covered only by a thin layer of granulation tissue.

In about 15% of cases of inflammatory bowel disease it is not possible to make a precise histological diagnosis as the features are not those of classical ulcerative colitis or Crohn's colitis. The term 'indeterminate colitis' is used to describe these appearances, but it is essentially a temporary classification. In most cases, subsequent clinical or pathological information allows a definitive diagnosis to be made.

Clinical features

Ulcerative colitis presents most commonly with bloody diarrhoea (Table 6.1), although this is not invariable, and blood may be absent from the stools. It is important to note that whilst 60% of children present with mild diarrhoea of insidious onset, with or without bleeding, 10% present with a fulminating colitis, possibly with toxic megacolon, and require emergency treatment when first seen (Werlin & Grand 1977). Nocturnal diarrhoea, marked tenesmus and urgency, colicky lower abdominal pain, anorexia and weight loss are signs of severe disease, whilst the presence of vomiting and severe pain and fever, indicate fulminating disease. On examination, there may be only minimal colonic tenderness in mild disease, whereas in severe cases the patient may be severely dehydrated, anaemic and febrile with marked tachycardia.

In children, the severity of fulminating colitis is easily underestimated by the inexperienced physician. The development of abdominal distension and tenderness, reduced or absent bowel sounds and persistent colonic gas shadows on a plain abdominal X-ray indicate the development of toxic megacolon. Surprisingly, the sedimentation rate may be normal in patients with fulminant colitis (Werlin & Grand 1977).

Diagnosis

Laboratory assessment

Stool culture is essential to exclude infection with an enteroinvasive organism, such as *Shigella, Salmonella, Campylobacter* or *Yersinia* as the cause of bloody diarrhoea. Microscopy of fresh stool for amoebae is indicated, together with assay of *C. difficile* toxin.

Haematological and biochemical investigation is useful in assessing disease severity; anaemia, erythrocyte sedimentation rate, leucocytosis, hypoalbuminaemia, hypokalaemia and hypomagnesaemia become more pronounced as the disease worsens.

Diagnostic imaging (Evers & Laufer 1983)

In mild and moderate disease, a plain film is usually normal, but in severe attacks, extensive ulceration, with thumbprinting created by oedematous mucosa may be seen, sometimes accompanied by colonic dilatation. In toxic megacolon the colon does not need to be grossly dilated and may be at its widest part (usually the transverse colon and splenic flexure) only 4 cm in diameter.

Barium enema. (See Table 5.2). A good double contrast enema is the procedure of preference whenever a barium enema is indicated. The barium enema should not be performed in a patient with active uncontrolled disease. In mild disease there may be no abnormality, or changes may be confined to the rectosigmoid region. Superficial mucosal ulceration is the earliest radiological lesion, but may be absent from the distal colon in patients receiving rectal steriods. Subsequently, loss of haustrations and deeper ulceration with mural thickening are seen, and the colon becomes shortened and tubular. In patients with pan-colitis, the last few centimetres of ileum may appear dilated and featureless, indicating a 'back-wash' ileitis.

Colonoscopy

Loss of the normal vascular pattern is the initial abnormality, followed by hyperaemia, granularity and contact bleeding. Subsequently, the haemorrhagic mucosa becomes patchily and superficially ulcerated, but without fissuring. Inflammatory polyposis, as distinct from the cobblestoning seen in Crohn's disease, is commonly seen in the colon. In contrast to Crohn's colitis, the disease is continuous and predominantly left-sided.

Differential diagnosis

Infective colitis, for example due to *Shigella, Salmonella, Campylobacter* or *Yersinia* is excluded by the identification of pathogens in the stool. Pseudomembranous colitis is uncommon in children (Buts et al 1977); almost always there is a history of previous exposure to antimicrobials and *C. difficile* toxin is found in the stools (Larsen & Price 1977). Endoscopy reveals raised, adherent, yellow-white mucosal plaques comprising crypt necrosis and replacement of the epithelium by a pseudomembrane of fibrin, mucous and inflammatory cells. Abdominal pain and bloody diarrhoea may accompany the haemolytic-uraemic syndrome, and colitis may dominate the clinical presentation and mimic ulcerative colitis (Tochen & Campbell 1977).

Ulcerative colitis may infrequently be associated with minimal gastrointestinal symptoms and present with chronic liver disease (Kane et al 1980).

Ulcerative colitis can be differentiated from Crohn's disease involving the colon in 85% of cases, on the basis of a combined clinical, radiological, endoscopic and histological assessment, as previously discussed (Tedesco 1980). Allergic colitis usually presents in infancy; where typically a strong family history of atopy, eosinophilia, raised total IgE and radioallergosorbent (RAST) titres, and positive skin prick tests. Although the appearance of the colon may be indistinguishable from ulcerative colitis, histology reveals a marked increase in eosinophils in the lamina propria (Jenkins et al 1984). Symptoms remit promptly with the institution of an allergen avoidance (usually cows milk and/or soya free) diet (see Ch. 23).

Complications

Intestinal

Anal fissures and intestinal strictures and fistulae occur much less frequently in ulcerative colitis than in Crohn's disease. Massive haemorrhage can occur during fulminating episodes (Werlin & Grand 1977), but the two most important local complications are toxic megacolon and carcinoma.

There is an increased incidence of carcinoma of the colon and rectum after 10 years of ulcerative pan-colitis. In a large retrospective study, the incidence of carcinoma complicating pan-colitis beginning in childhood was found to be 20% per decade after the first 10 years, (Devroede et al 1971). These data were obtained, however, when colectomy was unusual and probably from a group of patients with severe colitis. The current risks are probably considerably less than this. Lennard-Jones et al (1977) reported an incidence of one in 200 for each year of disease between 10 and 20 years, and one in 60 thereafter. In patients with a left-sided colitis or proctitis, the risks appear to be considerably smaller (Butt et al 1980).

Commonly, epithelial dysplasia precedes the development of invasive carcinoma, and, although dysplastic lesions are often patchy, carcinoma without associated dysplasia is rare (Morson & Dawson 1979, Butt et al 1980). When carcinoma does complicate colitis, the outlook is the same as that for colorectal carcinoma in general (Butt et al 1980), although the younger patient has a substantially poorer prognosis than the older.

Extraintestinal (Greenstein et al 1976)

Joint, skin and eyes. Asymmetric arthritis of the large joints in the lower limbs is the most common extraintestinal manifestation in ulcerative colitis (Lindsley & Schaller 1974). It occurs in about one quarter of patients, usually during exacerbations of disease. Spondylitis occurs in about 4% of patients with ulcerative colitis and is usually in association with HLA-B27. Erythema nodosum and pyoderma gangrenosum are the most frequent skin manifestations and occur in about 5% of patients. Stomatitis and ocular disorders occur in 4% although the incidence of asymptomatic uveitis may be as high as 30%, particularly in boys (Daum et al 1979).

Liver Disease. The incidence and the spectrum of liver disease occuring in ulcerative colitis are very similar to those in Crohn's disease (Dew et al 1979). Proctocolectomy may result in arrest or regression of the liver disease, but surgery is rarely indicated on this basis alone (Eade et al 1970).

Nephrolithiasis. Renal stones occur in about 5% of patients but the incidence is increased following colectomy and ileostomy, possibly as a result of the reduced urinary volume which follows colectomy (Singer et al 1973). Urate stones have been reported following ileostomy in ulcerative colitis, presumably because of intestinal loss of alkali and the consequent urinary acidification (Brewer et al 1970).

Growth retardation. Short stature occurs in children with ulcerative colitis, but less frequently than in Crohn's disease and affects less than one fifth of patients at presentation (Berger et al 1975). When present, the same treatment should be instituted as discussed above for growth failure in children with Crohn's disease. Proctocolectomy, in the prepubertal child with growth failure due to ulcerative colitis, should be curative and followed by return to genetic growth potential (Berger et al 1975).

Medical management

The aims of medical therapy in mild to moderate disease are to induce and to maintain remission. The aim in fulminating colitis is to save life, by colectomy if necessary.

Mild attack

Patients with diarrhoea and abdominal pain but little bleeding or systemic upset, usually respond to sulphasalazine. (30–50 mg/kg/24 h) and do not require systemic corticosteroids. Those children with distal disease confined to the rectum or when proctitis is severe causing marked tenesmus, may respond to a topical steroid preparation. Although hydrocortisone foam is more easily retained than a liquid preparation, it penetrates only as far as the sigmoid colon. There is no evidence that dietary manipulation aids the induction of remission in ulcerative colitis but it is sensible to avoid foods, usually those high in residue, which exacerbate diarrhoea. An agent which reduces motility, such as loperamide, is often helpful in reducing frequency of bowel movements and urgency.

Moderate attack

Patients with bloody diarrhoea, passed more than six times per 24 hours, associated with colicky abdominal pain, tenesmus, mild constitutional upset, anorexia, weight loss, low-grade fever, leucocytosis and mild anaemia should be admitted to hospital and require oral corticosteroids. Prednisone or prednisolone (1–2 mg/kg/24 h) are equally effective when given either as a single daily dose or in four divided doses (Powell-Tuck et al 1978). The dose of corticosteroids is reduced progressively after one or two weeks, by which time clinical improvement, if it is to take place, has occurred.

A recent study has suggested that adrenocorticotrophic hormone (ACTH) given daily over 8 hours by intravenous infusion is more efficacious in controlling an attack of ulcerative colitis when it is given for a first episode or when the patient has been off corticosteroid therapy for some time (Meyers et al 1983).

Anticholinergics, opioids and their analogues, such as loperamide, are contraindicated as they may precipitate the development of a toxic megacolon (Binder et al 1974). In addition to corticosteroids, correction of fluid, electrolyte, nutrient and blood deficits is of great importance. Serum concentrations of albumin should not be allowed to fall below 25 g/l or haemoglobin below 9 g/dl. Magnesium deficiency is an important complication of any diarrhoeal disorder including colitis (Grand & Colodny 1972). Because total body magnesium status is only poorly reflected in plasma levels, deficiency is not always accompanied by hypomagnesaemia (Harris & Wilkinson 1971), and diagnosis rests upon the urinary excretion of less than 40% of a test dose of parenteral magnesium in 24 hours (Harris & Wilkinson 1971).

There is good evidence from controlled trials that sulphasalazine has a prophylactic as well as a therapeutic effect in ulcerative colitis (Misiewicz et al 1965). Thus, once an improvement on corticosteroids has begun, sulphasalazine may be given in the hope of accelerating and then maintaining remission when corticosteroids are reduced. Patients who might be susceptible, (non-Caucasians and Mediterraneans) should have a preliminary red cell glucose-6-phosphate dehydrogenase screen before starting treatment, and all patients on long-term sulphasalazine should have regular haematological tests to detect the presence of blood dyscrasias, which are sometimes associated with its use. Because sulphasalazine is associated with impaired folate absorption (Reisenauer & Halsted 1981) it seems sensible to prescribe folic acid (1.0 mg/24 h) concurrently.

Whilst 70–80% of patients with active disease will respond to corticosteroids and go into remission, the role of corticosteroids in prophylaxis seems limited. Moderate doses (15 mg/24 h of prednisolone) are no better than placebo in maintaining remission in adults (Lennard-Jones et al 1965), with some patients developing symptoms as soon as the high dose of corticosteroids is reduced, often at about 10–15 mg prednisolone/24 h. Although larger doses may have a role, it is only at the expense of unacceptable side effects, even when dosage occurs on an alternate day basis. If sulphasalazine and topical steroids are already being used in such steroid-dependent patients, there may be a role for azathioprine, which has a steroid-sparing effect in chronic active ulcerative colitis (Kirk & Lennard-Jones 1982). However, a child requiring long-term doses of corticosteroids sufficiently high to produce significant side effects or to require azathioprine, may benefit more from colectomy than from immunosuppressives. The long-term effects of immunosuppressives are unknown, but may include an increased incidence of malignancy (Kinlen et al 1979).

Early encouraging reports regarding the use of disodium cromoglycate in ulcerative proctitis and colitis (Heatley et al 1975), have not been supported by controlled studies (Buckell et al 1978).

A controlled trial of parenteral nutrition in patients with moderate or severe disease failed to show any benefit compared with steroids (Dickinson et al 1980). The correction of malnutrition is however mandatory in all patients.

Fulminating attack

This is a grave, easily underestimated, medical emergency. The features are listed in Table 6.5. Referral to a centre experienced in its management and

Table 6.5 Characteristics of fulminating colitis (after Werlin & Grand 1977)

Major features

Severe bloody diarrhoea > 5/day
Oral temperature > 38° during first hospital day
Tachycardia (pulse > 90)
Anaemia (haematocrit < 30%) allowing for transfusion
Hypoalbuminaemia (< 3.0 g/100 ml)
Toxic megacolon

Associated features

Leucocytosis
Raised erythrocyte sedimentation rate (ESR)
Hypokalaemia
Hypomagnesaemia

the adoption of a team approach, with the involvement of physicians, surgeons, nurses, psychiatrists and social workers is highly desirable.

Intravenous correction of fluid and electrolyte deficits will be necessary in all patients, and most will require blood transfusions and frequent albumin infusions. Major emergency surgery in children in the presence of a low serum albumin and hence a low circulating plasma volume, is a particularly hazardous undertaking. All patients require parenteral corticosteroids, given as hydrocortisone 10 mg/kg/24 h, or alternatively as prednisolone 2.0 mg/kg/24 h, which produces less sodium retention. Most patients receive parenteral broad-spectrum antibiotics empirically (e.g. penicillin, gentamicin and metronidazole). Many patients are markedly catabolic and parenteral nutrition is usually indicated on these grounds alone. The importance of frequent haematological and biochemical monitoring and clinical observation cannot be overemphasized. Development of abdominal distension with increasing tachycardia, fever and leucocytosis are signs of a developing toxic megacolon, and erect and supine plain abdominal X-rays, performed twice daily, are essential. Frequent changes of bed position with or without a long nasoenteric suction tube may reduce the risk of toxic megacolon (Present et al 1981)

About one third of children respond to medical treatment within 12 days; a much smaller proportion respond thereafter and continuing medical treatment beyond 12 days is associated with a substantially increased incidence of complications (Werlin & Grand 1977). Over half the patients require early surgery (within 2 months) because of failed medical treatment, massive bleeding, colonic perforation or toxic megacolon. The majority of children who respond to medical treatment, come to colectomy within 2 years (Werlin & Grand 1977).

Toxic megacolon

With increasingly severe fulminating colitis, the development of a toxic megacolon is indicated by abdominal distension and tenderness, paucity or absence of bowel sounds and the persistence of colonic gas shadows on plain abdominal X-rays, sometimes with isolated islands of oedematous mucosa. The patient appears ill, febrile and marked hypoalbuminaemia and electrolyte disturbances are almost invariably present. Gram-negative septicaemia and massive haemorrhage may occur. Colonic perforation is indicated by increased distension and tenderness, and confirmed by free intraperitoneal gas on a lateral decubitus film. The clinical signs of this life-threatening complication may be masked by concomitant corticosteroid therapy. In the series by Werlin & Grand (1977), a toxic megacolon developed in 3 out of 19 patients with severe colitis. Initial management is as outlined for fulminating colitis, bearing in mind the need for regular plain abdominal X-rays and the possibility of perforation.

It is essential not to persist with medical management unless there is unequivocal and objective evidence of rapid improvement. Prolonged medical treatment is associated with a 30% mortality, and of those dying under medical management, there is a 33% incidence of perforation which carries an 82% mortality without surgery. Even if surgery is performed following perforation, the mortality is 51% (Kirsner 1974). Early colectomy (within 48 to 72 hours) is therefore indicated in the absence of rapid improvement following the institution of intensive medical treatment. Most children who develop a toxic megacolon come to early colectomy, and it is therefore important to prepare parents and child for this eventuality early in the course of a fulminating illness.

Surgery (Telander et al 1981)

The indications for surgery are summarized in Table 6.6.

Table 6.6 Indications for surgery in ulcerative colitis

Emergency
Fulminating colitis with no response to intensive medical treatment, within 2 weeks
Toxic megacolon, not improving within 48–72 hours of intensive medical treatment, or manifest deterioration following initiation of medical therapy
Massive haemorrhage
Colonic perforation

Elective
Failed medical treatment (chronic ill health, unacceptable steroid-induced side effects, substantial loss of schooling, growth failure)
Patients with relatively quiescent pan-colitis of 10 or more years duration in whom long-term colonoscopic follow-up is not possible or where colectomy is preferred by the patients
Severe colonic dysplasia persisting over several months, present at multiple sites or associated with lesions
Severe extraintestinal manifestations, intractable to medical therapy

Emergency

In emergencies, subtotal colectomy with mucous fistula and terminal ileostomy is the procedure of choice. The simultaneous removal of the rectum in these circumstances increases mortality and morbidity considerably and complications in the retained rectum in the immediate postoperative period are few. The retained rectum may, however, subsequently be the site of continuing inflammation, with a purulent or mucous discharge from the anus or mucous fistula. When symptoms persist for longer than 6–12 months, proctectomy is advisable particularly as the retained rectum remains a potential site for development of carcinoma. Furthermore, the extraintestinal manifestations of ulcerative colitis may continue until both colon and rectum are excised (Alexander-Williams & Buchmann 1980). Removal of the rectum may be followed later by the construction of a continent Kock ileostomy or an ileal reservoir and anal anastomosis. There is however little experience of ileoanal anastomosis in childhood.

An occasional patient may have such mild rectal disease following sub-total colectomy that an ileorectal anastomosis is possible.

Elective

The precise timing of elective surgery should take into account not only the symptoms and the complications of chronically active disease but also important milestones in the child's educational and psychosocial development. It is very important to prepare the child and parents psychologically before colectomy and a decision should be made in the light of advice from physician, surgeon, psychiatrist and stoma therapist, all of whom should be experienced in the management of inflammatory bowel disease in children.

The choices of surgical procedures are as follows.

1. Proctocolectomy with terminal ileostomy

Although this operation is curative and has been used with great success, it involves loss of the rectum and a permanent ileostomy. The ileal mucosa adapts following colectomy and the volume of effluent decreases in the weeks after surgery, but the loss of about 500 ml fluid per day containing sodium (100–130 mmol/l), predisposes the patient to dehydration and renal calculi; proteolytic enzymes within the ileostomy effluent may also cause skin soreness and ulceration unless stoma care is scrupulous. With modern surgical techniques, impotence in the male and dyspareunia in the female are much less common than previously. Provided that appropriate preparation is made, the psychosocial adjustment of children and adolescents with a stoma is very good (Hyams et al 1982).

2. Proctocolectomy and continent ileostomy (Kock pouch)

This procedure is curative. A conventional terminal ileostomy is replaced by a pouch of terminal small intestine with a nipple valve on the efferent loop which renders the stoma continent (Kock 1973). The pouch is emptied three to four times a day by means of a catheter. The quality of life with this ileostomy is better than with the standard type (Telander et al 1981).

3. Proctocolectomy with ileal reservoir and anal anastomosis (Parks pouch)

In this procedure, which has not yet been widely used, all the diseased large bowel mucosa is removed but the anal sphincter is preserved. A small intestinal pouch is constructed within the pelvis and exteriorized by means of an endoanal anastomosis (Parks et al 1980). Spontaneous, controlled evacuation is the aim, but about half of the patients require catheterization. The operation has the advantage of not requiring an abdominal stoma.

4. Colectomy with rectal mucosectomy and endorectal pull-through

This procedure utilizes the fact that ulcerative colitis is a mucosal disease. In addition to colectomy, the diseased rectal mucosa is removed, but the anorectal musculature preserved. The terminal ileum is then placed inside the retained muscular wall of the rectum and anastomosed to the anus (Martin et al 1977). As a result, all diseased mucosa is resected, while at the same time anorectal continence is preserved. This procedure, although still relatively new, has been performed with extremely encoraging results in young patients (Martin et al 1977, Fonkalsrud et al 1979, Telander & Perrault 1981), a good result being obtained in 70 to 90%. Nearly all patients are able to distinguished between flatus and fluid, have good anal sphincter tone and experience voluntary rectal control. Because the rectal musculature is left in situ, the risk of impotence in the male, or bladder dysfunction, is virtually eliminated. The formation of a neorectum by either the use of a balloon catheter to dilate the terminal ileum (Telander & Perrault 1981) or by the construction of an internal ileal reservoir (Fonkalsrud 1980) appears to decrease the frequency of stooling. The frequency of bowel actions diminishes gradually during the first year, to about 5–6 times per day, and once or twice at night. (Telander & Perrault 1981). Although in early series postoperative complications were fairly frequent, these are now considerably less, but the procedure remains surgically demanding and the question of whether any unresected islands of rectal mucosa constitute a risk of cancer remains unanswered.

Prognosis

Although 10% of patients with ulcerative colitis with onset in childhood or adolescence will experience only one episode, the rest will have further symptoms. About 20% have only intermittent symptoms and remain well between flare-ups, 50% have chronic but not incapacitating disease, while the remaining 20% have chronically active incapacitating disease (Michener et al 1979). One third of patients require a colectomy (Michener et al 1979) and provided the rectal mucosa is also removed, subsequent life expectancy is normal (Devroede et al 1971). In disease confined to the rectum or distal colon, the prognosis is good in 90%, with only 10% experiencing progression to pan-colitis. In 75% the disease resolves completely, and in 15% intermittent symptoms continue (Farmer 1981).

The long-term risks of colorectal carcinoma in patients with colitis have been discussed. The advent of colonoscopy makes it possible to examine the entire colon, both by direct inspection and microscopically. There is therefore an argument in favour of sigmoidoscopy and biopsy every 6–12 months, and colonoscopy every 2 years, in place of colectomy for patients with pan-colitis of 8–10 years duration. In addition to the detection of frank carcinoma, regular examination with biopsies makes it possible to detect precancerous mucosal dysplasia. Severe dysplasia persisting over several months should be regarded as precancerous, as should severe dysplasia present at multiple sites, or in association with a macroscopic lesion (Butt et al 1980). Proctocolectomy should then be advised. At present, the question of regular, long-term surveillance versus prophylactic colectomy is unanswered. In the younger patient with 10 years of pan-colitis, prophylactic surgery may be preferable in view of the very prolonged follow-up necessary, uncertainties about the efficiency of colon-oscopy in detecting precancerous changes, the recent availability of conti-nent ileostomies or mucosal proctectomy and ileal pull-through operations, and the facility with which young patients adapt to a stoma (Hyams et al 1982).

Psychosocial support (Farmer 1981)

Inflammatory bowel disease in childhood often presents the child and family with many years of chronic ill health, and multiple visits to hospital. In Crohn's disease in particular, the disease is often at its most aggressive in the years immediately after onset and it is under these circumstances that a team approach should be adopted, with physician, psychiatrist, social worker, clinical psychologist and nursing staff pooling their resources in order to support the child and his family. Not only will this type of approach improve the patient's sense of well-being, but it may also reduce the number of relapses in ulcerative colitis. While there is no good evidence that psychological factors are aetiologically important, symptoms are often worse at times of stress, and patients and their families often need help in dealing with this. At present, however, psychological intervention has not been shown to alter the long-term course of inflammatory bowel disease.

Self-help groups
The following is a list of self-help groups:
National Association for Colitis and Crohn's Disease, 3 Thorpefield Close, Marshalswick, St. Albans, Herts, UK
Crohn's in Childhood Research Appeal, 48 Ewell Down's Road, Ewell, Epsom, Surrey KT17 3BN, UK
Ileostomy Association, Amblehurst House, Chobham, Woking, Surrey GU24 8PZ, UK
National Foundation for Ileitis and Colitis, 444 Park Avenue South, New York, 10016, USA

REFERENCES

Aggett P J, Harries J T 1979 Current status of zinc in health and disease states. Archives of Disease in Childhood 54: 909–917
Alexander-Williams J, Buchmann P 1980 Criteria of assessment for suitability and results of ileorectal anastomosis. Clinics in Gastroenterology 9: 409–417
Bartnik W, Shorter R G 1980 Inflammatory bowel disease: Immunologic developments. In: Berk J E (ed) Developments in digestive diseases. Lea and Febiger, Philadelphia. 3: 109–127
Beeken W L 1973 Absorptive defects in young people with regional enteritis. Pediatrics 53: 69–74
Beeken W L, Kanich R E 1973 Microbial flora of the upper small bowel in Crohn's disease. Gastroenterology 65: 390–397
Berger M, Gribetz D, Korelitz B I 1975 Growth retardation in children with ulcerative colitis: the effect of medical and surgical therapy. Pediatrics 55: 459–467
Betts P R, Magrath G 1974 Growth pattern and dietary intake of children with chronic renal insufficiency. British Medical Journal 2: 1017–1021
Binder S C, Patterson J F, Glotzer D J 1974 Toxic megacolon in ulcerative colitis. Gastroenterology 66: 1088–1090
Brandt, Bernstein L H, Boley S J, Frank M S 1982 Metronidazole therapy for perirectal Crohn's disease: a follow-up study. Gastroenterology 83: 383–387

Brewer R I, Gelzayd E A, Kirsner J K 1970 Urinary crystalloid excretion in patients with inflammatory bowel disease. Gut 11: 314–318

Buchmann P, Alexander-Williams J 1980 Classification of perianal Crohn's disease. Clinics in Gastroenterology 9: 323–330

Buckell N A, Gould S R, Day D W, Lennard-Jones J E, Edwards A M 1978 Controlled trial of disodium cromoglycate in chronic persistent ulcerative colitis. Gut 19: 1140–1143

Burbige E J, Huang S S, Bayless T M 1975 Clinical manifestations of Crohn's disease in children and adolescents. Pediatrics 55: 866–871

Buts J P, Weber A A, Roy C C, Morin C L 1977 Pseudomembranous enterocolitis in children. Gastroenterology 78: 823–827

Butt J H, Lennard-Jones J E, Ritchie J K 1980 A practical approach to the risk of cancer in inflammatory bowel disease. Medical Clinics of North America 64: 1203–1220

Campbell C A, Walker-Smith J A, Hindocha P, Adinolfi M 1982 Acute phase proteins in chronic inflammatory bowel disease in childhood. Journal of Pediatric Gastroenterology and Nutrition 1: 193–200

Cave D R, Mitchell D N, Kane S P, Brooke B N 1973 Further animal evidence of a transmissible agent in Crohn's disease. Lancet ii: 1120–1122

Cave D R, Mitchell D N, Brooke B N 1976 Preliminary evidence of an agent from ulcerative colitis tissue. Lancet i: 1311–1314

Cooke W T, Mallas E, Prior P, Allan R N 1980 Crohn's disease: course, treatment and long term prognosis. Quarterly Journal of Medicine 49: 363–384

Daniels G E 1948 Psychiatric factors in ulcerative colitis. Gastroenterology 10: 59–62

Daum F, Gould H B, Gold D, Dinari G, Friedman A H, Zucker P, Cohen M I 1979 Asymptomatic transient uveitis in children with inflammatory bowel disease. American Journal of Diseases of Children 133: 170–171

Devroede G J, Taylor W F, Sauer W, Jackman R G, Stickler G B 1971 Cancer risk and life expectancy of children with ulcerative colitis. New England Journal of Medicine 285: 17–21

Dew M J, Thompson H, Allan R N 1979 The spectrum of hepatic dysfunction in inflammatory bowel disease. Quarterly Journal Medicine 48: 113–135

Dickinson J R, Ashton M G, Axon A T R, Smith R C, Yeung C K, Hill G L 1980 Controlled trial of intravenous hyperalimentation and total bowel rest as an adjunct to the routine therapy of acute colitis. Gastroenterology 79: 1199–1204

Dobbins J W, Binder H J 1977 Importance of the colon in enteric hyperoxaluria. New England Journal of Medicine 296: 298–301

Drife J O 1982 Drugs and sperm. British Medical Journal 284: 844–845

Driscoll R H, Rosenberg I H 1978 Total parenteral nutrition in inflammatory bowel disease. Pediatric Clinics of North America 62: (1) 185–201

Eade M N, Cooke W T, Brooke B N 1970 Liver disease in ulcerative colitis. II. The long term effect of colectomy. Annals of Internal Medicine 72: 489–497

Evers K, Laufer I 1983 Ulcerative colitis: radiology. In: Allan R N et al (eds) Inflammatory Bowel Diseases. Churchill Livingstone, Edinburgh, pp 177–193

Eyer S, Spadaccini C, Walker P, Ansel H, Schwartz M, Sumner H W 1980 Simultaneous ulcerative colitis and Crohn's disease. American Journal of Gastroenterology 73: 345–349

Farmer R G, Michener W M 1979 Prognosis of Crohn's disease with onset in childhood or adolescence. Digestive Diseases and Sciences 24: 752–757

Farmer R G, Michener W M, Mortimer E A 1980 Studies of family history among patients with inflammatory bowel disease. Clinical Gastroenterology 9: 271–278

Farmer R G 1981 Factors in the long-term prognosis of patients with inflammatory bowel disease. American Journal of Gastroenterology 75: 97–103

Fonkalsrud E W 1980 Total colectomy and endorectal ileal pull-through with internal ileal reservoir for ulcerative colitis. Surgery 150: 1–8

Fonkalsrud E W, Ament M E, Byrne W J 1979 Clinical experience with total colectomy and endorectal mucosal resection for inflammatory bowel disease. Gastroenterology 77: 156–160

Foster K J, Karran S J 1980 The role of hormones in intravenous feeding. In: Karran S J, Alberti K G, (eds) Practical Nutritional Support. Pitman Medical, London. pp 149–159

Freese D, Latimer J S, Gilberstadt S, Kane W, Sharp H 1980 Therapeutic response of the pericholangitis in the liver lesion associated with inflammatory bowel disease (IBD). Gastroenterology 78:1168A.

Gazzard B G, Price H L, Libby G W, Dawson A M 1978 The social toll of Crohn's disease. British Medical Journal 2: 1117–1119

Gilat T 1982 Metronidazole in Crohn's disease. Gastroenterology 83: 702–704

Gilat T 1983 Indicence of inflammatory bowel disease: going up or down? Gastroenterology 85: 196–197

Ginsburg C, Dambrauskas J T, Ault Ka, Falchuk Z M 1983 Impaired natural killer cell activity in patients with inflammatory bowel disease: evidence for a qualitative defect. Gastroenterology 85: 846–51

Golden M N H, Golden B E 1981 Trace elements: potential importance in human nutrition with particular reference to zinc and vanadium. British Medical Bulletin 37: 31–36

Goode A, Hawkins T, Teggetter J G W, Johnston I D A 1976 Use of an elemental diet for long term nutritional support in Crohn's disease. Lancet I: 122–124

Gordon I, Vivian G 1984 Radiolabelled leucocytes: a new diagnostic tool in occult infection/inflammation. Archives of Disease in Childhood 59: 62–66

Grand R J, Colodny A H 1972 Increased requirement for magnesium during parenteral therapy for granulomatous colitis. Journal of Pediatrics 81: 788–790

Greenstein A J, Janowitz H D, Sachar D B 1976 The extra-intestinal complications of Crohn's disease and ulcerative colitis: a study of 700 patients. Medicine 55: 401–412

Gryboski J D, Spiro H M 1978 Prognosis in children with Crohn's disease. Gastroenterology 74: 807–817

Gryboski J D, Hillemeier C 1980 Inflammatory bowel disease in children. Medical Clinics of North America 64: 1185–1202

Harries A D, Fitz Simons E, Fifield R, Dew M J, Rhodes J 1983 Platelet count: a simple measure of activity in Crohn's disease. British Medical Journal 286:1476

Harris I, Wilkinson A W 1971 Magnesium depletion in children. Lancet 2: 735–736

Heatley R V, Calcraft B J, Rhodes J, Owen E, Evans B K 1975 Disodium cromoglycate in the treatment of chronic proctitis. Gut 16: 559–563

Helzer J E, Chammas S, Norland C C, Stillings W A, Alpers D H 1984 A study of the association between Crohn's disease and psychiatric illness. Gastroenterology 86: 324–330

Hodgson H J F, Potter B J, Jewell D P 1977 Immune complexes in ulcerative colitis and Crohn's disease. Clinical and Experimental Immunology 29: 87–196

Holdsworth C D 1981 Sulphasalazine desensitisation. British Medical Journal 282:110

Homer D R, Grand R J, Colodny A 1977 Growth, course and prognosis after surgery for Crohn's disease in children and adolescents. Pediatrics 59: 717–725

Hyams J S, Grand R J, Colodny A H, Schuster Sr, Eraklis A 1982 Course and prognosis after colectomy and ileostomy for inflammatory bowel disease in childhood and adolescence. Journal of Pediatric Surgery 17: 400–405

Jenkins H R, Pincott J R, Soothill J F, Milla P J, Harries J T 1984 Food allergy: the major cause of infantile colitis. Archives of Disease in Childhood 59: 326–329

Jones J H, Lennard-Jones J E 1966 Corticosteroids and corticotrophin in the treatment of Crohn's disease. Gut 7: 181–187

Kane W, Miller K, Sharp H L, 1980 Inflammatory bowel disease presenting as liver disease during childhood. Journal of Pediatrics 97: 775–778

Kelts D G, Grand R J, Shen G, Watkins J B, Werlin S L, Boehme C 1979 Nutritional basis of growth failure in children and adolescents with Crohn's disease. Gastroenterology 76: 720–727

Khojasteh A, Haghshenass M, Haghighi P 1983 Immunoproliferative small intestinal disease. New England Journal of Medicine 308: 1401–1405

Kinlen L J, Sheil A G R, Peto J, Doll R 1979 Collaborative United Kingdom-Australasian study of cancer in patients treated with immunosuppressive drugs. British Medical Journal 2: 1461–1466

Kirk A P, Lennard-Jones J E 1982 Controlled trial of azathioprine in chronic ulcerative colitis. British Medical Journal 284: 1291–1292

Kirschner B S, Klich J R, Kalman S S, de Favaro M V, Rosenberg I H, 1981 Reversal of growth retardation in Crohn's disease with therapy emphasising oral nutritional restitution. Gastroenterology 80: 10–15

Kirsner J B, 1974 Toxic megacolon complicating ulcerative colitis: current therapeutic perspectives. Gastroenterology 66: 1088–1090

Kirsner J B, Shorter R G 1982 Recent developments in nonspecific inflammatory bowel disease. New England Journal of Medicine 306: 837–848

Kock N G 1973 Continent ileostomy. In: Allgower M, Bergents S E, Calne R Y (eds) Progress in Surgery. Karger, Basel. 12: 180–201

Korelitz B I, Gribetz D, Kopel F B 1968 Granulomatous colitis in children: a study of 25 cases and comparison with ulcerative colitis. Pediatrics 42: 446–457

Krawitt E L, Beeken W L, Janney C D 1976 Calcium absorption in Crohn's disease. Gastroenterology 71: 251–254

Larsen H E, Price A B 1977 Pseudomembranous colitis: presence of clostridial toxin. Lancet ii: 1312–1314

Layden T, Rosenberg J, Nemchausky B, Elson C. Rosenberg I 1976 Reversal of growth arrest in adolescents with Crohn's disease after parenteral alimentation. Gastroenterology 70: 1017–1021

Lee J R 1983 The radiological features of Crohn's disease. In: Allan R N, Keighley M R B, Alexander-Williams J, Hawkins C (eds) Inflammatory Bowel Diseases. Churchill Livingstone, Edinburgh. pp 376–391

Lennard-Jones J E, Morson B C, Ritchie J K, Shove D C, Williams C B 1977 Cancer in colitis: an assessment of the individual risk by clinical and histological criteria. Gastroenterology 73: 1280–1289

Lennard-Jones J E, Misiewicz J J, Connell A M, Baron J H, Avery-Jones F 1965 Prednisone as maintenance treatment for ulcerative colitis in remission. Lancet i: 188–189

Lindsley C B, Schaller J G 1974 Arthritis associated with inflammatory bowel disease in children. Journal of Pediatrics 84: 16–20

Lloyd-Still J D, Green O C 1979 A clinical scoring system for chronic inflammatory bowel disease in children. Digestive Diseases and Sciences 24: (8) 620–624

McClain C, Soutor C, Zieve L 1980 Zinc deficiency: a complication of Crohn's disease. Gastroenterology 78: 272–279

Martin L W, Le Coultre C, Schubert W K 1977 Total colectomy and mucosal proctectomy with preservation of continence in ulcerative colitis. Annals of Surgery 186: 477–480

Mendeloff A I, Mark M, Siegel C, Lilienfeld A M 1970 Illness experience and the stresses in patients with irritable colon and ulcerative colitis. New England Journal of Medicine 282: 14–17

Merritt R J, Blackburn G L 1981 Nutritional assessment and metabolic response to illness of the hospitalised child. In: Suskind R M (ed) Textbook of Pediatric Nutrition. Raven Press, New York. pp 285–308

Meyers S, Sachar D B, Goldberg J D, Janowitz H D 1983 Corticotrophin versus hydrocortisone in the intravenous treatment of ulcerative colitis. A prospective, randomised double-blind clinical trial. Gastroenterology 85: 351–357

Michener W M, Farmer R G, Mortimer E A 1979 Long-term prognosis of ulcerative colitis with onset in childhood or adolescence. Journal of Clinical Gastroenterology 1: 301–305

Misiewicz J J, Lennard-Jones J E, Connell A, Baron J H, Avery-Jones F 1965 Controlled trial of sulphasalazine in maintenance therapy for ulcerative colitis. Lancet i: 185–188

Moriarty K J, Hegarty J E, Clarke M, Fairclough P D, Dawson A M 1981 A comparison of the relative nitrogen-sparing properties of whole protein, protein hydrolysate, and the equivalent amino acid mixture in man. Gastroenterology 80:1234

Morin C L, Roulet M, Roy C C, Weber A 1980 Continuous elemental enteral alimentation in children with Crohn's disease and growth failure. Gastroenterology 79: 1205–1210

Morson B C, Dawson I M P 1979 Gastrointestinal Pathology. Blackwell, Oxford, 293–312, 523–551

Motil K J, Grand R J, Maletskos C J, Young V R 1982a The effect of disease, drug and diet on whole body protein metabolism in adolescents with Crohn's disease and growth failure. Journal of Pediatrics 101: 345–351

Motil K J, Grand R J, Matthews D E, Bier D M, Maletskos C S, Young V R 1982b Whole body leucine metabolism in adolescents with Crohn's disease and growth failure during nutritional supplementation. Gastroenterology 82: 1359–1368

Nolan D J 1981 Barium examination of the small intestine. Gut 22: 682–694

O'Donoghue D P, Dawson A M 1977 Crohn's disease in childhood. Archives of Disease in Children 52: 627–632

O'Morain C A, Segal A W, Levi A J 1984 Elemental diets in the treatment of acute Crohn's disease: a controlled study. British Medical Journal 288: 1859–1862

Parks A G, Nicholls R J, Belliveau P 1980 Proctocolectomy with ileal reservoir and anal anastomosis. British Journal of Surgery 67: 533–538

Poley J R, Hoffman A F 1976 Role of fat maldigestion in pathogenesis of steatorrhoea in ileal resection. Gastroenterology 71: 38–44

Powell-Tuck J, Brown R L, Lennard-Jones J E 1978 A comparison of oral prednisolone given as single or multiple daily doses for active proctocolitis. Scandinavian Journal of Gastroenterology 13: 833–837

Powell-Tuck J, Garlick P J, Lennard-Jones J E, Waterlow J C 1984 Rates of whole body protein synthesis and break down increase with the severity of inflammatory bowel disease. Gut 25: 460–464

Present D H, Korelitz B I, Wisch N, Glass J L, Sachar D B, Pasternack B S 1980 Treatment of Crohn's disease with 6-mercaptopurine. New England Journal of Medicine 302 (18): 981–987

Present D H, Wolfson D, Gelernt I M, Rabin P H, Bauer J, Chapman M L 1981 The medical management of toxic megacolon. Gastroenterology 80:1255A

Puntis J, McNeish A S, Allan R N 1984 Long-term prognosis of Crohn's disease with onset in childhood and adolescence. Gut 25: 329–336

Reisenauer A M, Halsted C H 1981 Human jejunal brush border folate conjugase. Characteristics and inhibition by salicylazosulfapyridine. Biochemica Biophysica Acta 659: 62–69

Sachar D B, Auslander M O, Walfish J S 1980 Aetiological theories of inflammatory bowel disease. Clinical Gastroenterology 9: 231–257

Savery Muttu S H, Peters A M, Lavender J P, Hodgson H J, Chadwick V S 1983 [111]Indium autologous leucocytes in inflammatory bowel disease. Gut 24: 293–299

Singer A M, Bennett R C, Carter N G, Hughes E S R 1973 Blood and urinary changes in patients with ileostomies and ileorectal anastomosis. British Medical Journal 3: 141–143

Strickland R G, Sachar D B 1977 The immunology of inflammatory bowel disease. In: Jerzy Glass (ed) Progress in Gastroenterology Volume III. GB. pp 821–838

Strobel C T, Byrne W J, Ament M E 1979 Home parenteral nutrition in inflammatory bowel disease. Pediatric Clinics of North America 62: (1) 185–201

Summers F W, Smitz D M, Sessions J T Jr, Becktel J M, Best W R, Kern F Jr, Singleton J W 1979 National Co-operative Crohn's disease study: Results of drug treatment. Gastroenterology 77: 847–869

Tedesco F J 1980 Differential diagnosis of ulcerative colitis and Crohn's ileocolitis and other specific inflammatory disease of the bowel. Medical Clinics of North America 64: 1173–1183

Telander R L, Smith S L, Marcinek H M, O'Fallon W M, Van Heerden J A, Perrault J 1981 Surgical treatment of ulcerative colitis in children. Surgery 90: 787–794

Telander R L, Perrault J 1981 Colectomy with rectal mucosectomy and ileoanal anastomosis in young patients. Archives of Surgery 116: 623–629

Tochen M L, Campbell J R 1977 Colitis in children with the hemolytic-uremic syndrome. Journal of Pediatric Surgery 12: 213–219

Weedon D D, Shorter R G, Ilstrup D M, Huizenga K A, Taylor W F 1973 Crohn's disease and cancer. New England Journal of Medicine 289: 1099–1103

Werlin S L, Grand R J 1977 Severe colitis in children and adolescents: diagnosis course and treatment. Gastroenterology 73: 828–832

Werlin S L, Grand R J 1978 Bloody diarrhoea — a new complication of sulfasalazine. Journal of Pediatrics 92: 450–451

Whittington P F, Barnes H V, Bayless T M 1977 Medical management of Crohn's disease in adolescence. Gastroenterology 72: 1338–1344

Williams C B et al 1982 Total colonoscopy in childhood. Archives of Disease in Childhood 57: 49–53

Functional and structural alterations of the small intestine during malnutrition

INTRODUCTION

The syndromes of protein and protein-energy malnutrition (marasmus and kwashiorkor) are almost always accompanied by diarrhoea (Lifshitz 1981, Mata 1982). Correa in 1908 described a disease known as 'culebrilla', that eventually became known as kwashiorkor, in which diarrhoea was the chief problem (Correa 1908). In some protected traditional societies where malnutrition is not associated with diarrhoea, a physiological stunting of growth occurs in comparatively healthy individuals (Mata 1978, Fagundes-Neto 1980). On the other hand, where malnourished children live under poor hygienic and sanitary conditions in a 'transitional' or 'developing' society, infectious processes, especially diarrhoea, lead to severe wasting, morbidity and mortality (Mata et al 1977, Mata 1982, Fagundes-Neto 1980, Lifshitz 1981).

In this chapter we discuss the consequences of malnutrition and diarrhoea on the structural and functional integrity of the small intestine. Several essential intestinal functions may be disrupted in patients with malnutrition and diarrhoea; these include the protective barrier to the external environment, homeostatic metabolic exchanges and nutrient absorption. In addition, the susceptibility of the malnourished intestine to injurious processes, the specific effects of bacterial proliferation and structural changes in the intestine induced by malnutrition, are considered. Data, predominantly from clinical studies but also where appropriate from experimental models, that attempt to focus on malnutrition per se, are reviewed.

FUNCTIONAL DEFECTS OF THE INTESTINE DURING MALNUTRITION

Barrier to infection and toxins

Because the gastrointestinal tract constitutes the largest contact area between the external and internal environment (the intestinal surface area is over 200 times greater than body surface area), its integrity is vital to protection from foreign organisms, toxigenic and antigenic substances. Malnourished children appear to have an increased susceptibility to intestinal infection, diarrhoea, and endotoxaemia (Klein et al 1977), although the factors permitting these processes require further study. The frequency of intestinal infections in malnourished children may in part result from compromised immunologic function (Gross & Newberne 1980); there is a reduction in the size of Peyer's patches and appendix, and depleted paracortical and germinal centres in gut-associated lymphoid tissue (Smythe et al 1971). Local secretory immunity that is S-IgA-mediated may be impaired while serum immunoglobulins are normal.

In addition to immunologic deficiencies, structural changes in the small intestine may also permit increased antigen and/or toxin penetration from lumen to blood (Worthington et al 1974, Teichberg et al 1981). For example, in long-term severely malnourished rats, there is an increased intestinal penetration of large molecules and even viral particles (Worthington et al 1974).

These immunological and structural changes seen in malnutrition could play a role in predisposing the malnourished child to infection, endotoxaemia, and dietary protein hypersensitivity leading to chronic diarrhoea (Chandra & Newberne 1977, Iyngkaran et al 1978).

Homeostatic metabolic exchange surface: water and electrolyte economy

The small intestine plays an important role in maintaining water, electrolyte and acid-base balance in body fluids. When this homeostatic capacity is exhausted, dehydration and metabolic acidosis can occur (Lugo de Rivera et al 1972). The intestinal route may account for a substantial proportion of bicarbonate losses, even in diseases primarily affecting another organ, such as the kidney (Schoeneman & Lifshitz 1974).

In malnutrition there is an increased frequency and severity of metabolic acidosis in association with diarrhoea (Lifshitz 1981). This metabolic acidosis is thought to occur in response to a sequence of events in which malabsorbed carbohydrates may play an important role. Carbohydrates are fermented by bacterial flora into short chain organic acids some of which can be efficiently absorbed in the colon conserving considerable energy (Perman et al 1981). Organic anions are, however, excreted leaving excess hydrogen ions in the intestine that are neutralized by bicarbonate, eventually resulting in acidosis (Lugo de Rivera et al 1972, Lifshitz 1981, Torres-Pinedo et al 1968).

In addition decreased sodium absorption, increased faecal potassium loss and colonic secretion leading to diarrhoea will result from the production of deconjugated bile salts, hydroxy fatty acids and the osmotic effect of malabsorbed carbohydrate. Faecal losses of sodium, potassium and chloride correlate with the amount of stool produced (Darrow 1946). Removal of any malabsorbed carbohydrate should ameliorate this process (Lifshitz 1981).

Most of the studies alluded to have been reported from clinical data on populations with a poorly defined marginal nutritional status. More precise studies need to be done on the compensating role of the colon during malnutrition.

In limited experimental studies, it has been suggested that the intestinal electrochemical gradient for Na^+ may be altered during extreme nutritional stress. Starvation of rats for 17 hours decreases jejunal (Na^+-K^+)-ATPase activity and a lack of Na^+ extrusion from the mucosal cell will decrease the $^+(Na^+)$ coupled active transport processes (Karasov & Diamond 1983). In erythrocytes and leukocytes of malnourished children with marasmus there is an abnormally elevated intracellular Na^+ concentration which in part, appears to result from a slowly functioning Na^+, K^+ pump (Patrick & Golden, 1977, Kaplay 1978). The effect of chronic malnutrition, in animal models or humans, on intestinal (Na^+-K^+)-ATPase activity and electrolyte gradients remains to be established.

Malnutrition and susceptibility of the intestine to injury

Clinical studies from Bangladesh suggest that nutritional status affects the duration, but not the frequency, of diarrhoea. The duration of diarrhoea was markedly prolonged in patients with the most severe wasting, while the incidence of diarrhoea was indistinguishable from the best nourished patients in that population (Black et al 1984). Thus, the intestine of malnourished children appears more susceptible to prolonged damage when an intestinal injury occurs. This may be due to an immunological defect, or to delayed recovery of the intestine. Evidence from experimental studies is compatible with this view. The small intestine of experimentally malnourished rats appears only mildly affected by protein-energy malnutrition, yet it appears to be more susceptible to damage than the intestine of well-nourished animals (Teichberg et al 1981). The jejunal cells of malnourished rats are also more sensitive to hyperosmolality showing an increased loss of protein and DNA and a greater secretion of sodium (Lifshitz 1981). They also generate more cyclic AMP (Lifshitz et al 1985).

In addition to the susceptibility of the malnourished intestine to injurious processes related to diarrhoeal disease, the ability to metabolize toxic and carcinogenic chemicals may also be defective. The intestine contains detoxication mechanisms similar to those found in the liver, which may act as a protective barrier. Experiments with purified diets and under conditions of starvation indicate a loss of the ability to hydroxylate polycyclic carcinogens (Wattenberg 1975).

Malnutrition and malabsorption

General

Nutrient malabsorption has been extensively studied under conditions of malnutrition. Infections play a major role in the pathophysiology of the malabsorption which is seen in children with protein-energy malnutrition. These perpetuate and worsen the abnormal nutritional status of the patient and are associated with diarrhoea (Lifshitz 1981, Scrimshaw 1977).

Malabsorption of nutrients is primarily related to pancreatic insufficiency which develops rapidly in malnutrition (Barbezat & Hansen 1968). This results in an impairment of the digestion and absorption of protein, carbohydrates, lipids, minerals, and lipid soluble vitamins (McCance et al 1970). Alterations in pancreatic function appear transitory and return to normal as soon as nutritional recovery begins (Schneider & Viteri 1974, Rossi et al 1983). Zinc deficiency has been shown to reduce the activities of intestinal disaccharidases and leucine aminopeptidase in the rat (Park et al 1985) and decrease net water and sodium transport (Ghishan 1984).

Fat malabsorption

Fat absorption is impaired in children with protein-energy malnutrition because of pancreatic insufficiency and a reduced intraduodenal capacity to form fat micelles as a result of bile salt insufficiency. The type of fat being consumed may also contribute to steatorrhoea as vegetable (i.e. unsaturated) fats are better tolerated than animal lipids (Dean 1952, Ashworth et al 1968). Reduced protein synthesis and in particular β-lipoprotein synthesis during protein malnutrition may also contribute to the fat malabsorption (Isselbacher & Budz 1963). Fat malabsorption may also result from carbohydrate intolerance associated with diarrhoea and malnutrition (Lifshitz & Holman, 1964), and a decrease in faecal fat excretion when disaccharides are eliminated from the diet of malnourished children has been documented (Bowie et al 1963). The osmotic effects of unabsorbed carbohydrates can result in dilution of bile acids to concentrations below the critical micellar concentration (Ringrose et al 1972). It has been demonstrated in the malnourished rat model that lipid transport is unaffected (Zeman & Fratzke 1976), whereas lipid absorption is reduced in the offspring of protein-deficient rats.

Carbohydrate malabsorption

Malnourished patients have decreased levels of intestinal disaccharidases (Bowie et al 1963) and a diminished capacity to absorb carbohydrates (James 1971). Disaccharidase deficiencies in these children may be due to deficient production of enzymes and/or tissue damage (Hirschhorn et al 1968, Lifshitz & Holman 1964, Sunshine & Kretchmer 1964) and may persist even after the acute stage of malnutrition. Lactase, sucrase, and maltase activities are reported to be lower in patients with marasmus than in those with kwashiorkor (James 1971).

The frequency of lactase deficiency has been correlated with the extent of mucosal damage (Brunser et al 1968, Stanfield et al 1965). Although it has been shown that feeding maltose and sucrose can regulate sucrase and maltase activity in the small intestine of normal human volunteers (Rosensweig & Herman 1968), the regulation of enzyme activity by substrate has not been studied in malnutrition. Some of the intestinal oligodisaccharidase deficiencies reported in marasmus and kwashiorkor could be due to lack of intake of the appropriate dietary substrate. The transport capacity for monosaccharides may also be sensitive to dietary carbohydrate levels and therefore, dietary intake itself may lead to the decreased glucose transport that is frequently noted (Karasov & Diamond 1983).

Carbohydrate malabsorption has been shown to contribute to the diarrhoea in malnourished patients (James 1971, Lifshitz et al 1971) and the deleterious effect of lactose in diarrhoeal disease among malnourished children has long been recognized (Bowie et al 1963, Dean 1952). Malabsorption of monosaccharides may also be an important feature of chronic malnutrition and diarrhoeal disease (Lifshitz et al 1970), and since carbohydrates provide 50% of dietary calories, it must be assumed that carbohydrate malabsorption plays an important role in the development and maintenance of malnutrition (Lifshitz 1981).

In contrast to human studies, most studies using malnourished animals have described increased intestinal transport rates for monosaccharides (e.g. Kershaw et al 1960, Younoszai & Lynch 1974), and increased disaccharidase activities (Adams & Leichter 1973, Solimano et al 1967, Hamilton et al 1983).

In animals with experimental osmotic diarrhoea, some disaccharidase loss can be prevented by feeding the corresponding carbohydrate. These data suggest that during osmotic diarrhoea specific disaccharidases are regulated by the corresponding disaccharides (Pergolizzi et al 1977). Thus, removal of specific carbohydrates from the diet during recovery from diarrhoea and malnutrition may perpetuate the deficiencies of intestinal disaccharidases. Unfortunately, administration of these carbohydrates may also lead to carbohydrate intolerance (Lifshitz et al 1971). Further studies remain to be done to ascertain the mechanisms of adaptation of the small intestine during the stress and recovery from malnurition and diarrhoea.

Protein and nitrogen malabsorption

Protein malabsorption is a frequent occurrence during malnutrition (Thompson & Trowell 1952) and approximately one-third of the nitrogen intake may be lost (Waterlow et al 1960). There is an altered absorption of amino acids, di- and tripeptides (Adibi & Allen 1970, Matthews & Adibi 1976), and intestinal peptide hydrolases are depressed (Gjessing et al 1977, Kumar et al 1971). These decreased enzyme levels can persist, even after nutritional recovery. The peptide hydrolase enzyme deficiencies are seen in morphologically damaged intestinal mucosa (Gjessing et al 1977).

Results from studies using malnourished animals are again at variance with human studies, showing an increased absorption of certain amino acids (Wapnir & Lifshitz 1974, Kershaw et al 1960). Experimental evidence of the effects of malnutrition on small peptide absorption is limited, although dipeptide hydrolysis is decreased in the jejunal mucosa (Mahboob & Zerman 1976).

Malabsorption of vitamins and minerals

Diarrhoea and steatorrhoea lead to malabsorption of other substances including vitamins and minerals. For example, there is impaired absorption of vitamin B_{12} and loss of bile salts in the stools (Alvarado et al 1973), both of which probably result from defective function of the ileum. Protein malnutrition may also result in mineral malabsorption (Wapnir 1985).

Bacterial proliferation and intestinal malfunction

Bacterial overgrowth in the small intestine is a striking feature of protein-energy malnutrition (Mata et al 1972). Gastric hypochlorhydria, intestinal hypotonia and hypomotility (James 1970), and immunological deficiencies (Bell et al 1976) are factors that may facilitate the colonization of the small bowel. These may occur simultaneously with the ingestion of large quantities of faecal bacteria, because of poor sanitary conditions (Mata et al 1971).

Nonspecific bacterial proliferation of faecal and colonic bacteria in the upper segments of the small bowel usually leads to diarrhoeal disease (Coello-Ramirez & Lifshitz 1972, Ramos-Alvarez & Olarte 1964). Although enteric microbial populations may cause the diarrhoea, bacterial overgrowth is usually a secondary phenomenon (Lifshitz 1977), and may result from the presence of free carbohydrates in the intestinal lumen (Coello-Ramirez & Lifshitz 1972). Anaerobes such as *Bacteroides* and *Veilonella*, are capable of causing deconjugation and 7-alpha dehydroxylation of primary bile salts in the intestinal lumen (Shimada et al 1969). They may also metabolize foodstuffs producing hydroxy fatty acids, short chain organic acids and alcohol. Elevated concentrations of these injurious factors in the jejunal lumen may induce glucose malabsorption, sodium and water secretion and also morphological abnormalities of the intestinal mucosa (Donaldson 1965, Gracey et al 1971). Proliferation of intestinal microflora in upper segments of the bowel has been reported as occuring in malnourished children even when they have no diarrhoea (Mata et al 1972). Further studies should be done to determine the quantitative and qualitative differences in small bowel microbial flora which may account for variation in the production of injurious factors to the small bowel and, therefore, of the presence or absence of diarrhoea.

In the colon, bacterial metabolism appears to play a beneficial role in relation to nonabsorbed carbohydrate. Colonic flora can convert mono- and disaccharides to absorbable short-chain organic acids and a large proportion Perman 1982). The effects of small intestinal colonization by faecal and colonic bacteria on the intestinal epithelium of malnourished rats has not been studied. However, studies in normal rats have shown deconjugation of bile salts, ultrastructural alteration in epithelial cells and diminished jejunal transport capacity (Lifshitz et al 1978, Berant et al 1981) which may suggest compounding of alterations already present in malnourished rats.

STRUCTURAL ALTERATIONS OF THE INTESTINE DURING MALNUTRITION

Morphological changes

The overlay of enteric and systemic infection which is practically ubiquitous among malnourished children of the underdeveloped world, greatly complicates an understanding of small intestinal morphological alterations caused by malnutrition. Clinical observations strongly suggest that infection plays an important role in producing the intestinal structural abnormalities during malnutrition. For example, there is a delayed improvement in the villous pattern when patients who are receiving an inadequate diet, are kept at home in a contaminated environment, whereas children kept in the relatively hygienic conditions of a hospital show a strikingly rapid improvement of the intestinal mucosa (Stanfield et al 1965). In some studies of malnourished children the morphological alterations observed in the intestine are more closely related to *diarrhoea* than malnutrition (Schneider & Viteri 1972). Nevertheless, the differences in the degree of damage to the intestinal mucosa and the similar prevalence of infection in kwashiorkor and marasmus suggests that the nutritional status is an important factor in cell damage.

There is a spectrum of alterations in malnourished patients ranging from severe damage to none at all (Brunser et al 1966, Stanfield et al 1965, Martins-Campos et al 1979). Histological changes are generally more dramatic with kwashiorkor than marasmus and include a flat sprue-like intestinal mucosa in as many as 10–60% of children, with a substantial lymphocytic infiltration, cuboidal epithelium, fat bodies within absorptive cells and elongated crypts (Brunser et al 1968, Brunser 1977, Stanfield et al 1965). The mitotic index, and thus the rate of cell renewal, is reported to be decreased. The severity of morphological damage in kwashiorkor may in part reflect a loss of nutrient-recycling mechanisms that further compromise the intestine (Viteri & Torun 1980). Not all cases of kwashiorkor show these severe alterations and much milder, and even normal mucosal architecture has been documented in some patients.

Marasmic patients have milder changes in small intestinal morphology (Brunser et al 1966, 1976, Brunser 1977, Martins-Campos et al 1979).

There are no epithelial fat bodies, villi may be moderately shortened and become broad, but there is rarely severe mucosal flattening. The epithelium is only slightly cuboidal, and there is only slight infiltration of the lamina propria with lymphocytes and other inflammatory cell types. The crypts appear morphologically normal; although the mitotic index is reduced to an even greater extent than in kwashiorkor. It has been suggested that this aberration is related to a deficit in the calories required for mitosis. Post mortem studies suggest that the ileum is more affected than the duodenum in both types of malnutrition (Passmore 1947). Macromolecular absorption appears to be enhanced in the jejunal mucosa of patients with malnutrition (Heyman et al 1984).

In experimental animal studies of malnutrition, architectural changes in intestinal structure are almost always milder than in clinical material (Hill et al 1968, Teichberg et al 1980), but cell production is altered (Hopper et al 1972).

Ultrastructural alterations

In both kwashiorkor and marasmus, blunting of the microvilli irregularly shaped nuclei and numerous autophagic lysosomes have been described (Shiner et al 1973, Thernon et al 1971). It is speculated that autophagia provides a mechanism for the reutilization of cellular nutrients (dipeptides, amino acids, fatty acids, etc), in the absence of an exogenous source. Since the intestinal epithelium is exposed to noxious agents that damage cell membranes through infectious processes, autophagia may also be a response to organelle damage. The epithelial cell basement membrane is also reported to be variably thickened and layered during malnutrition (Brunser et al 1976, Martins-Campos et al 1979).

In plasma cells of the lamina propria of patients with severe kwashiorkor there is a diminished rough endoplasmic reticulum (site of antibody production), and little material (antibodies) appears to accumulate in the cisternae of the endoplasmic reticulum (Shiner et al 1975). Limited studies on marasmic patients indicate that the plasma cells have normal amounts of rough endoplasmic reticulum, but the cisternae of the reticulum are collapsed and not filled with immunoglobulins (Martins-Campos et al 1979). Although most earlier reports on the microvillous brush border of experimental rats reported no effect due to malnutrition, our recent morphometric studies suggest there is a decrease in the absorptive surface area (Ribeiro et al 1987). The increased numbers of lysosomes reported from clinical material may be related to infectious status. Intestinal goblet cell mucin is also depleted during malnutrition thereby increasing susceptibility to infection (Sherman et al 1985).

Membrane alterations

There is some evidence to suggest that the cellular membranes of malnourished individuals may be altered in their biochemical constituents and in the amounts produced. Studies in nonintestinal tissue of malnourished patients indicate for example that the cholesterol:phospholipid ratio in the erythrocyte plasma membrane is increased during protein-calorie malnutrition (Brown et al 1978). Since the enzymatic activities of membrane proteins depend in part on their hydrophobic interactions, this could have a broad effect. The details concerning the effect of malnutrition on the chemical characteristics of enterocyte membranes are not known. Data on glomerular epithelial surface area in malnourished rats (Ichikawa et al 1980) indicate a decreased production of epithelial cell plasma membrane, and a similar process appears to occur in the intestine (Wehman et al 1978). The alterations in membrane structure and function during malnutrition therefore require more investigation.

REFERENCES

Adams J L, Leichter J 1973 Effect of protein-deficient diets with various amounts of carbohydrates on intestinal disaccharidase activity in the rat. Journal of Nutrition 193:1716

Adibi S A, Allen E R 1970 Impaired jejunal absorption rates of essential amino acids induced by either dietary caloric or protein deprivation in man. Gastroenterology 58:404

Alvarado J, Vargas W, Diaz N, Viteri F E 1973 Vitamin B_{12} absorption in protein-calorie malnourished children and during recovery: influence of protein and of diarrhoea. American Journal of Clinical Nutrition 26:595

Ashworth A, Bell R, James W P T, Waterlow J C 1968 Caloric requirements of children recovering from protein-calorie malnutrition. Lancet ii:600

Barbezat G O, Hansen J D L 1968 The exocrine pancreas and protein-caloric malnutrition. Pediatrics 42:77

Bell R G, Turner J, Gracey M, Suharjo A, Suroto 1976 Serum and small intestinal immunoglobulin levels in undernourished children. American Journal of Clinical Nutrition 29:393

Berant M, Lifshitz F, Bayne M A, Wapnir R A 1981 Jejunal cAMP activated sodium secretion and deconjugated bile salts and fatty acids. Biochemical Medicine 25:327

Black R E, Brown K H, Becker S 1984 Malnutrition is a determining factor in diarrheal duration, but not incidence, among young children in a longitudinal study in rural Bangladesh. American Journal of Clinical Nutrition 37:87

Bond J H, Currier B E Buchwald H, Levitt M D 1980 Colonic conservation of malabsorbed carbohydrate. Gastroenterology 78:444

Bowie M D, Brinkman G L, Hansen J D L 1963 Diarrhea in protein-caloric malnutrition. Lancet ii:550

Brown K H, Suskind R M, Lubin B, Kulapongs P, Leitzman C, Olsen R E 1978 Changes in red blood cell membrane in protein caloric malnutrition. American Journal of Clinical Nutrition 31:574

Brunser O 1977 Effects of malnutrition on intestinal structure and function in children. Clinics in Gastroenterology 6: 341–353

Brunser O, Reid A M, Mockeberg F, Maccioni A, Contreras D 1966 Jejunal biopsies in infant malnutrition with special reference to mitotic index. Pediatrics 38:605

Brunser O, Reid A, Mockeberg F, Maccioni A, Contreras I 1968 Jejunal mucosa in infantile malnutrition. American Journal of Clinical Nutrition. 21:976

Brunser O, Castillo C, Araza M 1976 Fine structure of the small intestinal mucosa in infantile marasmic malnutrition. Gastroenterology 70:495

Chandra R K, Newberne P M 1977 Nutrition, immunity, and infection. Mechanisms of intractions. Plenum, New York.

Coello-Ramirez P, Lifshitz F 1972 Enteric microflora and carbohydrate intolerance in infants with diarrhea. Pediatrics 49:233

Correa 1908 Revista Medica Yucatan 3(6) In: Wheaton B, Howells G, Phillips I 1968 Diarrhea in kwashiorkor. British Medical Journal 4:608

Darrow D C 1946 The retention of electrolytes during recovery from severe dehydration due to diarrhea. Journal of Pediatrics 28:515

Dean R F A 1952 The treatment of kwashiorkor with milk and vegetable proteins. British Medical Journal 2:791

Donaldson R M Jr 1965 Studies of the pathogenesis of steatorrhea in the blind loop syndrome. Journal of Clinical Investigation 44:1815

Fagundes-Neto U 1980 Malnutrition and the intestine. In: Lifshitz F (ed) Clinical Disorders in Pediatric Gastroenterology and Nutrition. Marcel Dekker, New York. p 249

Ghishan F K 1984 Transport of electrolytes, water and glucose in zinc deficiency. Journal of Pediatric Gastroenterology and Nutrition. 3:608

Gjessing E C, Villanueva D, Duque E, Bolanos E, Mayoral L G 1977 Dipeptide hydrolase activity of the intestinal mucosa from protein-malnourished adult patients and controls. American Journal of Clinical Nutrition 30:1044

Gracey M, Burke V, Oshin A 1971 Bacteria, bile salts, and intestinal monosaccharide malabsorption. Gut 12:683

Gross R L, Newberne P M 1980 Role of nutrition in immunologic function. Physiological Reviews 60:188

Hamilton J R, Guiraldes E, Rossi M 1983 Impact of malnutrition on the developing gut: studies in suckling rats. Journal of Pediatric Gastroenterology and Nutrition 2:S151

Heyman M, Boudraa G, Sarrut S et al 1984 Macromolecular transport in jejunal mucosa of children with severe malnutrition: A quantitative study. Journal of Pediatric Gastroenterology and Nutrition 3: 357–363

Hill R B Jr, Prosper J, Hirschfield J S, Kern F Jr 1968 Protein starvation and the small intestine. I. The growth and morphology of the small intestine in weanling rats. Experimental and Molecular Pathology 8:66

Hirschhorn N, Soba J R, Siddiquea A 1968 Jejunal disaccharidase activities in acute diarrhea and convalescence. Gastroenterology 54:1244

Hopper A F, Rose P M, Wannemacher R W 1972 Cell population changes in the intestinal mucosa in protein depleted or starved rats. II changes in cell migration rates. Journal of Cellular Biology 53:225

Ichikawa I, Pinkerton M L, Klahr J C, Troy M, Martinez-Maldonado M, Brenner B 1980 Mechanism of reduced glomerular-filtration rate in chronic malnutrition. Journal of Clinical Investigation 65:982

Isselbacher K J, Budz D M 1963 Synthesis of lipoproteins by rat intestinal mucosa. Nature 200:364

Iyngkaran N, Robinson M J, Sumithran E, Lam S K, Puthucheary S D, Yadow M 1978 Cow's milk protein sensitive enteropathy: an important factor in prolonging diarrhea of acute infective enteritis in early infancy. Archives of Disease in Childhood 53:150

James W P T 1970 Sugar absorption and intestinal motility in children when malnourished and after treatment. Clinical Science 39:305

James W P T 1971 Effects of protein calorie malnutrition on intestinal absorption. Annals of the New York Academy of Sciences 176:244

Kaplay S 1978 Erythrocyte membrane sodium and potassium activated ATPase in protein-calorie malnutrition. American Journal of Clinical Nutrition 31:479

Karasov W H, Diamond J M 1983 Adaptive regulation of sugar and amino acid transport by vertebrate intestine. American Journal of Physiology 245:S443

Kershaw T G, Meame K D, Wiseman G 1960 the effect of semistarvation on absorption by the rat small intestine in vitro and in vivo. Journal of Physiology (London) 152:182

Klein K, Suskind R M, Kulapongs P, Mertz G, Olson R E 1977 Endotoxemia, a possible cause of decreased complement activity in malnourished Thai children. In: Suskind R M (ed) 'Malnutrition and the Immune response'. Raven, New York. p 321

Kumar V, Ghai V P, Chase H P 1971 Intestinal dipeptide hydrolase activities in undernourished children. Archives of Disease in Childhood 46:801

Lifshitz F 1977 The enteric flora in childhood disease-diarrhea. American Journal of Clinical Nutrition 30:1811

Lifshitz F 1981 Effects of diarrhea on infant nutrition. In: Lebenthal E (ed) Textbook of Gastroenterology and Nutrition. Raven Press, New York. p 1003

Lifshitz F, Holman G H 1964 Disaccharidase deficiencies with steatorrhea. Journal of Pediatrics 64:34

Lifshitz F, Coello-Ramirez P, Gutierrez-Topete G 1970 Monosaccharide intolerance and hypoglycemia in infants with diarrhea. II. Metabolic studies in 23 infants. Journal of Pediatrics 77:604

Lifshitz F, Coello-Ramirez P, Gutierrez-Topete G, Cornado-Cornet M D 1971 Carbohydrate malabsorption in infants with diarrhea. Journal of Pediatrics 79:760

Lifshitz F, Wapnir R A, Wehman H J, Pergolizzi R, Hawkins R L, Dias-Bensussen S 1978 The effects of small intestinal colonisation by fecal and colonic bacteria on intestinal function in rats. Journal of Nutrition 108:1913

Lifshitz F, Teichberg S, Wapnir R A 1985 Cyclic AMP mediated jejunal secretion in lactose fed malnourished rats. American Journal of Clinical Nutrition 41:1265

Lugo de Rivera C, Rodriguez H, Torres-Pinedo R 1972 Studies on the mechanism of sugar malabsorption in infantile infectious diarrhea. American Journal of Clinical Nutrition 25:1248

McCance R A, Rutishausen D H E, Boozer C N 1970 Effect of kwashiorkor on absorption and excretion of N, fat and minerals. Archives of Disease in Childhood 45:410

Mahboob S, Zeman F J 1976 Intestinal dipeptidase in the intestine of the prenatally protein-deprived rat. Nutrition Reports International 14:423

Martins-Campos J V, Fagundes-Neto U, Patricio F R S, Wehba J, Carvalho A A, Shiner M 1979 Jejunal mucosa in marasmic children. Clinical pathological and fine structural evaluation of the effect of protein-energy malnutrition and environmental contamination. American Journal of Clinical Nutrition 32:1575

Mata L 1978 The children of Santa Maria Cauque. A prospective field study of health and growth. MIT Press, Cambridge, Mass.

Mata L 1982 Child feedings in less developed countries: induced breast feeding in a transitional society. In: Lifshitz F (ed) Pediatric Nutrition, Infant Feedings, Deficiencies, and Diseases. Marcel Dekker, New York. p 35

Mata L J, Urrutia J J, Lechtig A 1971 Infection and nutrition of children of a low socioeconomic rural community. American Journal of Clinical Nutrition 24:249

Mata L J, Jimenez F, Cordon M 1972 Gastrointestinal flora of children with protein-caloric malnutrition. American Journal of Clinical Nutrition 25:1118

Mata L J, Kronmal R A, Urrutia J J, Garcia B 1977 Effect of infection on food intake and the nutritional state: perspectives as received from the village. American Journal of Clinical Nutrition 30:1215

Matthews D M, Adibi S A 1976 Peptide absorption. Gastroenterology 71:151

Park J H Y, Grandjean C J, Antonson D L, Vanderhoof J A 1985 Effects of short-term isolated zinc deficiency on intestinal growth and activities of several brush border enzymes in weanling rats. Pediatric Research 19:1333

Passmore R, 1947 Mixed deficiency diseases in India. A clinical description. Transactions of the Royal society of Tropical Medicine and Hygiene 41:189

Patrick J, Golden M 1977 Leukocyte electrolytes, and sodium transport in protein energy malnutrition. American Journal of Clinical Nutrition 30:1478

Pergolizzi R, Lifshitz F, Teichberg S, Wapnir R A 1977 Interaction between dietary carbohydrates and intestinal disaccharidases in experimental diarrhea. American Journal of Clinical Nutrition 30:484

Perman J A 1982 Carbohydrate intolerance and the enteric microflora. In: Lifshitz F (ed) Carbohydrate Intolerance in Infancy. p 137

Perman J A, Modler S, Olson A C 1981 Role of pH in production of hydrogen from carbohydrates by colonic flora: studies in vivo and in vitro. Journal of clinical Investigation 67:643

Ramos-Alvarez M, Olarte J 1964 Diarrheal disease of children: occurrence of enteropathogenic viruses and bacteria. American Journal of Diseases of Children 107:218

Ribeiro H da Costa, Teichberg S, McGarvey E, Lifshitz F 1987 Quantitative alterations in the structural development of jejunal absorptive epithelial cells and their subcellular organelles in protein-energy malnourished rats: a stereological analysis (in press)

Ringrose R E, Thompson J B, Welsh J D 1972 Lactose malabsorption and steatorrhea. American Journal of Digestive Diseases 17:533

Rosensweig N S, Herman R H 1968 Control of jejunal sucrose or fructose in man. A model for the study of enzyme regulation in man. Journal of Clinical Investigation 47:2253

Rossi T M, Lee P C, Lebenthal E 1983 Effect of feeding regimens on the functional recovery of pancreatic enzymes in postnatally malnourished weanling rats. Pediatric Research 17:806

Schneider R E, Viteri F E 1972 Morphological aspects of the duodenojejunal mucosa in protein-caloric malnourished children and during recovery. American Journal of Clinical Nutrition 25:1092

Schneider, R E, Viteri F E 1974 Luminal events of lipid absorption in protein-calorie malnourished children: relationship with nutritional recovery and diarrhea. II. Alterations in bile acid content of duodenal aspirates. American Journal of Clinical Nutrition 27:788

Schoeneman M, Lifshitz F 1974 The transport of bicarbonate by the small intestine of a patient with proximal renal tubular acidosis. Pediatric Research 8:735

Scrimshaw N S 1977 Effect of infection on nutrient requirement. American Journal of Clinical Nutrition 30:1536

Sherman P, Forstner J, Roomi N, Kharti I, Forstner G 1985 Mucin depletion in the intestine of malnourished rats. American Journal of Physiology 348:G418

Shimada K, Bricknell K S, Finegold S M 1969 Deconjugation of bile acids by intestinal bacteria: review of the literature and additional studies. Journal of Infectious Diseases 119:273

Shiner M, Redmond A O B, Hansen J D L 1973 The jejunal mucosa in protein-calorie malnutrition. A clinical histological and ultrastructural study. Experimental and Molecular Pathology 19:61

Shiner M, Redmond A O B, Hansen J D L 1975 Protein energy malnutrition and the immune system of the gut. In: Goldstein F (ed) Proceedings of the Bockus International Society of Gastroenterology. Donaldson Printing Co., Philadelphia. pp 125–134

Smythe P M, Breteton-Stiles G G, Grace H J 1971 Thymolymphatic deficiency and depression of cell-mediated immunity in protein-calorie malnutrition. Lancet ii:939

Solimano G, Burgess E A, Levin B 1967 Protein-calorie malnutrition: effect of deficient diets on enzyme levels of jejunal mucosa of rats. British Journal of Nutrition 21:55

Stanfield J P, Hutt M S R, Turricliffe R 1965 Intestinal biopsies in kwashiorkor. Lancet ii:519

Sunshine P, Kretchmer N 1964 Studies of small intestine during development. III. Infantile diarrhea associated with intolerance to disaccharides. Pediatrics 34:38

Teichberg S, McGarvey E, Lifshitz F 1980 Quantitative morphology of the rat jejunum during protein-energy malnutrition. Federation Proceedings 39:767

Teichberg S, Fagundes-Neto U, Bayne M A, Lifshitz F 1981 Jejunal macromolecular absorption and bile salt deconjugation in protein-energy malnourished rats. American Journal of Clinical Nutrition 34:1281

Thernon J J, Wittmann W, Pinaloo J G 1971 The fine structure of the jejunum in kwahshiorkor. Experimental and Molecular Pathology 14:184

Thomson M D, Trowell H C 1952 Pancreatic enzyme activity in duodenal contents of children with a type of kwashiorkor. Lancet i:1031

Torres-Pinedo R, Conde E, Robillard G, Maldonado M 1968 Studies on infant diarrhea. III. Changes in composition of saline and glucose-saline solutions instilled into the colon. Pediatrics 42:303

Viteri E, Torun B 1980 Protein-caloric malnutrition. In: Goodhart R S, Sohilo M E (eds) Modern Nutrition in Health and Disease, 6th edn. Lea and Febiger, Philadelphia. p 697

Wapnir R A 1985 The rate of protein breakdown products in the absorption of essential trace elements. In: Lifshitz F (ed) Nutrition for special needs in infancy — protein hydrolysates. Marcel Dekker Inc, New York. p 37

Wapnir R A, Lifshitz F 1974 Absorption of amino acids in malnourished rats. Journal of Nutrition 104:843

Waterlow J C, Cravioto J, Stephen J M L 1960 Protein malnutrition in man. Advances in Protein Chemistry 15:131

Wattenberg L 1975 Effects of dietary constituents on the metabolism of chemical carcinogens. Cancer Research 35:3326

Wehman H J, Lifshitz F, Teichberg S 1978 Effects of enteric microbial overgrowth on small intestinal ultrastructure in the rat. American Journal of Gastroenterology 70:249

Worthington B S, Boatman E S, Kenny G C 1974 Intestinal absorption of intact proteins in normal and protein deficient rats. American Journal of Clinical Nutrition 27:276

Younoszai M K, Lynch A 1974 In vivo intestinal absorption of hexose in growth retarded suckling rat pups. Journal of Nutrition 104: 671

Zeman F J, Fratzke M L 1976 Lipid absorption in the young of protein deficient rats. Lipids 11:652

Small intestinal enteropathies

The term small intestinal enteropathy describes the presence of a morphological abnormality of the small intestinal mucosa. It may be found in a wide variety of disorders, and appears to occur chiefly in the proximal small intestine. However, the enteropathy associated with infective enteritis in infancy may be variable in distribution and on occasions affect the ileal mucosa predominantly. This information is at present based only on post mortem findings (Walker-Smith 1972) and studies in the experimental animal. Indeed there is a paucity of information available concerning the morphology of the distal small intestine in children with many of the enteropathies described in this chapter.

In the proximal small intestine the enteropathy may be of uniform severity as in untreated coeliac disease, or patchy, as in cow's milk sensitive enteropathy and postenteritis enteropathy (Manuel et al 1979). In some enteropathies the changes are subtle and contained within the mucosa without gross disruption of normal architecture, e.g. eosinophilic material in the crypt lumina as found in cystic fibrosis, whereas in others there are severe changes with gross alteration of structure, e.g. the flat mucosa characteristic of coeliac disease. Table 8.1 lists those disorders in childhood where a small intestinal enteropathy has been described, based upon biopsy and autopsy studies as well as observation of specimens obtained at laparotomy.

Table 8.1 Causes of proximal small intestinal enteropathies in childhood

Coeliac disease
Transient food sensitive enteropathies cow's milk, fish, soy, chicken meat, gluten, rice, egg
Bacterial and viral enteritis, postenteritis syndrome
Parasitic infestation: giardia cryptosporidia strongyloides
Intractable diarrhoea of infancy
Congenital microvillous atrophy
Autoimmune enteropathy
Tropical sprue
Intestinal lymphangiectasia
Cystic fibrosis
Eosinophilic gastroenteritis
Histiocytosis X
Nonspecific enterocolitis
Crohn's disease
Drugs, e.g. methotrexate
Radiation enteritis
Lymphoma
Protein-energy malnutrition

COELIAC DISEASE

This condition was first described in the second century A.D. by Aretaeus the Cappadocian, who wrote of the 'coeliac affection' in adults (Dowd & Walker Smith 1974). Nearly 800 years later Samuel Gee (1888) described a similar disorder in children, giving a vivid and accurate clinical account of the condition as we now recognize it. In 1950 Dicke made the discovery that dietary gluten was the toxic factor and that withdrawal of gluten led to a complete clinical remission. Seven years later Sakula & Shiner (1957) reported the first small intestinal biopsy in a child with coeliac disease, describing the typical flat appearance of the mucosa which is now recognized to be characteristic of this disorder. Despite these major advances the basic pathophysiology operating in coeliac disease remains uncertain.

Definition

Coeliac disease may present in childhood or adult life and results from gluten-induced enteropathy which predominantly affects the proximal small intestinal mucosa leading to malabsorption, and associated biochemical and clinical abnormalities. Withdrawal of dietary gluten results in complete remission, but the intolerance to gluten is permanent.

Aetiology

Gluten is a storage protein in the endosperm of wheat, barley and oats. Gluten from wheat and rye is toxic to all patients with coeliac disease, the response to other glutens such as barley and oats is, however, less clearly established. Gluten is a large complex molecule and consists of a mixture of four heterogeneous classes of proteins: gliadins, glutenins, albumins and globulins. Techniques such as gel electrophoresis have shown the gliadin fraction to contain about 40 different components, and most interest has centred around the α-gliadin fraction which has been shown to be the most toxic component (Kendall et al 1972) but other gliadin fractions are also toxic. Enzymatic degradation of gluten or gliadin suggests that the toxic portion of the gliadin molecule is a polypeptide with a molecular weight of less than 15 000 (Kowlessar 1967, Dissanayake et al 1974a). As gliadin is present in variable amounts in different wheats, it is possible that some wheats are more toxic than others.

Controversy exists regarding the basic mechanism by which gluten induces mucosal abnormalities, and there are two schools of thought.

Biochemical theories

A number of hypotheses have been advanced involving cellular metabolism or structure. Frazer (1956) proposed a primary deficiency of a cytoplasmic peptidase which resulted in the accumulation of a toxic peptide. Later studies produced no evidence to support this view (Douglas & Booth 1970). Along similar lines Phelan et al (1974) demonstrated that some carbohydrases abolished the toxicity of gliadin and that there was a deficiency of these enzymes in coeliac disease. This observation remains unconfirmed. Hekkens (1978) and Weiser & Douglas (1976, 1978) have suggested that enterocyte membrane structure is different in coeliac disease, particularly with regard to the binding of wheat glutens to a hypothetical receptor site in a manner analagous to other plant lectins. At present there seems to be little evidence to support any of the above hypotheses.

Immunological abnormalities

In recent years a great deal of evidence, both direct and indirect, has accumulated indicating that a variety of immunological abnormalities are present in patients with coeliac disease, but whether the toxic effects of gluten are mediated by a primary immune process remains controversial.

Amongst the direct evidence is the demonstration of disturbances in humoral reactivity, with elevated titres of circulating antibodies to various dietary proteins and reticulin, abnormalities of serum immunoglobulin and plasma-containing immunoglobulin cell concentrations in the lamina propria, and evidence of complement activation. Serum IgG (Immunoglobulin G) and IgM concentrations are usually reduced, whereas IgA levels are raised (Kenrick & Walker-Smith 1970, Asquith et al 1969), but there is considerable variation in the frequency of these abnormalities. Unsworth et al (1981) have associated IgA class anti-gliadin antibody almost exclusively with coeliac disease whereas antibodies of IgG class are less disease-specific and may be associated with other gastrointestinal diseases. Both the elevated levels of dietary protein antibodies and the abnormalities of serum immunoglobulins return to normal following treatment. Data on the quantification of immunoglobulin-containing plasma cells in the lamina propria are variable according to the age of the patient and the state of treatment (Savilahti 1972, Lancaster Smith et al 1974, Kilby 1975). Local IgA production is probably stimulated initially in both children and adults, to become exhausted only later. The current hypothesis is that IgA blast cells are stimulated within gut-associated lymphoid tissue. These committed blast cells then migrate to the lamina propria where they secrete immunoglobulin. Low numbers of isolated mucosal lymphoid follicles in untreated coeliac disease in childhood compared to increased numbers found in postgluten challenges, would indirectly support the proposal that IgA production is initially stimulated but becomes exhausted with time. Shiner & Ballard (1972) found antibody, mainly IgA, in the basement membrane of the small intestinal epithelial cells after gluten challenge in children; in addition they observed deposition of complement and immune complexes in the lamina propria. Within 1–6 hours of gluten challenge in adults, there is evidence of serum complement consumption, and complement binding immune complexes appear in the serum (Doe et al 1974).

Using in vitro culture techniques, Falchuk et al (1974) have studied the pathogenesis of gluten toxicity in biopsy specimens from patients with coeliac disease. Their data suggests that gluten peptides are not directly toxic but that activation of an endogenous effector mechanism is first required; and propose this to be a local immune system. Activation results in the elaboration of a humoral material, which in turn, reacts with gluten peptides, the complex mediating the toxic effects of gluten. Falchuk et al (1974) suggest that the humoral material is a locally produced gluten antibody. Finally, Ezoke et al (1974) have described lymphocyte-dependent serum antibodies which can co-opt lymphocytes known as K or killer cells to attack gluten-labelled targets in vitro.

Direct evidence of abnormalities in cellular reactivity include increased numbers of intraepithelial lymphocytes in the small intestinal mucosa of untreated and challenge patients (Ferguson & Murray 1971) (Figure 8.1) and gluten stimulation of lymphocytes (Holmes et al 1972). There is clear evidence that the majority of intraepithelial lymphocytes are cytotoxic suppressor cells in adults (Selby et al 1983). In untreated coeliac disease in adults, intraepithelial lymphocytes have been reported to have an elevated mitotic index (Marsh 1982). Leigh et al (1985) have since proposed, on the basis of 'mini challenges' with a gliadin fraction, that the coeliac lesion is due to an intense inflammatory reaction triggered by T-lymphocyte-gluten interactions within the lamina propria. The presence within the lamina propria of numerous DR+ macrophages and T4 helper cells would provide the cellular basis for the subsequent lymphokine-induced inflammatory and cellular changes.

More general evidence for an immune abnormality includes the

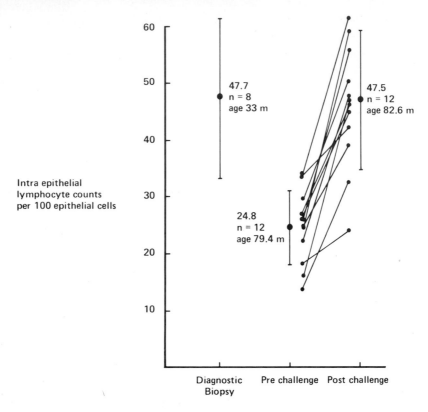

Fig. 8.1 Intraepithelial lymphocyte counts in children with coeliac disease, at diagnosis, pre-challenge on a gluten-free diet and after a relapse following a positive challenge.

occasional report of gluten shock and the improvement in the mucosal abnormality following steroid therapy (Wall et al 1970).

Genetic and environmental factors

Coeliac disease only occurs in those parts of the world where gluten is ingested, such as Britain, Europe, North and South America, Australia and the Punjab region of the Indian subcontinent; it has not yet been clearly documented in the Chinese, Japanese, or black Africans, nor in West Indians or American Negroes. A partial explanation for this geographical distribution may be related to the predisposition of people possessing the histocompatibility antigen HLA-B8 to develop coeliac disease, since nearly all countries from which coeliac disease has been reported have a high frequency of this antigen (McNeish et al 1974). Recent studies have shown a stronger association with the HLA (human leukocyte antigen) D/DR locus. Indeed it has been shown that susceptibility to coeliac disease is primarily associated with the DC locus of the HLA D region (Tosi et al 1983).

The reported incidence of coeliac disease within the British Isles shows considerable variation, ranging from between one in 2000 and one in 6000 in England (Carter et al 1959) to one in 300 in the west of Ireland (Mylotte et al 1973). In the 1980's reports have appeared of a declining incidence of coeliac disease presenting in childhood (Dossetor et al 1981). It remains to be established if this is a real phenomenon, and if it represents a delay in age of presentation of coeliac disease rather than a true decline in its incidence. It is of interest that in Britain in 1983 the numbers of new children with coeliac disease registered with the Coeliac Society showed no significant fall from previous years (Crossed Grain 1984).

The familial occurrence of coeliac disease is well known, susceptibility to a number of environmental factors being inherited by polygenic variation (McCrae 1969). It has also been suggested that the condition is inherited as a dominant gene with incomplete penetrance, yet the reported discordance for the condition in some monozygotic twins, argues strongly against such a mode of inheritance. However, the difficulties in excluding coeliac disease in an asymptomatic monozygotic twin have now become apparent. Kamath et al (1983) have reported such a child where the small intestinal mucosa which was previously normal (Walker-Smith 1973) became abnormal (a flat mucosa), and confirmed by gluten challenge and appropriate biopsies that the child suffered from coeliac disease. It is clear that monozygotic twins both possess the coeliac trait.

However, whilst the predisposition to coeliac disease is genetically controlled, other stimuli are necessary to trigger the innate susceptibility in both adults and children. At the cellular level it seems likely that a specific interaction between gluten DR compatible macrophages and T-helper lymphocytes occurs within the lamina propria. Following activation of antigen-specific lymphocytes the subsequent events are all nonspecific and mediated through lymphokines. Lymphokines may attract other lymphocytes, induce B-lymphocyte antibody production and activate mast cells, producing a wide range of enzymatic vasoactive and chemotactic factors which could result in many of the observed features of coeliac disease.

Pathology

The proximal small intestinal mucosa is abnormal whereas the distal mucosa is usually normal. However, the direct instillation of gluten into the ileum induces mucosal abnormalities in patients with coeliac disease but not in normal individuals (Rubin et al 1960), indicating that the whole length of the small intestinal mucosa is sensitive to gluten. The proximal distribution of the mucosal abnormality accords with the concept of a noxious agent in the diet becoming completely hydrolysed in the gut lumen, so that by the time it reaches the ileum it is no longer toxic. The observation of Kamath et al (1983) that the mucosa is normal prior to the clinical manifestation of

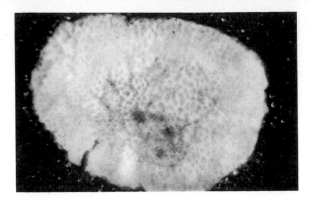

Fig. 8.2A Dissecting microscopic appearances of proximal small intestinal mucosa in untreated coeliac disease, showing flat mosaic appearance.

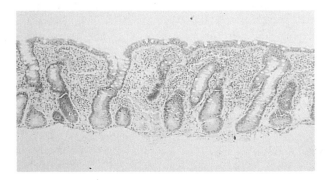

Fig. 8.2B Light microscopic appearance of proximal small intestinal mucosa in untreated coeliac disease (Haematoxylin and eosin stain, magnified). The normal villous architecture is lost and the mucosa is flat; the surface epithelial cells are abnormal and there are increased numbers of plasma cells in the lamina propria.

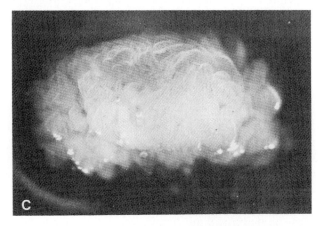

Fig. 8.2C Dissecting microscope appearances of the proximal small intestinal mucosa in treated coeliac disease showing normal leaf and finger-shaped villi.

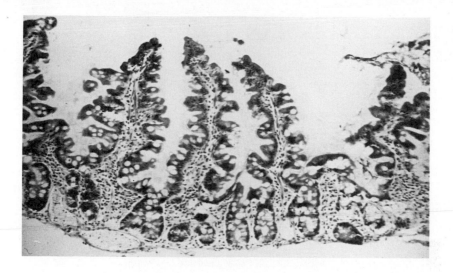

Fig. 8.2D Normal light microscope appearances of proximal small intestinal mucosa in treated coeliac disease (Haematoxylin stain, magnified).

coeliac disease suggests that some environmental trigger may render the mucosa susceptible to gluten.

The characteristic dissecting and light microscopic appearances of the proximal small intestinal mucosa in untreated coeliac disease are shown in Figures 8.2A and B; with treatment the mucosal lesion usually reverts completely to normal in children (Figs. 8.2C and D). Kinetic studies have shown that the turnover rate of the epithelial cells is increased in untreated coeliac disease especially in children (Wright et al 1973). The increased loss of epithelial cells from the villi into the lumen is accompanied by a compensatory increase in crypt cell replication, which ultimately results in villous atrophy and elongated hyperplastic crypts, i.e. crypt hyperplastic villous atrophy. When examined under the dissecting or stereomicroscope the mucosa of children with coeliac disease is completely flat or featureless, or it may have a flat mosaic appearance with irregular areas divided by grooves. Normal 'fingers, leaves or ridges' cannot be seen (Fig. 8.2A). When examined histologically under the light microscope the mucosa has an appearance described as subtotal or total villous atrophy, with loss of the normal villous architecture and elongated hyperplastic crypts. The normally columnar surface epithelial cells with their basally located oval nuclei may become pseudostratified or cuboidal with spherical and pyknotic nuclei. These changes are accompanied by a quantitative increase in lamina propria plasma cells with a concomitant decrease of lymphocytes, and an increase in intraepithelial lymphocytes (Fig. 8.2B) with an elevated mitotic index. This raised index has been reported as of predictive value for the diagnosis of coeliac disease (Marsh 1982).

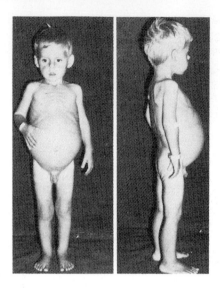

Fig. 8.3 Classical clinical features of untreated coeliac disease with muscle wasting and abdominal distension.

The severity of the proximal mucosal lesion has generally been regarded as uniform, but studies in adults suggest that the lesion may be 'patchy' with areas of flat mucosa adjacent to less abnormal mucosa. In untreated children the lesion is typically uniform whereas it may be patchy following gluten challenge (Manuel et al 1979). At present the finding of anything but a flat biopsy in a child who presents with suspected coeliac disease should alert the physician to the possibility of an alternative diagnosis. There is no natural recovery of the mucosal lesion by present definitions. The time required for the mucosa to return to normal following the institution of a gluten-free diet in an individual child may sometimes be surprisingly long, up to a year for example, many perhaps longer.

Clinical features

The majority of children present before the age of 2 years. The interval between the introduction of gluten-containing foods and the development of symptoms, however, is variable and although most children become symptomatic within 6 months of starting cereals, others may present in late childhood. In young infants acute symptoms such as diarrhoea and vomiting may occur soon after the first ingestion of gluten and mimic the clinical picture of acute infective enteritis. Since the publication in 1974 by the DHSS of the booklet 'Present-day Practice in Infant Feeding', gluten has been introduced at a later, more appropriate age (6 months or more) to infants in Britain. It is thus becoming very uncommon to see infants presenting with coeliac disease under the age of one year.

The classical features of abnormal stools, anorexia, vomiting, abdominal distension, and muscle wasting (Fig. 8.3) occur in approximately half the children presenting before the age of 2 years; frequently there is a history of irritability, apathy and delay or regression of motor development, and hypotonia may be present.

A diagnosis of coeliac disease should never be dismissed because of the absence of classical features since the condition has a wide spectrum of presentation. The bowel pattern may vary from bouts of explosive watery diarrhoea in the young infant to bulky offensive stools in the older child. Episodes of diarrhoea may alternate with constipation and occasionally constipation may be a presenting feature. The typical irritability and fretfulness may be absent. Older children may present with symptoms of more insidious onset, such as persistent iron deficiency anaemia, short stature or delayed puberty and may or may not have a history of gastrointestinal symptoms. In this age-group there is often little to find on physical examination apart from shortness of stature.

Investigations

Peroral small intestinal biopsy, prior to starting a gluten-free diet, with subsequent gluten challenge is mandatory for the diagnosis of coeliac disease. It should only be performed in centres with experience in the preparation and interpretation of mucosal specimens. The only rare exception when diagnostic biopsy should be deferred, is the acutely ill child with a dilated small bowel (i.e. 'coeliac crisis'), when biopsy is more likely to be complicated by bleeding and/or perforation. However, these two complications are now exceptionally uncommon. A number of screening tests such as serum iron and folate, red cell folate, serum reticulin antibodies, quantification of faecal fat, and urinary xylose following an oral load have been recommended but are far from ideal. Rolles et al (1973) have applied the one-hour blood xylose test as a screening test and reported a high degree of discrimination between children with and without coeliac disease. Lamabadusuriya et al (1975), using a somewhat different oral loading dose of xylose, did not find the test as reliable and reported three chilren with a flat mucosa due to coeliac disease who had a normal one-hour blood xylose concentration. A more appropriate test may be screening for antigliadin antibody. Unsworth et al (1981) have reported such an antibody in 100% of untreated children with coeliac disease but it was also present in children with other gastrointestinal problems. Whether this 100% accuracy will be found in larger series awaits evaluation. No test at present preempts the use of small intestinal biopsy for diagnosis in every case.

A clinical suspicion of coeliac disease is the single most important indication for biopsy. The early performance of this investigation avoids time-consuming, expensive and discomforting investigations, and reduces the duration of hospitalization to a minimum by providing a rapid diagnosis.

Diagnostic criteria

The demonstration of a flat small intestinal mucosa followed by a clinical response to dietary withdrawal of gluten used to be considered an adequate basis for a definitive diagnosis of coeliac disease. The recognition of other causes of a flat mucosa (see Table 8.2) and the existence of a syndrome of transient gluten intolerance have necessitated stricter diagnostic criteria. A definitive diagnosis of coeliac disease (i.e. permanent gluten intolerance) can be made only when gluten-induced mucosal abnormalities have been demonstrated following initial diagnosis and treatment. A scheme for such a diagnostic programme is illustrated in Figure 8.4 and we have applied this to 32 chilren with a past diagnosis of coeliac disease (Walker-Smith et al 1978). In 23 of the patients the diagnosis had been based on a flat mucosal biopsy and a clinical response to a gluten-free diet; in the remaining nine children biopsy had not been performed. After returning to a normal diet vague symptoms were common and unreliable in predicting which children developed mucosal abnormalities; such symptoms are probably related to the anxiety associated with returning to the 'toxic' gluten-containing diet. After two years of returning to a normal diet, four of the children who had initial flat biopsies, and two of the nine patients who did not have initial biopsies also had normal biopsies, i.e. appeared not to have coeliac disease. This study emphasizes the necessity of applying strict diagnostic criteria for coeliac disease.

Even when a 2-year follow-up is applied, some unanswered problems arise that will only be resolved by very long-term follow-up. A positive gluten challenge is used to indicate permanence of the intolerance, whereas it only proves persistence of the abnormality. Furthermore, it is possible that clinical (and possibly histological) expressions of the disease, including the degree of gluten sensitivity, may vary at different ages. Three cases (Schmitz et al 1978) have already been reported in whom a positive gluten challenge was later followed by apparent gluten tolerance, as indicated by spontaneous remission of the small intestinal mucosal lesion on a gluten-containing diet. These cases were older and the period of gluten intolerance was much longer than cases of 'transient' intolerance hitherto reported (McNeish et al 1979).

Table 8.2 Established causes of a flat small intestinal mucosa

---

Coeliac disease
Cow's milk protein intolerance
Soy protein intolerance
Acute viral and bacterial enteritis and postenteritis syndrome
Autoimmune enteropathy
Protein-energy malnutrition
Tropical sprue
Giardiasis

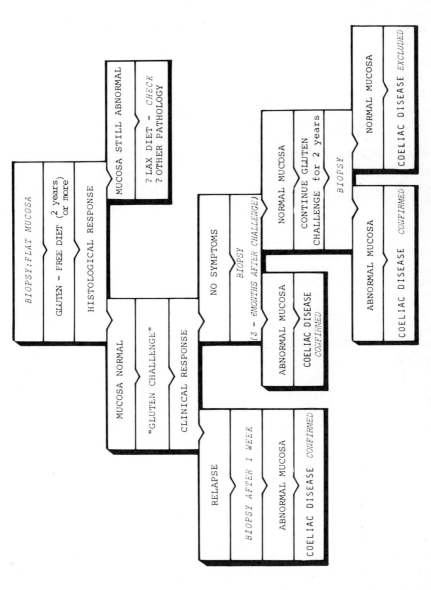

Fig. 8.4 Schema for diagnostic criteria and investigatory regime for coeliac disease.

Complications

Retarded growth and development

Severe growth retardation and delayed puberty are less common complications than formerly but may still occur as a mode of presentation (Groll et al 1980). Vanderschueren-Lodeweyckx et al (1973) found evidence of growth hormone deficiency in nine out of 13 children with coeliac disease. Thus coeliac disease should be considered as a diagnostic possibility in children of short stature who have growth hormone deficiency. A low serum somatomedin level has been described in such children and it has been suggested that there is limitation of somatomedin generation unrelated to a defect of growth hormone secretion in some children.

Skeletal abnormalities

Rickets and osteoporosis are now uncommon complications of coeliac disease.

Hypoproteinaemia

Hypoalbuminaemia, hypogammaglobulinaemia and hypoprothrombinaemia may all occur. Hypoalbuminaemia occurs in about one-third of cases and mainly results from intestinal loss of protein. Hypoprothrombinaemia is secondary to malabsorption of vitamin K and can be rapidly corrected with intramuscular vitamin Kl (1 mg) which should be done prior to diagnostic biopsies.

Anaemia

Iron deficiency anaemia is quite common. Although serum and/or red cell folate levels are often reduced, megaloblastic anaemia is most unusual. The combination of iron and folate deficiency should suggest the possibility of coeliac disease.

Milk intolerance

Intolerance to the lactose or protein moieties of cow's milk may occasionally be present at the time of diagnosis in infants (Young & Pringle 1971; Visakorpi and Immonen 1967). More recently a prolonged intolerance to both cow's milk protein and gluten has been reported. Both proteins, either separately or together, apparently inducing sub-total villous trophy (Watt et al 1983). In our experience this occurs uncommonly. Withdrawal of dietary disaccharides and/or cow's milk protein should only be considered if gastrointestinal symptoms persist following the institution of a gluten-free diet. Reduced activity of mucosal disaccharidases is an almost invariable finding in untreated coeliac disease and is not by itself an indication for a disaccharide-free diet; clinical intolerance is the only indication for such diets.

Neoplastic disease

Untreated adult coeliac disease may be complicated by lymphoma and carcinoma (Harris et al 1967). The risk of children developing neoplastic disease is not known.

Associated diseases

Diabetes mellitus

The association between diabetes mellitus and coeliac disease is now well documented and in one patient hyperthyroidism was also present (Chambers 1975). Autoimmune thyroiditis has also been reported in coeliac disease (MacLaurin et al 1972). HLA studies strongly suggest a common genetic predisposition to coeliac disease and insulin-dependent diabetes. It has been shown that both are individually associated with HLA-DR3 but the frequency of this finding in patients with both disorders does not differ significantly from those with either condition alone (Shanahan et al 1982). Recent descriptions of patients with an autoimmune enteropathy and a polyendocrinopathy (Savage et al 1985) (see page 204) indicate the necessity for strict diagnostic criteria in coeliac disease.

Isolated IgA deficiency

An association betwen IgA deficiency and coeliac disease has been described. Unlike the other abnormalities of serum immunoglobulins described in children with coeliac disease, this is not influenced by a gluten-free diet (Savilahti et al 1971). Thus IgA deficiency appears to be a disorder that predisposes to coeliac disease but only a small proportion of children with this deficiency develop the disorder (Savilahti 1974).

Dermatitis herpetiformis

Although there is an association between dermatitis herpetiformis and coeliac disease, it is uncommonly seen in childhood. The severity of the enteropathy in dermatitis herpetiformis varies from patient to patient and may be patchy in any one individual patient (Brow et al 1971). Both the enteropathy and the skin lesions may respond to withdrawal of dietary gluten (Kumar et al 1973).

Other associations

Cystic fibrosis and alpha-1-antitrypsin deficiency have been reported in children with coeliac disease, but the significance of these associations is uncertain. Both occur sufficiently freqently for the apparent association to be by chance alone.

Management

The specific treatment for coeliac disease is a gluten-free diet. Such a diet is generally regarded as one which is free of wheat, rye, oats and barley; maize (sweetcorn) and rice are harmless. The evidence that wheat and rye are toxic in childhood coeliac disease is well established, but the effect of oats and barley is controversial. Dissanayake et al (1974b) have provided some evidence that oats are not toxic in adults, but their period of observation following challenge with oats was far too short to draw firm conclusions. A survey of coeliac children in Britain showed that 12% were upset by oats (Segall 1974).

Elimination of dietary gluten often leads to a rapid clinical response within a few days, although in some children obvious improvement may be delayed. The first sign of improvement is often a change of mood, the child becoming less irritable, clinging and withdrawn. There follows a gain in weight with further symptomatic relief such as improvement in diarrhoea. Anxiety, depression and preoccupation with the child and their illness are common in the mother and usually disappear rapidly as the child begins to recover (Gardiner et al 1972). In the majority of patients a gluten-free diet is all that is required, and only in a minority is it necessary to temporarily exclude disaccharides and/or cow's milk protein. Ideally, treated patients should be followed up by a centre experienced in coeliac disease and their progress and diet checked at regular intervals. The necessity for a life-long diet depends on fulfilling the diagnostic criteria previously discussed.

TRANSIENT FOOD SENSITIVE ENTEROPATHIES

This group of clinical syndromes results from the sensitization of an individual to one or more dietary proteins and are of variable duration in childhood. Clinically the reaction to these, and other foods, may be quick, i.e. within one hour, or slow, occurring hours or days after food ingestion. In some cases acute anaphylactic reactions have occurred. Abnormalities of the small intestinal mucosa have been reported in cow's milk protein, soy protein, gluten, eggs, chicken, rice and fish intolerances. The enteropathy is not usually as severe as that seen in coeliac disease, although a flat mucosa may be seen, and usually resolves by the age of 18 months to 2 years.

The mucosal abnormalities which occur in transient protein intolerance are generally considered to result from an allergic reaction following the transient sensitization to dietary antigens. The precise mechanisms which cause the enteropathy remain unclear although the application of the Gell & Coombs (1968) classification of hypersensitivity reaction provides a basis for investigation. For the reactions to occur the offending antigen must enter the mucosa in appropriate amounts to cause sensitization. There are two hypotheses regarding this process: firstly, sensitization caused from an overstimulation of the immune system by excess antigen entry, or secondly, a minimal entry of antigen sufficient to stimulte a reaginic response, rather than its suppression, as in the normal course of events. It is likely that both hypotheses are correct in different circumstances. The latter occurs in atopic individuals and the former following enteric infection or in an IgA-deficient individual. An increased entry of antigen may occur both during (Gruskay & Cook 1955) and after (Jackson et al 1983) an enteric infection. It remains to be established whether small intestinal mucosal damage due to food ingestion occurs in adults, other than in patients with coeliac disease.

Cow's milk protein intolerance

Cow's milk ingestion may cause a variety of extraintestinal features in infancy such as eczema and asthma but this account will be confined to those disorders where milk has caused small intestinal mucosal damage, i.e. cow's milk sensitive enteropathy.

Pathogenesis

It is probable that there are two syndromes, a primary disorder of immunological origin and a secondary disorder, following mucosal damage which in turn produces an immunological abnormality. It seems probable that abnormal handling of dietary antigens across the intestinal mucosa occurs in infants with this disorder. This may be related to a temporary immunodeficiency state such as transient IgA-deficiency (Taylor et al 1973), or to non-specific mucosal damage from any cause. There is evidence that acute enteritis may be followed not only by lactose intolerance, but by more persistent and longer lasting cow's milk protein intolerance (Harrison et al 1975, 1976).

Unlike coeliac disease HLA status is normal in this disorder, suggesting that environmental factors are more important than genetic factors (Kuitunen et al 1975). Evidence of complement activation and of abnormalities in local B and T cell mediated function suggests that more than one reaction may participate in this disorder.

Pathology

In the vast majority of patients with slow onset of symptoms after cow's milk ingestion, the architecture of the proximal small intestinal mucosa is abnormal. The severity of the enteropathy is variable. In some early reports the mucosa was flat and indistinguishable from that seen in coeliac disease (Kuitunen et al 1975) but more recently from the same centre less severe mucosal damage has been characteristic. Typically the mucosa in untreated cow's milk-sensitive enteropathy is thin (Maluenda et al 1984) and the pathological changes are patchy (Manuel et al 1979). The intraepithelial lymphocytes are increased although not to the levels found in untreated coeliac disease (Phillips et al 1979). The mucosa rapidly returns towards normal on withdrawal of milk, only to relapse following challenge with milk (Walker-Smith 1975).

Clinical features

Presentation may be acute with vomiting and diarrhoea, or as a chronic syndrome characterized by less severe vomiting and diarrhoea, with failure to thrive. The majority present with acute symptoms under the age of 6 months and have features indistinguishable from acute infective enteritis; lactose intolerance may accompany protein intolerance but is of relatively short duration.

There is usually a latent interval between the introduction of cow's milk and the onset of symptoms, but occasionally violent reactions, such as anaphylactoid shock, may immediately follow the infant's first contact with cow's milk. The chronic syndrome may present in a very similar fashion to coeliac disease with loose stools and failure to thrive. Cow's milk protein intolerance may also be associated with iron deficiency anaemia due to intestinal blood loss (either occult or overt). This is related to an endoscopic colitis (Gryboski 1967, Jenkins et al 1984) which is discussed in more detail elsewhere (Ch. 6 and 16).

Diagnostic criteria

Because of its transient nature it may be difficult to fulfil all the diagnostic criteria for cow's milk sensitive enteropathy but nevertheless accurate diagnosis is important. It is important to exclude an infective cause of the enteropathy. As with all dietary protein intolerances, diagnosis is based upon the response, as judged by serial biopsies, to withdrawal and reintroduction of the offending protein. The finding of a patchy enteropathy with a thin mucosa in a cow's milk-fed infant, who responds rapidly to a cow's milk elimination diet provides firm presumptive evidence for this diagnosis. Such children may be described as having a milk elimination responsive enteropathy. The transient nature of this disorder as well as the desire to avoid early milk challenge (because of the potential risk of acute anaphylaxis) leads in practice to a late milk challenge at the age of 9 months to one year at which time the children may no longer be milk intolerant. Milk provocation in such circumstances merely establishes normal tolerance to milk.

Management

Treatment involves the substitution of cow's milk feeds with commercially available cow's milk, protein-free formulae (see Francis 1987). Cow's milk substitutes fall into four categories based on (i) casein hydrolysate (Pregestimil®), and for infants over 6 months, Nutramigen® (peferred option); (ii) soya protein (Cow & Gate formula S, Prosobee® liquid, Prosobee® powder, Wysoy®); (iii) comminuted chicken which requires supplementation with the complete range of vitamins and minerals, and for children over 6 months, a boiled diet based on comminuted chicken plus vitamins and minerals; and (iv) for children over 1 year, boiled goat's milk plus vitamins A, D, C, B_{12} and folic acid tablets containing lactose. Only those formulae which are nutritionally complete (if necessary with vitamin supplementation) are recommended and those with a low osmolality should be chosen for young infants or infants with small bowel disease. It is important to ensure that both liquid and solid feeds are free of cow's milk proteins. Disaccharide intolerance may accompany the protein intolerance, and in such circumstances disaccharides should also be withdrawn from the diet. The necessity for dietary treatment is always temporary, and reintroduction of a normal diet is usually possible by the age of 1 to 2 years. This is usually achieved in the home, but a history of severe reactions, such as urticaria or anaphylactoid shock, is an absolute indication for reintroduction of a normal diet under very close medical supervision.

Soy protein intolerance

It has been shown that soy protein can induce a small intestinal enteropathy which resolves with soy elimination and which reappears when soy protein is reintroduced into the diet (Ament & Rubin 1972). These workers described a flat mucosal lesion indistinguishable to that found in coeliac disease, but more usually the damage is less severe and is similar to cow's milk sensitive enteropathy (Perkkio et al 1981). The frequency of soy protein intolerance may well be increasing with the more wide-spread use of soy protein-based infant feeds.

Transient gluten intolerance

Firm evidence for a syndrome of transient gluten intolerance based upon serial small intestinal biopsies related to dietary elimination and challenge has only been described in one patient (Walker-Smith & Phillips 1979). However, a number of children have been reinvestigated following a diagnosis of coeliac disease (based on the finding of a flat mucosa and a clinical response to a gluten-free diet), who have remained clinically well with a normal small intestinal mucosa for more than 2 years after the reintroduction of a gluten-containing diet (Lindberg & Meeuwisse 1973, McNicholl et al 1974). Proof of a temporary gluten toxicity can only be established by early reinvestigation with the demonstration of gluten toxicity and the finding that such toxicity disappears after a time interval. Such early reintroduction is not routine practice, hence there is still controversy regarding this entity. This emphasises the necessity to reinvestigate, by means of gluten challenge and intestinal biopsy, infants diagnosed as having coeliac disease before recommending a life-long diet.

Other food sensitive enteropathies

It has now been established by serial biopsy and dietary elimination and challenge, that egg protein (Iyngkaran et al 1982), rice, chicken and fish (Vitoria et al 1982) may all temporarily damage the small intestinal mucosa in infancy. In the latter study all were infants under the age of 6 months who were also cow's milk intolerant.

BACTERIAL AND VIRAL ENTERITIS AND POST-ENTERITIS SYNDROME

Infective enteritis is a major problem in childhood throughout the world and is considered in detail elsewhere (see Ch. 15). Discussion here will therefore be limited to the morphological appearances of the small intestinal mucosa in acute enteritis and in the 'post-enteritis syndrome' (i.e. persistently loose stools and/or failure to thrive for longer than 2 weeks following an acute episode of diarrhoea with or without vomiting). In early studies proof of an infecting agent asssociated with the acute illness was often not established. Later studies using electron microscopy, specialized culture techniques and toxin testing procedures, have provided evidence for the presence of specific organisms at the time of acute gastroenteritis. Some of these organisms are recognized to be pathogenic in man, e.g. rotavirus, Norwalk agent, and *Campylobacter* species; others await general acceptance of their pathogenicity in man e.g. calicivirus, astrovirus, coronavirus and cryptosporidia.

Acute disease

The evidence that a small intestinal enteropathy may accompany acute

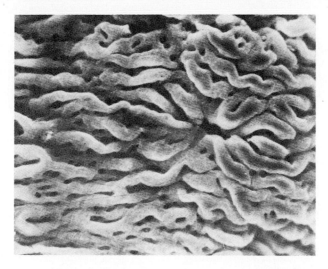

Fig. 8.5 Dissecting microscope appearances of autolysed small intestinal mucosa, showing short thick ridges, from an infant who died as a sequel to acute gastroenteritis.

enteritis is derived from autopsy studies and from peroral biopsies performed during the acute phase of disease.

Using a modification of the technique described by Creamer & Leppard (1965), autopsy studies in children dying during the acute phase were first reported by Walker-Smith (1972). Morphological abnormalities were found in seven of the ten patients studied (see Fig. 8.5) and the severity and extent of the abnormalities were variable. In the majority the enteropathy was proximal, but in one patient the whole of the small intestine was affected, and in another the ileum was chiefly involved. The mucosal lesions tended to be patchy in individual patients. Barnes & Townley (1973) in a series of 31 infants with acute enteritis made similar findings. The interpretation of single biopsies as a guide to the overall state of the proximal small intestinal mucosa must however be cautious in the light of the studies discussed above (Walker-Smith 1972).

Viral infections

This section will refer only to reports of small bowel morphology in human viral infections.

Norwalk agent

In adult volunteer studies patchy proximal small intestinal mucosal lesions were reported following oral administration of Norwalk agent, however Norwalk agent was not detected within the biopsies (Schreiber et al 1973).

Rotavirus

Bishop et al (1976) described the presence of rotavirus particles within the epithelium of the severely abnormal mucosae from some of the patients with acute gastroenteritis reported earlier by Barnes & Townley (1973). Rotavirus is the most frequently detected virus in the stools of children with acute gastroenteritis and is now accepted as a cause of small intestinal mucosal damage in childhood.

Other viruses

Adenovirus has been found within the severely abnormal mucosa of patients dying from acute gastroenteritis (Phillips 1981). Astrovirus has been detected within the proximal small intestinal mucosa of biopsy samples in association with a patchy enteropathy (Phillips et al 1982)

Bacterial infections

It has been reported that in certain human infections with classical EPEC (enteropathogenic *Escherichia coli*) serotypes there is a morphologically characteristic appearance within the small and large bowel associated with adhesion of *Escherichia coli* (*Esch. coli*) to the mucosal surface (Ulshen & Rollo 1980, Phillips 1981). This appearance includes a crypt hyperplastic villous atrophy and adhesion of *Esch. coli* to pedestal-like protrusions of the enterocyte apical membrane with loss of microvilli and disruption of the terminal web. All cases involved infants with protracted diarrhoea. Following antibiotic therapy and necessary dietary management the *Esch. coli* infections resolved with concomitant improvement in bowel morphology (see Ch. 15).

Chronic disease

Mucosal abnormalities have been well documented in a proportion of children who developed protracted diarrhoea following an acute episode of enteritis (Burke et al 1965, Boyce et al 1974), the degree of abnormality ranging from a completely flat mucosa to lesser degrees of abnormality.

The pathogenesis of the enteropathy in both acute and chronic diarrhoea in infancy is not known; infective agents and various dietary proteins may play an individual and/or collective pathophysiological role. The above aspects are considered in more detail in Chapter 16.

PARASITIC INFECTIONS

Giardiasis

Infestation with this flagellate protozoan is dealt with more fully elsewhere (see Ch. 10), and this discussion will be confined to the morphology of the small intestinal mucosa.

Giardiasis may be accompanied by gastrointestinal symptoms in both adults and children in the absence of recognizable immunodeficiency. Clinical symptoms, however, are variable and both asymptomatic carriage and frank malabsorption may be associated with the presence of the parasite. Histological features are similarly variable; Wright & Tomkins (1978) have shown a relationship between the severity of the enteropathy and the degree of malabsorption. Other reported small bowel abnormalities in giardiasis include increased isolated mucosal lymphoid follicles, reduced disaccharidase activities, increased lamina propria inflammatory cells, and increased intraepithelial lymphocytes (Farthing, et al 1983). The mucosal abnormalities associated with giardiasis, whether in the immunodeficient (Ochs et al 1972) or the immunocompetent subject, (Ogilvie & Harries 1977) improve on eradication of the parasite.

Cryptosporidia

This coccidian parasite is becoming implicated as a cause of acute gastroenteritis in childhood and as a potential cause of the postenteritis syndrome. Its presence in the small bowel is associated with a mild enteropathy and a characteristic method of mucosal adhesion.

CONGENITAL MICROVILLOUS ATROPHY

Davidson et al (1978) described a syndrome of familial intractable diarrhoea from birth with hypoplastic villous atrophy on small intestinal biopsy which was usually fatal. Jejunal epithelium of three of the five described patients was examined with the electron microscope and in one of these a distinct ultrastructural abnormality of the microvilli was reported. Similar observations were made by Schmitz et al (1982) who called the syndrome 'congenital microvillous atrophy' because of the appearance of the exposed surface epithelium of the small intestinal mucosa, which was characterized by depletion and shortening of the microvilli with instances of microvilli within involutions of the apical membrane (Fig. 8.6). By contrast the crypt epithelium was preserved with microvilli which was not as affected as the villous epithelium but possessed increased numbers of secretory granules. Using polyacrylamide gel electrophoresis of the microvillous membrane it has been shown in one case that there is an absent myosin band (Carruthers et al 1985). It is possible that this disorder is a lesion of the cytoskeleton but whether this is a truly congenital or an acquired lesion remains an open question.

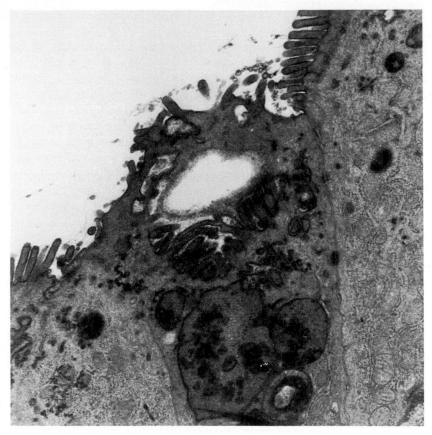

Fig. 8.6 Congenital microvillous atrophy. Electron micrograph, magnified × 24 000, showing typical microvillous involution

AUTOIMMUNE ENTEROPATHY

A syndrome has now been recognized which presents as intractable diarrhoea in infancy with an abnormal small intestinal mucosa which may be flat and indistinguishable from untreated coeliac disease. There is however no response to gluten restriction, but there is evidence of autoimmune disease, i.e. the presence of circulating autoantibodies and/or an associated polyendocrinopathy. A highly characteristic feature is the gut enterocyte autoantibody (Unsworth et al 1982, Savage et al 1985). The antibody reported in the above cases was a complement-fixing IgG which reacted preferentially with a cytoplasmic antigen in villous tip enterocytes. These cases are similar to the patient described by McCarthy et al (1978). At present treatment is very unsatisfactory. Some, but not all, are steroid-responsive. Some have survived on a regime of intermittent intragastric feeding with a comminuted chicken meat formula and one has responded to a hypoallergenic diet (Savage et al 1985). (See also Ch. 16).

TROPICAL SPRUE

This poorly-understood disorder is relatively uncommon in children as compared to adults and is characterized by diarrhoea, megaloblastic anaemia, and malabsorption of vitamin B_{12}, folic acid and fat (Lindenbaum 1973). The pathogenesis of this disorder is not known, but infection with bacterial overgrowth of the small intestine is of probable importance in the development of the condition. There is a nonspecific enteropathy which affects the whole length of the small intestine; occasionally the mucosa is flat but usually the lesion is less severe. The condition responds to folic acid and/or antibiotic therapy. The diagnosis should be considered in children in nontropical countries who have recently lived in an area endemic for tropical sprue.

EOSINOPHILIC GASTROENTERITIS

This syndrome is a disorder involving the stomach and/or small intestine and is characterized by eosinophilic infiltration of the gastrointestinal tract wall, eosinophilia and the development of gastrointestinal symptoms following the ingestion of certain specific dietary foods. Improvement follows withdrawal of the offending dietary constituent(s) and/or corticosteroid therapy (Greenberger & Gryboski 1973, Gryboski 1967). The pathogenesis is not clearly understood but an allergic or immunological basis seems likely. Cow's milk protein intolerance may present as an eosinophilic gastroenteropathy. The disorder can be classified according to the extent of the eosinophilic infiltration: (1) primary mucosal involvement with malabsorption and protein loss, (2) muscle layer disease with obstructive features or (3) subserosal disease with eosinophilic ascites. Eosinophilic gastroenteritis as seen in childhood is almost invariably a primary mucosal disease. The small intestinal mucosal enteropathy varies in severity. There may be mild eosinophilic infiltration of the lamina propria with preservation of villous pattern, or at the other extreme, a severe infiltrative lesion with a flat mucosa. The mucosal lesion is patchy and, when using multiple biopsy techniques, varying degrees of severity may be found in an individual patient. Some support for an allergic pathogenesis has come from the finding of marked mast cell degranulation in the epithelial glands of the stomach in a patient with eosinophilic gastritis (Phillips & Lewis 1982).

HISTIOCYTOSIS X

Histiocytic infiltration of the small intestine may be present in infants with disseminated histiocytosis X (Letterer-Siwe syndrome). In an autopsy review of 12 cases (Keeling & Harries 1973) the small intestine was found to be involved in six cases, four of whom had developed diarrhoea during the course of their illness; the ileum was most commonly affected but changes in the duodenum and jejunum were also found. The abnormalities include infiltration of the lamina propria with abnormal histiocytes and multinucleate giant cells. The villous architecture and epithelium were normal in all but one case, in whom there was loss of the normal villous pattern. The cellular infiltration may impair intestinal function resulting in malabsorption.

OTHER ENTEROPATHIES

Small intestinal lymphomas, radiation enteritis, acute necrotizing enterocolitis, chronic inflammatory bowel disease, iron-deficiency anaemia, intractable diarrhoea of unknown origin and the administration of certain drugs may be associated with a small intestinal enteropathy and gastrointestinal symptoms. Although gastrointestinal symptoms commonly follow the administration of a variety of drugs, in only a few instances have small intestinal mucosal abnormalities been demonstrated. Methotrexate and high doses of neomycin may induce mucosal lesions (Dobbins 1968) although there is no evidence that therapeutic doses of neomycin produce mucosal damage. With increasingly aggressive cytotoxic drug requirements in the treatment of malignant disease and organ transplantation it is likely that small intestinal enteropathies from both the drugs themselves and graft versus host disease will be encountered (see Ch. 22). Mild mucosal changes have been reported in association with iron-deficiency anaemia, but whether the iron deficiency is primary in the pathogenesis of the muscosal lesions has not been established.

REFERENCES

Ament M E, Rubin C E 1972 Soy protein — another cause of the flat intestinal lesion. Gastroenterology 62:227
Asquith P, Thompson R A, Cooke W T 1969 Serum immunoglobulins in adult coeliac disease. Lancet ii:129
Barnes G L, Townley R R W 1973 Duodenal mucosal damage in 31 infants with gastroenteritis. Archives of Disease in Childhood 48:343
Bishop R F, Cameron D J S, Barnes G P, Holmes I H, Ruck B J 1976 The aetiology of diarrhoea in newborn infants. Ciba Foundation Symposium 42 (new series) Acute diarrhoea in childhood. Elsevier Excerpta Medica North, Holland
Boyce M J, France N E, Walker-Smith J A 1974 Small intestinal morphology in a group of infants and young children with delayed recovery after acute diarrhoea and vomiting. Gut 15:827
Brow J R, Parker F, Weinstein W M, Rubin C E 1971 The small intestinal mucosa in dermatitis herpetiformis I: Severity and distribution of the small intestinal lesion and associated malabsorption. Gastroenterology 60: 355–361
Burke V, Kerry K R, Anderson C M 1965 The relationship of dietary lactose in refractory diarrhoea in infancy. Australian Pediatric Journal 1:147
Carruthers L, Phillips A D, Dourmashkin R, Walker-Smith J A 1985 Biochemical abnormality in brush border membrane protein of a patient with congenital microvillus atrophy. Journal of Pediatric Gastroenterology and Nutrition 4: 902–907
Carter C, Sheldon W, Walker C 1959 The inheritance of coeliac disease. Annals of Human Genetics 23:266
Chambers T L 1975 Coeliac disease, diabetes mellitus hyperthyroidism. Archives of Disease in Childhood 50: 162–164

Creamer B, Leppard P 1965 Post mortem examination of a small intestine in the coeliac syndrome. Gut 6:466

Davidson G P, Cutz E, Hamilton J R, Gall D G 1978 Familial enteropathy: a syndrome of protracted diarrhoea from birth, failure to thrive, and hypoplastic villous atrophy. Gastroenterology 75:783

Department of Health and Social Security 1974 Present-day Practice in Infant Feeding. HMSO, London

Dicke W K 1950 Coeliakie. M D Thesis, University of Utrecht

Dissanayake A S, Jerrome D W, Offord R E, Truelove S C, Whitehead R 1974a Identifying toxic fractions of wheat gluten and their effect on the jejunal mucosa in coeliac disease. Gut 15:931

Dissanayake A S, Truelove S, Whitehead R 1974b Lack of harmful effect of oats on small intestinal mucosa in coeliac disease. British Medical Journal 4:189

Dobbins W O 1968 Drug-induced steatorrhoea. Gastroenterology 54:1193

Doe W F, Henry K, Booth C C 1974 Complement in coeliac disease. In: Hekkens W, Pena A (eds) Coeliac Disease. Proceedings of the 2nd International Coeliac Symposium, Stenfert Kroese, Leiden. p 189

Dossetor J F B, Gibson A A M, McNeish A S 1981 Childhood Coeliac disease is disappearing. Lancet i:322

Douglas A P, Booth C C 1970 Digestion of gliadin peptides by normal human jejunal mucosa and by mucosa from patients with adult coeliac disease. Clinical Science 38:11

Dowd B, Walker-Smith J A 1974 Samuel Gee, Aretaeus and the coeliac affection. British Medical Journal 2:45

Ezoke W, Ferguson N, Fakhri O, Hekkens W, Hobbs J R 1974 Antibodies in the sera of coeliac patients which can co-opt K cells to attack gluten-labelled targets. In: Hekkens W, Pena A (eds) Coeliac Disease. Proceedings of the 2nd International Coeliac Symposium, Stenfert Kroese, Leiden. p 176

Falchuk Z M, Gebhard R L, Strober W 1974 The pathogenesis of gluten sensitive enteropathy (coeliac sprue): organ culture studies. In: Hekkens W, Pena A (eds) Coeliac Disease. Proceedings of the 2nd International Coeliac Symposium. Stenfert Kroese, Leiden. p 107

Farthing M J G, Chong S K F, Walker-Smith J A 1983 Acute allergic phenomena in giardiasis. Lancet ii:1428

Ferguson A, Murray D 1971 Quantitation of intra-epithelial lymphocytes in human jejunum. Gut 12:988

Francis D E M 1987 Diets for Sick Children. 4th edn. Blackwell, Oxford

Frazer A C 1956 Growth defect in coeliac disease. Proceedings of the Royal Society of Medicine 49:1009

Gardiner A, Porteous N, Walker-Smith J A 1972 The effect of coeliac disease on the mother child relationship. Australian Paediatric Journal 8:39

Gee S J 1888 On the coeliac affection. St. Bartholomew's Hospital Reports 24: 17–20

Gell P G H, Coombs R R A 1968 Classification of allergic reactions responsible for hypersensitivity and disease. In: Gell P G H, Coombs R R A (eds) Clinical Aspects of Immunology. Blackwell, Oxford. p 575

Greenberger N, Gryboski J D 1973 Allergic disorders of the intestine and eosinophilic gastroenteritis. In: Sleisenger, Fordtran (eds) Gastrointestinal Disease. Saunders, Philadelphia. p 1066

Groll A, Candy D C A, Preece M A, Tanner J M, Harries J T 1980 Short stature as the primary manifestation of coeliac disease. Lancet ii: 1097–1099

Gruskay F L, Cook R E 1955 The gastrointestinal absorption of unaltered protein in normal infants and in infants recovering from diarrhoea. Pediatrics 16:763

Gryboski J D 1967 Gastrointestinal milk allergy in infants Pediatrics 40:354

Harris O D, Cooke W T, Thompson M, Waterhouse J A H 1967 Malignancy in adult coeliac disease and idiopathic steatorrhoea. American Journal of Medicine 42:899

Harrison M, Wood C B S, Walker-Smith J A 1975 Sugar malabsorption in cow's milk protein intolerance. Archives of Disease in Childhood 50:746

Harrison B M, Kilby A, Walker-Smith J A, France N E, Wood C B S 1976 Cow's milk protein intolerance: a possible association with gastroenteritis, lactose intolerance and IgA deficiency. British Medical Journal 1:1501

Hekkens W 1978 Protein chemistry and toxicity overview. In: McNicholl B,

McCarthy C F, Fottrell P F (eds) Perspectives in Coeliac Disease. Third International Coeliac Symposium. MTP Press, Lancaster. p 3

Holmes G K T, Asquith P, Cooke W T 1972 Cell mediated mechanisms in adult coeliac disease. Gut 13:324

Iyngkaran N, Abidin Z, Meng L L, Yadav M 1982 Egg-protein-induced villous atrophy. Journal of Pediatric Gastroenterology and Nutrition 1:29

Jackson D, Walker-Smith J A, Phillips A D 1983 Macromolecular absorption by histologically normal and abnormal small intestine mucosa in childhood: An in vitro study using organ culture. Journal of Pediatric Gastroenterology and Nutrition 2: 235–248

Jenkins H R, Pincott J R, Soothill J F, Milla P J, Harries J T 1984 Food Allergy: the major cause of infantile colitis. Archives of Disease in Childhood 59:326

Kamath K E, Dorney S F A 1983 Is discordance for coeliac disease in monozygotic twins permanent? Pediatric Research 17:422

Keeling J W, Harries J T 1973 Intestinal malabsorption in infants with Histiocytosis X. Archives of Disease in Childhood 48:350

Kendall M J, Schneider R, Cox P S, Hawkins C E 1972 Gluten subfractions in coeliac disease. Lancet ii:1065

Kenrick K G, Walker-Smith J A 1970 Immunoglobulins and dietary protein antibodies in childhood coeliac disease. Gut 11:635

Kilby A, Walker-Smith J A, Wood C B S 1975 Small intestinal mucosa in cow's milk allergy. Lancet i:53

Kowlessar O D 1967 Effect of wheat proteins in coeliac disease. Gastroenterology 52:893

Kuitunen P, Visakorpi J K, Savilahti E, Pelkonen P 1975 Malabsorption syndrome with cow's milk intolerance: clinical findings and course in 54 cases. Archives of Disease in Childhood 50:351

Kumar P J, Silk D B A, Marks R, Clark M L, Dawson A M 1973 Treatment of dermatitis herpetiformis with corticosteroids and a gluten free diet: a study of jejunal morphology and function. Gut 14:280

Lamabadusuriya S P, Packer S, Harries J T 1975 Limitations of xylose tolerance test as a screening procedure in childhood coeliac disease. Archives of Disease in Childhood 50:34

Lancaster-Smith M, Kumar R P, Clark M L 1974 Immunological phenomena following gluten challenge in the jejunum of patients with adult coeliac disease and dermatitis herpetiformis. In: Hekkens W, Pena A (eds) Coeliac Disease. Proceedings of the 2nd International Coeliac Symposium. Stenfert Kroese, Leiden. p 173

Leigh R J, Marsh M N, Crowe P, Kelly C, Garner V, Gordon D 1985 Studies of intestinal lymphoid tissue IX. Dose-dependent, gluten-induced lymphoid infiltration of coeliac jejunal epithelium. Scandinavian Journal of Gastroenterology 6: 715–719

Lindberg T, Meeuwisse G 1973 Transient coeliac disease — does it exist? Acta Paediatrica Scandinavica, Supplement 236:56

Lindenbaum J 1973 Tropical enteropathy. Gastroenterology 64:637

McCarthy D M, Katz S I, Ganzze L, Waldmann T A, Nelson D L 1978 IgA deficiency associated with total villous atrophy of the small intestine and an organ-specific anti-epithelial antibody. Journal of Immunology 120: 932–938

McCrae W N 1969 Inheritance of coeliac disease. Journal of Medical Genetics 6:129

MacLaurin B P, Mathews N, Kilpatrick J A 1972 Coeliac disease associated with autoimmune thyroiditis, Sjogern's syndrome and a lymphocytotoxi serum factor. Australian and New Zealand Journal of Medicine 4:401

McNeish A S, Rolles C J, Nelson R, Kyaw Myit T O, Mackintosh P, Williams A F 1974 Factors affecting the differing racial incidence of coeliac disease. In: Hekkens W, Pena A (eds) Coeliac Disease. Proceedings of the 2nd International Coeliac Symposium. Stenfert Kroese, Leiden. p 330

McNeish A S, Harms H K, Rey J, Shmerling D H, Visakorpi J K, Walker-Smith J A 1979 The diagnosis of coeliac disease — a commentary on the current practices of members of the European Society for Paediatric Gastroenterology and Nutrition Archives of Disease in Childhood 54: 783–786

McNicholl B, Egan-Mitchell B, Fottrell P F 1974 Varying susceptibility in coeliac disease. In: Hekkens W, Pena A (eds) Coeliac Disease. Proceedings of the 2nd International Coeliac Symposium. Stenfert Kroese, Leiden. p 413

Maluenda C, Phillips A D, Briddon A, Walker-Smith J A 1984 Quantitative analysis of small intestinal mucosa in cow's milk sensitive enteropathy. Journal of Pediatric Gastroenterology and Nutrition. 3: 349–356

Manuel P, Walker-Smith J A, France N E 1979 Patchy enteropathy. Gut 20:211

Marsh M N 1982 Studies of intestinal lymphoid tissue. IV — The predictive value of raised mitotic indices among jejunal epithelial lymphocytes in the diagnosis of gluten-sensitive enteropathy. Journal of Clinical Pathology 35:517

Mylotte J M, Eagan-Mitchell B, Fottrell P F, McNicholl B, McCarthy C F 1973 Incidence of coeliac disease in the West of Ireland. British Medical Journal 60:703

Ochs H D, Ament M E, Davis S D 1972 Giardiasis with malabsorption in X-linked agammaglobulinaemia. New England Journal of Medicine 287:341

Ogilvie, Harries 1977 Small Intestinal Enteropathies. In: J T Harries (ed) Essentials of Paediatric Gastroenterology. Churchill Livingstone, Edinburgh

Perkkio M, Savilahti E, Kuitunen P 1981 Morphometric and immunochemical study of jejunal biopsies from children with intestinal soy allergy. European Journal of Pediatrics 137: 63–69

Phelan J J, McCarthy C F, Stevans F M, McNicholl B, Fottrell P F 1974 The nature of gliadin toxicity in coeliac disease: a new concept. In: Hekkens W, Pena A S (eds) Coeliac Disease. Proceedings of the 2nd International Coeliac Symposium Stenfert Kroese, Leiden. p 60

Phillips A D 1981 Small intestinal mucosa in childhood in health and disease. Scandinavian Journal of Gastroenterology 16: Supplement 70, 65

Phillips A D, Lewis D C 1982 Intraepithelial mast cells in the gut. Pediatric Research 16:1044

Phillips A D, Rice S J, France N E, Walker-Smith J A 1979 Small intestinal lymphocyte levels in cow's milk protein intolerance. Gut 20:509

Phillips A D, Rice S J, Walker-Smith J A 1982 Astrovirus within human small intestinal mucosa. Gut 23:A293

Rolles C J, Kendall M J, Nutter S, Anderson C M 1973 One hour blood xylose screening test for coeliac disease. Lancet ii:1043

Rubin C E, Brandborg L L, Phelps P A, Taylor H C 1960 Studies of coeliac sprue. Gastroenterology 38:28

Sakula J, Shiner M 1957 Coeliac disease with atrophy of the small intestine mucosa. Lancet ii:876

Savage M O, Mirakian R, Wozniak E R et al 1985 Specific autoantibodies to gut epithelium in two infants with severe protracted diarrhoea. Journal of Pediatric Gastroenterology and Nutrition. 4:187

Savilahti E 1972 Intestinal immunoglobulins in children with coeliac disease. Gut 13:958

Savilahti E 1974 Immunofluorescence in coeliac disease. In: Hekkens W, Pena A (eds) Coeliac Disease. Proceedings of the 2nd International Coeliac Symposium, Stenfert Kroese, Leiden. p 163

Savilahti E, Pelkonen P, Visakorpi J K 1971 IgA deficiency in children. A clinical study with special reference to intestinal findings. Archives of Disease in Childhood 46:665

Schmitz J, Jos J, Rey J 1978 Transient mucosal atrophy in confirmed coeliac disease. In: McCarthy, McNicholl (eds) Perspectives in Coeliac Disease. Proceedings of the Third International Coeliac Symposium, Galway. MPT Press, Lancaster. p 259

Schmitz J, Ginies J L, Arnaud-Battandier F et al 1982 Congenital microvillous atrophy, a rare cause of neonatal intractable diarrhoea. Pediatric Research 16:1041

Schreiber D S, Blacklow N R, Trier J S 1973 The mucosal lesion of the proximal small intestine in acute infectious nonbacterial gastroenteritis. New England Journal of Medicine 288:1318

Segall E 1974 Oats and coeliac disease. British Medical Journal 4:589

Selby W S, Janossy G, Bofill M, Jewell D P 1983 Lymphocyte subpopulations in the human small intestine. The findings in normal mucosa and in the mucosa of patients with adult coeliac disease. Clinical and Experimental Immunology 53: 219–228

Shanahan F, McKenna R, McCarthy C F, Drury M I 1982 Coeliac disease and diabetes mellitus: a study of 24 patients with HLA typing. Quarterly Journal of Medicine 203:329

Shiner M, Ballard J 1972 Antigen-antibody reactions in the jejunal mucosa in childhood coeliac disease after gluten challenge. Lancet i:1202

Taylor B, Norman A P, Orgel H A, Stokes C R, Turner M W, Soothill J F 1973 Transient IgA deficiency and pathogenesis of infantile atopy. Lancet ii:111

Tosi R, Vismara D, Tanigaki N et al 1983 Evidence that coeliac disease is primarily associated with a DC locus allergic specificity. Clinical Immunology and Immunopathology 28: 395–404

Ulshen M H, Rollo J L 1980 Pathogenesis of *Escherichia coli* gastroenteritis in man — another mechanism. New England Journal of Medicine 302:99

Unsworth D J, Kieffer M, Holborow E J, Coombs R R A, Walker-Smith J A 1981. IgA anti-gliadin antibodies in coeliac disease. Clinical and Experimental Immunology 46:286

Unsworth D J, Hutchins P, Mitchell J et al 1982 Flat small intestinal mucosa and autoantibodies against the gut epithelium. Journal of Pediatric Gastroenterology and Nutrition 1:503

Vanderschueren-Lodeweyckx M, Wolter M, Molla A, Eggermont E, Eeckels R 1973 Plasma growth hormone in coeliac disease. Helvetica Paediatrica Acta 28:349

Visakorpi J K, Immonen P 1967 Intolerance to cow's milk and wheat gluten in the primary malabsorption syndrome in infancy. Acta Paediatrica Scandinavica 6:49

Vitoria J C, Camarero C, Sojo A, Ruiz A, Rodriguezsoriano J 1982 Enteropathy related to fish, rice and chicken. Archives of Disease in Childhood 57: 44–48

Walker-Smith J A 1972 Uniformity of dissecting microscope appearances in proximal small intestine. Gut 13:17

Walker-Smith J A 1973 Discordance for childhood coeliac disease in monozygotic twins. Gut 14:374

Walker-Smith J A 1975 Cow's milk protein intolerance; transient food intolerance of infancy. Archives of Disease in Childhood 50:347

Walker-Smith J A, Phillips A D 1979 The pathology of gastrointestinal allergy. In: Pepys J, Edwards A M (eds) The Mast Cell: its role in health and disease. p 629

Walker-Smith J A, Kilby A, France N E 1978 Reinvestigation of children previously diagnosed as coeliac disease. In: McNicholl B, McCarthy C F, Fottrell P F (eds) Perspectives in Coeliac Disease. MTP Press Limited, Lancaster. p 267

Wall A J, Douglas A P, Booth C C, Pearse A G E 1970 Response of the jejunal mucosal in adult coeliac disease to oral prednisolone. Gut 11:7

Watt J, Pincott J R, Harries J T 1983 Combined cow's milk protein and gluten-induced enteropathy: common and rare. Gut 24: 165–170

Weiser M M, Douglas A P 1976 An alternative mechanism for gluten toxicity in coeliac disease. Lancet i:567

Weiser M M, Douglas A P 1978 Cell surface glycosyl-transferases of the enterocyte in coeliac disease. In: McCarthy, McNicholl (eds) Perspectives in Coeliac Disease. Third International Coeliac Symposium, MPT Press Limited, Lancaster. p 451

Wright S G, Tomkins A M 1978 Quantitative histology in giardiasis. Journal of Clinical Pathology 31:712

Wright N, Watson A, Morley A, Appleton D, Marks J, Douglas A 1973 The cell cycle time in the flat (avillous) mucosa of the human small intestine. Gut 14:603

Young W, Pringle E M 1971 110 children with coeliac disease. Archives of Disease in Childhood 46:421

Selective inborn errors of absorption

INTRODUCTION

The selective inborn errors of absorption are not commonly encountered in clinical practice, but nevertheless represent an important group of disorders. Their early diagnosis and the institution of treatment may be life-saving. A correct diagnosis is essential for informed genetic counselling. Because of the selective nature of the absorptive defects, detailed investigations in patients with a number of these disorders have provided important information about the normal physiological processes involved in absorption and have enabled the physiological roles of a number of dietary nutrients to be elucidated.

The conditions may be classified according to the microlocalization of the defect or according to the dietary constituents affected. For most practical purposes we believe the latter is a more helpful approach and such a classification is shown in Table 9.1.

In order to fully understand the selective inborn errors of absorption it is necessary to have a knowledge of the normal physiological processes. It is not, however, possible in this chapter to discuss in detail these processes, and the reader will therefore be referred to recent reviews.

CARBOHYDRATES

Physiology (see Gray 1975, Kimmich 1981)

Starch is hydrolysed within the gut lumen by salivary and pancreatic

211

Table 9.1   Classification of selective inborn errors of absorption and digestion

Carbohydrates	Lactase deficiency a. Caucasian type b. Non-caucasian type Sucrase-isomaltase deficiency Trehalase deficiency Glucose-galactose malabsorption
Lipids	Abetalipoproteinaemia Familial hypobetalipoproteinaemia a. Heterozygous b. Homozygous Primary bile acid malabsorption Cystic fibrosis
Proteins and amino acids	Trypsinogen deficiency Enterokinase deficiency Hartnup disease Cystinuria Lysinuric protein intolerance Blue diaper syndrome Oast house syndrome Iminoglycinuria Lowe's syndrome
Water and electrolytes	Congenital chloridorrhoea Lethal familial protracted diarrhoea
Vitamins	Selective vitamin B_{12} malabsorption Transcobalamin II deficiency Congenital folate malabsorption
Minerals	Acrodermatitis enteropathica Primary hypomagnesaemia Familial hypophosphataemic rickets

amylase to give maltose, maltotriose and α-limit dextrins which, together with sucrose and lactose, are then hydrolysed at the brush border to yield the monosaccharides glucose, fructose and galactose. Brush border hydrolysis is carried out by the oligosaccharidases lactase, maltase and sucrase-isomaltase, which are large glycoproteins with pH optima of approximately 6.0 (Gray 1975, Semenza 1981). Their maximal activity is in the enterocytes of the proximal jejunum (Newcomer and McGill 1966).

Following hydrolysis, the monosaccharides are translocated across the brush border membrane by carrier-mediated systems, and it is likely that the surface oligosaccharidases are located immediately adjacent to the carriers. Glucose and galactose share the same sodium-coupled, energy dependent, electrogenic transport system.

It has been suggested (Crane 1965, Kimmich 1973) that the brush border carrier has two binding sites, one for glucose and galactose, and one for the monovalent cations sodium and potassium. Sodium binding increases the carrier's affinity for the monosaccharides, whereas potassium has the reverse effect. The intracellular concentration of sodium is kept low as a result of active extrusion of the ion out of the enterocyte into the lateral intercellular spaces by membrane-bound Na^+K^+ ATPase, the energy being derived from the hydrolysis of ATP. The net result is the generation of a sodium gradient between the intestinal lumen and the interior of the enterocyte, allowing sodium to diffuse passively down an electro-chemical gradient into the enterocyte. Intracellular hexose enters the intercellular spaces and then the portal vein by diffusion down a concentration gradient, almost certainly via a carrier-mediated system. The absorption of fructose appears to be carrier-mediated but is independent of energy or sodium (Holdsworth & Dawson 1965, Schultz & Strecker, 1970, Gray 1975).

Lactase deficiency

Caucasian type

Congenital lactase deficiency was first reported by Holzel et al in 1959. Patients present with profuse watery diarrhoea soon after the introduction of milk feeds, and the condition is fatal unless an early diagnosis is established and lactose withdrawn from the diet. A presumptive diagnosis can be made on the basis of a careful clinical history but a definitive diagnosis requires the demonstration of an isolated deficiency or absence of lactase activity (Levin et al 1970, Asp & Dahlquist 1974).

Monosaccharide absorption is unaffected and, therefore, treatment with a lactose-free formula containing monosaccharides is highly effective. This rare condition must be distinguished from the temporary lactase deficiency which often complicates enteric infections and is found in various enteropathies.

Non-caucasian type

From infancy onwards, lactose malabsorption is the commonest form of carbohydrate intolerance. In most populations brush border lactase activity declines in childhood. This may be regarded as physiologically normal and it occurs in most mammalian species. The extent to which lactase-deficient subjects can tolerate lactose varies considerably (Bayless et al 1975). Symptoms are, however, generally mild and do not occur until the age of two to three years. The condition is inherited as an autosomal dominant (Ransome-Kuti et al 1975).

Sucrase-isomaltase deficiency

Congenital sucrase-isomaltase deficiency was first described in 1960 by Weijers et al, and although it is generally considered to be a rare condition, it may occur in as many as 0.2% of North Americans (Peterson and Herber

1967) and in 10% of Greenland Eskimos (McNair et al 1972). The prevalence of the heterozygous state varies from 9–43%.

The severity of symptoms varies from severe diarrhoea in infancy, to intermittent, bothersome symptoms in the older child (Antonowicz et al 1972, Ament et al 1973). The correct diagnosis may, therefore, be missed for several months or years, with symptoms being attributed to conditions such as 'toddler diarrhoea' or 'maternal anxiety'. The diagnosis is established by the demonstration of deficient sucrase and isomaltase activities in a morphologically normal jejunal biopsy. Maltase (α-glucosidase) activity is also reduced, since sucrase accounts for a large proportion of the total maltase activity. As with the other congenital disorders of carbohydrate absorption, dietary withdrawal of the offending sugars results in prompt symptomatic improvement.

The basic molecular defect in sucrase-isomaltase deficiency may vary in different patients (Harries 1982) but whatever the basic defect, sucrase-isomaltase deficiency appears to be inherited in an autosomal recessive fashion.

Trehalase deficiency

Trehalose (α-D-glucopyranoside) is a non-reducing disaccharide which occurs in plants such as mushrooms, some microorganisms, many insects, and in *Ascaris lumbricoides* and *Artenia salina*. Trehalase deficiency has been documented in a family who developed symptoms following the ingestion of mushrooms (Madzarovova-Nohejlova 1973). An autosomal dominant type of inheritance was suggested.

Glucose-galactose malabsorption

This condition was first described in 1962 by Lindquist & Meeuwisse. In many patients clinical tolerance to the offending carbohydrates improves with age despite the fact that the enzyme deficiency and transport defect persists (Ament et al 1973, Elsas & Lambe 1973, Fairclough et al 1978). In vivo and in vitro studies have shown markedly impaired or absent sodium-coupled mucosal uptake of glucose, and impaired uptake has also been documented in one or both parents (Meeuwisse & Dahlquist 1968).

Wozniak et al (1984) have recently shown that there are at least two molecular variants of the transport defect. One results from deletion of the transport site which does not change with age. In the other there is a reduced number of normally functioning transport sites which appear to increase in number with age. Absorption of fructose, xylose, leucine and alanine is intact (Schneider et al 1966, Phillips & McGill 1973, Wimberley et al 1974, Hughes & Senior 1975). The finding that amino acid absorption and Na^+K^+ ATPase activity are normal suggests that alterations in the sodium gradient are not involved in the pathophysiology of this condition.

Pathogenesis of gastrointestinal symptoms in carbohydrate absorption

If unabsorbed sugars accumulate in the lumen of the small intestine, an osmotic gradient is created which results in bulk movement of fluid and electrolytes from plasma to lumen. In addition, the physiological drive which glucose and galactose provide for absorption of fluid and electrolytes is dissipated. These factors result in excessive amounts of fluid and sugars entering the large intestine, where bacterial metabolism of the sugars generates short-chain organic acids (e.g. acetic, butyric and propionic acids), carbon dioxide and hydrogen. This in turn generates a second osmotic gradient between plasma and lumen with further movement of fluid into the lumen. These events lead to colicky abdominal pain and distension, watery acid stools containing increased amounts of electrolytes and sugars and perianal excoriation as a result of an increased H^+ ion concentration. Body losses of fluid and electrolytes, particularly in young infants, may lead to severe dehydration. Thus, the need for early diagnosis and treatment cannot be overemphasized.

LIPIDS

Lipids are by definition hydrophobic or non-polar compounds which are insoluble in water, but soluble in organic solvents. They, therefore, differ from the other nutrients discussed in this chapter which are water-soluble, and as a result the requirements for their efficient absorption are also different. The major barrier to the absorption of water-soluble compounds is the lipid-rich membrane of the enterocyte, but lipids are able to cross the membrane by a passive, energy-independent process. Lipids, however, must be rendered miscible or solubilized within the aqueous environments of both the gut lumen and the intracellular contents of the enterocyte. Thus, when considering the congenital defects of the enterocyte in relation to lipid absorption, the major problems are concerned with intracellular events and the exit of lipid from the enterocyte.

Physiology (see Friedman & Nylund 1980, Thomson & Dietschy 1981)

The principal dietary lipid is triglyceride, which is first hydrolysed by lipases within the gut lumen to form free fatty acids and monoglycerides. Bile salts above a certain concentration (critical micellar concentration) aggregate to form micelles which are able to solubilize the products of lipolysis and transport them to the brush border of the enterocyte (Carey & Small 1972) which they enter by passive diffusion across the lipid microvillus membrane. Since this is a passive process, no congenital defects involving entry of lipid into the enterocyte have been described. In health the bile salts are conserved by a highly efficient enterohepatic circulation

(Heaton 1972, Hofmann 1977), and are absorbed principally by an active carrier-mediated, sodium-dependent transport system in the ileum.

Within the enterocyte, the fatty acids are first reesterified to triglyceride and then packaged into lipoprotein particles (predominantly chylomicrons) for transport in the aqueous environment of the lymphatic system and bloodstream.

Abetalipoproteinaemia (ABL)

The clinical features of ABL were first described by Bassen & Kornzweig in 1950, and approximately 50 cases have now been reported in the world's literature (Herbert et al 1978). In 1960, three laboratories independently demonstrated the total absence of beta-lipoprotein (low density lipoprotein) from the plasma of affected individuals (Lamy et al 1960, Mabry et al 1960, Salt et al 1960).

In 1971, Gotto et al showed that apoprotein B (the major apoprotein of betalipoprotein) was undetectable in plasma of patients with ABL. The primary abnormality is not known, but the most likely defect is a failure to synthesize apoprotein B, although defects in the intracellular assembly of lipoproteins containing apoprotein B or in their secretion are also possible. The condition is inherited as an autosomal recessive, with affected individuals being homozygous for the condition.

The major clinical and biochemical features of abetalipoproteinaemia are listed in Table 9.2. The steatorrhoea and spiky red cells (acanthocytes) are present from birth, and the condition commonly presents in early infancy as a result of the fat malabsorption and failure to thrive. The other clinical features of neuropathy and retinopathy tend to develop towards the end of the first decade or early teens, and some patients present at this stage. The absence of low density lipoproteins, very low density lipoproteins and chylomicrons from the serum reflects the necessity of apoprotein B for their

Table 9.2   Biochemical and clinical features of abetalipoproteinaemia

Present from birth

Absence of apoprotein B
Absence of low density lipoproteins
Absence of very low density lipoproteins
Absence of chylomicrons
Greatly reduced concentrations of serum lipids
Malabsorption of fat
Acanthocytosis

Typically develop in later childhood or adolescence

Pigmentary retinopathy
Ataxic neuropathy

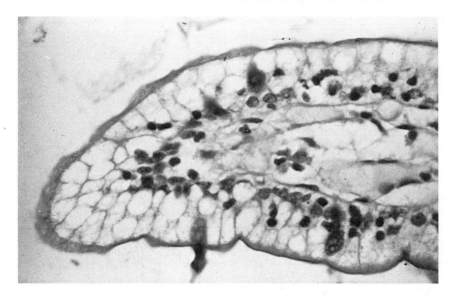

Fig. 9.1 Jejunal biopsy showing villus tip from a patient with abetalipoproteinaemia stained with PAS. The cytoplasm of the epithelial cells appears foamy and vacuolated due to accumulation of unstained lipid which also displaces nuclei to the basal region of the cells (×420) (Courtesy Blackwell Scientific Publications).

formation and results in the markedly reduced concentrations of the serum lipids.

The gastrointestinal symptoms are characterized by poor appetite, vomiting, failure to thrive and large, loose stools. These symptoms have led to the correct diagnosis by the age of four weeks (Lloyd 1968).

The activities of pancreatic amylase, lipase and trypsin, and the concentrations of bile salts in duodenal juice are normal (e.g. Salt et al 1960), which suggests that there is no abnormality in the intraluminal phase of fat absorption. Studies on intestinal mucosa obtained by peroral biopsy have localized the absorptive defect within the enterocyte. The biopsy has a characteristic 'white sea-anemone' appearance under the dissecting microscope. Under light microscopy the villus architecture is normal but the cells are distended and vacuolated. Histochemical techniques show the vacuolation to be due to lipid accumulation within the mucosal cells, which is particularly evident at the villus tip (Fig. 9.1). Studies using both light and electron microscopy have suggested that fat droplets are not transported through the endoplasmic reticulum to the Golgi apparatus, and are not 'packaged' and secreted into the lymphatics in the normal way. These observations, together with the lack of chylomicrons in the serum and the failure of serum triglyceride concentrations to rise after a fat meal, provide evidence that apoprotein B is essential for the synthesis of chylomicrons and the efficient transport of fat away from the enterocyte. Despite the inability to form chylomicrons, 50–80% of dietary fat is absorbed, which implies the existence of an alternative absorptive pathway.

It is generally agreed that symptoms related to steatorrhoea improve with age in patients with ABL. This may in part reflect acquired adaptive mechanisms, but is more likely to be related to unconscious dietary changes. If measures are instituted to correct the fat malabsorption in the young child, normal physical growth potential can be achieved (Muller et al 1977).

The diagnosis should be suspected in all patients with unexplained malabsorption, particularly if the symptoms date from birth, and in older children and young adults who have atypical retinitis pigmentosa or an ataxic neuropathy similar to that of Friedreich's ataxia. The finding of acanthocytes in a fresh, wet, undiluted blood film, together with abnormally low serum cholesterol and triglyceride concentrations, is virtually diagnostic. The absence of apoprotein B-containing lipoproteins can then be confirmed by immunochemical, ultracentrifugal and electrophoretic techniques. The appearance of the jejunal mucosa both under the dissecting and electron microscope, although not pathognomonic, is highly characteristic of the condition.

An hypothesis to explain the pathogenesis of the neurological and retinal lesions is that they result from a prolonged deficiency of a fat-soluble compound normally transported by the lipoproteins which are absent in this condition. Vitamin E, which normally depends on chylomicrons for its absorption and the low density lipoproteins for its transport, is such a substance and is undetectable from birth in serum of patients with ABL (Kayden et al 1965, Muller et al 1974). This condition, therefore, provides an ideal model for studying the effects of vitamin E deficiency in man. We have treated eight patients with ABL for up to 18 years on very large oral doses of vitamin E (approximately 100 mg/kg/day). When given in such large amounts vitamin E became detectable in the serum of all patients, and in vitro red cell haemolysis, an indicator of tissue concentrations of the vitamin, became normal (Muller et al 1974).

The long-term effects of oral vitamin E therapy in the eight patients have been reported in detail (Muller at al 1977, Muller & Lloyd 1982, Muller et al 1983). The patients who first received oral vitamin E supplements by the age of 18 months are now aged from 14 to 18 years and are completely normal. The three older patients already showed some neurological dysfunction before supplementation with vitamin E in childhood. The condition of two of them has remained essentially unchanged. The third patient is now 29 years of age. He was diagnosed at the age of 7 years and first received vitamin E at the age of 10, by which time he already had marked ataxia, absent tendon reflexes, delayed motor nerve conduction velocities, pigmentary retinopathy and abnormal retinal function. Within two years of starting vitamin E his gait, motor nerve conduction velocities, electroretinogram and electro-oculogram had improved, although his fundal appearance remained unchanged and his tendon reflexes absent. Over the following 17 years there has been further improvement in his gait, and his motor nerve conduction velocities and retinal function tests have returned to normal. Other investigators have also reported similar beneficial effects of large oral doses of vitamin E in ABL (Azizi et al 1978, Herbert et al 1978, Miller et al 1980). These long-term studies in patients with ABL indicate that vitamin E is important for normal neurological function and this has been confirmed by three other lines of evidence. Firstly, patients with other chronic disorders of fat absorption and a severe deficiency of vitamin E have been reported, who have similar neurological features to those found in ABL. Some of these patients have also responded to vitamin E supplementation. Secondly, patients have been reported with neurological disease associated with a selective deficiency of vitamin E in whom there was no evidence of generalized fat malabsorption (Harding et al 1985). Thirdly, the neuropathological changes observed in vitamin E-deficient states in man, including ABL, are similar to those found in the vitamin E-deficient rat and monkey (Nelson et al 1981). The evidence relating vitamin E and neurological function has recently been reviewed (Muller et al 1983).

The currently recommended treatment for patients with ABL is a restriction of dietary fat to control the fat malabsorption and supplements of the fat-soluble vitamins (Lloyd & Muller 1972). Normally, 15 000–20 000 IU/24 h of vitamin A is required to maintain normal plasma levels and sufficient vitamin K is given to maintain a normal clotting time. Massive doses of vitamin E (100 mg/kg/24 h) are recommended to maintain an adequate vitamin E status.

Familial hypobetalipoproteinaemia

This condition has been reviewed in detail by Herbert et al (1978) and is thought to be a genetic disorder distinct from classical ABL. It appears to be transmitted as an autosomal dominant trait and both heterozygotes and homozygotes for the condition have been described.

Heterozygous condition

Fredrickson et al (1972) proposed three diagnostic criteria for the heterozygous condition:

1. abnormally low concentrations of low-density lipoprotein, which are nonetheless present and identifiable immunochemically, together with normal concentrations of very low-density and high-density lipoproteins
2. no secondary cause for the hypobetalipoproteinaemia
3. similar lipoprotein and lipid findings in a first-degree relative

The majority of the affected individuals from the 17 families reported with heterozygous hypobetalipoproteinaemia have been fit and healthy without any features of ABL. Patients have, however, been reported with some of the features of classical ABL (Herbert et al 1978, Scott et al 1979). Heterozygous individuals have been shown to have greatly reduced concentrations of apoprotein B, whereas the concentrations of the other apoproteins fall within the normal range (Alaupovic et al 1980). Studies by Levy et al (1970) and Sigurdsson et al (1977) in a total of five patients have suggested that the reduced low-density lipoprotein concentrations result from reduced synthesis rather than increased catabolism of low-density lipoproteins.

Homozygous condition

Patients with the homozygous form of the condition are very rare, with only four cases reported in the literature. They are clinically and chemically indistinguishable from subjects with classical ABL and can only be distinguished from them by the finding of a reduced serum cholesterol and low-density lipoprotein concentration in a first-degree relative (i.e. a heterozygote for the condition).

PROTEIN AND AMINO ACIDS

Physiology (see Silk 1982)

Protein digestion is initiated in the stomach by the enzyme pepsin, and continued in the lumen of the small intestine. The principal intraluminal proteolytic enzyme is trypsin, which is secreted by the pancreas as trypsinogen which is an inactive precursor of zymogen. Activation is by the action of enterokinase which is present in the brush border membrane of the proximal small intestine. Intraluminal protein digestion yields a mixture of free amino acids and small peptides of 2–6 amino acid residues (Gray & Cooper 1971). The larger peptides undergo further hydrolysis by brush border bound peptidases until only free amino acids and di- and tripeptides are presented for absorption.

There are two major mechanisms for the absorption of the products of luminal digestion of protein at the brush border membrane of the enterocyte: a) the transport of free amino acids by group-specific, active, electrogenic, Na^+-coupled, co-transport systems (Schultz & Curran 1970) and b) the transport of unhydrolysed peptides (Silk 1974, Matthews 1975, Matthews & Adibi 1976).

There is little information regarding exit of amino acids from the cell, but the available evidence points to facilitated diffusion (Danisi et al 1976, Mircheff et al 1980). The recent description of a defect in lysine transport at the basolateral membrane of the enterocyte in lysinuric protein intolerance (Desjeux et al, 1980) suggests that special exit mechanisms are present, that they are group-specific, and that the basolateral translocation mechanisms are under different genetic control from those involved at the brush border. Inborn errors of protein absorption may occur either at the level of protein digestion or of amino acid transport. The majority of defects of amino acid transport are, however, of theoretical rather than practical importance, since the normal absorption of amino acids as peptides ensures that nutritional deficiencies are unusual. Thus, the defective amino acid absorption in cystinuria (Morin et al 1971) and iminoglycinuria (Goodman et al 1967) are not of clinical importance and these conditions will not, therefore, be considered any further.

Studies of intestinal function in patients with these conditions have, however, helped to elucidate the pathways of absorption of both free amino acids and peptides.

Trypsinogen deficiency

The two patients described by Townes et al (1967) presented in early infancy with failure to thrive, oedema, hypoproteinaemia, anaemia and neutropaenia. Feeding with a protein hydrolysate formula resulted in rapid improvement. Addition of exogenous trypsin to the duodenal juice of the patients induced activation of all proteolytic enzymes except trypsin.

Enterokinase deficiency

The infants reported by Tarlow et al (1970) presented in a similar way to those with trypsinogen deficiency except for the presence of steatorrhoea, the mechanism of which is not known. Treatment with pancreatic extract was highly effective. Addition of exogenous enterokinase to duodenal juice, or incubation of juice with normal duodenal mucosa resulted in activation of all the proteolytic enzymes. Enterokinase was undetectable in both the mucosa and duodenal juice of the affected children. Since exogenous trypsin may not activate trypsinogen, it is possible that the infants reported with trypsinogen deficiency were in fact lacking enterokinase and not the zymogen.

Hartnup disease

This condition results from a transport defect of the free neutral amino acids in the proximal renal tubule and the small intestine (Milne 1964). Patients are able, however, to maintain a reasonable state of nutrition when on an adequate diet with no obvious intestinal disturbances. The unexpectedly good state of nutrition most likely results from the fact that absorption of small peptides, when presented either as a large oral load of individual dipeptides (Asatoor et al 1970) or as a more physiological mixture of small peptides of 2–3 residues (Leonard et al 1976) is unaffected by the transport defect.

The onset of the condition is in early childhood with a pellagra-like rash, mental retardation and/or a dementing psychiatric disturbance similar to that seen in pellagra. Less often, there is a reversible cerebellar ataxia.

These clinical manifestations are, however, intermittent and variable, with the skin rash being the primary cause of referral to hospital. The pellagra results from the abnormally small proportion of dietary tryptophan available for the nutritionally important kynurenine-nicotinamide pathway. Unabsorbed free tryptophan is metabolized by intestinal bacteria to produce metabolites such as indoles, some of which may be potent inhibitors of the kynurenine-nicotinamide pathway and may, therefore, further decrease the already diminished production of nicotinamide (Milne et al 1960). As tryptophan can be absorbed in the form of di- and tripeptides, it is perhaps surprising that clinical symptoms occur at all. However, all clinical attacks are associated with an inadequate or irregular diet, and this may well result in insufficient absorption of peptide-bound tryptophan. The metabolism of the other neutral amino acids in this disorder does not seem to present the same difficulties.

The attacks of pellagra grow milder with age, presumably because of decreased requirements for nicotinamide when growth has ceased. The biochemical lesion is, however, always present. The key biochemical finding is an aminoaciduria and aminoacidorrhoea which is restricted to the neutral amino acids. Plasma neutral amino acid concentrations fail to rise following an oral load of free amino acids and bacterial degradation products of the unabsorbed amino acids are found in the stool and urine.

There is no specific treatment for the condition other than supplements of nicotinamide (25–50 mg/24 h). Monoamine oxidase inhibitors are contraindicated. The ultimate prognosis is good, with amelioration of the condition in adult life.

Lysinuric protein intolerance

Lysinuric protein intolerance (LPI) unlike Hartnup disease and cystinuria, presents with severe symptoms which include marked failure to thrive, diarrhoea, vomiting, protein intolerance, hepatic splenomegaly and often mental retardation (Perheentupa & Visakorpi 1965). Onset is in infancy commencing at the time of weaning from the breast to a cow's milk-containing formula. After the first year of life protein aversion is common and symptoms ameliorate with a decreased protein intake. If a high protein intake is maintained, hyperammonaemia, hepatosplenomegaly and sometimes coma develop. LPI is a defect of dibasic amino acid transport which is inherited as an autosomal recessive trait. The transport defect has been demonstrated in the small intestine (Desjeux et al 1980), liver (Simell 1975), and proximal renal tubules (Simell et al 1975). Oral load studies have shown impaired intestinal absorption of lysine, ornithine and arginine, with normal absorption of citrulline. In contrast to the situation in cystinuria and Hartnup disease, no significant absorption of dipeptide-bound lysine occurs (Rajantie et al 1980a, 1980b). These findings suggested that a defect of lysine transport may be present at the basolateral border of the enterocyte and this has been confirmed by in vitro studies of initial uptake, cellular accumulation and steady-state transepithelial fluxes, in jejunal mucosa obtained by peroral biopsy in patients with LPI (Desjeux et al 1980).

The pathognomonic features are increased faecal and urinary excretion, and decreased plasma concentrations of the dibasic amino acids with hyperammonaemia following a protein load. An intravenous alanine load (6.6 mmol/kg body weight) in 5% w/v aqueous solution produces hyperammonaemia which is prevented by the addition of ornithine (1.1 mmol/kg body weight) to the infusion; the provision of a urea cycle intermediate allows the alanine to be metabolized. Liver function is mildly deranged and may be associated with portal hypertension.

The cornerstone of treatment is a low protein diet of 1.5 g/kg body weight. Early attempts at preventing hyperammonaemia with arginine or ornithine supplements were not entirely successful, presumably because of poor intestinal absorption (Simell et al 1975). Diarrhoea occurs if more than 22 g of arginine is given as a single dose. However, the use of a urea cycle intermediate did allow the use of a low protein diet and resulted in catchup growth. Rajantie et al (1980a) have shown that another urea cycle intermediate, citrulline, is absorbed entirely normally and is capable of preventing the ornithinopenic hyperammonaemia in LPI. This may allow a higher intake of dietary protein to be used.

Blue diaper syndrome

Blue diaper syndrome results from the isolated malabsorption of tryptophan and is associated with an increased absorption of calcium. It is inherited as an autosomal recessive trait and presents in the neonatal period with failure to thrive, recurrent pyrexia, irritability, constipation and a blue discoloration of the nappies (Drummond et al 1964). The stools contain large quantities of indoles, tryptophan, tryptamine and indolic acid. The blue discoloration results from the presence of indigotin (indigo blue), an oxidation product of urinary indicans. Malabsorption of tryptophan was assumed on the basis of low plasma tryptophan concentrations following oral loading tests with tryptophan and an increased faecal and urinary excretion of indoles following oral neomycin. Hypercalcaemia and nephrocalcinosis were presumed to result from an increased Ca^{++} absorption. There is no evidence that this disorder affects renal tubules, and urinary excretion of amino acids is normal.

Thier & Alpers (1969) have suggested that it is a specific tryptophan transport system which is defective in blue diaper syndrome, rather than the group-specific system which is affected in Hartnup disease. It would seem unlikely, however, that such a severe clinical problem would occur if the group-specific system was intact. A more likely explanation is that a basolateral membrane transport defect is present in an analogous way to lysinuric protein intolerance.

Oast-house syndrome (methionine malabsorption)

This very rare condition, so-called because of the patients' odour, presents with convulsions, diarrhoea and severe mental retardation (Hooft et al 1964). An isolated defect of methionine transport in both intestine and kidney has been demonstrated. In the patient described by Hooft et al (1964), α-hydroxybutyric acid (a bacterial breakdown product of methionine) was found in both urine and faeces following oral loads of methionine and was responsible for the characteristic odour. On treating the patient with a methionine-free diet, the symptoms improved. It is interesting to speculate that this condition may be another example of a basolateral membrane defect.

Lowe's syndrome

Lowe's syndrome unlike the other conditions mentioned above, is inherited as a sex-linked trait and is characterized by mental retardation, cataracts and renal tubular acidosis with aminoaciduria. Defective absorption of lysine and arginine has been demonstrated (Bartsocas et al 1969) but the significance of this is not clear.

WATER AND ELECTROLYTES

Inherited defects involving the active transport of electrolytes are rare, but are of physiological importance because of the information they provide regarding the normal process of intestinal water and electrolyte transport.

Congenital chloridorrhoea is the only defect of intestinal electrolyte transport which has been clearly defined. Infants with familial lethal protracted diarrhoea have been described and may be examples of as yet undefined defects of electrolyte transport (Fordtran 1967, Davidson et al 1978, Candy et al 1981). This condition(s) is considered in chapter 16.

Physiology (see Schultz & Frizzell 1972)

The principal site for the absorption of water and electrolytes is the proximal jejunum. The major driving force for water absorption is provided by the osmotic gradients set up by the active absorption of solutes. In the proximal jejunum, the most important mechanism is that of Na^+-coupled co-transport of a wide variety of water soluble organic solutes which include D-hexoses, L-amino acids, di- and tripeptides and some vitamins (Schultz & Curran 1970). The intestinal mucosa is, however, a complex epithelium in which absorption and secretion occur simultaneously. Absorption takes place primarily in the villous cells, and it is here that Na^+-coupled co-transport systems are most highly developed, whereas secretion is thought to occur in crypt cells (Field 1981, Welsh et al 1982). The ileum and colon act as a functional unit conserving water and electrolytes and in both, Na^+

and Cl⁻ are absorbed against considerable electrochemical gradients. Chloride is, however, absorbed more rapidly than Na⁺, suggesting that it is not simply the accompanying anion to Na⁺.

There are three mechanisms postulated for electrolyte absorption in the ileum in addition to the Na⁺-coupled co-transport of organic solutes.

1. Uncoupled electrogenic Na⁺ absorption (Schultz et al 1974)
2. Neutral coupled NaCl co-transport (Frizzell et al 1979)
3. Double anion cation exchange (Turnberg et al 1970)

The colon transforms liquid ileal effluent into solid stool and in so doing creates large ionic concentration gradients. Active electrogenic transport is the major mechanism of Na⁺ absorption and the paired ion exchanges postulated for the ileum either do not take place or are of lesser importance, although Cl⁻ is actively absorbed and HCO_3 secreted by closely related processes.

Congenital chloridorrhoea (CCD)

In 1945 Darrow, and Gamble et al simultaneously described an unusual form of severe watery diarrhoea with hypokalaemia, hypochloraemia and metabolic alkalosis. A unique and striking feature of the condition was the high concentration of Cl⁻ in stools (often as high as 150 mmol/l) which exceeded the sum of the Na⁺ and K⁺ concentrations. To date, more than 40 cases have been reported, half of which have come from Finland (Holmberg et al 1977a). The condition is inherited as an autosomal recessive trait.

Investigation of patients with CCD using in vivo perfusion techniques (Turnberg 1971, Bieberdorf et al 1972, Rask-Madsen et al 1976) has shown that the principal defect is of active Cl^-/HCO_3 transport and that the defect is restricted to the ileum and colon. Secretion of Cl⁻ by the stomach and renal Cl⁻ transport are normal (Pearson et al 1973). Studies of jejunal transport show normal absorption of glucose, sodium, water and bicarbonate (Turnberg 1971, Pearson et al 1973, Rask-Madsen et al 1976). Na⁺ and Cl⁻ are secreted into the lumen of the intestine. Cl⁻ enters at a faster rate than Na⁺ and the ionic balance is maintained by the absorption of HCO_3 which leads to a fall in luminal pH (Turnberg 1971, Rask-Madsen et al 1976). In a study of the colon of three patients with CCD and their healthy siblings, Holmberg et al (1975) showed that Na⁺ transport was intact but absorption was dependent on the luminal presence of HCO_3. The condition is apparent in fetal life and has so far always been associated with maternal hydramnios (Holmberg et al 1977a) (Fig. 9.2). The infants are all born prematurely. Growth is appropriate for the period of gestation and the abdomen is often distended at birth as shown in Figure 9.3.

The abdominal distension is associated with a paralytic ileus which may last several weeks, and which is unrelated to K⁺ secretion. It is, however,

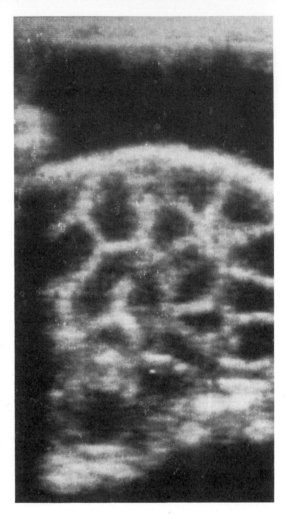

Fig. 9.2 Abdominal ultrasound of fetal abdomen in congenital chloridorrhoea showing dilated fluid-filled loops of intestine (Courtesy Blackwell Scientific Publications).

known that the excitatory adrenergic stimulation of smooth muscle cells is dependent on a change in Cl$^-$ membrane conductance and that the magnitude is directly related to the extracellular Cl$^-$ concentration (Szurszewski & Bulbring 1973). Thus, in the Cl$^-$ depleted state found in CCD, a paralytic ileus might be expected. Although diarrhoea and an absence of meconium is often recognized on the first day of life, it may be mistaken for urine and therefore go unnoticed. The majority of affected infants become hypernatraemic and hypochloraemic in the first week of life, but not hypokalaemic or alkalotic and this may result from the degree of functional development of the ileum and colon in early life.

In the neonatal period, acidosis is the rule rather than alkalosis and the

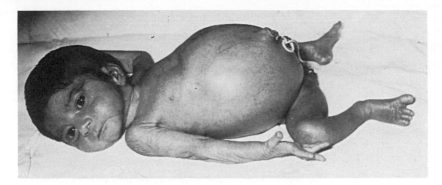

Fig. 9.3 An infant with congenital chloridorrhoea with distended abdomen (Courtesy Blackwell Scientific Publications).

original name of the disease 'congenital alkalosis with diarrhoea' is a misnomer. During this period, jaundice is common and presumably is aggravated by a combination of acidosis, dehydration and prematurity. If adequate electrolyte replacement is not instituted, severe alkalosis will develop over a period of a few weeks. In the 18 families studied by Holmberg et al (1977a), 7 previous infants had died, almost certainly from CCD, and there was one death of a known patient as a result of inadequate intravenous replacement therapy.

Infants who present later invariably have a history of diarrhoea or the passage of unformed stools since birth, with moderate to severe growth retardation. If inadequate replacement therapy is prolonged, osteoporosis may develop, which is thought to result from excessive urinary phosphate loss. As discussed above, the diagnosis may be suspected in utero by the presence of maternal hydramnios. After the first few months of life, stool electrolytes (i.e. Cl^- concentration >90 mmol/l which exceeds the sum of Na^+ and K^+ concentrations) confirms the diagnosis. Urine from these patients contains little or no Cl^- (Holmberg et al 1977a). Investigations show that infants who present after the neonatal period are markedly hypochloraemic and hypokalaemic, with metabolic alkalosis, but their serum Na^+ concentration is normal. These changes, compared to those found in the neonatal period, are due to secondary hyperaldosteronism, resulting in normal plasma Na^+ concentrations but low plasma K^+ concentrations.

Treatment, initially, consists of intravenous replacement therapy and later, oral electrolyte replacement, with full oral feeding being achieved by the age of one month in some infants. Many of the early patients were treated with KCl supplements only. Although this corrected the hypokalaemia and hypochloraemia, normal plasma Na^+ concentrations were only achieved by marked and persistent hyperaldosteronism. This caused juxtaglomerular hyperplasia, with increased angiotensin II activity resulting in vascular changes, and the hyperaldosteronism in turn causing hypokalaemic alkalosis and the predisposition to nephrocalcinosis. Although these patients were clinically well, renal changes consisting of hyalinized glomeruli, juxtaglomerular hyperplasia, calcium deposits and hypertensive vascular changes were present on biopsy (Pasternack et al 1967). Similar vascular changes were also present in muscle (Pasternack & Perheentupa 1966). As excess K^+ and low Na^+ are known to stimulate aldosterone production, and children with CCD lose Na^+ in their stools, Holmberg et al (1977b) have recommended that oral replacement solutions should contain both NaCl and KCl in the smallest dose that would maintain urinary chloride excretion (0.7% NaCl and 0.3% KCl for infants, and after the age of three years, 1.8% NaCl and 1.9% KCl). With this regime, the previously described renal and arteriolar changes have not occurred, acute episodes of dehydration have been less frequent and less severe, and growth has been normal. Mental retardation, which occurred in some patients treated solely with potassium, has not developed in those treated with full replacement therapy (Holmberg et al 1977a).

VITAMINS

Vitamin B_{12} (For Absorption, see Seetharam & Alpers 1982)

Selective vitamin B_{12} Malabsorption (Imerslund-Grasbeck syndrome)

In 1960, both Imerslund, and Grasbeck et al independently described an autosomal disorder with megaloblastic anaemia associated with proteinuria; to date, more than 100 such cases have been described. The age of presentation has varied from 2 to 15 years of age. The clinical features are pallor, weakness, irritability and loss of appetite in almost all patients, often associated with vomiting, pyrexia, glossitis and constipation. There may also be evidence of diminished vibration sense, extensor plantars and mental retardation. Older children often present with the signs and symptoms of anaemia. Approximately 90% of reported cases have proteinuria in the absence of any other abnormalities of renal function, which persists after treatment.

Malabsorption of vitamin B_{12} occurs in these patients and is not improved by the addition of gastric intrinsic factor (GIF). Gastric and intestinal function are normal in all other respects and serum concentrations of transcobalamin II are also normal. Mackenzie et al (1972) described uptake studies of free B_{12} and the B_{12}-GIF complex, using ileal biopsy homogenates from a patient with congenital B_{12} malabsorption and from controls. The results were similar in the patient and controls, with GIF causing a marked stimulation of B_{12} uptake. It was, therefore, concluded that the receptor was present and functioning normally in this condition, and that the defect was at some point beyond the attachment of the

B_{12}-GIF complex to the receptor, but before the vitamin was bound to transcobalamin II.

The condition is treated by monthly injections of 250 μg of hydroxocobalamin, which must be continued for life.

Deficiency of transcobalamin II

The deficiency of transcobalamin II is a very rare condition with less than 10 patients having been reported (Hakami et al 1971, Hitzig et al 1974, Chanarin 1982). Patients have generally presented during the first few weeks of life with failure to thrive. The blood shows severe anaemia, leucopenia and thrombocytopenia, and the marrow shows severe megaloblastic haemopoiesis. The diagnosis is dependent on the demonstration of an absence of transcobalamin II. Serum concentrations of vitamin B_{12} are normal. This apparent anomaly results from sequestration of the vitamin in the bloodstream because in the absence of transcobalamin II it is unavailable for tissue uptake.

Vitamin B_{12} is malabsorbed in this condition; studies in two children using whole body counting after an oral load of radio-labelled B_{12} showed virtually zero absorption (Chanarin 1982). This indicates that transcobalamin II is necessary for the transport of vitamin B_{12} away from the enterocyte and that this carrier protein is normally synthesized by the enterocyte. Direct evidence for the intestinal synthesis of transcobalamin II is not available, although Chanarin et al (1978) have provided indirect evidence for this hypothesis by following plasma binding of newly absorbed radio-labelled B_{12} after the saturation of available binding sites by an intramuscular injection of the unlabelled vitamin.

Treatment is by regular and very large injections of vitamin B_{12} (1 mg of hydroxocobalamin twice weekly), a small proportion of which is able to enter cells by passive diffusion.

Folate (for Absorption see Rosenberg (1981))

Congenital folate malabsorption

Congenital folate malabsorption is a rare condition (Luhby et al 1961, Lanzkowsky et al 1969, Santiago-Borrero et al 1973) in which patients develop a megaloblastic anaemia and other manifestations of folate deficiency (Chanarin 1982) as a result of a specific defect in folate absorption. All other parameters of intestinal function are normal. This condition presents the most convincing evidence for a specific intestinal transport mechanism for folate.

The clinical management of patients with congenital folate malabsorption is by regular parenteral folate sufficient to maintain health.

MINERALS

Acrodermatitis enteropathica

Acrodermatitis enteropathica (AE) is inherited in an autosomal recessive fashion. The clinical features were first described by Brandt in 1936 and the entity was later given its name by Danbolt & Closs (1942). In 1973, Moynahan & Barnes made the observation that all the manifestations of AE were a direct consequence of zinc deficiency, and that the administration of zinc supplements led to rapid and complete remission.

The available evidence indicates that the zinc deficiency in AE is a direct consequence of defective intestinal absorption. Lombeck et al (1975) measured whole body retention of ^{65}Zn, and their findings suggested that the net absorption of zinc was impaired. Balance studies have shown net intestinal secretion of zinc when AE patients were not receiving therapy, with reversion to absorption following oral zinc supplements (Aggett et al 1978). The first direct evidence for a defect in mucosal uptake of zinc came from the studies of Atherton et al (1979), who demonstrated a marked defect in the in vitro uptake of zinc by jejunal biopsies obtained from patients with AE. The histological appearance by light microscopy was entirely normal and uptake of zinc was equally defective whether or not the patients were receiving zinc supplements, thereby excluding the possibility that the defect was a nonspecific phenomenon secondary to zinc deficiency.

The classical clinical features of AE are dramatic, and include skin rashes, diarrhoea, failure to thrive, infections, alopecia, nail dystrophy, psychological and behavioural problems, stomatitis, glossitis, blepharitis, conjunctivitis and photophobia. The skin lesions are distributed at acral and

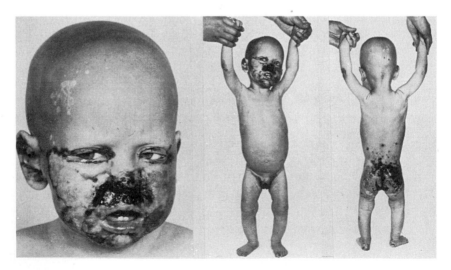

Fig. 9.4 Acrodermatitis enteropathica: before treatment (Courtesy Blackwell Scientific Publications).

mucocutaneous regions of the body and are vesicular, eczematoid and/or pustular, and in the acute stage the rash may become generalized and very disfiguring (Fig. 9.4). Hyperkeratotic skin flux may develop in the chronic stages (Fig 9.4). Typically, the skin lesions develop following the transition from breast to formula feeding, and may resolve if breast milk is reintroduced. Since this cannot be explained on the basis of the zinc content of the breast milk, it has been suggested that ligands present in breast milk facilitate zinc absorption. The condition was frequently fatal in childhood until the fortuitous discovery that the antifungal agent 5,7-di-iodo-8-hydroxyquinolone (Diodoquin®) could induce a complete clinical remission (Dillaha et al, 1953). Subsequently, Diodoquin® was shown to act as an

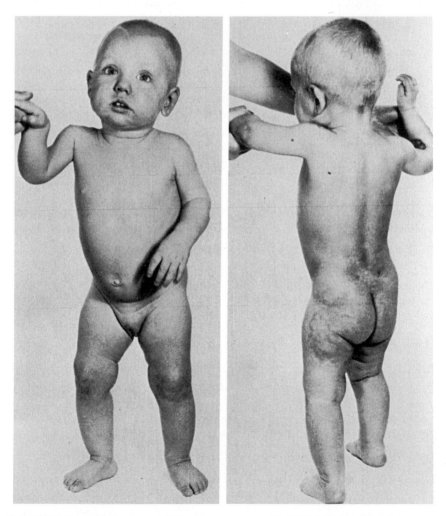

Fig. 9.5 Acrodermatitis enteropathica: after treatment with Zn^{++} (Courtesy Blackwell Scientific Publications).

ionophore, enhancing zinc absorption (Aggett et al 1979), and thereby capable of reversing net intestinal secretion of zinc to absorption (Aggett et al 1978).

There are reports of three women who survived to adulthood without zinc therapy, and two of these had children with fatal congenital malformations similar to those seen in the offspring of zinc-deficient rats. This suggests that zinc deficiency may be teratogenic in the human (Hambidge et al 1975). Subsequently, plasma zinc concentrations were carefully monitored during two pregnancies in a patient with AE treated with oral zinc supplements (Brenton et al 1981). The offspring had no congenital abnormalities and developed normally.

The diagnosis of AE is made essentially on clinical grounds, documentation of zinc deficiency and the prompt and dramatic resolution following zinc supplementation (Fig 9.5). The primary defect is permanent and, therefore, the diagnosis can only be made with certainty by discontinuing zinc therapy following a prolonged remission, and inducing a relapse. A combination of determining serum zinc concentrations and the activity of a zinc-dependent enzyme (e.g. alkaline phosphatase) is probably at present the most useful way of assessing total body zinc status. Great care is necessary in collecting samples, since contamination can lead to spuriously high zinc concentrations. Samples must be collected into plastic containers, and on no account should rubber stoppers be used. An important cause of sample contamination is the use of zinc containing ointments.

Oral zinc supplementation has now superseded Diodoquin® as the treatment of choice and should be continued on an indefinite basis. It is crucial to carefully monitor body zinc status during growth and pregnancy, and to adjust the dose of zinc as necessary.

Primary hypomagnesaemia

Primary hypomagnesaemia is probably inherited in an autosomal recessive fashion. The condition presents in early infancy with convulsions and/or tetany, and the biochemical features are hypomagnesaemia and hypocalcaemia.

Balance studies (Paunier et al 1968) and steady-state perfusion studies of the small gut (Milla et al 1979) have demonstrated that the pathogenesis of the magnesium deficiency is related to a primary defect in magnesium transport. Milla et al (1979) showed that net loss of magnesium into the lumen occurred when low concentrations (1 and 2 mmol/l) of magnesium were perfused, whereas at high concentrations (10 mmol/l) net absorption was observed which was similar to that of controls. Kinetic studies suggested that the primary abnormality in this condition is a defect in a carrier-mediated transport system which is saturated at a low intraluminal concentration. The normal absorption of magnesium from higher intraluminal concentrations probably occurs by simple passive diffusion, and accounts for the fact that hypomagnesaemia can be corrected by large oral doses of magnesium. Patients generally present at the age of a few weeks with generalized convulsions and tetany, but sometimes the clinical onset is delayed until later in infancy. Hypotonia may be marked and the convulsions fail to respond to conventional anti-convulsant drugs. Hypoproteinaemia and a peripheral oedema secondary to a protein-losing enteropathy, which improved with magnesium therapy, has been reported in one patient (Milla et al 1979).

The diagnosis is established by the demonstration of severe hypomagnesaemia and hypocalcaemia which cannot be explained by an acquired deficiency, and by the prompt biochemical and clinical response to magnesium therapy. It must also be shown that permanent therapy is required.

Magnesium (1–2 mmol/kg/24 h), given orally as one of the soluble salts, usually has a rapid effect in controlling convulsions and tetany, as well as correcting plasma magnesium and calcium levels. Higher doses may be necessary in some cases and can be associated with diarrhoea. Conventional anti-convulsant therapy and calcium supplements may be required during the early stages of treatment.

Familial hypophosphataemic rickets

Familial hypophosphataemic rickets (vitamin D-resistant hypophosphataemic rickets) is usually inherited in an X-linked fashion, but occasionally transmission may be autosomal dominant (Harrison & Harrison 1979). The major abnormality is a defect in the renal tubular reabsorption of phosphate (Rasmussen & Anast 1978), but intestinal absorption of phosphate and calcium is also impaired.

Initially, growth is normal but is impaired later and often clinical signs of rickets are not noticed until the patient is 1–3 years old, or more. The association of hypophosphataemia, a raised alkaline phosphatase, and radiological evidence of rickets and osteomalacia, suggests the diagnosis. Calcitriol (1,24-dihydroxy-D_3), together with phosphate supplements, is the treatment of choice (Glorieux et al 1980). Careful and frequent monitoring of serum calcium and phosphate, and urinary phosphate is important.

REFERENCES

Aggett P J, Atherton D J, Delves H T et al 1978 Studies in acrodermatitis enteropathica. In: Kirchgessner M (ed) 3rd International Symposium on Trace Element Metabolism in Man and Animals. Freising-Weihenstephan. pp 418–422

Aggett P J, Delves H T, Harries J T, Bangham A D 1979 The possible role of diodoquin as a zinc ionophore in the treatment of acrodermatitis enteropathica. Biochemical and Biophysical Research Communications 87: 513–517

Alaupovic P, Connor W E, Wolff O H, McGonathy W J, Illingworth D R 1980 Personal communication

Ament M E, Perera D R, Esther L J 1973 Sucrase-isomaltase deficiency — a frequently misdiagnosed disease. Journal of Paediatrics 83: 721–727

Antonowicz I, Lloyd-Still J D, Khaw K T, Shwachman H 1972 Congenital sucrase-isomaltase deficiency. Observations over a period of six years. Pediatrics 49: 847–853

Asatoor A M, Clegg B, Edwards K D G et al 1970 Intestinal absorption of two dipeptides in Hartnup disease. Gut 11: 380–387

Asp N-G, Dahlquist A 1974 Intestinal β-galactosidases in adult low lactase activity and in congenital lactase deficiency. Enzymes 18: 84–102

Atherton D J, Muller D P R, Aggett P J, Harries J T 1979 A defect in zinc uptake by jejunal biopsies in acrodermatitis enteropathica. Clinical Science 56: 505–507

Azizi E, Zaidman J L, Eshchar J, Szeinberg A 1978 Abetalipoproteinaemia treated with parenteral and oral vitamin A and E and with medium chain triglycerides. Acta Paediatrica Scandinavica 67: 797–801

Bartsocas C S, Levy H L, Crawford J D, Thier S O 1969 A defect in intestinal amino acid transport in Lowe's syndrome. American Journal of Diseases of Children 117: 93–95

Bassen F A, Kornzweig A L 1950 Malformation of the erythrocytes in a case of atypical retinitis pigmentosa. Blood 5: 381–387

Bayless T M, Rothfield B, Massa C, Wise L, Paige D, Bedine M S 1975 Lactose and milk intolerance: clinical implications. New England Journal of Medicine 292: 1156–1159

Bieberdorf F A, Gorden P, Fordtran J S 1972 Pathogenesis of congenital alkalosis with diarrhoea. Journal of Clinical Investigation 51: 1958–1968

Brandt T 1936 Dermatitis in children with disturbances of the general condition and absorption of food elements. Acta Dermatologica Venereologica 17: 513–546

Brenton D P, Jackson M J, Young A 1981 Two pregnancies in a patient with acrodermatitis enteropathica treated with zinc sulphate. Lancet ii: 500–502

Candy D C A, Larcher V F, Cameron D J S et al 1981 Lethal familial protracted diarrhoea. Archives of Disease in Childhood 56: 15–23

Carey M C, Small D M 1972 Micelle formation by bile salts. Physical-chemical and thermodynamic considerations. Archives of Internal Medicine 130: 506–527

Chanarin I 1982 Disorders of vitamin absorption. Clinics in Gastroenterology 11:(1), 73–85

Chanarin I, Muir M, Hughes A V, Hoffbrand A 1978 Evidence for an intestinal origin of transcobalamin II during vitamin B_{12} absorption. British Medical Journal i: 1453–1455

Crane R K 1965 Na^+-dependent transport in the intestine and other animal tissues. Federation Proceedings 24: 1000–1006

Danbolt N, Closs K 1942 Acrodermatitis enteropathica. Acta Dermatalogica Venereologica 23: 127–169

Danisi G, Tai Y H, Curran P F 1976 Mucosal and serosal fluxes of alanine in rabbit ileum. Biochimica et Biophysica Acta 455: 200–213

Darrow D C 1945 Congenital alkalosis with diarrhoea. Journal of Pediatrics 26: 519–532

Davidson G P, Cutz E, Hamilton J R, Gall D G 1978 Familial enteropathy: a syndrome of protracted diarrhoea from birth, failure to thrive and hypoplastic villous atrophy. Gastroenterology 75: 783–790

Desjeux J F, Rajantie J, Simell O, Dumontier A M, Perheentupa J 1980 Lysine fluxes across the jejunal epithelium in lysinuric protein intolerance. Journal of Clinical Investigation 65: 1382–1387

Dillaha C J, Lorinez A L, Aavik O R 1953 Acrodermatitis enteropathica: a review of the literature and report of a case successfully treated with diodoquin. Journal of the American Medical Association 152: 509–512

Drummond K N, Michael A F, Ulstrom R A, Gould R A 1964 The blue diaper syndrome: familial hypercalcemia and nephrocalcinosis and indicanuria. American Journal of Medicine 37: 928–948

Elsas L J, Lambe D W 1973 Familial glucose-galactose malabsorption. Remission of glucose intolerance. Journal of Pediatrics 83: 226–232

Fairclough P D, Clark M L, Dawson A M, Silk B D A, Milla P, Harries J T 1978 Absorption of glucose and maltose in congenital glucose-galactose malabsorption. Pediatric Research 12: 1112–1114

Field M 1981 Secretion of electrolytes and water by mammalian small intestine. In: Johnson L R (ed) Physiology of the gastrointestinal tract. Raven Press, New York. 2: 963–982

Fordtran J S 1967 Speculations on the pathogenesis of diarrhoea. Federal Proceedings 26: 1405–1414

Fredrickson D S, Gotto A M, Levy R I 1972 Familial lipoprotein deficiency. In:

Stanbury J B, Wyngaarden J B, Fredrickson D S (eds) The Metabolic Basis of Inherited Disease, 3rd edn, McGraw-Hill, New York. pp 493–530

Friedman H I, Nylund B 1980 Intestinal fat digestion, absorption and transport. A review. American Journal of Clinical Nutrition 33: 1108–1139

Frizzell R A, Field M, Schultz S G 1979 Sodium-coupled chloride transport by epithelial tissues. American Journal of Physiology 236: F1–8

Gamble J L, Fahey K R, Appleton J, MacLachlan E 1945 Congenital alkalosis with diarrhea. Journal of Pediatrics 26: 509–518

Glorieux F H, Marie P J, Pettifor J M, Delvin E E 1980 Bone response to phosphate salts, ergocalciferol and calcitriol in hypophosphatemic vitamin D-resistant rickets. New England Journal of Medicine 303: 1023–1031

Goodman S I, McIntyre C A, O'Brien D 1967 Impaired intestinal transport of proline in a patient with familial iminoaciduria. Journal of Pediatrics 71: 246–249

Gotto A M, Levy R I, John K, Fredrickson D A 1971 On the nature of the protein defect in abetalipoproteinaemia. New England Journal of Medicine 284: 813–818

Grasbeck R, Gordin R, Kantero I, Kuhlback B 1960 Selective vitamin B_{12} malabsorption and proteinuria in young people. A syndrome. Acta Medica Scandinavica 167: 289–296

Gray G M 1975 Carbohydrate digestion and absorption. Role of the small intestine. New England Journal of Medicine 292: 1225–1230

Gray G M, Cooper H L 1971 Protein digestion and absorption. Gastroenterology 61: 535–544

Hakami N, Neiman P E, Canellos G P, Lazerson J 1971 Neonatal megaloblastic anemia due to inherited transcobalamin II deficiency in two siblings. New England Journal of Medicine 285: 1163–1170

Hambidge K M, Neldner K H, Walravens P A 1975 Zinc, acrodermatitis enteropathica and congenital malformations. Lancet i:577

Harding A E, Matthews S, Jones S, Ellis C J K, Booth I W, Muller D P R 1985 Spinocerebellar degeneration associated with a selective defect of vitamin E absorption. New England Journal of Medicine 313: 32–35

Harries J T 1982 Disorders of carbohydrate absorption. Clinics in Gastroenterology 11: 117–30

Harrison H E, Harrison H C 1979 Disorders of calcium and phosphate metabolism in childhood and adolescence. In: Major Problems in Clinical Pediatrics. Saunders, Philadelphia. p 219

Heaton K W 1972 The enterohepatic circulation. In: Bile Salts in Health and Disease. Churchill Livingstone, Edinburgh. pp 58–81

Herbert P N, Gotto A M, Fredrickson D S 1978 Familial lipoprotein deficiency. In: Stanbury J B, Wyngaarden J B, Fredrickson D S (eds) The Metabolic Basis of Inherited Disease, 4th edn. McGraw-Hill, New York, pp 544–588

Hitzig W H, Dohmann U, Pluss H J, Vischer D 1974 Hereditary transcobalamin II deficiency: clinical findings in a new family. Journal of Pediatrics 85: 622–628

Hofmann A F 1977 The enterohepatic circulation of bile acids in man. In: Paumgartner G (ed) Clinics of Gastroenterology. Saunders, London. 6:(1), 3–24

Holdsworth C D, Dawson A M 1965 Absorption of fructose in man. Proceedings of the Society of Experimental Biology & Medicine 118: 142–145

Holmberg C, Perheentupa J, Launiala K 1975 Colonic electrolyte transport in health and in congenital chloride diarrhoea. Journal of Clinical Investigation 56: 302–310

Holmberg C, Perheentupa J, Launiala K, Hallman N 1977a Congenital chloride diarrhoea. Archives of Disease in Childhood 52: 255–267

Holmberg C, Perheentupa J, Pasternack A 1977b The renal lesion in congenital chloride diarrhoea. Journal of Pediatrics 91: 738–743

Holzel A, Schwarz V, Sutcliffe K W 1959 Defective lactose absorption causing malnutrition in infancy. Lancet i: 1126–1128

Hooft C J, Timmermans J, Snoeck J, Antener I, Van den Hende C 1964 Methionine malabsorption in a mentally defective child. Lancet ii: 20–21

Hughes W S, Senior J R 1975 The glucose-galactose malabsorption syndrome in a 23-year-old woman. Gastroenterology 68: 142–145

Imerslund O 1960 Idiopathic chronic megaloblastic anemia in children. Acta Pediatrica 49: supplement 119

Kayden H J, Silber R, Kossmann C E 1965 The role of vitamin E deficiency in the abnormal autohemolysis of acanthocytosis. Transactions of the Association of American Physicians 78: 334–342

Kimmich G A 1973 Coupling between Na$^+$ and sugar transport in small intestine. Biochimica et Biophysica Acta 300: 31–78

Kimmich G A 1981 Intestinal absorption of sugar. In: Johnson L R (ed) Physiology of the gastrointestinal tract. Raven Press, New York, 2: 1035–1061

Lamy M J, Frézal J, Polonovski J, Rey J 1960 L'absence congenitale de betalipoproteins. Comptes Rendus des Séances de la Société de Biologie (Paris). 154: 1974–1978

Lanzkowsky P, Erlandson M E, Bezan A I 1969 Isolated defect of folic acid absorption associated with mental retardation and cerebral calcification. Blood 34: 452–465

Leonard J V, Marrs T C, Addison J M et al 1976 Intestinal absorption of amino acids and peptides in Hartnup disorder. Pediatric Research 10: 246–249

Levin B, Abraham J M, Burgess E A, Wallis P G 1970 Congenital lactose malabsorption. Archives of Disease in Childhood 45: 173–177

Levy R I, Langer T, Gotto A M, Fredrickson D S 1970 Familial hypobetalipoproteinaemia, a defect in lipoprotein synthesis. Clinical Research 18:539A

Lindquist B, Meeuwisse G W 1962 Chronic diarrhoea. caused by monosaccharide malabsorption. Acta Paediatrica Scandinavica 51: 674–685

Lloyd J K 1968 Disorders of the serum lipoproteins. I. Lipoprotein deficiency states. Archives of Disease in Childhood 43: 393–403

Lloyd J K, Muller D P R 1972 Management of abetalipoproteinaemia in childhood. In: Peeters H (ed) Protides of the Biological Fluids. Pergamon Press, Oxford. p 331–335

Lombeck I, Schnippering H G, Ritzl F, Feinendegen L E, Bremer H J 1975 Absorption of zinc in acrodermatitis enteropathica. Lancet i:855

Luhby A L, Eagle F J, Roth E, Cooperman J M 1961 Relapsing megaloblastic anemia in an infant due to a specific defect in gastrointestinal absorption of folic acid. American Journal of Diseases in Children 102: 482–483

Mabry C C, Di George A M, Auerbach V H 1960 Studies concerning the defect in a patient with acanthocytosis. Clinical Research 8:371A

Mackenzie I L, Donaldson R M Jr, Trier J S, Mathan V I 1972 Ileal mucosa in familial selective vitamin B$_{12}$ malabsorption. New England Journal of Medicine 286: 1021–1025

McNair A, Gudmand-Hoyer E, Jarman S, Orrild L 1972 Sucrose malabsorption in Greenland. British Medical Journal ii: 19–21

Madzarovova-Nohejlova J 1973 Trehalase deficiency in a family. Gastroenterology 65: 130–133

Matthews D M 1975 Intestinal absorption of peptides. Physiological Reviews 55: 537–608

Matthews D M, Adibi S A 1976 Peptide absorption. Gastroenterology 71: 151–161

Meeuwisse G W, Dahlquist A 1968 Glucose-galactose malabsorption: a study with biopsy of the small intestinal mucosa. Acta Paediatrica Scandinavica 57: 273–280

Milla P J, Aggett P J, Wolff O H, Harries J T 1979 Studies in primary hypomagnesaemia: evidence for defective carrier-mediated small intestinal transport of magnesium. Gut 20: 1029–1033

Miller R G, Davis C J F, Illingworth D R, Bradley W 1980 The neuropathy of abetalipoproteinemia, Neurology 30: 1286–1291

Milne M D 1964 Disorders of amino acid transport British Medical Journal i:327

Milne M D, Crawford M A, Girao C B, Loughridge L W 1960 The metabolic disorder in Hartnup disease. Quarterly Journal of Medicine 29: 407–421

Mircheff A K, van Os C H, Wright E M 1980 Pathways for alanine transport in intestinal baso-lateral membrane vesicles. Journal of Membrane Biology 52: 83–92

Morin C L, Thompson M W, Jackson S H, Sass-Korlsak A 1971 Biochemical and genetic studies in cystinuria: Observations on double heterozygotes of genotype I/II. Journal of Clinical Investigation 50: 1961–1976

Moynahan E J, Barnes P M 1973 Zinc deficiency and a synthetic diet for lactose intolerance. Lancet i: 676–677

Muller D P R, Lloyd J K 1982 Effect of large oral doses of vitamin E on the neurological sequelae of patients with abetalipoproteinaemia. Annals of the New York Academy of Sciences 393: 133–144

Muller D P R, Harries J T, Lloyd J K 1974 The relative importance of the factors involved in the absorption of vitamin E in children. Gut 15: 966–971

Muller D P R, Lloyd J K, Bird A C 1977 Long-term management of abetalipoproteinaemia. Possible role for vitamin E. Archives of Disease in Childhood 52: 209–214

Muller D P R, Lloyd J K, Wolff O H 1983 Vitamin E and neurological function. Lancet i: 225–228

Nelson J S, Fitch C D, Fischer V W, Brown G O, Chow A C 1981 Progressive neuropathological lesions in vitamin E deficient rhesus monkeys. Journal of Neuropathology and Experimental Neurology 40: 166–186

Newcomer A D, McGill D B 1966 Distribution of disaccharidase activity in the small bowel of normal and lactase deficient subjects. Gastroenterology 51: 481–488

Pasternack A, Perheentupa J 1966 Hypertensive angiopathy in familial chloride diarrhoea. Lancet ii: 1047–1049

Pasternack A, Perheentupa J, Launiala K, Hallman N 1967 Kidney biopsy findings in familial chloride diarrhoea. Acta Endocrinologica 55: 1–9

Paunier L, Radde I C, Kooh S W, Fraser D 1968 Primary hypomagnesemia with secondary hypocalcemia in an infant. Pediatrics 41: 385–402

Pearson A J, Sladen G E, Edmonds C J, Tavill A S, Wills M R, McIntyre N 1973 The pathophysiology of congenital chloridorrhoea. Quarterly Journal of Medicine 42: 453–466

Perheentupa J, Visakorpi J 1965 Protein intolerance with deficient transport of basic amino acids; another inborn error of metabolism. Lancet ii: 813–816

Peterson M L, Herber R 1967 Intestinal sucrase deficiency. Transactions of the Association of American Physicians 80: 275–283

Phillips S F, McGill D B 1973 Glucose-galactose malabsorption in an adult: perfusion studies of sugar, electrolyte and water transport. American Journal of Digestive Diseases 18: 1017–1024

Rajantie J, Simell O, Perheentupa J 1980a Intestinal absorption in lysinuric protein intolerance: impaired for diamino acids, normal for citrulline. Gut 21: 519–524

Rajantie J, Simell O, Perheentupa J 1980b Basolateral membrane transport defect for lysine in lysinuric protein intolerance. Lancet i: 1219–1221

Ransome-Kuti O, Kretchmer N, Johnson J D, Gribble J T 1975 A genetic study of lactose digestion in Nigerian families. Gastroenterology 68: 431–436

Rask-Madsen J, Kamper J, Oddsson E, Krog E 1976 Congenital chloridorrhoea, a question of reversed brush border processes and varying junctional tightness. Scandinavian Journal of Gastroenterology 11: 377–383

Rasmussen H, Anast C 1978 Familial hypophosphatemic (vitamin D-resistant) rickets and vitamin D-dependent rickets. In: Stanbury J B, Wyngaarden J B, Fredrickson D S (eds) The Metabolic Basis of Inherited Disease, 4th edn, McGraw-Hill, New York. pp 1537–1562

Rosenberg I M 1981 Intestinal absorption of folate. In: Johnson L R (ed) Physiology of the Gastrointestinal Tract, Raven Press, New York, 2: 1221–1230

Salt H B, Wolff O H, Lloyd J K, Fosbrooke A S, Cameron A H, Hubble D V 1960 On having no betalipoprotein — a syndrome comprising abetalipoproteinaemia, acanthocytosis and steatorrhoea. Lancet ii: 325–329

Santiago-Borrero P J, Santini R Jr, Perez-Santiago E, Maldonado N, Millan S, Coll-Camalez G 1973 Congenital isolated defect of folic acid absorption. Journal of Pediatrics 82: 450–455

Schneider A J, Kinter W B, Stirling C E 1966 Glucose-galactose malabsorption. New England Journal of Medicine 274: 305–312

Schultz S G, Curran P F 1970 Coupled transport of sodium and organic solutes. Physiological Reviews 50: 637–718

Schultz S G, Frizzell R A 1972 An overview of intestinal absorptive and secretory processes. Gastroenterology 63: 161–170

Schultz S G, Strecker C K 1970 Fructose influx across the brush border of rabbit ileum. Biochimica et Biophysica Acta 211: 586–588

Schultz S G, Frizzell R A, Nellans H N 1974 Ion transport by mammalian small intestine. Annual Review of Physiology 36: 51–91

Scott B B, Miller J P, Losowsky M S 1979 Hypobetalipoproteinaemia — a variant of the Bassen-Kornzweig syndrome. Gut 20: 163–168

Seetharam B, Alpers D H 1982 Absorption and transport of cobalamin (vitamin B_{12}). Annual Reviews of Nutrition 2: 334–349

Semenza G 1981 Molecular pathophysiology of small-intestinal sucrase-isomaltase. Clinics in Gastroenterology 10:(3), 691–706

Sigurdsson G, Nicoll A, Lewis B 1977 Turnover of apolipoprotein-B in two subjects with familial hypobetalipoproteinaemia. Metabolism 26: 25–31

Silk D B A 1974 Peptide absorption in man. Gut 15: 494–501

Silk D B A 1982 Disorders of nitrogen metabolism. Clinics in Gastroenterology 11:(1), 47–72

Simell O 1975 Diamino acid transport into granulocytes and liver slices of patients with lysinuric protein intolerance. Pediatric Research 9: 504–508

Simell O, Perheentupa J, Rapola J, Visakorpi J K, Eskelin L E 1975 Lysinuric protein intolerance. American Journal of Medicine 59: 229–240

Szurszewski J, Bulbring E 1973 The stimulant action of acetylcholine and catecholamine on the uterus. Philosophical Transactions of the Royal Society, London, Series B, 265: 149–156

Tarlow M J, Hadorn B, Arthurton M W, Lloyd J K 1970 Intestinal enterokinase deficiency. Archives of Disease in Childhood 45: 651–655

Thier S O, Alpers D H 1969 Disorders of intestinal transport of amino acids. American Journal of Disease of Childhood 117: 13–23

Thomson A B R, Dietschy J M 1981 Intestinal lipid absorption: major extracellular and intracellular events. In: Johnson L R (ed) Physiology of the Gastrointestinal Tract. Raven Press, New York. 2: 1147–1220

Townes P L, Bryson M F, Miller G 1967 Further observations on trypsinogen deficiency disease: report of a second case. Journal of Pediatrics 71: 220–224

Turnberg L A 1971 Abnormalities in intestinal electrolyte transport in congenital chloridorrhoea. Gut 12: 544–551

Turnberg L A, Fordtran J S, Carter N W, Rector F C 1970 Mechanism of bicarbonate absorption and its relationship to sodium transport in the human jejunum. Journal of Clinical Investigation 49: 557–567

Weijers H A, Van de Kamer J H, Mossel D A A, Dicke W K 1960 Diarrhoea caused by deficiency of sugar splitting enzymes. Lancet ii: 296–297

Welsh M J, Smith P L, Fromm M, Frizzell R A 1982 Crypts are the site of intestinal fluid and electrolyte secretion. Science 218: 1219–1221

Wimberley P D, Harries J T, Burgess E A 1974 Congenital glucose-galactose malabsorption. Proceedings of the Royal Society of Medicine 67: 755–756

Wozniak E, Fenton T R, Walker-Smith J A, Milla P J 1984 Glucose absorption in congenital glucose-galactose malabsorption: a kinetic basis for clinical remission. Paediatric Research 18:1063

10

S. G. Wright

Parasitic infections

A vast number of the world's population is infected with parasites, e.g. 1.3×10^9 individuals have ascariasis, but the eradication of these infections is not an achievable goal. The extent to which parasites harm the host is difficult to determine. It would seem probable that parasites in the gut lumen or adhering to the gut mucosa would affect digestion and absorption of nutrients with eventual deterioration in nutritional status and that if this were the case infants and children in the endemic areas would be at greatest risk (Keusch 1982).

A great deal more work is needed however to produce valid measures of the effects of intestinal parasitoses on nutritional status. The following review draws attention to the clinical diseases caused by these intestinal parasitic infections in man.

PROTOZOA

Giardia lamblia

Giardia lamblia is a flagellate protozoan parasite which inhabits the small intestine (Figs. 10.1 and 10.2). It has a worldwide distribution but is most common in the tropics where infection rates of up to 40% have been reported. It is also common in Eastern Europe and the Mediterranean. Giardiasis is the most common parasitic infection reported by the Public Health Laboratory Service in England and Wales where it is not uncommon in communities living in overcrowded accommodation in inner city areas.

Infection occurs by ingesting cysts of the parasite from contaminated food or water. Person-to-person spread occurs especially in young children (Black et al 1977) and the retarded. Ingestion of 100 cysts will consistently

Fig. 10.1

Fig. 10.2

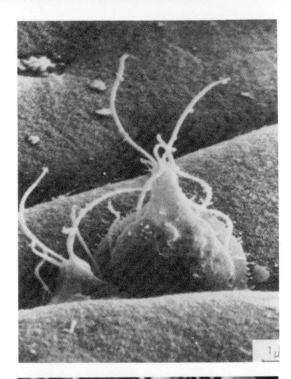

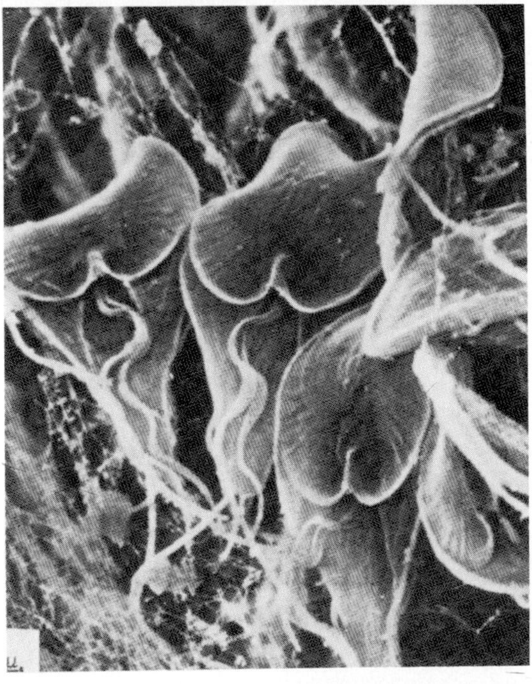

Figs 10.1 and 2   Scanning electron microscopic appearances of the trophozoic stage of *Giardia lamblia* attached to the surface of small intestinal mucosa

cause infection and as few as ten cysts may cause infection. Acceptable levels of water chlorination will not kill cysts and filtration is the usual way of cleansing municipal water supplies of cysts and ova. Heating water to over 50°C kills cysts rapidly. Cysts hatch in the duodenum liberating trophozoites which divide asexually. In the human the pattern of infestation is not known but it is probably similar to murine giardiasis where there is a rapid rise in trophozoite numbers, reaching a peak by 2 weeks after infection, followed by a progressive decline. Changes in parasite populations in acute human giardiasis may show a similar pattern. The time before faecal cyst excretion starts is sometimes longer than the incubation period and so several stool samples may need to be examined over one to two weeks before the diagnosis can be made.

Clinical features

The median incubation time is about seven days with a range of two to 28 days prior to the onset of an acute diarrhoeal illness. Anorexia, nausea, lethargy, abdominal distension, abdominal discomfort, flatulence and diarrhoea with loose to watery, yellow, foul-smelling stools are usual clinical features. Weight loss is usual. Spontaneous improvement in symptoms occurs after two to four weeks with ultimately complete resolution of the illness. The patient may eradicate the infection completely or remain an asymptomatic cyst excreter. The duration of asymptomatic cyst excretion has not been well studied but may last up to a year in some cases. A small proportion of patients remain symptomatic for weeks or months with continuing weight loss or failure to thrive in children. Infection which is frequently persistent is well recognized in immunodeficient patients.

Investigations have mainly been in adults (Wright et al 1977) but it is likely that similar changes occur in children. Patients often have impaired absorption of fat, d-xylose and vitamin B_{12} with secondary hypolactasia resulting in lactose intolerance. Folate deficiency is encountered in infections of long duration. Jejunal biopsies show a crypt hyperplastic partial villous atrophy and an increase of plasma cells and lymphocytes in the lamina propria. Subtotal villous atrophy is uncommon even in patients with severe malabsorption associated with giardiasis and a gluten-sensitive enteropathy must be borne in mind when this feature is seen in a biopsy. Follow-up with a repeat biopsy is essential so that a gluten-sensitive enteropathy is not missed.

Diagnosis and treatment

The diagnosis is made by finding cysts of the parasite in faecal samples following formol-ether concentration. Cyst excretion can vary considerably (Danciger & Lopez 1975) and several samples may be required before the parasites are found. Where stool samples do not contain cysts and the diagnosis is likely, the upper gastrointestinal tract can be sampled by jejunal aspiration, jejunal biopsy and by the Enterotest capsule. Jejunal mucosa obtained at biopsy should be imprinted on a culture plate and trophozoites may be found in these samples (Kamath & Murugasu 1974), or in fluid stools.

Metronidazole syrup is given in a dose of 3 mg/kg three times a day for 14 days. Alternatively it can be given as a high dose regimen (depending on the age of the child) over three days; children over 10 years receiving 2.0 g as a single daily dose with food; 7 to 10 years 1.0 g/day; 3 to 7 years 600–800 mg/24 h; 1 to 3 years 500 mg/24 h. Tinidazole may be used in single doses of 25 to 30 mg/kg with food, but it is not available as a syrup and it is difficult to get children to swallow crushed tablets because of the very bitter taste. Mepacrine is effective in doses of 1.5 mg/kg three times a day for 5 to 10 days. Dietary restrictions are not usually necessary apart from advising a low lactose diet in those with lactose intolerance.

Cytosporidium

These organisms are sporozoan parasites which cause enteritis in a number of animals. Human cryptosporidiosis was initially regarded as an opportunistic infection in immunosuppressed patients (Meisel et al 1976) but enteritis due to cryptosporidiosis in normal humans has now been recognized (Jokipii et al 1983, Tzipori 1983)

It is not known for certain if the parasite is intracellular or extracellular. Infection occurs by the ingestion of oocysts which are disrupted in the intestine liberating four sporozoites which adhere to the microvillus of the enterocytes, where they develop into mature trophozoites and then divide asexually into eight merozoites. Merozoites may continue the asexual cycle or enter the sexual cycle to produce oocysts by union of gametes. Oocysts are passed in the faeces and the diagnosis is made following the staining of faecal smears with Giemsa stain or a modified Ziehl-Nielsen method. The parasite can also be found in mucosal biopsies from the duodenum, jejunum or rectum.

Diarrhoea, abdominal pain, and flatulence were prominent symptoms in one series of cases (Jokipii et al 1983). The median duration of disease was 10 days before spontaneous resolution occurred. No specific treatment is available.

Leishmania donovani

This organism causes visceral leishmaniasis characterized by hepatosplenomegaly and prolonged fever. The parasites are found within macrophages in many tissues of the body, particularly bone marrow and spleen. The occasional patient has diarrhoea, and jejunal biopsies have shown abnormal villous architecture and macrophages which contain parasites in the lamina

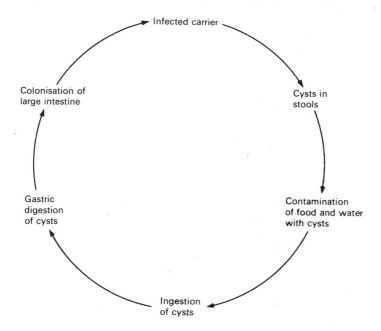

Fig. 10.3   Life cycle of *Entamoeba histolytica*

propria (Muigai et al 1983). Treatment with daily intravenous sodium stibogluconate (20 mg antimony/kg) for a minimum of 21 days usually eradicates the infection.

Entamoeba histolytica

This organism has a worldwide distribution but is common in the tropics. Low standards of personal and public hygiene favour faecal-oral transmission of the infection. Recent work has shed light on the pathogenicity of the organism (Sargeaunt et al 1982). Isoenzyme patterns have been defined for clones of amoebae, and 19 different patterns (zymodemes) are presently recognized of which only seven have been associated with clinical disease, i.e. amoebic dysentery, amoeboma and amoebic liver abscess. The pathogenic strains are resistant to serum and complement-mediated lysis (Reed et al 1983). These findings suggest that not all amoebae are pathogenic and that infection can only be transmitted by cysts from a person with, or recovering from, invasive amoebic disease.

Trophozoites of the non-pathogenic zymodemes are presumed to live commensally on the luminal surface of the colonic epithelium especially the caecum and ascending colon. Periodically trophozoites encyst and cysts are passed in the faeces as shown in Figure 10.3. Trophozoites and cysts of pathogenic and non-pathogenic zymodemes are indistinguishable on morphological grounds.

Amoebic dysentery

There is a considerable range in the severity of amoebic dysentery. Mild disease is associated with abdominal discomfort and increased frequency of bowel action with bloodstained mucus or frank blood with the stools. At the other extreme, there can be severe dysenteric diarrhoea with considerable abdominal pain, watery stools which are uniformly bloodstained, and severe abdominal tenderness.

Proctosigmoidoscopy should be performed cautiously in patients with severe colitic symptoms. The typical appearances are scattered elliptical ulcers with surrounding mucosal erythema on an otherwise normal mucosa. A diffusely inflamed, ulcerated mucosa indistinguishable from severe bacillary dysentery or nonspecific ulcerative colitis may be seen. Barium enema examinations show a granular, ulcerated mucosa in affected areas. The rectum and caecum are areas of predilection.

Severe disease may be associated with anaemia, electrolyte losses, hypoproteinaemia and a raised sedimentation rate. Complications of severe amoebic dysentery include haemorrhage, perforation, toxic megacolon and sloughing of varying amounts of colonic mucosa.

The diagnosis is made by finding motile trophozoites containing ingested red cells on microscopy of faecal smears, scrapings from ulcerated mucosa and flecks of bloodstained mucus in faeces. The cellular exudate in invasive amoebiasis mainly consists of red cells. Amoebae can be found in sections of rectal biopsies stained with haematoxylin and eosin where they are seen in the advancing edge of ulcers and in the basal slough. Serological tests for amoebiasis are only positive in 65% of patients with amoebic dysentery and therefore a negative test does not exclude the diagnosis. In contrast, these tests are positive in over 95% of patients with amoebic liver abscess or amoeboma. Cysts of *Entamoeba histolytica* are found in the stools of asymptomatic cyst excreters and some patients with amoebic liver abscess.

Amoeboma

Amoeboma is a late and uncommon complication of invasive amoebiasis occurring after amoebic dysentery has resolved. There may be one or more amoebomae in the colon and the caecum is often involved. The pathological changes comprise granulation tissue in which amoebae are difficult to find. Abdominal pain, change in bowel habit, often with blood in the stools and one or more tender abdominal masses are usual findings. Barium enema shows an irregular narrowing of the affected colon and in adults these appearances may be difficult to distinguish from a carcinoma of the colon. Positive serological tests for amoebiasis and rapid improvement on treatment with metronidazole indicate the parasitic aetiology of the lesion.

Amoebic liver abscess

Amoebic liver abscesses (ALA) are uncommon in children but do occur. Amoebae are carried to the liver in portal blood and there they produce one or more expanding regions of liver cell necrosis which may or may not intercommunicate. ALA may arise in individuals: i) during amoebic dysentery; ii) without a history of previous dysentery; iii) with or without cysts in the stool. The pathogenic zymodemes have been incriminated in ALA (Sargeaunt et al 1982).

The symptoms and signs relate to the site and size of the abscess. Most are single and are in the right lobe of the liver. Fever, anorexia, night sweats and lethargy are the usual constitutional symptoms. Abscesses in the lower part of the right lobe produce right hypochondrial pain.

A normochromic, normocytic anaemia with a neutrophil leucocytosis and a raised sedimentation rate are usually found. Plasma albumin levels fall while total globulin increases. There may be a minor elevation of plasma transaminases with a normal bilirubin and commonly a marked elevation of alkaline phosphatase levels. Serological tests for amoebiasis are almost invariably positive at high titre. When an initial test is negative with an ALA, seroconversion to positive occurs within a week. Chest radiographs may show an elevated hemidiaphragm often with a localized bulge over the abscess, and atelectasis, consolidation or pleural effusion.

Recent advances in imaging techniques have allowed very accurate definition of the site and size of ALAs, with ultrasound scanning being the most useful. Aspiration of abscesses can be done under ultrasound control. The need for aspiration of the abscess must be considered in all cases. Liver aspiration by the percutaneous route is a safe procedure and should be performed at the outset if the abscess is very large or there is any indication that rupture is imminent. Aspiration may also be indicated during the course of drug treatment if the patient's general condition, physical signs and vital signs have not improved within 48 hours of starting treatment. Occasionally it is necessary to change the drug regimen to include chloroquine or emetine but this is uncommon.

Treatment

Metronidazole is usually used at a dose of 40 mg/kg/24 h in three divided doses for 10 days. Rapid improvement occurs within 48 hours in dysentery, amoeboma and liver abscess. This should be followed by diloxanide furoate 8 mg/kg three times a day for 10 days to eradicate luminal amoebae not killed by metronidazole. Diloxanide furoate is also given to cyst excreters because there is no ready means of determining whether encysted amoebae belong to pathogenic or non-pathogenic zymodemes.

Transfusion of blood or plasma, nutritional support and antibiotics may be needed by patients with severe amoebic dysentery. Steroids must not be given as this allows the infection to progress more rapidly.

Balantidium coli

This is the largest of man's protozoan parasites (40–154μm long) and is visible to the naked eye. The infection is acquired from pigs by ingestion of cysts and is usually a commensal in man. Occasional cases of balantidiasis associated with invasion of the distal ileum and colon have been described with abdominal pain and dysenteric diarrhoea. Trophozoites are found in the stools of symptomatic and asymptomatic patients. Treatment with metronidazole, nitrimidazine or paromomycin is effective.

HELMINTHS

Hookworm

Man is the definitive host of two species of hookworm, *Ancylostoma duodenale* and *Necator americanus*. They both have a wide geographical distribution in areas of the world where the climate is sufficiently warm and moist to allow development of free living infective larvae in the soil. The adults live in the upper small intestine, firmly attached to the mucosa by their mouth parts (Fig. 10.4), and ingest blood from the host. They move from site to site and this causes bleeding from sites where they have been attached. Nutrients are absorbed from blood during its transit through the worm gut, and the rest passes into the host's gut where it can be digested and absorbed. Adult females lay eggs which are passed in the faeces.

In warm moist soil the eggs hatch and the larvae develop to the infective stage. In the case of *N. americanus*, man is infected by larval penetration of the skin and there is then a stage of migration to the right heart and lungs via blood vessels. The larvae enter the air spaces of the lungs and travel up the bronchial tree to the hypopharynx where they are swallowed to reach the small bowel lumen. Infection with *A. duodenale* occurs both by larval penetration of the skin and by ingestion of larvae. The larvae mature in the gut lumen without a stage of tissue migration. Adults and children who go barefoot are at risk, particularly in subsistence farming areas, where night soil is used as fertilizer. The eggs of the two species are indistinguishable.

Clinical features

Most infected individuals have no symptoms. Abnormalities of intestinal structure and function tend to occur in individuals who are heavily infected. Iron deficiency anaemia occurs when, in addition to heavy hookworm infection, iron stores are low and diets are deficient in available iron. Patients with severe iron deficiency anaemia may present in high output cardiac failure with gross congestive features, which may progress to low output failure which has a high mortality.

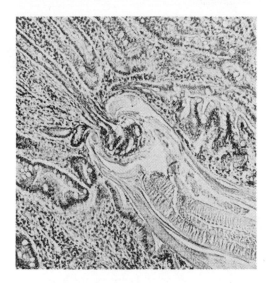

Fig. 10.4   Adult hookworm firmly attached to small intestinal mucosa

Diagnosis and treatment

The diagnosis is made by finding eggs of the parasite in faecal samples. Tetrachlorethylene in a dose of 0.1 ml/kg body weight to a maximum single dose of 4 ml is an effective and cheap treatment. Bephenium hydroxyna-phthoate is also effective; children up to 2 years receive 2.5 g and those over 2 years 5.0 g. A single dose is effective for *A. duodenale* but daily doses for 3 days are required for *N. americanus*. When hookworm and ascariasis coexist it is recommended that the ascariasis be treated first, as either of the above drugs may stimulate migration of ascarids into the bile or pancreatic duct. Mebendazole, 100 mg twice daily for 3 days, is effective against hookworm and ascariasis, as is albendazole, 100 mg twice daily for one day.

The management of severe anaemia with cardiac failure requires cautious transfusion of packed cells with concurrent use of diuretics. Later the hook-worm infection is treated and body stores of iron are repleted using the oral or occasionally the parenteral route.

Ascariasis

Ascaris lumbricoides has a world-wide distribution in the hot, humid areas of the world. Vast numbers of people are infected but the adverse conse-quences of this infection are still being debated (Schultz 1982).

Infection occurs by ingesting eggs in contaminated food and water. Pica may be important in children. Larvae hatch in the gut lumen and penetrate the mucosa to enter blood vessels or lymphatics. After an extensive migration the larvae reach the lungs, enter the air spaces and pass up the bronchial tree where they are swallowed and reach the lumen of the small intestine. The adult maintains its position in the gut by its own motility and lives for approximately one year.

Clinical features

Symptoms related to the migration of larvae through the lungs are uncommon. In countries where there is a short wet season, pneumonitis, thought to be associated with larval migration, has been reported. Pulmonary manifestations occur when man is infected with the pig ascarid *Ascaris suum* (Phills et al 1972).

Parasites in the gut lumen rarely cause symptoms. Occasionally adult worms are passed in vomit or faeces, and may be incidental findings on barium follow-through films. Small intestinal obstruction with all the usual features occurs when a large, knotted bolus of adult worms obstructs the gut lumen. Adult worms may obstruct the bile or pancreatic duct by migrating through the ampulla of Vater to cause pain and obstructive jaundice or pancreatitis. Ascarids may perforate the bowel wall to cause peritonitis and may migrate through suture lines of intestinal anastomoses. In exceptional cases, multiple liver abscesses can develop around adult worms that have migrated to the liver. Eosinophilia occurs during the phase of tissue migration but is absent in established luminal infections.

Diagnosis and treatment

Eggs are usually seen in faecal smears. Piperazine salts have been the mainstay of treatment for many years; a single dose regimen of piperazine hydrate elixir (750 mg of the hydrate per 5 ml) is effective, as follows: children under 2 years 120 mg/kg body weight; 2–4 years 10 ml; 5–6 years 15 ml; 6–10 years 20 ml; and children over 10 years 30 ml. Underweight children should be given a dose worked out on the basis of 120 mg/kg. Mebendazole can be given to children over 2 years, 100 mg twice a day for 3 days. Albendazole is effective in doses of 100 mg twice a day for 1 day.

Strongyloides stercoralis

Adult worms live in the small bowel lumen where they cling to intestinal villi. The females lay eggs which promptly hatch into rhabditiform larvae. These larvae are passed in the faeces and in warm, moist soil conditions develop either into infective filariform larvae which can penetrate exposed skin on the human host to maintain the cycle, or into free living adults which can in turn produce rhabditiform larvae. Infective filariform larvae in the host travel via the venous system to the right heart, and then via the lung and bronchial tree to the gut lumen.

Most infected persons are asymptomatic. A malabsorption syndrome occasionally occurs but the factors responsible are poorly understood. Studies in infants in Papua New Guinea have associated heavy infection with a *Strongyloides fulleborni*-like worm with abdominal distension, respiratory distress, diarrhoea and oedema (Vince et al 1979).

Rhabditiform larvae may mature to the infective filariform stage during transit down the gut. These filariform larvae invade the mucosa of the rectum, the anal canal or the perianal skin and then follow the usual path of migration, often appearing beneath the skin over the trunk or buttocks to cause a serpiginous, itching urticaria that lasts about an hour. This is known as 'larvae currens' to distinguish it from cutaneous 'larva migrans' which meander about very slowly. When the larvae reach the gut they mature into adults to maintain the infection. Diagnosis of strongyloidiasis is delayed unless the peculiar urticaria is recognized by the physician.

Very rarely, massive autoinfection by infective filariform larvae occurs, resulting initially in abdominal pain, vomiting, ileus and constipation (Rivera et al 1970). Treatment may halt the process or there may be progression to diarrhoea, pneumonitis, meningeal signs and septicaemia. There is a high mortality. Massive autoinfection may occur in immunodeficiency or in individuals immunosuppressed by drugs such as steroids and cytotoxic agents. Occasional cases are seen in apparently healthy persons not receiving any medication. Strongyloides larvae are found in gastric aspirate, faeces and sputum. Eosinophilia is absent as a result of the immunosuppression. Intensive supportive therapy including ventilatory support, treatment of septicaemia and treatment of the strongyloidiasis are necessary. Treatment for presumed strongyloidiasis should be considered in patients from or in the tropics, prior to administration of cytotoxic or immunosuppressive drugs.

Rhabditiform larvae are usually found in the faeces but may also be found in fluid aspirated from the jejunum.

Treatment

Thiabendazole in doses of 25 mg/kg up to a maximum single dose of 1.5 g is given twice a day for 3 days in most cases. In the massive autoinfection syndromes the dose is calculated as above and is given for 2 weeks although this is very nauseating. Albendazole is also effective at a dose of 400 mg twice a day for 3 days. It is well absorbed from the gut and causes less side effects, and may prove to be a better drug in the massive autoinfection syndrome.

Capillaria philippinensis

This nematode infection of man was first described from the Philippines in the 1960s. It is limited in geographical extent to coastal regions of the island of Luzon and some coastal areas of Thailand.

Severe dehydrating diarrhoea with electrolyte depletion, protein loss into the gut, steatorrhoea and weight loss are usual features, but jejunal biopsy changes are minimal. The adult worms are readily found in the gut lumen and vast numbers of eggs are passed daily in the faeces.

Children over 2 years old are treated with mebendazole, 400 mg/24 h for up to 28 days. The disease improves rapidly on treatment, with resolution of symptoms and a decline in egg output. Thiabendazole can also be used but often causes marked nausea. Further courses of medication are given if relapse occurs.

Trichuris trichiura

This is the whipworm which attaches itself to the mucosa by its long slender anterior portion. The caecum and colonic mucosa are parasitized. Most infections are asymptomatic and the diagnosis is made when *Trichuris* ova are found in faecal samples. Severe infections with large numbers of worms are seen occasionally in children who are poorly nourished. They have dysenteric diarrhoea and often rectal prolapse. The worms can be seen on the rectal mucosa at proctoscopy. It is difficult to know whether the heavy worm infection causes the malnutrition, as has been suggested in a study from Malaysia (Gilman et al 1983), or whether malnourished children have impaired ability to clear worms from the gut.

Infection occurs by ingesting *Trichuris* ova which hatch in the gut lumen. The larvae migrate down the intestine to the caecum and colon where the adults are found. Eggs are easily identified in faecal smears. Mebendazole in a dose of 100 mg twice a day for 3 days eradicates the infection.

Enterobius vermicularis

Threadworms are one of the commonest infestations of children. Eggs are ingested and the liberated larvae migrate down the gut to the colonic lumen. Gravid females migrate out onto the perianal skin where they deposit their ova, which are very sticky and adhere to the skin and to fingers which scratch the perianal skin in response to the marked local pruritus evoked by the oviposition. Eggs are therefore easily transferred to the mouth to reinfect the host. Eggs which adhere to bedclothes, underclothes and towels may infect other members of the family. A mother may be infected by getting eggs on her fingers while examining the perianal skin of her infected child. Rarely, appendicitis and granulomas of the female genital tract have been caused by *Enterobius*.

The parasitological diagnosis is made either by identifying the adult worm or by obtaining ova by swabbing the unwashed perianal skin. The swab is then placed in a small amount of saline and the centrifuged deposit is examined for ova. This is one of the most difficult helminthic infections to eradicate. Personal hygiene should be stressed in an effort to break the cycle of autoinfection via the fingers to mouth route. Careful hand-washing with brushing of the finger nails first thing in the morning should be encouraged. A variety of drugs can be used. Mebendazole in a dose of 100 mg repeated after two weeks is effective. Piperazine hydrate can also be used; children over 12 years should be given 2 g/24 h in 2 divided doses; those aged 6–12 years, 1.5 g/24 h; children aged less than 6 years, 250 mg per year of age. Dosage is continued for seven days and the course may be repeated after a seven-day interval.

Toxocariasis

Toxocara canis and *T. cati* are nematode parasites of the dog and cat. When humans ingest the eggs the larvae hatch, penetrate the gut mucosa and migrate via vascular or lymphatic channels. The parasite is in the wrong host and so the migration is aimless. First infections are thought to sensitize the host without causing significant disease but subsequent infections are associated with granuloma formation around larvae. The severity of disease depends on the number of migrating larvae and the site of granuloma formation. Young children playing in parks and gardens are at risk of infection, particularly if there is a history of pica.

Fever, hepatosplenomegaly, eosinophilia and pulmonary infiltrates occur in the syndrome of visceral larva migrans. Granuloma formation in the eye can cause monocular blindness. It has been suggested that toxocariasis can lead to cerebral granuloma formation and epilepsy.

An enzyme-linked immunoabsorbent assay (ELISA) for *Toxocara* antibodies is a sensitive diagnostic test using a secretory antigen from the parasite gut. The worm does not develop to the adult stage in man and eggs are not found in the faeces.

Treatment is aimed at killing any larvae which are migrating. Diethylcarbamazine (maximum 3 mg/kg) is given 3 times a day for 3 weeks after starting at a low dose and building up to the maximum dose over a week. Clinical improvement is fairly rapid in visceral larva migrans. The eosinophil count falls to normal levels though the ELISA test remains positive for prolonged periods.

TAPEWORMS

Tapeworms have a scolex which grips onto the gut mucosa by suckers, hooks or sucking gooves and distal to that, segments (proglottids) which become increasingly mature. These segments are hermaphroditic and self-fertile. Mature gravid segments break off from the distal end of the worm and are either passed to the exterior intact in varying lengths or disintegrate in the gut lumen so that eggs are passed in the faeces.

Taeniasis

When the intermediate hosts, pigs (*Taenia solium*) or cattle (*T. saginata*) ingest the eggs, embryos hatch and invade the mucosa of the gut wall and migrate to muscle (particularly the tongue, diaphragm and heart) causing cysticercosis cellulosae in pigs and cysticercosis bovis in cattle. Cysticerci are bladder-like structures with the scolex inverted into the bladder. Man is infected by eating raw or inadequately cooked meat containing cysticerci. The surrounding tissue is digested away and the scolex is evaginated. It fixes to the mucosa of the small intestine by hooks and suckers (*T. solium*) or by suckers (*T. saginata*). Proglottids develop and when they are mature they break off from the worm and are passed in the faeces. The occurrence of symptoms attributable to these species is difficult to assess but abdominal discomfort, weight loss, nausea and urticaria have all been reported.

Diagnosis and treatment

The parasitological diagnosis is made by examining segments which have been passed in the faeces. A mature segment is pressed between two microscope slides and the number of lateral branches of the uterus is counted. There are about nine in *T. solium* and about 20 in *T. saginata*.

Niclosamide is used in the treatment of both infections. Children over 6 years are given 4 tablets; 2 to 6 years, 2 tablets, and those under 2, one tablet. Half the dose is given before, and the other half after breakfast. The tablets must be thoroughly chewed before they are swallowed. In *T. solium* infections a drastic purge is given 2 hours after the second dose of tablets in order to ensure rapid expulsion of the worm and prevent cysticercosis cellulosae (see below). Praziquantel is effective for both species in a single dose, 10 mg/kg. Both drugs destroy the scolex. If no segments have been passed by 4 months after treatment, the infection has been eradicated.

Taeniasis is controlled by condemning measly pork and beef, by freezing meat to −10°C for 10 days or by thorough cooking of the meat.

Complications

Cysticerci of *T. solium* can be found in human tissues (cysticercosis cellulosae) i.e. the human can be infected with both the intermediate and adult stages of the parasite. This could arise in one of two ways. If the eggs are ingested, they hatch liberating the oncosphere which invades the gut wall and is carried by vascular or lymphatic routes to some distant site. Alternatively, autoinfection can occur as a result of regurgitation of gravid proglottids into the stomach where eggs are liberated and hatch to release oncospheres which invade the gut wall and are carried away as above. The exact means is not known but the former mechanism appears more likely. Almost any tissue in the body may be affected. Subcutaneous nodules may indicate spread to superficial tissues. Calcified cysticerci may be seen on X-ray in skeletal muscles. Cysticerci commonly affect the brain causing epilepsy and raised intracranial pressure in endemic areas.

There is some evidence that praziquantel will kill cysticerci. Botero & Castaño (1982) gave 10 mg/kg 3 times a day for 6 days to patients with subcutaneous cysts which disappeared after treatment. This regimen was given twice, with an interval of one to two months between courses, to patients with cerebral cysticercosis. Latterly, the dose was increased to 50 mg/kg/24 h in 3 divided doses for 10 days, with dexamethasone 0.1 mg/kg 4 times a day beginning one day before, and continuing for 3 days after, praziquantel. Further studies are required in this area. Cysticerci cannot resolve when they are calcified.

Diphyllobothriasis

Man is the definitve host of *Diphyllobothrium latum* but there are two intermediate hosts. The adult worm produces up to 1 000 000 eggs daily, which when deposited in fresh water, hatch to liberate a ciliated miracidium. This can only survive for 2 days and must be ingested by a copepod such as cyclops. The proceroid develops in the body cavity of the cyclops which must then be eaten by a freshwater fish. The proceroid larvae are then released into the gut of the fish, where they penetrate the gut wall and develop into plerocercoids. Large fish can become infected by eating infected smaller fish and human infection occurs by eating raw or under-cooked fish.

The adult worm may cause no symptoms even though it may reach 10 m in length and survive for 25 years. Occasionally vitamin B_{12} deficiency causing megaloblastic anaemia arises as a result of the worm absorbing and using the vitamin and thus denying it to the host (von Bonsdorff 1977). The parasitological diagnosis is made by finding eggs in the stools.

The drugs used for taeniasis are effective in the same doses.

Echinococcosis (Hydatid disease)

Man can be an intermediate host in the life cycle of the dog tapeworm *Echinococcus granulosus* in which sheep, goats, cattle etc, are the usual intermediate hosts. Man can also occasionally be infected with the intermediate form of the tapeworm of voles and foxes, *E. multilocularis*, this is rare and has a very poor prognosis.

Infection occurs by ingestion of eggs. The eggs hatch and release an oncosphere which penetrates the intestinal mucosa and enters a branch of the portal vein. The oncosphere is carried to the liver (the organ most commonly affected), where it develops into a cyst lined internally by a germinal epithelium from which daughter cysts bud. The lung is the second most common site for hydatid disease. The peritoneal cavity can be involved when a liver cyst ruptures. Multiple cysts may develop and are felt (per abdomen and per rectum) as smooth rounded intra-abdominal masses. Eosinophilia and positive serological tests for hydatid are usual but not invariable findings. Residence in endemic areas which include Welsh and Scottish sheep-farming areas, Cyprus, the Middle East and Australasia is a useful reminder of the possibility of this diagnosis when investigating unexplained hepatomegaly.

Ultrasound scanning and computerized axial tomography are helpful in assessing the number, position and size of the cysts.

Echinococcus multilocularis progressively spreads through the affected tissue by external budding of daughter cysts. The infection is not localized by a cyst wall. There is no drug treatment of proven value. Mebendazole in high doses, 12 mg/kg three times a day for one to three months, seems to have been effective in some cases, particularly where there is pleural or peritoneal involvement. Preliminary studies have shown that albendazole, which is much better absorbed than mebandazole, may be more effective (Morris & Dykes 1983). Most of these studies have involved adults and little information is available for the paediatric age group.

When cysts are very large, or are causing symptoms and when rupture is likely, surgical removal is necessary. Operative techniques for this have been reviewed (Saidi 1979).

Hymenolepiasis

Hymenolepis nana is a small tapeworm measuring up to 40 mm in length with 200 proglottids. Gravid segments are disrupted in the gut lumen and eggs are passed in faeces. There is no intermediate host and man is infected by ingesting the eggs. The oncosphere is liberated from the eggs and penetrates a villus to become a cysticercoid. After four days the cysticercoid enters the gut lumen to develop into the adult worm which grips the mucosa with hooks and suckers. The cycle takes 30 days from the ingestion of eggs to the passage of eggs in the faeces. Heavy infections (over 2000 worms) have been associated with abdominal pain and diarrhoea. Treatment with niclosamide is effective; children over six years take 4 tables on the first day and then 2 tablets daily for 6 days; children from two to six, 2 tablets on the first day and then one per 24 h for 6 days; children under 2 years take one tablet on the first day and half a tablet daily for 6 days. Praziquantel, 20 mg/kg, given as a single dose, is also effective.

Hymenolepia diminuta measures 300 to 600 mm by 4 mm with up to 1000 proglottids. The adult worm has suckers on the scolex which grip the mucosa. Eggs are shed in the faeces and the cysticercoid stage is found in insects, e.g. *Xenopsylla cheopis* (the rat flea), *Tribolium confusatum* (the flour beetle). Rats and children become infected when they eat the insects. Heavy infections are associated with diarrhoea. Treatment with niclosamide as for *H. nana* is effective.

SCHISTOSOMES

The two most common species which affect the gut of man are *Schistosoma mansoni* and *S. japonicum*. The distribution of *S. mansoni* includes the Middle East, particularly Egypt; east, central and west Africa; some islands of the Caribbean, particularly St. Lucia; and South America, notably Brazil. *S. japonicum* has been eradicated from Japan but is endemic in China and the islands of Luzon, Leyte, Samar, Nindoro, Mindanao and Bohol in the Philippines, with a localized focus in Malaysia. A separate species, *S. mekongi*, causes outcrops of disease in Thailand, Laos and Cambodia.

Life cycle

Eggs of the parasites are shed in faeces and hatch only in fresh water, liberating the ciliate miracidium which must find a fresh water snail of the appropriate genus, *Bulinus* for *S. mansoni* and *Oncomelania* for *S. japonicum*, within 48 hours of hatching. The miracidium develops into a mother sporocyst from which daughter cysts bud. These release cercariae which are able to survive in water for up to 12 hours and during this time must invade the skin of a suitable host. The cercaria loses its tail and becomes a schistosomule which may be retained in the skin for several days and evoke a localized papular eruption (swimmer's itch).

The schistosomule enters peripheral veins and migrates through the vascular system to reach the branches of the portal vein in the liver. Paired worms with the female lying in the gynaecophoric canal of the male migrate out to the peripheral branches of the portal vein. *S. mansoni* tends to be found mainly in the colonic venules while *S. japonicum* is found in venules surrounding the small and large intestine.

Eggs are laid by the female and may embolize through the portal vein to impact in presinusoidal branches in the liver or enter the submucosal tissues of the gut. Eggs in the gut wall may pass through the mucosa to be shed in the faeces, or be retained in the gut wall.

Pathology

The pathological changes in the host relate to eggs and not to adult worms. Granulomas comprising macrophages, lymphocytes, plasma cells and eosinophils form around eggs and are immunologically mediated responses to protein antigens that leak out of the eggs. These antigens are probably proteolytic enzymes produced by the miracidium. When there is no granuloma formation an area of tissue necrosis is found around the eggs. It is likely that both humoral and cell-mediated responses are important in localizing these cytotoxic substances. Granulomas resolve with fibrosis when the eggs have been destroyed. The intensity of fibrosis will depend to a large extent on the intensity of ovideposition.

The gross effects of these changes are seen in the intestine and liver. Focal deposition of eggs in the gut wall produces polypoid lesions. Granulomas in the presinusoidal branches of the portal vein can cause congestive hepatosplenomegaly. These granulomas in the gut and the liver may resolve but prolonged localized ovideposition in the gut can eventually cause irreversible fibrotic polyps and strictures. Prolonged embolization of eggs to the liver can cause schistosomal hepatofibrosis (Symmer's clay pipe stem fibrosis) which is irreversible and causes portal hypertension. This condition should not be classed as a cirrhosis as there are no regenerating nodules and the lobular architecture of the liver is well preserved.

Clinical features

Swimmer's itch heralding the development of schistosomiasis is very uncommon. When infection with a large number of schistosomules occurs at the same time, a febrile illness with dyspnoea, pulmonary infiltrates, weakness, sweats and peripheral blood eosinophilia can follow. This is uncommon but does occasionally occur in expatriates (Stuiver 1984). Most infected persons are symptom-free. Surveys comparing a range of gastrointestinal symptoms between children in high and low prevalence villages show very little difference, though among white populations in central and southern Africa lethargy in a child is commonly ascribed to schistosomiasis. Abdominal pain, diarrhoea and the passing of blood in the stools are not common.

Granulomatous polyps have been found in Egyptian patients in association with anaemia, hypoalbuminaemia and protein loss into the gut. The polyps and these abnormalities resolved following treatment of S. mansoni. Longstanding fibrotic polyps and strictures are rare but do occur among adults. Polyps were not found in infected patients in a large post-mortem study from Brazil (Cheever & Andrade 1967). Colonic cancer has been described in longstanding S. japonicum infections in China.

Hepatosplenomegaly is common in heavily infected children. With increasing age a proportion of these children will progress to the stage of schistosomal hepatofibrosis with hypersplenism and variceal bleeding as possible complications. Liver function is relatively well preserved and portosystemic-encephalopathy is not usual after bleeding.

Diagnosis and treatment

The diagnosis is made by finding lateral spined eggs of *S. mansoni* or the smaller, rounder eggs with a rudimentary lateral spine of *S. japonicum* in faecal concentrates. When eggs are not found in faeces they may be found in rectal snips. A proctoscope is introduced to its full length and three or four small fragments of mucosa are avulsed using a small curette. These fragments are separately squashed between two microscope slides for immediate microscopy. Living eggs can be distinguished by the flickering movements of their flame cells. Eggs that appear black are calcified and dead. Rectal biopsies which are fixed and processed by standard techniques show eggs within granulomas.

Serological tests using a variety of schistosome antigens have been used. These only indicate that the host has had contact with schistosomes. The tests do not distinguish between nonhuman schistosomes and the usual species found in man. The circum-oval precipitin test and the more recently developed schistosome ELISA both detect antibodies to egg antigens and therefore indicate that ovideposition has occurred. A strongly positive ELISA test may be grounds for recommending treatment with the newer nontoxic drugs, whereas a positive test using a schistosome worm antigen should prompt a further search for eggs. Eosinophilia in the peripheral blood is common in schistosomiasis.

Praziquantel is now the drug of first choice. A variety of drug regimens have been used but a single dose of 40 mg/kg gives good results with a low incidence of side effects. Nausea and dizziness beginning an hour after treatment and lasting up to three hours are the usual side effects. Praziquantel is effective against both species but has a slightly higher efficacy against *S. mansoni* than against *S. japonicum*. Oxamniquine is effective against *S. mansoni* in doses of 15 mg/kg for three days. Episodes of fever five days after treatment with oxamniquine are the most notable side effects.

If after three months of treatment no viable eggs are found in stools or rectal snips, the infection is cured. Serological tests take over a year to revert to negative and are not useful in evaluating treatment.

TREMATODES

Fasciola hepatica

Fascioliasis is mainly a disease of herbivores, particularly sheep, but man can be infected. The complex life cycle involves the deposition of eggs in water which hatch liberating miracidia. The miracidium invades the foot-piece of fresh water snails (*Lymnaea*) and within the snail a sporocyst develops. Cercariae are produced by the sporocyst and these reach fresh water by rupture of the sporocyst onto the external surface of the snail. The cercariae encyst either on aquatic vegetation, for example wild water cress, or free in fresh water. The definitive host ingests the encysted cercariae and these are released by the digestive processes of the host. The larvae migrate through the duodenal wall and cross the peritoneal cavity to the surface of the liver which they enter to reach intrahepatic bile ducts by burrowing through liver parenchyma. The adult hermaphroditic worms mature and start to lay eggs which are carried down the biliary tract to the gut lumen, to be passed in the faeces.

When small numbers of adult worms are present there may be no symptoms attributable to the infection. The diagnosis may be made by finding eggs on stool microscopy carried out for some unrelated reason. Upper abdominal pain, hepatomegaly, vomiting and diarrhoea have all been associated with heavy infections and hepatosplenomegaly, cholangitis, obstructive jaundice and haemobilia have been reported in very heavy infections. Eggs are easily found in the stools and duodenal aspirates in heavier infections. Eosinophilia in the peripheral blood is usually present. Longstanding infections are not associated with cholangiocarcinoma.

Treatment with bithionol (40 mg/kg in 2 divided doses after food on alternate days for 15 days), is effective.

Clonorchiasis and opisthorciasis

Clonorchis sinensis snd *Opisthorcis viverrini* are very similar and will be considered together. Clonorchiasis is common in China, Korea, Japan and south east Asia, and opisthorciasis is common in Thailand.

Eggs of the parasites are deposited in fresh water and hatch to release a miracidium. The miracidium enters the tissues of a fresh water snail forming a sporcyst from which cercariae develop which are released into the surrounding water. Cercariae enter the tissues of various species of freshwater fish. Man is infected by eating raw, smoked or pickled fish as these treatments do not kill the encysted cercariae. The larval forms of the parasites are released by digestion and migrate through the ampulla of Vater to enter the biliary tree where the hermaphroditic adults mature and lay eggs. The adults are found in both intrahepatic and extrahepatic branches of the biliary tree and in the pancreatic ducts. Bile-filled dilatations are found proximal to adults in the smaller intrahepatic ducts.

Upper abdominal pain, diarrhoea, vomiting, gall stones and hepatomegaly have been associated with both infections. Obstructive jaundice, cholangitis and septicaemia occur in very heavy infections. Infections with both agents can cause cholangiocarcinoma. This may relate to adenomatous hyperplasia in the bile duct wall, but other environmental or genetic factors may also be involved.

The diagnosis is made by finding eggs in the faeces or in fluid aspirated from the duodenum. Treatment with praziquantel in doses of 25 mg/kg three times a day for one day has superseded all other drugs.

REFERENCES

Black R E, Dykes A C, Sinclair S F, Wells J G 1977 Giardiasis in day care centres: evidence of person to person transmission. Pediatrics 60: 486–491

von Bonsdorff B 1977 Diphyllobothriasis in man. Academic Press, London

Botero D, Castāno S 1982 Treatment of cysticercosis with praziquantel in Colombia. American Journal of Tropical Medicine & Hygiene 31: 810–821

Cheever A W, Andrade Z A 1967 Pathological lesions associated with *Schistosoma mansoni* infection in man. Transactions of the Royal Society of Tropical Medicine & Hygiene 61: 626–639

Danciger M, Lopez M 1975 Numbers of giardia in the feces of infected children. American Journal of Tropical Medicine & Hygiene 24: 237–242

Gilman R H, Chong Y H, Greenberg B, Vivik H K, Dixon H B 1983 The adverse consequences of heavy *Trichuris* infection. Transactions of the Royal Society of Tropical Medicine & Hygiene 77: 432–438

Jokipii L, Pohjola S, Jokipii A M M 1983 Cryptosporidium: a frequent finding in patients with gastrointestinal symptoms. Lancet ii: 358–361

Kamath K R, Murugasu R 1974 A comparative study of four methods of detecting *Giardia lamblia* in children. Gastroenterology 66: 16–21

Keusch G T (ed) 1982 The Biology of Parasitic Infection. Reviews of Infectious Diseases 4: 735–911

Meisel J L, Perera D R, Meligro C, Rubin C E 1976 Overwhelming watery diarrhea associated with a cryptosporidium in an immunosuppressed patient. Gastroenterology 70: 1156–1160

Morris D L, Dykes P W W 1983 Albendazole in hydatid disease. Gut 24:A985

Muigai R, Gatei D G, Shaunak S, Wozniak A, Bryceson A D M 1983 Jejunal function and pathology in visceral leishmaniasis, Lancet ii: 476–479

Phills J A, Harrold A J, Whiteman G V, Perelmutter L 1972 Pulmonary infiltrates, asthma and eosinophilia due to *Ascaris suum* infestation in man. New England Journal of Medicine 286: 965–970

Reed S L, Sargeaunt P G, Braude A I 1983 Resistance to lysis by human serum in pathogenic *Entamoeba histolytica*. Transactions of the Royal Society of Tropical Medicine & Hygiene 77: 199–204

Rivera E, Maldonado N, Velez-Gracia E, Grillo A J, Malaret G 1970 Hyperinfection syndrome with *Strongyloides stercoralis*. Annals of Internal Medicine 72: 199–204

Saidi F 1979 Surgery of Hydatid disease. Saunders, London

Sargeaunt P G, Jackson T S H G, Simjee A 1982 Biochemical homogeneity of *Entamoeba histolytica* isolates especially those from liver abscess. Lancet i: 1386–1388

Schultz M G 1982 Ascariasis: nutritional importance. Review of Infectious Diseases 4: 815–823

Stuiver P C 1984 Acute schistosomiasis (Katayama Fever). British Medical Journal 288: 221–222

Tzipori S 1983 Cryptosporidiosis in animals and humans. Microbiological Reviews 47: 84–96

Vince J D, Ashford R W, Gratten M J, Bana-Kori J 1979 Strongyloides species infection in young infants of Papua New Guinea: association with generalised oedema. Papua New Guinea Medical Journal 22: 120–127

Wright S G, Tomkins A M, Ridley D S 1977 Giardiasis: clinical and therapeutic aspects. Gut 18: 343–350

Protein-losing enteropathies

INTRODUCTION

Protein-losing enteropathy is a syndrome characterized by an excessive loss of plasma proteins into the gastrointestinal tract. Although its causes are numerous, the consequences of the protein loss on the metabolism of plasma proteins and the procedures necessary to prove it are similar and will be considered first.

CONSEQUENCES OF THE PROTEIN-LOSING ENTEROPATHY ON THE METABOLISM OF PLASMA PROTEINS

Loss of plasma proteins through the intestinal epithelium into the lumen is a physiological process. Albumin has been shown by autoradiography to pass from central lacteals and extracellular spaces through the epithelial basal membrane, and to enter intercellular spaces and epithelial cells by a process of pinocytosis. Thus albumin is either metabolized by the enterocytes or lost into the lumen at the apex of the villi as epithelial cells are extruded (Brooks & Dobbins 1972). It has been estimated that approximately 10% of albumin catabolism occurs in the gut, representing a loss of about 1 g per day in adults (Rossing 1967, Rothschild et al 1972). Such a small quantity of protein is easily digested by the pancreatic proteases; the constituent amino acids and peptides are then absorbed and reutilized. The rate of synthesis of the liver is similar in children and adults (Krasilnikoff et al 1966) (Table 11.1): Increased albumin synthesis has been shown to be triggered by decreased colloid content of the hepatic interstitial space. However, the most important factor regulating albumin synthesis is the nutritional state of the subject, and primarily the amino acid supply. In man

Table 11.1 Albumin metabolism in normal children

	Weight (kg)	Albumin concentration (g/l)	Rate of synthesis (g/kg/day)	Fractional catabolic rate[1] (%/day)	Distribution ratio[2] (%)
<1 month (n = 2)	2.9	36	0.30	17.2	33
1 year (n = 3)	10	42	0.21	10.3	43
3 years (n = 1)	15.3	42	0.16	9.3	51
6 years (n = 3)	20	45	0.16	9.4	47
8 years (n = 1)	26	50	0.13	6.3	46
adults	mean	43	0.16	8.4	42
(n = 27)	range	(38–49)	(0.10–0.21)	(6.8–10.4)	(37–55)

Adapted from Krasilnikoff et al, 1966.
[1] fractional catabolic rate = % of intravascular mass degraded per day
[2] distribution ration = intravascular mass/total body mass of albumin.

the half time of survival of albumin molecules is 20 days (Rothschild et al 1972).

Contrary to albumin synthesis, synthesis of IgG, IgA and IgM by plasma cells is triggered only by antigen stimulus (Wells 1976) (Table 11.2).

In protein-losing enteropathies all serum proteins are lost into the intestinal lumen at the same rate, irrespective of their molecular weight (Waldmann 1966). Half-lives of survival of albumin, immunoglobulin, and ceruloplasmin are markedly reduced; half-life of albumin may be decreased to 3 days. Patients may lose 10 to over 50% of their plasma albumin pool each day (Waldmann 1966). As soon as the protein loss amounts to more than twice normal, hypoproteinaemia develops since albumin synthesis cannot be more than doubled and immunoglobulin synthesis is not triggered by their low levels. However, the reduction in serum protein concentrations is not identical for the various proteins. Those with the longest half-life (albumin, IgG) are the most severely depressed; transferrin, IgM, ceruloplasmin, and fibrinogen retain normal or only slightly reduced plasma concentrations (Waldmann 1966).

DIAGNOSTIC PROCEDURES

Since 1957, when Citrin et al first demonstrated the gastrointestinal loss of protein by recovering intravenously administered ^{131}I-labelled albumin from the gastric juice of a patient with giant hypertrophy of the gastric mucosa, a number of other radioactive substances have been used to study the metabolism of plasma proteins and their catabolism in the gastrointestinal tract. Because of its stability, ^{131}I-labelled albumin has been found to be most useful in determining the total body albumin pool, its rate of degradation and synthesis. A number of markers including ^{131}I-polyvinyl pyrrolidone, ^{59}Fe-labelled iron dextran and [67]Cu-labelled ceruloplasmin have been used to estimate protein loss from the gastrointestinal tract, but ^{51}Cr-albumin remains the most widely used. It has an apparent half-life of survival of only 3 to 10 days, is neither digested nor reabsorbed in the

Table 11.2 Immunoglobulin metabolism in human subjects

Class	Serum concentration (g/l)	Rate of synthesis (mg/kg/day)	Fractional catabolic rate[1] (%/day)	Plasma half-time (days)	Distribution ratio[2] (%)	Plasma pool (mg/kg/day)
IgG						
mean	9.9	36	6.9	21	52	500
range	6–16	20–60	4.3–9.8	14–28	32–64	280–820
IgA	2.3	24	24	5.9	55	101
IgM	1.0	2.2	10.6	5.1	74	23

Adapted from Wells 1976
1,2 as in Table 11.1

intestinal lumen, and has proved to be the most suitable for obtaining an accurate estimate of protein loss (Waldmann 1966).

The serious limitations imposed on the routine use of these substances in paediatrics by their radioactivity may now be overcome by the measurement of the faecal concentration or clearance of α_1-antitrypsin, which has recently been proposed as a test to estimate enteric protein loss, α_1-antitrypsin, which is better designated as α_1-proteinase inhibitor since its physiological role is to control the elastolytic activity secreted primarily by neutrophils, is a glycoprotein of approximately 55 000 daltons molecular weight synthesized by the liver and has a half-life of 4 days (Travis & Salvesen 1983). It inactivates virtually all mammalian serine proteinases, including pancreatic trypsin, chymotrypsin and elastase. Thus, contrary to all the other plasma proteins, it is not digested in the gut lumen, nor is it reabsorbed. It is easily assayed in the stools by immunological methods and recent studies have validated the determination of faecal α_1-proteinase inhibitor clearance as a valuable tool for the quantitation of faecal protein loss. There is good correlation between ^{51}Cr-albumin clearance and α_1-proteinase inhibitor clearance in adults and children (Florent et al 1981, Hill et al 1981). Faecal α_1-proteinase inhibitor clearance (faecal concentration $\times$ daily stool weight/serum concentration), which necessitates a 3–4 day stool collection, varies widely in normal children where it should not exceed 13 ml/day (Hill et al 1981, Thomas et al 1983). A random determination of faecal alpha$_1$-proteinase inhibitor (normal value <3.4 mg/g dry stool), has been found to correlate closely to α_1-proteinase inhibitor clearance, and may be used in ambulatory patients as a screening test for mucosal disorders with an excessive loss of protein in the intestinal lumen (Thomas et al 1981, 1983).

PROTEIN-LOSING ENTEROPATHIES (Table 11.3)

Protein-losing enteropathies may be grouped according to two basic pathological processes (Rothschild et al 1972). In the first group of conditions, the loss of protein is essentially secondary to increased gut permeability to plasma or interstitial fluid, while in the second group it is mainly due to altered intestinal and mesenteric flow. In the latter case proteins are lost together with other lymph constituents such as lipids (chylomicrons) and lymphocytes. In certain cases both mechanisms may be involved, as in Crohn's disease, radiation enteritis and the nephrotic syndrome.

Protein-losing enteropathies secondary to increased mucosal permeability

The first conditions considered here are those in which protein-losing enteropathy is the main feature, with conspicuous oedema and marked hypoproteinaemia, such as hypertrophic gastritis, allergic gastroenteropathy and several types of polyposis.

Table 11.3 Main conditions associated with excessive gastrointestinal loss of protein in childhood

---

Increased mucosal permeability to protein

Hypertrophic gastritis
Allergic gastroenteropathy or eosinophilic gastroenteritis
Polyposis
Coeliac disease, tropical sprue
Cow's milk protein intolerance
Hypogammaglobulinaemia
Graft-versus-host disease
Contaminated small bowel syndrome
Ulcerative colitis
Granulomatous enterocolitis (Crohn's disease)
Enterocolitis
Radiation enteritis
Nephrotic syndrome

Altered lymph flow

Primary intestinal lymphangiectasia
Aquired intestinal lymphangiectasia
    impaired venous flow: congestive heart failure, constrictive pericarditis
    organic obstruction: mesenteric panniculitis, pancreatitis, lymphoma, tuberculosis,
    Hodgkin's disease

Hypertrophic gastritis

Hypertrophic gastritis is a rare entity (less than 20 cases published), generally affecting children between 3 and 10 years of age. Anorexia, nausea and vomiting, abdominal pain rapidly followed by generalized oedema are the main symptoms. Plasma proteins are low because of loss from the stomach. Upper gastrointestinal tract X-rays and endoscopic examination show enlarged, succulent gastric rugae throughout the fundus. Biopsy specimens from enlarged folds reveal a polymorph inflammatory infiltrate of the lamina propria with oedema and epithelial hyperplasia. Contrary to the disease described in 1888 by Ménétrier in adults, hypertrophic gastritis is usually a completely reversible condition after several weeks. It has been associated either with viral infection by cytomegalovirus or with gastrointestinal allergy as a familial history of allergy and raised eosinophils in the blood are often noticed. Albumin perfusions may be necessary during the acute phase of the disease (Chouraqui et al 1981, Kraut et al 1981).

Allergic enteropathy

Allergic gastroenteropathy (Waldmann et al 1967), or eosinophilic gastroenteritis, was first reported as a cause of excessive loss of protein in the gastrointestinal tract. It usually presents with oedema as the major symptom, growth retardation, severe hypoalbuminaemia, hypogammaglob-ulinaemia, anaemia, and peripheral blood eosinophilia, and is often associated with manifestations of allergy. An excessively high number of eosinophils in the lamina propria is the only abnormal finding in an other-wise normal intestinal mucosa. Waldmann et al (1967) showed that the half-life of ^{131}I albumin could be as short as 3 days with a normal milk-containing diet, but returned to more normal values when milk was with-drawn or when corticosteroids were administered. Katz et al (1977) reported that the stomach may also be involved and was also infiltrated with eosinophils. In certain cases, marked thickening of the mucosa has been reported as resulting in pyloric obstruction in adults as well as in infants (Colon et al 1983). Although exclusion of cow's milk protein from the diet often leads to regression of all symptoms, a strict exclusion diet omitting proteins known to be antigenic has not always been of therapeutic value (Katz 1977, Colon et al 1983). In these cases corticosteroid therapy may be required.

Polyposis

Severe protein-losing enteropathy associated with chronic blood loss and resulting eventually in cachexia and even death has been described with both adenomatous polyps and generalized juvenile polyposis in children and in infants (Gourley et al 1982).

Miscellaneous

In all other conditions in which a protein-losing enteropathy may be considered to be a consequence of an increased permeability of the gastroin-testinal mucosa, loss of protein is usually only a minor or transient symptom, for example in acute gastrointestinal infections (Ghadimi et al 1973) or in parasitic infestations (Sherman & Liebman 1980).

Protein loss may, however, be part of a more serious condition. This is the case in chronic diseases such as coeliac disease, tropical sprue, hypo-gammaglobulinaemia, with the resulting chronic infections and/or infestations, graft-versus-host disease (Weisdorf et al 1983), the contaminated small bowel syndrome, or cow's milk protein intolerance, in which the intestinal mucosa shows partial to subtotal villous atrophy. It is also true in ulcerative colitis, granulomatous enterocolitis (Crohn's disease), and enterocolitis, where the loss of protein related to mucosal inflammation is made worse by an increased loss of desquamated cells (Waldmann 1966, Thomas et al 1981). In all these situations, malabsorption, malnutrition and chronic infection often lead to inadequate amino acid supply and defective albumin synthesis (Jeejeeboy et al 1969) which may be unable to compensate for even a modest degree of protein loss (Rothschild 1972). Thus, in most of these diffuse diseases, the severity of the enteric loss of protein cannot be assessed by serum albumin alone.

Protein-losing enteropathy secondary to altered lymph flow

In most tissues lymph drainage is important for maintaining the interstitial fluid volume within the normal range. There are two aspects of this function: removal of fluid and removal of proteins. The fluid which is removed represents the difference between the fluid flowing out of arterial capillaries under hydrostatic pressure and fluid reabsorbed in venous capillaries under oncotic pressure (2–4 l/day). The oncotic pressure is maintained by the continuous removal of tissue proteins leaking from the capillaries of the lymphatic system (Nicoll & Taylor 1977).

Intestinal lymph flows from the blind central lacteals of intestinal villi, to collecting ducts of increasing diameter, ultimately reaching the thoracic duct, which receives lymph from the body below the diaphragm. In the main lymphatic trunks, lymphoid cells circulate in the lymphatic system from peripheral lymph nodes via specialized post-capillary venules, leave the lymph nodes by their efferent lymphatic channels and return to the main circulation by the thoracic duct. It has been well documented that 80% of these lymphoid cells trafficking in the lymphatic system are long-lived, recirculating, thymus-derived T-lymphocytes. T cells homing to the intestinal mucosa probably do not recirculate. Since triglyceride-rich chylomicrons leaving the enterocytes cannot enter capillaries and are removed from the interstitial space by the central lacteals, mesenteric lymph, particularly following a meal, also contains lipids. Intestinal lymph fluid and protein flow increase simultaneously. Although glucose, saline or fat increase lymph flow to a similar extent, fat is responsible for a much greater flux of protein in lymph (Borgstrom & Laurell 1953, Granger & Taylor 1978).

Lymph flow may be hindered by congenital abnormalities of the lymphatic ducts or by any process which causes an obstruction, whether inflammatory or tumoral, or an increased venous pressure. In the latter cases, hydrostatic pressure will increase in the central lacteals which become dilated and lymphangiectasia results.

Primary lymphangiectasia

Intestinal lymphangiectasia was first described by Waldmann et al in 1961 and is usually thought to be primary when it presents in childhood or infancy, but is probably part of a systemic lymphatic dysplasia (Waldmann 1966).

Symptoms usually appear before 3 years of age but may be delayed until adolescence. Diarrhoea and/or oedema are most often the first and these remain the main symptoms of the disease, but may be intermittent. Steatorrhoea is moderate. Nausea and vomiting and abdominal pain are less frequent symptoms. Oedema may be symmetrical, as a consequence of hypoproteinaemia, or asymmetrical because of associated lymphoedema. Both pleural and peritoneal chylous effusions are frequent. In young children failure to thrive is the rule (Waldmann 1966, Vardy et al 1975). Antenatal diagnosis has been possible by ultrasound (Munck et al 1986).

Hypoproteinaemia with hypoalbuminaemia and hypogammaglobulin-aemia is a consequence of the excessive loss of proteins into the gastro-intestinal tract, as has been repeatedly shown by the greatly increased clearance of labelled macromolecules or α_1-protease inhibitor. The half life of albumin may be reduced to 3–4 days. Hypocalcaemia associated with hypoalbuminaemia may be responsible for symptoms of tetany and plasma lipids may be lowered by the malabsorption of fat.

Plasma lymphocytes are usually below 1500/ml and often between 500 and 1000/ml. This decrease affects mainly T lymphocytes (the predominant lymphocytes in the thoracic duct) which are reduced to 20% of normal. Nevertheless, there are sufficient T lymphocytes for normal B cell regulation so that although immunoglobulins are low, antibody production remains normal. On the other hand, the decreased number of circulating T lymphocytes is responsible for a high percentage of negative skin tests for delayed hypersensitivity, impaired lymphoblastic proliferation in the presence of nonspecific mitogens and a greatly increased tolerance to skin grafts (Weiden et al 1972). Infections are, however, more frequent or severe than in normal children. Intestinal biopsies if taken from an affected area show gross dilatation of the lymphatics of the lamina propria, which is the pathognomonic lesion of the disorder. These frequently distort and enlarge individual villi although there is no villous atrophy (Vardy 1975). A considerable degree of interstitial oedema may distend the mucosal and submucosal layers (Mistilis 1965).

A small bowel barium examination can be normal but usually shows the following features: 1) enlargement of the intestinal folds of both jejunum and ileum; 2) distal dilution of the barium column, while 3) there is no or minimal dilatation of the bowel. Although pedal lymphangiography does not usually allow visualization of the lymphatic ducts, it does document in a majority of cases abnormal lymphatics in the lower extremities (hypoplasia of lymph vessels or dilated lymphatics) or less frequently, partial obstruction of the thoracic duct. In rare cases it shows contrast reflux into the mesenteric lymphatics (Shimkin 1970) (Fig. 11.1).

The natural course of the disease may be relatively mild, consisting of bouts of diarrhoea and oedema with hypoproteinaemia or, when large areas of the intestine are involved, it may be much more severe leading to severe growth retardation, and even intractable diarrhoea and death. Treatment is usually medical and is limited to a low fat diet, the main effect of which is probably not to decrease mesenteric lymph flow but to prevent engorgement of the intestinal lymphatics and hence a rise in lymph hydrostatic pressure (Jeffries et al 1964; Mistilis et al 1965). Medium chain triglycerides

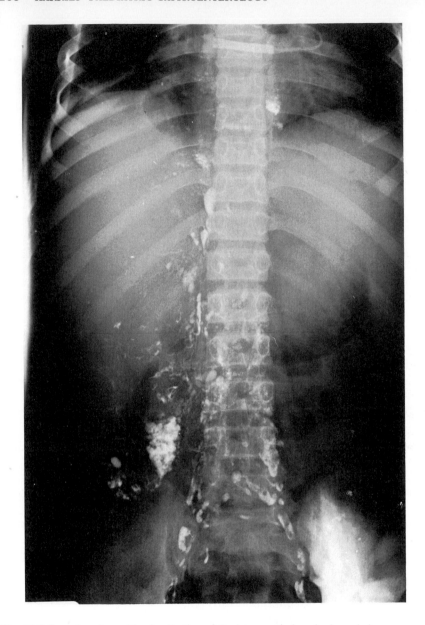

Fig. 11.1 Lymphangiographic visualization of the lateroaortic lymph channels in a severe case of primary lymphangiectasia. Note the absence of the thoracic duct which is replaced by numerous hypoplastic ducts, and the absence of lymph flow in the thorax and reflux of contrast material in mesenteric lymphatics in the lower right part of the abdomen. Increased density of the left innominate bone is suggestive of melorrheostosis as has been previously reported (Mistilis et al 1965) (by courtesy of Dr. C. Ricour).

may be used to replace long chain triglycerides since fatty acids with <12 carbon atoms are not reesterified in the enterocytes and enter the general circulation directly through the portal vein. The diet must also be supplemented with fat soluble vitamins. Some patients may require long-term diuretics to control oedema. Following the institution of a low fat diet (<10 g/24 h) diarrhoea ceases, plasma albumin concentrations rise progressively to normal or near normal, and the oedema disappears. Immunoglobulin levels and lymphocyte counts seldom return to strictly normal values; several months may be necessary before a stable condition is reached. Finally growth rate improves. Although tolerance to fat may increase as the child grows, a diet restricted in fat is probably necessary for life (Tift & Lloyd 1975).

In the few cases where the lymphatic anomaly is limited to a particular segment of intestine a resection may provide a cure. A lympho-venous anastomosis has been performed with success on one occasion (Mistilis & Skyring 1966). More recently peritoneo-venous shunts have been used in chylous ascites (Man & Spitz 1985).

Acquired intestinal lymphangiectasia

Impaired lymph flow may be functional as a consequence of congestive heart failure and constrictive pericarditis. This has been looked for systematically since clinical, biochemical and histological features of secondary lymphangiectasia are identical with those of congenital lymphangiectasia. On lymphangiography the thoracic duct may appear tortuous and dilated. When heart failure is treated or pericardectomy is performed the intestinal lymphangiectasia and protein-losing gastroenteropathy resolve and immune function returns to normal (Nelson et al 1975).

Impaired lymph flow may also result from mechanical obstruction of the lymphatics in the abdomen, as in mesenteric panniculitis, pancreatitis or tumour of the pancreas, and diseases of the mesenteric lymph nodes such as tuberculosis, lymphoma and Hodgkin's disease.

Although in children, intestinal lymphangiectasia most often results from a primary lymphatic abnormality, these other acquired causes of lymphatic obstruction have to be kept in mind, since their treatment may cure the protein-losing enteropathy.

REFERENCES

Borgström B, Laurell C B 1953 Studies on lymph and lymph-proteins during absorption of fat and saline by rats. Acta Physiologica Scandinavica 29: 264–280
Brooks S G, Dobbins W O 1972 Autoradiographic localization of I-125 labelled albumin in the intestine of guinea pigs: a light and electron microscopic study. Gastroenterology 62: 1001–1012
Chouraqui J P, Roy C C, Brochu P, Gregoire H, Morin C L, Weber A M 1981 Menetrier's disease in children: report of a patient and review of sixteen other cases. Gastroenterology 80: 1042–1047

Citrin Y, Sterling K, Halsted J A 1957 The mechanism of hypoproteinemia associated with giant hypertrophy of the gastric mucosa. The New England Journal of Medicine 257: 906–912

Colón A R, Sorkin L F, Stern W R, Lessinger V S, Hefter L G, Hodin E 1983 Eosinophilic Gastroenteritis. Journal of Pediatric Gastroenterology and Nutrition 2: 187–189

Florent C, L'Hirondel C, Desmazures C, Aymes C, Bernier J J 1981 Intestinal clearance of α_1-antitrypsin, a sensitive method for the detection of protein-losing enteropathy. Gastroenterology 81: 777–780

Ghadimi H, Kumar S, Abaci F 1973 Endogenous amino acid loss and its significance in infantile diarrhea. Pediatric Research 7: 161–168

Gourley G R, Odell G B, Selkurt J, Morrissey J, Gilbert E 1982 Juvenile polyps associated with protein-losing enteropathy. Digestive Diseases and Sciences 27: 941–945

Granger D N, Taylor A E 1978 Effects of solute-coupled transport on lymph flow and oncotic pressures in cat ileum. American Journal of Physiology 235(4): E429–E436

Hill R E, Hercz A, Corey M L, Gilday D L, Hamilton J R 1981 Fecal clearance of α_1-antitrypsin: a reliable measure of enteric protein loss in children. The Journal of Pediatrics 99: 416–418

Jeejeebhoy K N, Samuel A M, Singh B, Nadkarni G D, Desai H G, Borkar A V, Mani L S 1969 Metabolism of albumin and fibrinogen in patients with tropical sprue. Gastroenterology 56: 252–267

Jeffries G H, Chapman A, Sleisenger M H 1964 Low-fat diet in intestinal lymphangiectasia. Its effect on albumin metabolism. The New England Journal of Medicine 270: 761–766

Katz A J, Goldman H, Grand R J 1977 Gastric mucosal biopsy in eosinophilic (allergic) gastroenteritis. Gastroenterology 73: 705–709

Krasilnikoff P A, Andersen S B, Rossing N 1966 Albumin metabolism in normal children. In: Peeters H (ed) Protides of the biological fluids, Elsevier, Amsterdam, vol 14, pp 315–317

Kraut J R, Powell R, Hruby M A, Lloyd-Still J D 1981 Menetrier's disease in childhood: report of two cases and a review of the literature. Journal of Pediatric Surgery 16: 707–711

Man D W K, Spitz L 1985 The management of chylous ascites in children. Journal of Pediatric Surgery 20: 72–75

Ménétrier P 1888 Des polyadenomes gastriques et de leurs rapports avec le cancer de l'estomac. Archives de Physiologie Normale et Pathologique 32: 236–262

Mistilis S P, Skyring A P, Stephen D D 1965 Intestinal lymphangiectasia, Mechanism of enteric loss of plasma-protein and fat. The Lancet i: 77–79

Mistilis S P, Skyring A P 1966 Intestinal lymphangiectasia. Therapeutic effect of lymph venous anastomosis. American Journal of Medicine 40: 634–641

Munck A, Foucaud P, Walti H, Dumez Y, Vaudour G, Navarro J 1986 Lymphangiectasies intestinales primitives à révélation anténatale. Archives Françaises de Pédiatrie 43: 195–196

Nelson D L, Blaese R M, Strober W, Bruce R M, Waldmann T A 1975 Constrictive pericarditis, intestinal lymphangiectasia, and reversible immunologic deficiency. The Journal of Pediatrics 86: 548–554

Nicoll P A, Taylor A E 1977 Lymph formation and flow. Annual Review of Physiology 39: 73–95

Rossing N 1967 The normal metabolism of ^{131}I-labelled albumin in man. Clinical Science 33: 593–602

Rothschild M A, Oratz M, Schreiber S S 1972 Albumin synthesis. The New England Journal of Medicine 286: 748–757, 816–821

Sherman P, Liebman W M 1980 Apparent protein-losing enteropathy associated with giardiasis. American Journal of Diseases of Children 134: 893–894

Shimkin P M, Waldmann T A, Krugman R L 1970 Intestinal Lymphangiectasia. American Journal of Roentgenology 110: 827–841

Thomas D W, Sinatra F R, Merritt R J 1981 Random fecal alpha-l-antitrypsin concentration in children with gastrointestinal disease. Gastroenterology 80: 776–782

Thomas D W, Sinatra F R, Merritt R J 1983 Fecal α_1-antitrypsin excretion in young people with Crohn's disease. Journal of Pediatric Gastroenterology and Nutrition 2: 491–496

Tift W L, Lloyd J K 1975 Intestinal lymphangiectasia. Long-term results with MCT diet. Archives of Disease in Childhood 50: 269–276

Travis J, Salvesen G S 1983 Human plasma proteinase inhibitors. Annual Review of Biochemistry 52: 655–709

Vardy P A, Lebenthal E, Shwachman H 1975 Intestinal lymphangiectasia: a reappraisal. Pediatrics 55: 842–851

Waldmann T A, Steinfeld J L, Dutcher J F, Davidson J D, Gordon R S Jr 1961 The role of the gastrointestinal system in "idiopathic hypoproteinemia". Gastroenterology 41: 197–207

Waldmann T A 1966 Protein-losing enteropathy. Gastroenterology 50: 422–443

Waldmann T A, Wochner R D, Laster L, Gordon R S Jr 1967 Allergic gastroenteropathy. A cause of excessive gastrointestinal protein loss. The New England Journal of Medicine 276: 761–769

Weiden P L, Blaese R M, Strober W, Block J B, Waldmann T A 1972 Impaired lymphocyte transformation in intestinal lymphangiectasia: evidence for at least two functionally distinct lymphocyte populations in man. The Journal of Clinical Investigation 51: 1319–1325

Weisdorf S A, Salati L M, Longsdorf J A, Ramsay N K C, Sharp H L 1983 Graft-versus-host disease of the intestine: a protein losing enteropathy characterized by fecal α_1-antitrypsin. Gastroenterology 85: 1076–1081

Wells J V 1976 Metabolism of immunoglobulins. In: Fudenberg H H, Stites D P, Caldwell J L, Wells J V (eds) Basic and clinical immunology. Lange Medical Publications, Los Altos USA. pp 195–203

The irritable bowel syndrome

The irritable bowel syndrome (IBS) encompasses a number of gastrointestinal symptoms, notably abdominal pain, constipation and loose stools for which no organic cause can be found. This syndrome is a major cause of industrial absenteeism in adult life (Almy 1967) and in childhood is probably the single most common problem encountered in a paediatric gastroenterology clinic. Despite the common nature of the problem, little is known of its pathogenesis in either adult or child. Studies of intestinal motor activity have suggested abnormalities of colonic function in adult patients with this syndrome. More recently attention has focussed on the small intestine (Thompson et al 1979). Horowitz & Farrer (1962) described abnormalities of jejunal motor activity that corresponded to bouts of pain in patients with IBS and Moriarty & Dawson (1982) have shown that pain can be reproduced in these patients by balloon distension of the small intestine at both upper and lower sites whilst Ritchie & Salem (1965) showed a significant decrease in overall small intestinal motor activity.

In childhood, patients fall into three main groups — those whose predominant symptom is abdominal pain, Apley's 'little belly achers' (Apley 1959), those whose main complaint is of loose frequent stools, and those who present with constipation.

RECURRENT ABDOMINAL PAIN (RAP)

Apley (1959) found that about 10% of schoolchildren suffer recurrent episodes (more than 3) of self-limiting abdominal pain for longer than 3 months which interfered with their activities and for which no cause could be found. In only 7% is an organic cause for the pain found. The pain is usually periumbilical and colicky in nature but may be dull and continuous and felt at other abdominal sites. There is a peak incidence at five years in both sexes and a further peak at puberty in girls. Complaints of abdominal pain are significantly commoner in the families of affected children and occur more frequently in 'highly strung', anxious children. Psychogenic factors are commoner than in control children, and there is more rapid relief of symptoms in those treated with informal psychotherapy. Careful study of the data, however, shows that approximately 40% of patients are unresponsive to psychotherapy.

The high proportion that appear unresponsive to psychotherapy might suggest that obscure organic disease is the cause of the symptoms. Food intolerance, including food allergy and lactose intolerance, have been claimed (McMichael et al 1965, Alun Jones et al 1982) to play a role in this syndrome. Some children do respond to elimination diets, especially the elimination of the commoner allergens of cows' milk, egg and wheat. A strong family and/or personal history of atopic related disease and gastrointestinal disturbance together with prompt response to an elimination diet suggests that allergy does play a role in some patients. There is clear evidence that food allergy accounts for many cases of migraine, in a proportion of which recurrent abdominal pain is also a feature (Egger et al 1983). However, earlier suggestions that lactose intolerance would explain many cases (McMichael et al 1965) has not been born out in practice. More recent studies have suggested that over half of the children with abdominal pain have symptoms that persist into adult life, and in about one-third a diagnosis of irritable bowel syndrome is ultimately made (Christensen & Mortenssen 1975). In addition to abdominal pain, some children experience intermittent fluctuating episodes of diarrhoea and constipation reminiscent of adults with IBS (Drossman et al 1977), together with other nonspecific symptoms including bloating, nausea and abdominal tenderness often over the descending and sigmoid colon (Apley 1959). The relationship between recurrent abdominal pain (RAP) and organic gastrointestinal disease in the developing countries and in immigrants to the developed parts of the world is more complex. For example, Gupta et al (1974) showed that 76% of children with RAP had associated intestinal infections; these observations cannot necessarily reflect a casual relationship between RAP and intestinal infestation since the incidence of bowel infestation in Indian children is particularly high.

Pathophysiology

The pathophysiological mechanisms operating in RAP with or without associated vomiting are not known, but a variety of mechanisms may be postulated. Attacks may represent the transient somatic correlates of anxiety, depression or anger mediated by the autonomic nervous system, or simply physiological responses to ingested material. Hyperactive colonic motor responses to cholinergic agonists have been found in children with recurrent abdominal pain which appear very similar to those seen in adults with IBS (Kopel et al 1967). Whilst the findings of disturbed colonic and small intestinal motor activity (Connel et al 1965, Horowitz & Farrer 1962) have led to speculation regarding the role of the psychogenic factors suggested by Apley, recent reports of the effects of neuropeptides in the central nervous system (CNS) on intestinal motor activity (Ewart & Wingate 1983) lends credence to the notion that centrally determined events may be important in this syndrome.

Diagnosis

Physical examination and laboratory investigations are usually unrewarding. It is our practice to arrange a full blood count, clean specimen of urine and abdominal ultrasound, where indicated skin prick testing, barium meal and follow-through and endoscopy are undertaken. The diagnosis of a functional syndrome is based on the association between a physical complaint and emotional or behavioural symptoms, which include too little as well as too much expression of feelings for the given circumstances, the context in which the circumstances occur and the attitudes of the child and parents to the symptoms. The absence of physical disease can only be taken as a pointer towards stress being a possible alternative cause. To justify a diagnosis of RAP as an emotional or stress disorder, there should be evidence to eliminate organic disease, together with evidence of an emotional disturbance; in addition, a relationship in time between pain and stress and the relief of pain with the reduction in stress both lend weight to the diagnosis (Apley 1959).

It should be emphasized that the stress is as perceived by the child, and not necessarily as seen by the doctor or parent. What is seen as trivial through adult eyes may be interpreted as world-shattering by a child; also some innocent event may be misinterpreted as of worrying significance by a young child of limited experience and understanding. Thus, in addition to careful medical history, examination and investigation, evidence on these psychosocial aspects should be requested from as many sources as relevant, but always from parents, teachers, family doctor and, equally importantly, the child.

Abdominal pain is more likely to be due to organic disease in the preschool child and in those over the age of 10 years, and in children with pain which is localized elsewhere than at the umbilicus (Marshall 1967) Urinary tract infections must always be excluded in patients with RAP.

Treatment

It is most important to reassure the parents that there is no serious organic pathology and that the condition will settle with increasing age. In those in whom atopy is clearly present a trial of an empirical exclusion diet such as a cows' milk protein, egg-free diet or, where indicated, another exclusion diet is very worthwhile. It is important, however that such a diet is controlled by an experienced paediatric dietitian if nutritional deficiencies are to be avoided.

The basis of treatment is the removal of any stressful factors which may be discovered, and an approach to the whole child and family is required. When the stress results from interactions in the family, therapy aimed to help the whole group may provide indirect relief to the symptom (Berger 1974). Simple explanatory models of the disorder given to both child and parents are sometimes helpful, though many parents continue to be symptomatic despite these simple measures (Apley & Hale 1973) Christensen & Mortensen 1975). A combined paediatric and psychiatric approach may offer longer lasting relief, though this is yet to be put to the test. The reader is referred to Green (1967) for a useful account of the diagnosis and management of recurrent organic abdominal pain in childhood.

If there is considerable family distress regarding the loose stools a trial of mebeverine or loperamide is often helpful. Drugs may, however, reinforce the parent's suspicions that underlying bowel disease is really present.

Prognosis

Two important prospective studies have provided information on the prognosis in children with RAP. Apley & Hale (1973) followed up 30 children for 10 to 14 years who had been treated by simple reassurance and explanations of, and discussions about, their symptoms. This group was compared with 30 untreated patients who had been previously followed up for eight to 20 years (Apley 1959). At the time of follow-up the patients were aged 15–28 years; nine patients in each group lost their pain and did not develop other symptoms, and nine of the untreated and ten of the treated groups lost their pain but developed other symptoms such as headaches, 'anxiety', or other pains or somatic symptoms. Only three cases, all untreated, developed migraine in adolescence or early adult life. Persistence of pain occurred more often in boys than girls, but more girls developed other symptoms. The younger the child at the onset of symptoms and the longer the delay in treatment the worse the prognosis.

Christensen & Mortensen (1975) studied 34 patients 30 years after they were first investigated and compared them with a randomly selected group of adult subjects who had not experienced RAP in childhood. They found abdominal pain to be a common complaint in the control group of adults (13 out of 45), but significantly less than in the group who had RAP in childhood (18 out of 34). Nongastrointestinal complaints were also more frequent in the patient group (11 out of 34), especially headache, back pain, 'bad nerves' and gynaecological symptoms; in the control group six out of 45 had similar symptoms. The main difference between the adults who had RAP in childhood compared to those who did not was a tendency to complain more of physical or nervous symptoms generally, and only somewhat more of abdominal pain. Out of the 94 cases of RAP in childhood reported in these two studies, only four were found to have organic abdominal disorders in adulthood; one had an ovarian cyst and the other three had duodenal ulcers. In general, therefore, there is a strong tendency for children with RAP to become adults who complain of a variety of gastrointestinal and other symptoms. When abdominal pain was associated with vomiting there is a tendency to develop migraine or severe headaches, and a proportion of children with RAP developed symptoms of an irritable colon type.

Symptoms may become conditioned somatic responses to stress; alternatively perpetuation of previously organically determined symptoms, or those with a psychological aetiology, may occur as a result of their reinforcement by the responses of parents or others. Hypochondrial concern by the child may be expressed by complaints of aches and pains, particularly if there are adult models of this type of behaviour in the family. In some children abdominal pain or vomiting can have the quality of hysterical conversion symptoms. In all cases, whatever the origin or mechanism, symptoms may achieve secondary and perhaps adaptive functions by diverting the attention, concern or interest of the child and those caring for him away from the external stress as perceived by the child and on to the physical complaint. The result is that the anxiety-provoking event for the child is curtailed or avoided and at the same time converted into a source of personal attention through the somatic symptom.

TODDLER DIARRHOEA

Although RAP is a common problem in general paediatic practice, it is the child with loose, frequent, foul-smelling stools that most commonly presents to the paediatric gastroenterologist. A condition known variously as toddler diarrhoea, chronic nonspecific diarrhoea and the irritable bowel syndrome of childhood. The condition occurs in children between the ages of one year and 5 years, and is more common in boys who are typically overactive and described as 'a handful', 'disruptive', and 'difficult to cope with'. The diarrhoea is intermittent and characterized by the precipitous passage of loose mucousy stools, often containing undigested food particles such as peas and carrots. The stools are only passed during waking hours and are often exacerbated by stress. Despite the abnormal stools, failure to thrive is *not* a feature of this syndrome. The condition appears to be self-limiting in over 90% of cases; however in one study a high incidence of constipation was found on follow-up (Davidson & Wasserman 1966). In the same study a marked familial tendency was shown; in 67% of patients at least one parent had a recurrent functional bowel disorder and of those with unaffected parents, 55% had a sibling with a similar condition. It seems clear that toddler diarrhoea is part of a spectrum of functional bowel disorders which is present just as frequently in childhood as in adult life.

Pathophysiology

Intestinal transport. The nature of this common apparently self-limiting condition is not clear. The diarrhoea is not associated with malabsorption, and in the adult with the diarrhoeal variant of the IBS, there is no evidence of abnormal secretion of water and electrolytes in the small intestine (Read et al 1980). Using a well validated double lumen jejunal perfusion technique (Milla et al 1978), we have been unable to show any difference in water, electrolyte or glucose absorption in the proximal jejunum of children with toddler diarrhoea or in those whose small intestinal function was being studied as part of the investigation of their short stature.

Mucosal enzymes Although the small intestinal mucosa is morphologically normal, Tripp et al (1980) found a significant increase in the specific activities of (Na^+K^+)-ATPase and basal adenylate cyclase in jejunal biopsies from children with toddler diarrhoea compared with those from children with the postenteritis syndrome. In the active phase of the postenteritis syndrome adenylate cyclase activity was normal and $Na^+K^+ATPase$ activity was reduced. However, during the recovery phase of the postenteritis syndrome, the activity of both enzymes was increased in a similar proportion to that found in toddler diarrhoea. These findings add credibility to the clinical impression that toddler diarrhoea may follow an acute enteric infection. Tripp et al (1980) suggested that the increase in specific enzyme activity was a response of normal villous cells to crypt cell secretion and that this might be mediated via prostaglandins.

Prostaglandins. Dodge et al (1981) determined plasma concentrations of prostaglandin E2 (PGE2) and prostglandin F (PGF) by radio-immunoassay (RIA) in 30 patients with toddler diarrhoea, and 26 healthy controls. PGF was raised in 17, and PGE2 raised in 4 of the patients. In a proportion of the patients there was a good clinical response to aspirin (a prostglandin synthetase inhibitor) or loperamide (an opiate analogue). Although sequential data is not given, it is stated that aspirin therapy resulted in a decrease in plasma levels of prostglandins but that loperamide had little effect. These observations may have important implications with respect to the pathogenesis of toddler diarrhoea as well as its treatment. For example, there is good experimental evidence that prostaglandins induce secretion in the small intestine (Matachansky & Bernier 1973) and that loperamide can partially block this effect (Sandhu et al 1981). However, studies both in children and in adults (described above) suggest that the small intestine is not in a secretory state, thus if excessive secretion is involved it might be taking place in either the lower small intestine or the colon.

Food intolerance. More recently, a study of adults with IBS suggested that in a proportion of patients unsuspected food allergy may play a role in the pathogenesis of the condition (Alun Jones et al 1982). It is certainly the case that some children do respond to elimination diets, especially of the commoner allergens such as cows' milk, egg and wheat proteins. However, these patients can nearly always be differentiated by their personal or close family history of atopy, peripheral blood eosinophilia, high IgE and positive radio-allergoabsorbent tests (RAST) or skin prick tests and ultimately by the response of their symptoms to the elimination followed by challenge with the suspected allergens. Abnormal breath hydrogen tests have suggested that lactose intolerance occurs commonly in IBS, however, few patients have demonstrated clear cut lactose intolerance (the production of watery stools containing reducing substances in response to a lactose load). Recently Savilahti et al (1985) showed that 6 in 21 patients with IBS had evidence of food allergy; all were atopic.

Intestinal motor activity. Whilst the abnormal breath hydrogen test may provide evidence of lactose malabsorption, it also provides a measure of small intestinal transit. Thus an abnormal breath test may result from the rapid delivery of a large quantity of lactose to the colon, because of reduced contact time in the proximal jejunum. It is of interest that Corbett et al (1981) have shown decreased small intestinal transit time in adults with IBS which is increased by treatment with loperamide. Thus the previously reported beneficial effects of loperamide may be related to an effect on small intestinal motility.

It had been known for many years, though largely ignored, that whole gut transit time was decreased in children with IBS. Davidson & Wasserman (1966) showed that 'starch intolerance', that is the presence of starch granules in the stool, was a manifestation of reduced whole gut transit time. The popular term 'peas and carrots' diarrhoea may be similarly explained. In our original studies of small intestinal absorption in toddler diarrhoea, transmural potential difference (PD) was monitored during the perfusions. It was repeatedly noted that in over 40% of the patients with toddler diarrhoea, wave forms of large amplitude between 8 and 13 mV occurred during perfusion with glucose, whereas in controls these waves appeared to be completely supressed during perfusion with glucose. Read et al (1977) reported the presence of these large amplitude waveforms, and later showed them to be associated with migrating motor complexes (MMC) in the small intestine (Read 1980). The recognition of the propulsive character of MMC in man (Vantrappen et al 1977) and the change to segmenting activity in the postprandial state which is initiated by the disruption of the MCC (Vantrappen et al 1977) prompted studies of small intestinal motility in children with IBS (Fenton et al 1983a). No differences in fasting activity could be found, but initiation of postprandial activity as shown by disruption of the MMC with intraduodenal dextrose was clearly defective in the patients with IBS. Further studies have since shown that in those patients in whom dextrose did not disrupt the motor complex there were abnormalities in postprandial activity induced by perfusion of the duodenum with soya milk (Fenton et al 1983b). Postprandial activity was weaker, short-lived and in a third of patients was punctuated by an MMC. It is of interest that failure of the MMC to be disrupted by food has been demonstrated in the experimental animal subjected to vagotomy (Diament et al 1980) and shortened postprandial motor activity has been noted in adult patients who have developed postvagotomy diarrhoea (Thompson et al 1982).

An attractive hypothesis can be put forward which accounts both for the previous isolated findings and for more recent studies of small intestinal motility (Fenton et al 1983a). Failure of the MMC to disrupt with food and a shortened period of postprandial activity may lead to a rapid transit of small intestinal contents to the colon. The small intestinal effluent dumped in the colon under those circumstances may well contain excess bile salts and partially digested food. Further degradation by colonic bacteria might yield secretagogues such as hydroxy fatty acids and unconjugated bile salts which could adversely affect colonic absorption of water and electrolytes. These substances may also be responsible for increased prostaglandin production which could play a role in the production of the patient's symptoms. Two recent studies provide some evidence that supports this hypothesis. Jonas & Diver Haber (1982) studied stool output and composition in a small group of patients with IBS, compared to children with malabsorption due to cystic fibrosis, bacterial overgrowth of the small gut and controls. Although total daily quantities of stool, fat and bile acids were no different to control values, the extractable water phase and sodium and bile acids in this phase were increased in children with IBS. These findings could reflect an effect of bile acids on the colonic handling of water and electrolytes. More recently, Alun Jones et al (1982) showed that in adult patients with IBS, prostaglandin concentration in rectal mucosa was increased when the patients were exposed to foods which precipitated their symptoms.

Treatment

It is most important to reassure the parents that there is no serious organic pathology and that the condition will settle with increasing age. In those whom atopy is clearly present a trial of an empirical exclusion diet such as cows' milk protein, egg free diet or, where indicated, another exclusion diet, is very worthwhile. It is important, however, that such a diet is controlled by an experienced paediatric dietitian if nutritional deficiencies are to be avoided.

If there is considerable family distress regarding the loose stools a trial of mebeverine or loperamide is often helpful. Drugs may, however, reinforce the parent's suspicion that underlying bowel disease is really present.

CONSTIPATION

In this section the term constipation is used to mean the infrequent passage of stools which may be hard and pellet-like or firm and very large. Associated with this there may be leakage of liquid faeces around compacted stools in a capacious rectum causing soiling due to secondary anal incontinence. Constipation should be clearly distinguished from encopresis which is the voluntary passage of a normal stool in an inappropriate way or place. Encopresis will not be considered here but is covered in Chapter 13. The average baby passes 4 +/− 1.8 stools per day during the first week of life which by one year has fallen to approximately 1.6 per day and then declines to 1 over the preschool years (Weaver 1983). Most children present around the age of 3 to 4 years with a history of some 6 to 24 months. Some are said to have always been constipated and others have never achieved bowel control.

Whilst patients with toddler diarrhoea and abdominal pain may be intermittently troubled with constipation, the majority of children presenting with constipation do not experience diarrhoea and do not have persistent or marked abdominal pain. Their symptoms are solely those of constipation or soiling secondary to overflow incontinence. However, those who present from birth, fail to pass meconium in the first 24 hours of life or experience persistent symptoms of episodic diarrhoea and abdominal pain require further investigation to exclude both classical Hirschsprung's disease and zonal colonic aganglionosis. Rectal biopsy from clearly defined levels using both conventional histology and histochemistry is the definitive investigation (Lake et al 1978) for Hirschsprung's disease and its variants but anorectal manometry (as described in Ch. 3) may also be useful (Aaronson & Nixon 1972). Cystic fibrosis should be excluded in those who did not pass meconium in the first 24 hours of life and where there is developmental and growth delay, hypothyroidism.

Pathophysiology

Children with constipation fall into two groups, the majority for whom no cause can be found, who may later develop idiopathic megacolon and for whom there is no demonstrable functional abnormality. Here the problem may stem from a number of factors including a bout of constipation associated with loss of appetite due to an acute infection, moving house or a holiday, pain from an anal fissure, or difficult toilet training either due to unpleasant lavatory facilities, e.g. inadequate privacy at school, or to a persistent negative developmental phase experienced by some toddlers.

Physiological studies have focussed mainly on the motility of the rectum and anal sphincters following the recognition of the altered anal sphincteric reflexes in Hirschsprung's disease. In patients with idiopathic megacolon (Aaronson & Nixon 1972), unlike those with Hirschsprung's, the internal sphincter relaxes with rectal distension.

Table 12.1 Organic causes of constipation

Acute	Changes of diet, e.g. breast to bottle feeds
	Lack of intake
	Anal fissure
	Intestinal obstruction

Chronic

    Gastrointestinal
                Anal malformations
                Disorders of nerves and ganglia
                        Hirschsprung's disease
                        Total and zonal aganlionosis
                        Abnormalities of the myenteric plexus
                Disorders of smooth muscle
                        Perinatal ischaemia
                        Hollow visceral myopathy
                Cystic fibrosis
                Coeliac disease
                Food allergy

    Extraintestinal
                Hypothyroidism
                Hypercalcaemia
                Lead poisoning
                Renal failure

A minority may, however, have potentially serious pathology which is summarized in Table 12.1.

In a recent study of anorectal physiology in 106 children with long-standing constipation (Clayden & Lawson 1976), 10 were found to have ultra short-segment Hirschsprung's disease (with failure of relaxation of the internal sphincter), 10 others had similar physiological abnormalities, but normal ganglia/nerves were found on biopsy. In the other 86 cases, the physiological findings were abnormal, with high amplitude rhythmic fluctuations of the internal sphincter; a high rectal distension pressure was required to induce relaxation of the internal sphincter, and a markedly increased critical volume (volume associated with urgent desire to defaecate). It was suggested that failure of the lower portion of the internal sphincter to relax caused functional obstruction and compensatory hypertrophy of the upper portion of the internal sphincter occurred. 39% of these patients had a dramatic response to a single anal dilation, and another 9% responded to repeated dilation and sphincterotomy.

Clearly, whether the physiological abnormalities are secondary or primary remains to be determined. Failure of some patients to produce an increase in colonic motility in response to acetyl choline (Davidson et al 1963) and subsequent failure to improve dramatically following an anal pull-through operation suggests that some form of dynamic test of colon motor activity may be a useful approach in children with chronic constipation, to distinguish those more resistant cases who have an abnormality of colonic motor function.

Treatment

In our experience the majority of children with idiopathic constipation respond to measures designed to empty and keep their rectum empty combined with a behavioural programme based on simple rewards. The majority of cases can be managed on an outpatient basis and are helped by an explanation of the problem and its prognosis. If a large megacolon is present, loss of normal rectal sensation and its consequences of loss of bowel habit and failure to appreciate when the bowels are open should be explained. The rationale of therapy, i.e. the need to get and keep the rectum empty, for large soft faeces and for a regular habit are then easily understood.

We recommend emptying the rectum with enemas and the concurrent use of laxatives, such as docusate sodium (Dioctyl®) and lactulose, and a stimulant aperient, senna. It is important that an effective dose of oral aperients and laxatives are used; we start with Senokot® syrup, 5 ml at night, and docusate sodium syrup, 5 ml three times daily; which is then continued for as long as is necessary. In addition to the above many children consume a diet which is low in fibre and attention to this is vital, either as a formal high fibre diet or with the addition of bran to cereals or soup.

In order to achieve a regular bowel habit the above is combined with a behaviour modification programme. Time must be available in family life for the child to go to the lavatory in a relaxed manner after each main meal but it must be explained that a bowel action is not expected on every occasion, the aim being for about one a day. A simple reward system is a useful reinforcing method and star charts provide a record of achievement. Targets should be achievable and a symbol used for the lowest level of cooperation required such as the use of the lavatory and for the voluntary opening of the bowels. Extra symbols might be used for greater success such as a whole day clean or several days clean.

The successful introduction of such a scheme will require follow-up at six week intervals and later, reduction of medications. On rare occasions a period of inpatient management may be required either because of difficulty in emptying the rectum or inability of the parents to institute and control such a scheme. A similar scheme is used as above but the nurses and doctors involved must be motivated to ensure successful supervision. The opportunity can, however, be taken for continued explanations to the parents and child and the use of other reinforcing manoeuvres such as weekend leave.

Those that do not respond to the above scheme should be carefully re-evaluated for organic disease and a full and formal psychological assessment should be performed. On rare occasions previously unrecognized organic causes may be found, and it has recently become clear that chronic constipation may be caused by food allergy (Chin 1983) and relieved by the appropriate exclusion diet.

Prognosis

Long-term prognosis is excellent. The short-term results with the above scheme are over 90% success in our hands. Relapses are not uncommon but can nearly always be managed along the same lines.

AETIOLOGICAL FACTORS

It has recently been shown that there are several different stages of development of intestinal motility in man (Wozniak et al 1983) which occur prenatally and in early infancy (Fenton & Milla 1984). Both control and effector systems are involved in the developmental and maturational process. Several lines of evidence suggest that autonomic reactivity patterns are established in early infancy, but it is not clear what effects organic (such as atopy and food allergy) mechanical factors or emotional stress have on the developing control systems of the infant's alimentary tract. It is possible that functional disorders of the gastrointestinal tract may start insidiously and be concurrent with the setting up of a deviant balance in the autonomic control of the infant's gut. Subsequently some of these minor deviations of function may be more prone to become exaggerated and develop into lasting symptomatic disorders as a result of the influence of environmental circumstances or events.

REFERENCES

Aaronson I, Nixon H H 1972 A Clinical Evaluation of Anorectal Pressure, Studies in the Diagnosis of Hirschsprung's Disease. Gut 13: 138–146

Almy T P 1967 Digestive Disease As A National Problem. Gastroenterology 53: 821–833

Alun Jones V, McLaughlin P, Shorthouse M, Workman E, Hunter J O 1982 Food Intolerance: A Major Factor in the Pathogenesis of Irritable Bowel Syndrome. Lancet ii: 1115–1117

Apley J, 1959 The Child With Abdominal Pains. Blackwell Scientific Publications, Oxford

Apley J, Hale B 1973 Children with Recurrent Pain. How Do They Grow Up? British Medical Journal 3: 7–9

Berger M G 1974 Somatic Pain and School Avoidance. Clinical Paediatrics (Philadelphia) 13: 815–818

Chin K C, Tarlow M J, Allfree A J 1983 Allergy to Cows Milk Presenting as Chronic Constipation. British Medical Journal 287:1593

Christensen M F, Mortenson O 1975 The Long Term Prognosis in Children with Reccurrent Abdominal Pain. Archives of Disease in Childhood 50: 110–114

Clayden G S, Lawson J O 1976 Investigation and Management of Long Standing Chronic Constipation in Childhood. Archives of Disease in Childhood 51: 918–920

Connel A M, Avery Jones F, Rowlands E N 1965 Motility of the Pelvic Colon, II. Abdominal pain associated with colonic hypermotility after meals. Gut 6: 105–112

Corbett C L, Thomas S, Read N W, Hobson N, Bergman I, Holdsworth C D 1981 Electrochemical Detector for Breath Hydrogen Determination: Measurement of Small Bowel Transit Time in Normal Subjects and Patients With Irritable Bowel Syndrome. Gut 22: 836–840

Davidson M, Wasserman R 1966 The Irritable Colon of Childhood (Chronic Non-specific Diarrhoea Syndrome). Journal of Pediatrics 69: 1027–1038

Davidson M, Kugler M M, Bauer C H 1963 Diagnosis and Management in Children with Severe and Protracted Constipation and Obstipation. Journal of Pediatrics 67: 261–275

Diament N F, Hall K, Muir H, El-Sharkawy T Y 1980 Vagal Control of the Feeding
Motor Patterns in the Lower Oesophageal Sphincter, Stomach and Upper Small Intestine
of Dogs. In: Christensen J (ed) Gastrointestinal Motility. Raven Press, New York.
pp 365–370

Dodge J A, Handi I A, Burns G M, Yamashiro Y 1981 Toddler Diarrhoea and
Prostglandins. Archives of Disease in Childhood 56: 705–757

Drossman D A, Powell D W, Sessions J T 1977 The Irritable Bowel Syndrome.
Gastroenterology 73: 811–822

Egger J, Carter C M, Wilson J, Turner M W, Soothill J F, 1983 Is migraine food allergy?
A double blind controlled trial of oligoantigenic diet treatment. Lancet ii: 865–869

Ewart W R, Wingate D L 1983 Central Representation and Opioid Modulation of Gastric
Mechanoreception Activity in the Rat. American Journal of Physiology 244: G27–32

Fenton T R, Milla P J 1984 Age Related Differences of the MMC. Paediatric Research
18:1061

Fenton T R, Harries J T, Milla P J, 1983a. Disordered Small intestinal motility: A
Rational Basis for Toddler's Diarrhoea. Gut 24: 897–903

Fenton T R, Harries J T, Milla P J 1983b Abnormalities of Postprandial Small Intestinal
Motor Activity in Childhood: Their Role in the Pathogenesis of the Irritable Bowel
Syndrome. In: Labo G, Bortolotti M (eds) Gastrointestinal Motility Verona. Cortina
International 207–213

Green M, 1967 Diagnosis and Treatment of Psychogenic recurrent abdominal pain.
Paediatrics 40:84

Gupta S, Agareval H C, Bhardwaj O P, Supta J P 1974 Reccurrent Abdominal Pain in
Children. Indian Paediatrics 11: 115–120

Horowitz L, Farrar J T 1962 Intraluminal Small Intestinal Pressures in Normal Patients
and in Patients with Functional Gastrointestinal Disorders. Gastrenterology 42: 455–464

Jonas A, Diver Haber A 1982 Stool Output and Composition in the Chronic Non-Specific
Diarrhoea Syndrome. Archives of Disease in Childhood 57: 35–39

Kopel F B, Kim J C, Barbero G J 1967 Comparison of Recto-sigmoid Motility in Normal
Children, Children with Recurrent Abdominal Pain and Children with ulcerative colitis.
Pediatrics 39: 539–545

Lake B D, Puri P, Nixon H H, Claireaux A E 1978 Hirschrung's Disease. An Appraisal of
Histochemically Demonstrated Acetylcholinesterase Activity in Section Rectal Biopsies as
an Aid to Diagnosis. Archives of Pathology and Laboratory Medicine 102: 244–247

McMichael H B, Webb J, Dawson A M 1965 Lactose Deficiency in Adults: Cause of
Functional Diarrhoea. Lancet i: 717–720

Marshall D G 1967 Recurrent Abdominal Pain in Children: A Surgeon's View Point.
Pediatrics 40: 1024–1026

Matuchansky C, Bernier J J 1973 Effect of Prostglandin E1 on Glucose Water and
Electrolyte Absorption in the Human jejunum. Gastroenterology 64: 1111–1118

Milla P J, Acherton D A, Leonard J V, Wolff O H, Lake B D 1978 Disordered Intestinal
Functions in Glycogen Storage Disease. Journal of Inherited Metabolic Disease
1: 155–157

Moriarty K J, Dawson A M 1982 Functional Abdominal Pain: Further Evidence That
Whole Gut is Affected. British Medical Journal ii: 1670–1672

Read N W 1980 The Migrating motor Complex and Spontaneous Fluctuations of
Transmural Potential Difference in the Human Small Intestine. In: Christensen J (ed)
Gastrointestinal Motility. Raven Press, New York. pp 299–306

Read N W, Small R H, Levin R J, Holdsworth C D, Brown B H 1977 Relationship
Between Changes in Intraluminal Pressure and Transmural potential Difference in the
Human and Canine Jejunun in vivo. Gut 18: 141–145

Read N W, Krejs G J, Read M G, Santa Ana C A, Morowski S J, Fordtran J S 1980
Chronic Diarrhoea of Unknown Origin. Gastroenterology 78: 264–271

Ritchie J A, Salem S M 1965 Upper Intestinal Motilty in Ulcerative Colitis, idiopathic
Steatorrhea and the irritable colon syndrome. Gut 6: 325–337

Sandhu B K, Tripp J H, Candy D C A, Harries J T 1981 Loperamide: Studies on its
Mechanism of Action. Gut 22: 658–662

Savilahti E, Simell O 1985 Chronic non-specific diarrhoea. Archives of Disease in
Childhood 60: 452–456

Thompson D G, Laidlow J M, Wingate D L 1979 Abnormal small bowel motility
demonstrated by radiotelemetry in a patient with irritable colon. Lancet ii: 1321–1323

Thompson D G, Ritchie H D, Wingate D L 1982 Patterns of small intestinal motility in duodenal ulcer patients before and after vagotomy. Gut 23: 517–523

Tripp J H, Muller D P R, Harries J T 1980 Mucosal (Na+-K+) ATPase and Adenylate Cyclase Activities in Children with Toddler Diarrhoea and Postenteritis Syndrome. Pediatric Research 14: 1382–1386

Vantrappen G, Janssens J, Hellemans J, Shoos Y 1977 The interdigestive motor complex of normal subjects and patients with bacterial overgrowth of the small intestine. Journal of Clinical Investigation 59: 1158–1166

Weaver L T 1984 The Bowel habit of young children. Archives of Disease in childhood 59: 649–652

Wozniak E R, Fenton T R, Milla P J 1983 The Development of Fasting Small Intestinal Motility in the Human Neonate. In: Roman C (ed) Gastrointestinal Motility. MTP Press, Lancaster. pp 265–270

Psychological aspects of gastrointestinal disorders

INTRODUCTION

The relationship between the gastrointestinal tract and the psyche has been the cause of much debate. Whilst most physicians readily accept that gastrointestinal disease can have unpleasant psychological sequelae such as anxiety, depression, resentment or despair, some remain sceptical about the possibility of stress or distress provoking physical symptoms and particularly physical disease. Indisputably, however, the gastrointestinal tract is often the target of behavioural or emotional problems. Examples include feeding disorders, constipation and encopresis.

In this chapter I shall consider the complex relationship between emotions, behaviour and the gastrointestinal tract, propose a model for understanding that relationship, consider some specific disorders, and review the available treatments.

PSYCHOLOGICAL EFFECTS OF GASTROINTESTINAL DISEASE

The unpleasantness of gastrointestinal disease is well recognized. Pain, nausea, vomiting, and diarrhoea, are all highly demoralizing. Necessary investigations can be frightening and painful. Treatment can be unpleasant and the enforced separation of children from their families because of hospitalization has its own sequelae. It is, therefore, hardly surprising that children with gastrointestinal disease can become anxious or frightened, sad or depressed, angry and resentful, and generally demoralized. The situation can be aggravated by the effects of the illness or its treatment, such as growth delay or altered body or facial appearance. Missed school can lead to educational failure, which creates its own anxieties. Being different from other children may lead to social isolation and further distress.

Chronic or recurrent ill-health can lead to an overacceptance of the illness and a giving-in. The child becomes so demoralized he makes little or no attempt to cope. He may refuse his medication or diet. The natural but powerful emotional reactions outlined may well aggravate the disease, so setting up and maintaining a vicious circle. Some children adopt an opposite strategy of denying the illness and trying to lead a normal life, despite the ill health. Such children often fail to comply with treatment as part of the denial, so aggravating their poor health.

In addition to the psychological effects on the child, his family are also affected. Parents may feel responsible for their child's ill health, worried about the future, resentful that fate should select them and spoil their lives, angry that doctors cannot cure their child, and depressed by the burden. Such reactions are common and natural and needless to say, they are distressing. Unfortunately, unless parents can come to terms with their own distress, they are likely to communicate it to their child and so impose an additional stress. Once more, the danger of a vicious circle arises.

EFFECTS OF STRESS ON THE GASTROINTESTINAL TRACT

The term stress is often used either vaguely or euphemistically. It is used here to mean any stimulus which is sufficiently intense to produce an emotional response. Consequently, this can include any form of stressful event, which in childhood might be family tensions, separation, major changes such as that of school or house, difficulty in peer relationships, or loss of important friends or relatives. It can be appreciated that such stresses may be acute, intermittent or chronic, overt or covert, minor or major. These are important concepts, as all too often significant stresses are overlooked simply because they are not major and obvious traumatic events. Stresses are often subtle, low-key, persistent and sometimes far from clear to the outsider. An obvious example would be unresolved marital conflict.

Many studies have been reported demonstrating the effect of stress or emotion on salivation (Bogdanoff et al 1961), oesophageal motility (Wolf & Almy 1949), gastric motility and secretion (Wolf 1981, Engel et al 1956, Thompson et al 1983), small bowel motility (Granata et al 1973, Wingate et al 1982, Cann et al 1983) and colonic motility (Almy et al 1949, Chaudhary & Truelove 1961).

It has further been suggested that different emotions have different effects. For example, fear and depression have been found to be associated with hypomotility and hyposecretion of the stomach (Wolf & Wolff 1947) and hypomotility in the small bowel and colon (Chaudhary & Truelove 1961), whilst resentment, anger and aggression have been found to be associated with enhanced motor activity and secretion (Cann et al 1983).

Emotional conflict has been shown to produce changes in motility,

secretion and vascularity in the colon of normal subjects, leading to pete-
chial haemorrhages and minute ulceration (Grace et al 1951). Changes in
motility may occur as a result of central effects (Wingate et al 1982) with
increased sympathetic nervous activity (Furness & Costa 1974) either by
direct action of catecholamines or indirectly via sympathetic stimulation of
glucagon release (Bloom et al 1973), or by vagal stimulation (Prugh 1983).
Conditioning may also play a part in the genesis of gastrointestinal symptoms. Highly anxious patients who have had certain symptoms in the past,
possibly organically determined, may be conditioned to produce such symptoms at times of stress (Chaudhary & Truelove 1962, Esler & Goulston
1973).

It has been suggested in the past that children with specific diseases,
including gastrointestinal disease, have certain personality characteristics.
For example, children with ulcerative colitis have been described as over-
dependent, passive, inhibited and showing compulsive tendencies
(McDermott & Finch 1967), whilst children with peptic ulcers have been
described as generally tense and overcompliant, and often passive and
dependent. Their mothers are reported to be dominant and overprotective,
and their fathers are often distant and passive, though occasionally rigid and
punitive (Coddington 1968). Many of these statements are overgeneraliz-
ations, contradictory, or hopelessly vague. There is no worthwhile evidence
to indicate that children with any gastrointestinal disorder, or their parents,
have particular personality features (Lask 1982b).

What does seem reasonably certain is that stress can aggravate preexisting gastrointestinal pathology such as peptic ulceration and inflammatory bowel disease. It is also possible, though yet to be proven, that
stress could produce gastrointestinal pathology in predisposed individuals
(MacDonald & Bouchier 1980), such as peptic ulceration in adult life. In
childhood, it may well be shown eventually that in certain individuals who
are genetically or immunologically programmed, stress can induce disease
(Lipowski et al 1977). Indeed, Apley has stated that the gastrointestinal
tract mirrors the emotions more often than any other body system, and has
claimed that stress is manifested as different gastrointestinal disorders at
different ages (Apley 1982).

There can be little doubt that stress can produce such difficulties as
feeding problems, cyclical vomiting, recurrent abdominal pain, constipation
and diarrhoea.

THE GASTROINTESTINAL TRACT AS A TARGET FOR
BEHAVIOUR PROBLEMS

I have discussed above ways in which stress can affect the gastrointestinal
tract via complex psychophysiological pathways. Children under stress or
in distress can also manifest this in a more direct way, although not
necessarily deliberately or consciously. An early example is that of stool-

withholding in toddlers, preschool children, and occasionally even older children, leading to constipation and eventually overflow-incontinence. It is recognized that in a minority of cases there is an organic precipitant such as an anal fissure. In the majority of cases, however, there is evidence of coercive toilet-training or other problems in the parent-child relationship (Hersov 1977).

Nonconstipated faecal soiling is a not uncommon manifestation of distress in the 3–8 years age-group. Such children almost invariably show evidence of emotional disturbance and there is usually also family dysfunction (Hersov 1977).

Feeding difficulties can occur in any age-group. Often they start in infancy and usually seem to be associated with a tense mother-baby relationship, but which comes first is not always clear. Toddlers usually pass through a stage of food fads and sometimes food refusal. Older children can be very finicky about food and more disturbed children may overeat to the point of obesity, or undereat as in anorexia nervosa (see p. 291).

Other gastrointestinal manifestations of behaviour problems include air-swallowing, rumination, self-induced vomiting, and laxative abuse.

A PRACTICAL MODEL LINKING PSYCHOSOCIAL AND ORGANIC ASPECTS OF GASTROINTESTINAL DISORDERS

It is clear from the above discussion that there is a complex interaction between psychosocial and organic aspects of gastrointestinal disorders. The issue of primacy — which comes first — is contentious and often not easily proven. Chronic constipation exemplifies this. I believe that to seek primacy is to miss the point, and so deprive the child of optimal care. The same argument applies in asking whether or not a particular disorder or symptom is 'psychosomatic'. It is far more useful to give careful consideration to the organic *and* psychosocial aspects of a problem, so ensuring that problems are not missed.

In the more primitive days of medical practice the physician's conceptualization of a problem could be portrayed as:

Organic pathology   ————————→Physical symptoms

More recently, it has been recognized that physical symptoms are distressing and can lead to stress and even behaviour problems, thus:

Behaviour problems

Organic pathology   ————————→ Physical symptoms

Stress and distress

Stress and distress can themselves produce physical symptoms and aggravate pre-existing organic pathology, whilst behaviour problems such as noncompliance with treatment or diet can aggravate the organic pathology and/or the physical symptoms. Thus:

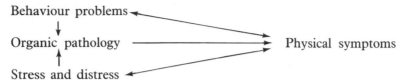

Stress and distress affect not only the child, but also his family. If the family cannot cope with their own reactions, it is likely that the child will develop further behavioural problems. This completes the cycle of interactions:

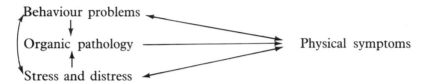

This model is applicable whatever the presenting problem, and allows for careful consideration of all relevant factors. Whether a child has vomiting, recurrent abdominal pain, constipation or soiling, peptic ulcer or inflammatory bowel disease, consideration of each component is likely to lead to comprehensive and therefore more effective care of the child and his family. As Booth & Harries (1984) have stated with reference to inflammatory bowel disease a comprehensive approach not only improves the patient's well-being, but may also reduce the number of relapses.

In the next section this model is applied in considering common gastrointestinal disorders.

SPECIFIC DISORDERS

Feeding problems

Feeding problems are very common, and often a cause of great concern.

Feeding problems in infancy and young children

Some babies are relatively easy to feed, others are particularly problematic. Some mothers take to feeding their babies with no difficulty, whilst others struggle. Developmental or physical problems in the baby, and ill health or emotional problems in the mother can aggravate these difficulties. Such problems in early life often set the tone for later childhood.

In assessing feeding difficulties physical aspects always receive full consideration. It is however just as important to give equal weight to the emotional side as many physical symptoms are extremely aversive and may readily provoke a food refusal syndrome. Where temperamental variation or developmental difficulties lead to feeding problems, the natural maternal response is one of anxiety, frustration and eventually resentment. On the other hand, if a mother is feeling in some way negative to her baby, or indeed simply anxious about feeding, her tension is liable to be communicated to the infant who may respond by rejecting feeds or behaving awkwardly during the feed. Marital problems may be detoured and expressed as difficulty in the mother-baby relationship, including the feeding aspect of this.

A vicious circle is readily initiated at a very early stage, and the paediatrician should give due consideration to all aspects of the problem from the beginning. If only the medical or physical aspects are considered, a complex emotional problem in mother-child interaction may well have taken hold by the time investigations have been completed. (Goldson et al 1985).

The same points apply at a later stage. Toddlers and young children can be notoriously fussy about their feeds. In turn, parents can be just as fussy about what they want their child to eat, and as he gets older, how he eats it. Undue rigidity or intense anxiety on the parental side is liable to create a backlash by the child if he is not endowed with an easygoing temperament. Equally, difficult behaviour from the child can test all but the most easygoing of parents.

Management of feeding difficulties should be focussed on all aspects of the problem. Changes of feeding schedule and content may have an important part to play, but no more important than helping a mother to cope with her own distress, loss of confidence and resentment.

In the early stages of a feeding problem, gentle reassurance, straightforward advice, and the provision of practical support may be sufficient. If not, however, then every effort should be made to provide comprehensive care (Bingley et al 1980) in order to prevent a more complex and long-lasting problem from arising. The skills and experience of a social worker, psychologist or psychiatrist should be sought when the paediatrician feels uncertain of how to explore and help alleviate emotional and behavioural difficulties. Involvement of the father is a valuable way of finding more support for a harassed, and distressed mother. Exploration of emotional problems either in the mother alone, in the marriage, or in the whole family is often very revealing.

Anorexia nervosa. This condition, affecting about 1 in 100 to 200 girls between the ages of 16–18 seems to be occuring increasingly frequently in young adolescents and even pre-pubertal children. It occurs about 10–20 times more commonly in adult females than males, although in the younger age-group the ratio is more like 5:1. The essential features are (a) a failure to gain weight at the time of expected growth-spurt or an actual loss of weight, (b) the presence of a determined food-avoidance accompanied by one or more of the following: a preoccupation with body weight and/or its control, fear of fatness, distorted body image, purging, self-induced vomiting, or excessive exercising, (c) the cessation of menstrual periods or the failure of these to commence at the expected age.

In the younger age-group there seems to be a wide variation in the clinical presentation. Rarely does the clinical picture fit with the classical description. Frequently there is an early history of feeding difficulties and not infrequently, the presentation may be more akin to that of school refusal, depression, psychogenic pains or vomiting (see below). In childhood there also seems to be far more variation of the clinical picture during the course of the illness. In particular, fluctuation between depression and anorexia nervosa often occurs. A vivid feature of the condition is the patient's determined control of those around her. Whilst initially appearing to be a sweet, gentle, friendly and sad child, she may soon also show herself to be manipulative, controlling and very aware of how to get her way. Splitting of family members and ward staff is common. This behaviour represents the child's attempt to control her environment in reaction to a strong sense of being controlled.

The differential diagnosis includes such conditions as Crohn's disease, but careful history-taking and clinical observation will always reveal the correct diagnosis.

The aetiology of anorexia nervosa is unknown. Many hypotheses have been put forward, but none have been shown to be universally applicable. Some, mostly emanating from psychoanalytic writers, are far-fetched or absurd. One of the most popular of these has been the equating by the patient of food ingestion with oral impregnation. Fortunately such thinking is gradually losing credibility.

Bruch (1978) sees the disorder as an attempt to gain personal effectiveness and autonomy through the control of weight. Crisp (1980) states that the illness represents a psychobiological regression to childhood in the form of mounting conflict in adolescence. Gore (1976) has suggested that food refusal may start for slimming purposes, but ultimately becomes an end in itself, reinforced by excessive parental attention and concern. Minuchin et al (1978) view the food-refusal as playing an important part in maintaining family stability — in particular the symptom acts as a detour from marital conflict, giving the parents a concern they can share.

More biologically-orientated explanations include the suggestion that these patients have disturbed perceptions of body feelings (such as hunger) and body image (size and shape); both suggestions are consistent with the findings that anorectic patients often perceive themselves as fatter than they are (Slade & Russell 1973) and misinterpret hunger pains (Silverstone & Russell 1967). Certainly after a sustained period of food-refusal, eating is uncomfortable and the associated pain can be aversive. The possibility of a primary hypothalamic disorder has been proposed but the few instances of proven hypothalamic dysfunction are just as likely to be due to self-starvation.

In a retrospective study of fifty early onset anorectics, we have found the most common premorbid features are an early history of feeding difficulties, severe family tensions with marital conflict, an over-involved relationship between the patient and her mother, and attempts by the patient to gain control over her environment. Common features of the illness in children are physical symptoms such as abdominal pain or nausea, depression, fear of fat and preoccupation with weight or calories. Distorted body image also frequently occurs.

Course and Management. The course is variable depending upon age at onset, length of illness before treatment is commenced, severity of symptoms, cooperation of parents and types of treatment used. Our experience is that in the younger age-group the sooner comprehensive treatment begins, the better the prognosis. Similarly the outlook improves when parents are able to modify their own behaviour.

Management issues are crucial. In all but the mildest cases admission is recommended. Combined approaches using both medical and psychological treatments are essential (Lask & Bryant 1986). Gradual refeeding should start immediately. If life is threatened, then nasogastric or intravenous feeding should not be delayed. Rewards for consistent weight gain are often helpful although care should be taken to ensure that the child does not manipulate these. The key issue here is that weight gain should be consistent for rewards to be earned. It is not unknown for anorectics to drink a pint of water or eat a large meal shortly before weighing, only to vomit or purge once the reward has been received. Weight gain should not be linked to parental visits, weekend leave or discharge. This may work well in adults (Crisp 1980) but children are often so ambivalent about such matters that for them to be used as rewards may be counter-productive.

Working with the family is an essential part of the management (Lask 1982a, 1982b). To send a recovering anorectic home to her still highly dysfunctional family is asking for an early relapse. Individual psychotherapy can be helpful (Bruch 1978) providing it is integrated with the family work. It is usually only helpful after some weight gain has been achieved. Psychotropic medication and appetite stimulants are of dubious value. Antidepressants are helpful only if there is associated depression.

It seems that a combination of gradual refeeding with rewards, individual and family psychotherapy is the most useful form of management. However, it is essential that the treatment team, which should consist of paediatricians, nurses, and psychiatrist or psychologist, is able to work constructively and harmoniously. They need to be alert to the anorectic's skill at splitting staff and manipulating her environment. Frequent meetings between all those concerned is the best way of ensuring the success of the treatment (Bingley et al 1980).

Overeating and obesity. These related problems are becoming increasingly frequent in childhood. As with other feeding disorders, overeating appears to start at an early age. In many, though not all cases, it seems that food has been used as a response to distress. The infant's cries have been (sometimes) misinterpreted as hunger, and have responded to feeding. It can be seen how a pattern can arise of a child learning to associate the resolution of distress with eating. As the child grows, he seeks comfort in food that may not otherwise be provided.

Overeaters not infrequently seem to be involved in an overclose relationship with their mothers, to the exclusion of other family members. Whilst this family pattern is by no means exclusive to childhood obesity, and not all obese children are involved in this way, it is striking how rigid and close that relationship often appears.

By the time such problems come to the paediatrician's attention, they have taken on the nature of an addiction. The child is addicted to food, and the family may be addicted to the way in which they have organized their relationships.

Management of severe overeating and subsequent obesity is remarkably difficult. In milder cases, advice about diet and exercise with warnings of the dangers of obesity are usually sufficient. In those cases that reach the paediatrician, it is likely that such measures have already been tried. Once more the only chance of success is the use of a comprehensive approach. Physical treatments are rarely sufficient. The main objective must be a change in eating habits which does not come from advice alone. Behaviour modification techniques (Brownell & Stunkard 1978) combined with treatment of family problems (Lask 1982a) holds most promise. It is often helpful to admit the obese child to hospital to initiate a change in eating behaviour and weight reduction. Unless a comprehensive approach is used, the child rapidly regains weight on discharge.

Disorders of defecation

Disorders of defecation are common problems in both paediatric and child psychiatric clinics.

From a psychiatric viewpoint these fall into three main types: constipation, primary encopresis, secondary encopresis and diarrhoea.

Constipation. The causes of constipation are not clearly understood. In some cases a fissure-in-ano seems to have been present. The pain on attempted defecation discourages the child from trying too often. The relief of pain by withholding then encourages him to further withold. A more common cause of constipation appears to be emotional disturbance. Coercive toilet training (just as with forced feeding) can lead to a backlash, in which the child refuses to cooperate — the battle of the bowel! The parent adopts a rigid and punitive approach, or alternatively, expects too much too soon. The child responds by depriving his parent. A pattern of witholding soon takes root. As with so many other problems, a vicious circle occurs: parental anxiety, distress or resentment leads to frenetic attempts to make the child perform; the more the parent tries the more the child refuses to cooperate.

The child may sit on the toilet, but be unable to defecate or he may refuse to sit on the toilet. A few such children are phobic of the toilet, but in most it is more a wilful refusal. Eventual overflow incontinence is often mistaken as diarrhoea or encopresis.

Primary encopresis. This term applies to children who have never gained bowel control. It is often associated with enuresis. Such children tend to come from disorganized and multi-problem families in which toilet training has been inconsistent or inadequate (Hersov 1977). There are often a variety of other behaviour problems, and usually other children in the family are also affected. Affected children are usually unaware that they are soiling and parental responses can aggravate the problem. Faeces tend to be of normal consistency.

Secondary encopresis These children have gained normal bowel control, but deposit their faeces in inappropriate places. Occasionally there may also be smearing. The faeces are usually of normal consistency. Almost always such behaviour is an expression of severe emotional disturbance arising from a background of family disharmony, marital conflict or coercive training (Hersov 1977). There are frequently associated behaviour problems.

Diarrhoea A few children are reported to have chronic or recurrent diarrhoea ('toddler' or 'functional' diarrhoea) for which no organic cause can be found (See Ch. 12).

Very rarely diarrhoea may be a result of laxative abuse or some other form of self-injury, the intention of which is either to produce weight-loss or give the impression of 'ill' health.

Management of disorders of defecation As with all other childhood psychiatric problems, a comprehensive approach is necessary, including attention being paid to organic, psychological and social factors. A careful history and physical examination almost always reveals the cause of the problem. Special investigations are rarely necessary and are only indicated where there is strong evidence of an organic disorder, or the condition has proved resistant to comprehensive treatment. The detailed investigation of constipation or encopresis is so intrusive and traumatic that it is likely to produce more problems than it solves.

Constipation should be managed by a combination of physical and behavioural measures as either alone is usually insufficient. Behavioural techniques include the institution of a toilet training programme. This involves the parents encouraging the child to sit on the toilet two or three times a day and rewarding him for doing so. Once he is used to sitting on the toilet, rewards are offered only for defecating. The reward programme is particularly important for those children who are toilet-phobic. Parents should be advised that the physical treatment may produce dramatic results, but that there are bound to be periods of relapse. A chronically constipated bowel takes some time to regain its tone, and the resultant failure to perform at the right time can be disappointing and worrying to the parents. If they are advised of this possibility, they seem to cope far better. It is advisable to continue the medical treatment for several weeks, gradually reducing the dose of laxatives, softeners, or whatever else is being used.

Primary encopresis requires the same toilet training programme as constipation, but medications are not of value. Rewards are particularly important for these children. Secondary encopresis requires a similar approach. When possible, it is best to advise the parents to ignore the soiling but to praise and encourage appropriate use of the toilet. In both forms of encopresis (and often in constipation too) there are family problems which require assessment and skilled treatment.

Functional diarrhoea occurs in anxious children. Relaxation techniques may help lower the level of emotional arousal (Furman 1973) and biofeedback has been successfully used in adults (Shuster 1974). There is little evidence for the value of psychotropic agents in such situations (Almy 1977).

Psychogenic abdominal pain and vomiting

Amongst the most common presenting problems in childhood are recurrent abdominal pain, vomiting, headache and limb pains which present either singly or in combination. This spectrum of symptoms seems to have collected an amazing series of diagnostic labels: periodic syndrome, recurrent abdominal pain, cyclical vomiting, irritable bowel syndrome, irritable colon, spastic colon, abdominal migraine, childhood migraine, psychogenic pains etc. This unhelpful confusion seems to arise from attempts by physicians to bulldoze a diagnostic label, so reinforcing the myth that a physical cause is a sine qua non for bodily symptoms (Apley 1982). Apley refers to the 'triple fallacy' that physical symptoms must be due to physical causes and must have physical treatments. Invariably such children are also physically investigated often to a dangerous degree.

Thorough history-taking and careful physical examination will in the vast majority of cases reveal the correct diagnosis of psychogenic pain or vomiting. The high incidence of psychogenic abdominal pain (between 1 in 9 and 1 in 6 children) (Apley et al 1978) should put this disorder at the top of the differential diagnosis list. It should be confidently excluded before embarking upon invasive or unpleasant investigations. Physicians need to balance their fears of overlooking serious progressive disease with the danger that they themselves may help to perpetuate the illness by well-meaning but never ending efforts to find a physical cause. In a long-term follow-up of 161 children with recurrent abdominal pain only 3 cases of organic disease were missed. Each should have been suspected on the grounds of weight-loss and anaemia. Other studies report similar findings (Stickler & Murphy 1979).

Children with psychogenic abdominal pain often present with episodes of severe pain, for which no precipitating factor or physical cause is obvious. The pain tends to occur in bouts, and is rarely continuous. It may occur as often as several times a day, or only once a week or less. The child can be in great distress, with pallor and tachycardia. Physical examination and special investigations reveal no organic pathology. Occasionally, a 'spastic colon' is reported on X-ray.

Psychogenic vomiting is less frequent, but still requires active consideration in any case of recurrent vomiting. It presents as bouts of vomiting which may occur regularly or irregularly, as often as daily, or as infrequently as once every few months. Bouts may last for a few hours or persist for several days, leading to dehydration, electrolyte imbalance, and eventually, if unchecked, coma and death. A precipitating cause is rarely found.

Recurrent headache and/or limb pains are occasional concomitants of psychogenic abdominal pain or vomiting. Either of these may also occur in isolation.

We have therefore a syndrome, which consists of one or more of the following symptoms: abdominal pain, vomiting, headache and limb pain. The disorder is usually psychogenic, in that although there are rarely obvious precipitating factors, careful and sympathetic psychosocial investigation invariably reveals areas of stress and distress. Organic pathology is nearly always absent.

If untreated, about one-third of patients with recurrent abdominal pain become symptom-free by adulthood; another third lose their abdominal pains by adult life but develop other symptoms such as recurrent headache; the final third continue to suffer from their pains and also develop other symptoms (Apley 1982). With psychiatric treatment the results are much better (Apley et al 1978, Berger et al 1977).

Treatment consists initially of careful psychosocial investigation. Stress factors are almost always uncovered, the most common being family difficulties, in particular marital conflict, and school-based problems. Such causes are not found unless they are carefully sought. Asking about them may occasionally lead to positive responses, though family disharmony is frequently denied. It is only when the family is interviewed (Bingley et al 1980) and school reports obtained that previously covert or denied problems are revealed.

The next step is to explain to the family how and why organic disease has been excluded. It is important not only to explain to the parents and child that the pains are real, and very painful, but also to ensure that they have understood this. Problems of cooperation arise far too frequently because explanations have been unclear, and the family have thought that they have been told that the child is imagining or making up the pain. It is sometimes helpful to use the analogy of tension headaches in adult-life.

When the problem is school-based, efforts should be made to remedy the situation. Discussion with the teacher may be sufficient, but if not, then the help of an educational psychologist or educational welfare officer should be sought. Most commonly, the problems are family-based and the most

effective treatment is family therapy (Lask 1982a). Individual psychotherapy for the child can also be helpful (Apley 1982). Teaching self-relaxation
works in some cases, and especially in older children, although this is
really only a form of symptom relief which does not tackle the root cause.
There is one exception and that is the anxious and oversensitive, or perfec-
tionist child, who sets himself (or has set for him) such high standards that
these are stressful to maintain. Psychotropic medication such as tranquil-
izers are of no value (British Medical Journal 1980b.) Beta-blockers have
been claimed to be of value for adults, but there is no useful information
on their value in childhood.

The same principles apply to psychogenic vomiting and also to headache
and limb pains. Clearly, physical treatments to restore hydration and electrolyte balance may be necessary. These should not, however, prevent the
initiation of a comprehensive management plan. These episodes may have
clear triggers such as infections or major life changes, but often the causes
are subtle and covert. Again, the most common are marital discord and
other family crises (Prugh 1983).

Psychiatric treatment follows the same pattern as for recurrent abdominal
pain. Without treatment symptoms tend to persist, whilst individual or
family psychotherapy usually leads to resolution of the difficulties (Bingley
et al 1980).

Inflammatory bowel disease

Such disorders often present the child and family with many years of
chronic ill health and many visits to hospital (Booth & Harries 1984), and
are discussed in detail in chapter 6. The emotional sequelae of such a
chronic and debilitating disorder have recently been reviewed (Bruce 1986).

Treatment of these diseases should always include both medical and
psychotherapeutic measures (Prugh 1983). Booth & Harries (1984) recommend the adoption of a team approach with the involvement of physician,
surgeon, psychiatrist, medical social worker, nurses and stoma therapist.
They state that not only does this approach improve the patient's sense of
well-being but may also reduce the number of relapses.

Stomas

A minority of children with inflammatory bowel disease require stoma
surgery. Whether or not the stoma is permanent, the psychosocial adjustment required by both child and family is enormous. In some children who
have been very ill for a long period, a stoma can come as a comparative
relief. In many however it is a shattering mutilation. Enormous anxieties
arise about what to tell people, how to mix with peers and how to cope with
physical relationships. In the early stages children have to learn to adjust

their diets, manage their stoma care, and cope with the devastating experience of ill-fitting bags with subsequent leaks and odours.

Despite all this, the majority of such children eventually adjust well to the stoma, and some seem to be psychologically healthier than those without stoma surgery. There is no evidence to indicate that stoma surgery should be avoided from a psychological viewpoint, but good preparation is important. The opportunity to meet other children with stomas preoperatively is valued, and clear descriptions of what is going to happen and why are appreciated. Diagrams are always helpful. Plenty of time should be set aside to discuss the operation whenever possible. Immediately following the operation and for several months afterwards, careful attention should be paid to the child's ability to cope. Once more, the use of the team approach is invaluable.

Peptic ulcer

High levels of emotional arousal in a child can produce changes in gastric and duodenal motility, secretion and engorgement through cortical-hypothalamic connections and vagal stimulation (Prugh 1983). The predisposing biological factors have not been identified. The potential stressful factors, and the resultant stresses are similar to those for the diseases already mentioned. The medical regimen should be combined with the psychosocial approach to ensure not only satisfactory resolution, but also minimization of the possibility of relapse.

Food allergy

The role of food allergy in the production of a variety of clinical syndromes remains controversial. It is however clear that food allergy may result in a variety of gastrointestinal symptoms (British Medical Journal 1980a).

There is very little doubt that whilst some children with gastrointestinal symptoms do suffer from food allergy, many in whom the condition is suspected do not. Parents or physicians, in a desperate attempt to find a physical diagnosis, latch on to the possibility of food allergy, and vigorously pursue it via investigation, dietary manipulation and other treatments. Sadly, many such children are suffering from much more common psychogenic disorders. The absurd and tragic extreme of this approach is the so-called 'total allergy syndrome' for which no medical evidence exists, and the allergy version of Meadow's syndrome (Warner & Hathaway 1984).

Where food allergy truly exists, the physician should ensure that the child is encouraged to lead as normal a life as possible — there need be only minimal limitation. In addition, it should be made clear that not all physical symptoms or indeed mood or behaviour variation is necessarily due to allergy. All children experience a variety of physical symptoms, and changes in mood and behaviour. To attribute all these to further allergy is bad medical practice.

When parents insist that their child's trouble is due to allergy although the physician is certain that this is not the case, they should receive a careful and sympathetic explanation for the physician's conviction. If this fails, the parents should be asked what would convince them that allergy is not to blame. Any reasonable tests or dietary manipulation might then be tried, providing a clear agreement is reached that once the trial is complete, no further allergen exploration will be attempted. This compromise is sometimes necessary because of the remarkable tenacity with which parents insist that allergy is to blame. The reasons for this are occasional ill-advised publicity in the media, the wish of the family to avoid exploration of psychological issues, and as Warner & Hathaway (1984) have pointed out, undue enthusiasm for allergy as an explanation amongst some physicians. Only when a comprehensive approach is adopted is it possible to resolve such problems.

CONCLUSIONS

There is a complex relationship between gastrointestinal disorders and psychosocial aspects of the child's life. Regardless of which is the primary problem, satisfactory resolution of the gastrointestinal symptoms is more likely to occur if attention is paid to both the physical and the psychosocial factors.

REFERENCES

Almy T 1977 Therapeutic strategy. Clinics in Gastroenterology 63: 709–721
Almy T, Kern F, Tulim M 1949 Alterations in colonic function in man under stress. Gastroenterology 12: 428–436
Apley J 1982 One Child. Apley J, Ounsted C (eds) Spastics International Medical Publications, London
Apley J, Mckeith R, Meadow R 1978 The child and his symptoms: a comprehensive approach, 3rd edn. Blackwell, Oxford
Berger H, Honig P, Liebman R 1977 Recurrent abdominal pain. American Journal of Diseases of Childhood 133: 486–490
Bingley E, Leonard J, Hensman S, Lask B, Wolff O 1980 Comprehensive care on a paediatric ward: — the family approach. Archives of Diseases in Childhood 55: 555–561
Bloom S, Edwards A, Vaughnan N 1973 The role of sympathetic innervation in the control of plasma glucagon concentrations in the calf. Journal of Physiology 233: 457–466
Bogdanoff M, Bogdanoff W, Wolf S 1961 Studies on salivary function in man. Journal of Psychosomatic Research 5: 170–174
Booth I, Harries J 1984 Inflammatory bowel disease in childhood. Gut 25: 188–202
British Medical Journal Leading Article 1980a How necessary are elimination diets in childhood? British Medical Journal 1: 138–139
British Medical Journal Leading Article 1980b Recurrent abdominal pain in childhood. British Medical Journal 1: 1096–1097
Brownell K, Stunkard A 1978 Behavioural therapy of obesity in children. American Journal of Diseases of Childhood 132: 403–412
Bruce T J R 1986 Emotional sequelae of chronic inflammatory bowel disease in children and adolescents. Clinical Gastroenterology 15: 89–104

Bruch H 1978 The golden cage: the enigma of anorexia nervosa. Open Books, London
Cann P, Read N, Brown C, et al 1983 Psychological stress and the passage of a standard meal in man. Gut 24: 236–240
Chaudhary N, Truelove S 1961 Human colonic motility: effect of emotions. Gastroenterology 40: 27–36
Chaudhary N, Truelove S 1962 The irritable colon syndrome. Quarterly Journal of Medicine 31: 307–322
Coddington R 1968 Peptic ulcer in children. Psychosomatics 9: 38–43
Crisp A 1980 Anorexia nervosa: let me be. Academic Press, London
Engel G, Reichsman F, Segal H 1956 A study of an infant with a gastric fistula. Psychosomatic Medicine 18: 374–398
Esler M, Goulston K 1973 Levels of anxiety in colonic disorders. New England Journal of Medicine 288: 16–20
Furman S 1973 Intestinal biofeedback in functional diarrhoea: a preliminary report. Journal of Behaviour Therapy and Experimental Psychiatry 44: 317–321
Furness J, Costa M 1974 The adrenergic innervation of the gastrointestinal tract. Ersebtich Physiologica 69: 1–51
Gore E 1976 Child psychiatry observed. Pergamon, Oxford
Grace W, Wolf S, Wolff H 1951 The human colon. Hoeber, New York
Goldson E, Milla P J, Bentovim A 1985 Failure to thrive: a transactional issue. Family Systems Medicine 3: 205–212
Granata L, Leone D, Paccione F 1973 Changes in jejunal motility during emotional reaction. Archives of Science and Biology 57: 87–97
Hersov L 1977 Faecal soiling in child psychiatry. Rutter M, Hersov L (eds) Blackwell, Oxford
Lask B 1982a Family Therapy in paediatric settings. In: Bentovim A, Gorell-Barnes J, Cooklin A (eds) Family Therapy. Academic Press, London
Lask B 1982b The child in the family. In: Apley J, Ounsted C (eds) One Child. S.I.M.P., London
Lask B, Bryant R 1986 Childhood onset anorexia nervosa. In: Meadow R (ed) Recent Advances in Paediatrics 8. Churchill Livingstone, London
Lipowski Z, Lipsitt D, Whybrown P 1977 Psychosomatic medicine. Oxford University Press, New York
MacDonald A, Bouchier I 1980 Non-organic gastrointestinal illness: a medical and psychiatric study. British Journal of Psychiatry 136: 276–283
McDermott J, Finch S 1967 Ulcerative colitis in children. Journal of the American Academy of Child Psychiatry 6:512
Minuchin S, Rosman B, Baker L 1978 Psychosomatic families. Anorexia nervosa in context. Harvard University Press
Prugh D 1983 The psychosocial aspects of paediatrics. Lea and Fediger, Philadelphia
Shuster M 1974 Operant conditioning in gastrointestinal dysfunctions. Hospital Practice 9:135
Silverstone T, Russell G 1967 Gastric "hunger" contractions in anorexia nervosa. British Journal of Psychiatry 113: 257–263
Slade P, Russell G 1973 Awareness of body dimensions in anorexia nervosa. Psychological Medicine 3: 188–189
Stickler G, Murphy D 1979 Recurrent abdominal pain. American Journal of Diseases of Children 131: 1340–134
Thompson D, Richelson E, Malagelada J-R 1983 Perturbation of upper gastrointestinal function by cold stress. Gut 24: 277–283
Warner J, Hathaway M 1984 Allergic form of Meadow's Syndrome (Munchausen by proxy). Archives of Disease in Childhood 59: 151–156
Wingate D, McRae S, Younger K, Thompson D 1982 Stress and jejunal motor activity. Gut 23: 404–409
Wolf S 1981 The psyche and the stomach. Gastroenterology 80: 605–614
Wolf S G, Almy T P 1949 Experimental observations on cardiospasm in man. Gastroenterology 13: 401–421
Wolf S, Wolff H G 1947 Human gastric function: an experimental study of a man and his stomach. 2nd edn. Oxford University Press, New York

Gut hormones and the adaptation to extrauterine nutrition

ADAPTATION TO EXTRAUTERINE NUTRITION

The newborn infant's adaptation to extrauterine nutrition involves major physiological changes, which are at least as complex in nature as the more obvious events that occur in the cardiovascular and respiratory system after birth.

The principal objective of this chapter is to examine the possible role of gastrointestinal hormones, released by enteral feeding, in stimulating adaptations to extrauterine nutrition. Other factors, including hormones outside the gut and hormones present in human milk, may also play a role and these will be considered briefly.

A body of data from experimental animals suggests that hormones from outside the gut, notably cortisol and thyroxin, influence gastrointestinal development (Lebenthal & Lee 1983). Administration of these two hormones results in gut mucosal development and increased brush border enzyme activities, and of interest in this context are the recent findings (Lucas et al, unpublished) that the type of diet employed in preterm infants influences the rate of postnatal elevation of circulating triiodothyronine concentrations.

Another potential set of factors that might influence postnatal development is the range of hormones present in human milk (Starkey & Orth 1977, Lucas & Mitchell 1980, Sack 1980, Werner et al 1982). Some hormones are present in milk, have high concentrations and appear to be secreted against concentration gradients. Calcitonin levels in milk are 20–90 times higher than the slightly raised maternal concentrations found in pregnancy and lactation (Werner et al 1982). Similar maternal serum-to-milk gradients have been shown for epidermal growth factor (Starkey & Orth 1977) and luteinizing hormone release hormone (LHRH). Concentrations of prostaglandins E and F are present at over 100 times the maternal plasma concentration (Lucas & Mitchell 1980). Mammary hormone secretion appears to be selective: in one study, calcitonin and neurotensin were measured simultaneously in maternal milk and plasma, and whereas levels of calcitonin in milk greatly exceeded those in plasma, the reverse was true for neurotensin (Werner et al 1982). The important question is whether these exogenous factors could influence postnatal adaptation. It is possible that protease inhibitors in milk may enhance the survival of peptide hormones in the gut for long enough to permit biological activity. Theoretically, ingested hormones could exert their effects 'topically' on the gut or systemically following absorption. Adrenocorticotrophic hormone (ACTH) and thyroid-stimulating (thyrotophic) hormone (TSH) have been shown to be absorbed from the gut in suckling rats, and to retain their physiological activity in terms of stimulating corticosterone and thyroxin release (Koldovsky et al 1980). Moreover, it is known that prostaglandins may be absorbed from the gut in human neonates with retention of biological activity. It is of note in this context that cortisol, thyroxin and prostaglandins have all been implicated in the development of the gastrointestinal tract (Giuraldes 1981, Vaucher et al 1982, Neu 1982). Furthermore, epidermal growth factor has been shown to produce hyperplasia of the gastrointestinal mucosa and pancreas (Dembinski et al 1982) and to stimulate ornithine decarboxylase activity in the stomach and duodenum in 8-day-old mice (Feldman et al 1978). The presence of hormones in breast-milk thus raises the interesting possibility that a mother may exert regulatory effects on the physiology of her progeny beyond the period of fetal development.

GUT HORMONES AND POSTNATAL ADAPTATION

Physiology of gut hormones: overview

The study of gut endocrinology started in 1902 with the discovery of the first hormone, secretin, by Bayliss and Starling. Gastrin was described shortly afterwards in 1905. Yet subsequent definition of the numerous peptides now isolated from the gut has proceeded slowly, largely because the gut is a 'diffuse' endocrine system defying the standard experimental

Table 14.1 Actions and distribution of hormones in the gut

Hormone	Principal location	Physiology
Gastrin	Antrum	Acid secretion, mucosal growth, gastric motility
Secretin	Duodenum	Pancreatic bicarbonate
CCK (cholecystokinin)	Jejunum	Gall bladder contraction stimulates pancreatic enzyme secretion
Motilin	Jejunum	GI motor activity
GIP (gastric inhibitory peptide)	Jejunum	Insulin release
Neurotensin	Ileum	Control of GI motility and secretion
Enteroglucagon	Ileum	Mucosal growth, inhibition of transit
PP (pancreatic polypeptide)	Pancreas	Inhibition of gall bladder and pancreatic enzymes

(Modified after S. R. Bloom, with permission)

endocrinological techniques of gland ablation and transplantation. The advent of radioimmunoassays and immunocytochemistry, together with advances in protein chemistry, has permitted localization and characterization of these peptides, together with their measurement in tissues and plasma in minute concentrations. Furthermore, the development and availability of cheap synthetic peptides that can be used for infusion in animals and man has permitted detailed study of gut hormone physiology in vivo.

In more recent years it has become apparent that the gut is a highly complex endocrine organ and the list of peptides secreted continues to increase. However, the accepted term 'gut hormones' used to describe these peptides is misleading: firstly, many of these peptides are not 'hormones' in the usual sense but are believed to be active locally ('paracrines') or are located in neurones and act as neurotransmitters; secondly, several 'gut' peptides are widely distributed in other organs, notably the brain. Eight peptides released from the gut are now thought to act as true circulating hormones: the locations of the endocrine cell lines secreting them and their known or proposed physiological actions are shown in Table 14.1. Other peptides (for review see Bloom & Polak 1981) are localized in both neural tissue and endocrine cells in the gut and may be found throughout the body in an extensive nonadrenergic, noncholinergic autonomic nervous system, the more prevalent components being neurones containing vasoactive intestinal peptide (VIP) and substance P (Bloom & Polak 1981). The investigation of the physiology of circulating hormones secreted by the gut has been easier than that of peptides acting as paracrines and neurotransmitters. They have been studied most in man and are those considered in this chapter.

Hypothesis: role of gut peptides in postnatal adaptation

It has been suggested that enteral feeding may trigger adaptations to postnatal feeding, at least in part, through the mediation of gut peptides. This hypothesis is shown diagramatically opposite:

Enteral feeding
↓
Gut hormone secretion
↓
Postnatal adaptive events
↓
including:
Gut growth
Changes in gut motility
Development of intestinal secretion
  and transport mechanisms
Initiation of the enteroinsular axis
Modulation of pancreatic endocrine function
Development of hepatic metabolism

The validation of this hypothesis requires a number of conditions to be met: the gut endocrine cell lines for these peptides should be present in the fetus; postnatally, gut hormones should be released by enteral feeding and not released in neonates deprived of nutrition by this route; gut peptide receptors should be responsive in the neonatal period; there should be a temporal relationship between postnatal gut hormone secretion and the adaptive changes proposed to be influenced by them; and finally there should be direct experimental evidence that either inhibition of endogenous hormone release or exogenous hormone administration would inhibit or induce respectively their proposed actions. This area of gut peptide physiology is a recent development and data required to support the above conditions are incomplete; therefore the role of gut peptides in the adaptation to extrauterine nutrition is speculative, although the body of data considered in the following sections is strongly supportive of such a role.

Gut hormones in the fetus

Regulatory peptides, together with their corresponding cell lines, have been identified in the human fetal gut from 6–16 weeks post-conception (Larsson & Jorgensen 1978, Chayvialle et al 1979, Lehy & Christina 1979, Buchan et al 1981). For most peptides examined, gut tissue concentrations rise to values found in the last 10 weeks of gestation, which are at least as high as those seen in adults (Buchan et al 1981), and since the gut is relatively large in the perinatal period, this may indicate a correspondingly larger gut endocrine cell mass for some lines in this period of development. There is a changing spectrum of molecular forms during fetal life and, indeed, certain peptides appear and disappear from different regions of the gut during development.

Recently, Aynsley Green and coworkers (reviewed by Aynsley Green 1985) obtained samples of fetal umbilical arterial and venous blood, maternal venous blood and amniotic fluid by fetoscopy prior to therapeutic termination of pregnancy at 18–21 weeks gestation in conscious, sedated mothers.

They found that concentrations of some hormones, e.g. gastrin and pancreatic peptide were greater in the maternal than the fetal circulation, whereas the reverse was the case for enteroglucagon and gastric inhibitory polypeptide (GIP). There was no significant difference between the maternal and fetal concentrations of glucagon.

Data from these fetal studies therefore satisfy the condition considered in the previous section that the gut endocrine system is well developed before birth, even if this occurs preterm. In addition, new questions are raised concerning the role of gut hormones in the fetus: in some instances these peptides are present in high circulating and tissue concentrations and their potential role in the ontogenesis of the fetal gut requires exploration, as does the possibility that gut peptides present in amniotic fluid might exert a direct 'topical' effect on the fetal gut and, perhaps, the fetal lung.

Gut peptide secretion at birth

Gastrointestinal peptides are found in significant concentrations in venous cord blood at birth at normal vaginal delivery as shown in Table 14.2. Most of the measured hormone concentrations at birth are similar to those seen in healthy fasting adults (see Fig. 14.1 for comparison), but it is of note that the concentrations of gastrin and vasoactive intestinal peptide (Lucas et al 1980b, 1982b) are significantly higher than fasting adult values. Hypergastrinaemia at birth has been reported also by Euler et al (1977), who suggested that gastrin might be released by vagal stimuli at delivery. This accords with the observation that plasma gastrin concentrations fall sharply towards fasting adult levels in the early hours postnatally, prior to the commencement of enteral feeding (Lucas et al 1980b, Aynsley Green et al 1977). These observations, which suggest gut peptide-releasing

Table 14.2 Enteroinsular hormone concentrations in venous cord plasma from normal deliveries compared with those from infants showing fetal distress (mean ± SEM)

Hormone	Normal Deliveries n = 20	Fetal Distress n = 8	P[1]
Motilin	34 ± 4	127 ± 24	<0.001
GIP	10 ± 2	28 ± 6	<0.01
Pancreatic polypeptide	13 ± 3	44 ± 10	<0.01
Pancreatic glucagon	4 ± 2	14 ± 4	<0.05
Neurotensin	33 ± 3	48 ± 4	<0.01
Enteroglucagon	77 ± 5	107 ± 10	<0.05
Gastrin	42 ± 5	39 ± 3	NS
Secretin	6 ± 1	5 ± 1	NS

[1] Mann Whitney rank sum test: NS = not significant

mechanisms may operate at birth, are further supported by the finding (see Table 14.2) that full term infants born following fetal distress show a selective venous cord plasma elevation of motilin, GIP, pancreatic polypeptide (PP), pancreatic glucagon, neurotensin and enteroglucagon (Lucas et al 1979). The rise in plasma motilin in fetal distress was especially marked (fivefold increase over values obtained in normal deliveries). It has been speculated that the release of motilin in fetal distress might account for the passage of meconium in this condition and that the failure of distressed preterm infants to pass meconium might relate in part to the lower concentrations of circulating motilin found at low gestational age.

Gut hormones and infant feeding

Rogers et al (1974) showed that gastrin and enteroglucagon increase in the plasma of human neonates during the first four days. That the early postnatal elevations in gastrin might be due to enteral feeding was shown by Lichtenberger & Johnson (1977) in neonatal rats and by Von Berger et al (1976) who found that this peptide rose in the plasma after the first feed in the human neonate. Aynsley Green et al (1977) examined the effects of the first feed of human milk in full term infants on several circulating peptides and noted a postprandial elevation in plasma gastrin, enteroglucagon and insulin, but not in GIP or pancreatic glucagon. All these changes except for the rise in enteroglucagon occurred after a first feed of 10% dextrose (Aynsley Green et al 1979). The lack of GIP response to the first feed accords with the findings of King et al (1977) who failed to identify an enteroinsular axis in the immediate postpartum period (vide infra). The absent response for pancreatic glucagon at the time of the first feed supports the view that the glucagon surge after birth (Sperling 1982), which is important in the initiation of glycogenolysis and gluconeogenesis, is likely to be independent of enteral feeding. Indeed, arguing teleologically, it makes good 'biological sense' for the newborn infant to achieve rapid regulation of blood glucose immediately after birth independently of the precise timing of the initiation of enteral feeding and to ensure that feeding at this stage does not diminish this glycaemic response by enhancing insulin release via the enteroinsular axis.

More recently, multiple gut hormonal surges in both term and preterm neonates have been discovered (Lucas et al 1980a, 1980b, 1980f). Figure 14.1 illustrates the time course of these postnatal hormonal surges during the first 24 days after birth in healthy preterm infants receiving enteral human milk feeds as intragastric boluses via a nasogastric tube. Plasma concentrations of motilin, GIP, enteroglucagon and PP all rose significantly above adult values. Plasma gastrin concentrations, which were raised briefly above the fasting adult level at birth, subsequently fell to adult values before the first feed at 2–6 hours of age (not shown on graph) and then increased fivefold to a peak on the sixth day.

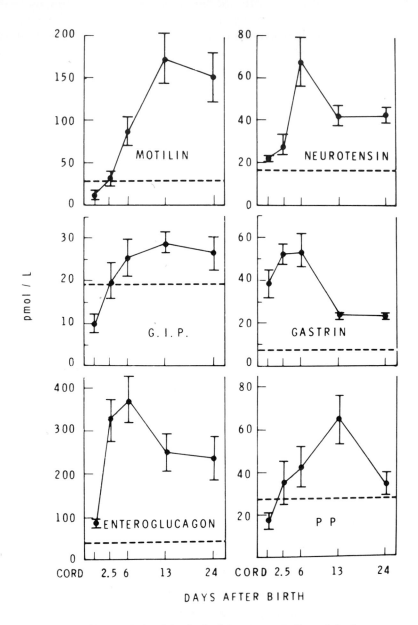

Fig. 14.1 Postnatal surges in basal (prefeed) plasma concentrations of gut hormones (pmol/l ± SEM) in preterm infants (mean gestation 33.5 weeks, birthweight 1950 g) at birth (cord blood, n = 6), 2.5 days (n = 8), 6 days (n = 10), 13 days (n = 12) and 24 days (n = 8). Cross-sectional data analysis, each infant contributing to one datum point only. Broken lines show mean adult fasting values. GIP: gastric inhibitory peptide; PP: pancreatic polypeptide.

In addition to the rise in basal hormonal concentrations, there are also progressive changes during the postnatal period in preterm infants in the effect of a feed on plasma concentrations of motilin, neurotensin, GIP, enteroglucagon, gastrin and secretin. In the early neonatal period responses to a feed are small or absent, whereas by 24 days the responses are marked. These changes are reported in detail elsewhere (Lucas et al 1980c, Lucas et al 1980f). The potential biological significance of the development of a GIP response to feeding in terms of the establishment of an enteroinsular axis is discussed below.

More limited data from term breastfed infants show that significant postnatal hormonal surges do occur but are smaller than those seen in preterm infants (Lucas et al 1982a). This difference might be explained by the fact that lactation takes some days to become established in breastfed infants and the fact that enteral feed volumes are smaller on a weight basis in term infants than those used for preterm neonates. However the rather more exaggerated postnatal gut peptide elevations in the preterm group require further exploration.

Possible biological effects of postnatal gut peptide secretion

Studies in animals and adult man demonstrate that gut hormones can induce some of the changes that are known to occur after birth in normally fed neonates. Thus, gastrin (Johnson 1976, 1977) and enteroglucagon (Gleeson et al 1971, Besterman et al 1978a, 1978b) may stimulate growth of the gastrointestinal mucosa, whereas cholecystokinin (Mainz et al 1973), pancreatic polypeptide (Greenberg et al 1977) and gastrin (Mayston & Barrowman 1971) may stimulate growth of the exocrine pancreas. It has been shown in neonatal rats (Lichtenberger & Johnson 1977) that feeding results in a rise in plasma gastrin which parallels the trophic changes in the gut induced by feeding.

It is tempting to speculate that the multiple hormonal surges which occur in human neonates might induce a variety of adaptive changes following the onset of enteral feeding. For example, motilin is thought to stimulate gastrointestinal motility (Ruppin et al 1976) and gastric emptying in adults. It is possible that the postnatal elevation in plasma motilin could contribute to the known increase in efficiency of gut motility that occurs during the neonatal period (Smith 1976). The rise in plasma enteroglucagon, gastrin and PP may be important factors in the increase in gut and pancreatic growth that occurs in enterally fed neonates. GIP may be the principal stimulus to insulin release via the enteroinsular axis (Dupre et al 1973, Creutzfeldt 1979, Lucas et al 1980d), a term coined to describe the transmission of signals from gut to pancreas. The presence of this axis explains the greater insulin response (described first in adults) to oral as opposed to intravenous glucose. Thus the postnatal surge in the basal GIP concentration, together with the development of the ability to elevate GIP even further following a feed, may result in the progressive enhancement of insulin release (Lowy & Schiff 1968) and glucose tolerance (Nakai et al 1976) described in the neonatal period.

Hormonal effects of deprivation of human neonates of enteral feeding

If the hypothesis is valid that enteral feeding is responsible for the postnatal gut hormone surges described above, then it would be predicted that infants deprived of enteral feeding should show no elevation in circulating gut hormones after birth; this is, indeed, the case. In a group of 10 preterm infants who, because of hyaline membrane disease received only intravenous fluids for the first six days after birth, there was no postnatal rise (above the cord blood level) during this period in the plasma concentrations of motilin, gastrin, enteroglucagon, GIP or neurotensin (Lucas et al 1983).

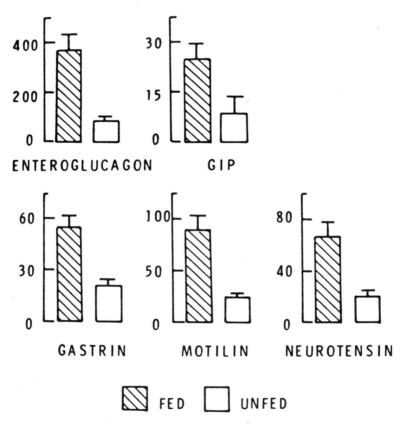

Fig. 14.2 Basal plasma concentrations of gut hormones (pmol/l ± SEM) on the sixth day in preterm infants who have been enterally fed since birth compared with those who, because of hyaline membrane disease, had been deprived of enteral feeding since birth and maintained on intravenous dextrose.

In contrast, levels of all these hormones increased markedly by the sixth day in preterm infants who had been fed orally (Fig. 14.2). Although the presence of hyaline membrane disease in the unfed group complicates the interpretation of the results, the study provides suggestive evidence that enteral feeding is likely to be the triggering mechanism for the gut hormone surges seen after birth. This is supported by unpublished data (Lucas et al) showing that gut hormone surges are delayed if enteral feeds are withheld for six to ten days.

Effects of route and nature of the diet on gut hormone secretion

There is considerable controversy over the most suitable type of enteral feed for preterm infants, and the route by which it should be given. With respect to the latter point, it should be noted that the data presented above apply largely to low birthweight infants who were fed with a bolus of milk given every three hours by syringe infusion over about five minutes into a nasogastric tube. Current feeding practices vary considerably: some authors recommend that nasogastric bolus feeds be instilled by gravity (rather than syringe infusion); such feeds may take 20 minutes or more to complete. In sick neonates especially, continuous intragastric infusion feeds are sometimes used, and other centres elect to feed transpylorically, bypassing the stomach. Most units do not encourage nonnutritive sucking during feeds, yet Bernbaum et al. (1983) have noted changes in gut motility and growth rates when the infant sucks on a pacifier during feeds. It is likely to be some time before the impact of these feeding practices on endocrine development is disentangled, but the recent findings of Aynsley Green et al (1982) suggest that whether an infant is fed by continuous intragastric infusion or by intermittent intragastric boluses over the first 13 days may influence the postnatal changes in some peptides: thus whereas there was little difference in the postnatal surges of motilin, neurotensin and enteroglucagon between the two groups, preprandial circulating concentrations of GIP, insulin and gastrin were lower at 13 days in the bolus fed group than those fed by intragastric infusion. In addition it should be noted that infants fed by intragastric infusion will have a relatively constant metabolic and endocrine milieu, whereas bolus fed infants will develop dynamic feeding responses. The latter type of response is arguably more 'physiological', at least for term infants, but it has never been established whether dynamic, feed-related changes in metabolism carry any benefits, for instance in terms of efficiency of utilization of nutrients.

Patterns of gut endocrine release also may be influenced by the mode of diet. In preterm infants, Calvert et al (unpublished) showed only minor effects on preprandial plasma gut hormone concentrations according to whether they were fed on a special preterm infant formula or human milk; small differences were observed in the secretion of GIP and PP. However, much greater differences have been observed in full term infants according

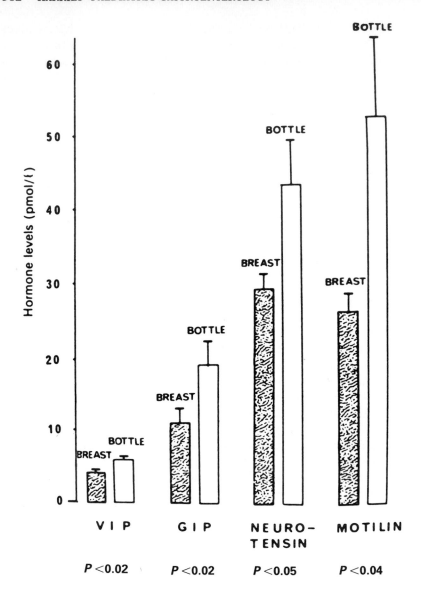

Fig. 14.3 Basal levels of gastric inhibitory peptide (GIP), vasoactive intestinal peptide (VIP), motilin and neurotensin in breast-fed (shaded bars) and bottle-fed (open bars) term infants on the sixth postnatal day (mean ± SEM).

to whether they were fed on a standard 'humanized' cow's milk-based formula or by breast (Lucas et al 1980e). Six-day-old breastfed and formula-fed infants differ markedly, not only in their basal circulating concentrations of several gut peptides (VIP, GIP, motilin, and neurotensin) (Fig. 14.3), but also in their dynamic hormonal responses to feeding, notably with respect to the release of insulin, motilin, neurotensin, entero-glucagon and PP. It has been speculated that these findings may account for differences in bowel motility patterns and subcutaneous fat deposition between breastfed and bottlefed infants. In a cohort study of 12–18-year-old adolescents, Kramer (1981) reported that breast feeding may protect against later obesity. This work raises the possibility that early dietary experience could influence the 'programming' of later metabolism. If such biochemical programming occurs, then it would be of considerable interest to investigate whether or not early differences in hormonal responses to feeding between breast and bottlefed infants could have persisting metabolic consequences. The hormonal differences between breast- and formula-fed infants had largely disappeared by 9 months of age (Aynsley Green 1984).

CLINICAL IMPLICATIONS: A CASE FOR ENTERAL FEEDING IN HIGH RISK NEONATES

Sick and low birthweight infants may be deprived of enteral feeding as part of their routine management. Such practices need to be reappraised in the light of our current knowledge of the physiology of postnatal adaptation. In many centres, for instance, infants of very low birthweight are fed routinely by the intravenous route during the early weeks of postnatal life: this policy has been defended partly on the grounds that this is the route by which the infant would have been fed had it remained in utero. Total parenteral nutrition (TPN) in this situation might be criticized on several grounds, for example, its potential for inducing serious metabolic compli-cations, the hazards of central venous lines, its expense, the need for inten-sive monitoring and the lack of protective effect against infection (compared with breast milk). A more biological objection however, would be that TPN may preclude possible beneficial effects of enteral feeding in terms of stimu-lating adaptation of the gut and intermediary metabolism to extrauterine nutrition. Experimental deprivation of enteral feeding is known to result in delay of gut development (Stoddart & Widdowson 1976).

Furthermore, in animal studies (reviewed by Hughes 1984) TPN results in rapid changes in the gut (within three days), which include marked mucosal atrophy, decrease in brush border enzyme activities and reduction of absorbtive surface as evidenced by diminished xylose absorption; indeed, xylose absorption is reduced also in TPN-fed human neonates.

In practice, after short periods of TPN, enteral feeds are usually tolerated within a few days. This accords with animal data showing reversal of TPN-induced changes by luminal nutrients (reviewed by Hughes 1984), and with the observation that enteral feeding in preterm infants, who have been deprived totally of this mode of nutrition for up to 10 days following delivery, is followed by gut hormone surges of normal magnitude. However in certain circumstances, for instance in extreme immaturity, and in

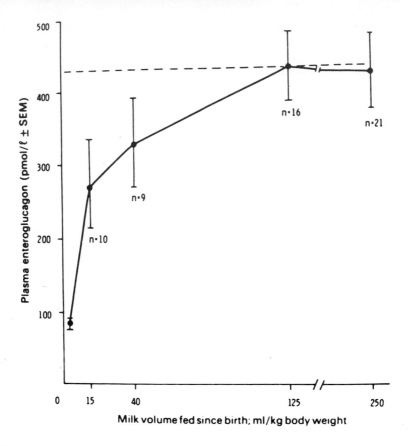

Fig. 14.4 Relationship between plasma enteroglucagon concentrations (pmol/l ± SEM) and the volume of milk consumed since birth (ml/kg body weight) in preterm infants. Rise after 15 ml/kg: $P < 0.001$.

particular, following surgery for congenital abnormalities of the gut, it may be necessary to employ TPN for prolonged periods from birth. Of some concern is the possibility that such a practice might have pathophysiological effects on the gut, other organs and perhaps intermediary metabolism. It is relevant to note in this context that by the end of the third trimester the fetus is swallowing amniotic fluid at the same 24 hour volume intake rate as that seen in a breast fed neonate; moreover, the daily enteral protein intake in the fetus is at least 25% of that provided by breast milk in the neonatal period (Friis Hansen 1982, Abbas & Tovey 1960). The possibility that prenatal enteral nutrition is important for maintaining the development of the gut in utero is being investigated currently by several groups: a naturally occurring human model for such research is the fetus with a high congenital block in the gut (duodenal atresia or oesophageal atresia without a fistula), in whom the intestine will not have received luminal nutrition during its development. If enteral nutrition in the fetus is shown to be of developmental significance for the gut, then the institution of TPN after birth could be regarded developmentally as a retrogressive step.

Recent data suggest a possible therapeutic solution. In some situations the infant undergoing TPN may be able to tolerate tiny quantities of enteral feed concomitantly. It is speculated that such 'minimal enteral feeding' might have a valuable biological role. Preliminary studies indicate that postnatal surges of some gastrointestinal hormones may be induced by surprisingly small quantities of intraluminal food. In Figure 14.4 the plasma concentration of enteroglucagon (which is thought to be trophic to the gut mucosa) is shown in relation to the total volume of milk (per kg body weight) consumed by the infant since birth. Within the range of intakes shown, enteroglucagon concentration was strongly correlated with postnatal milk intake and there was no correlation between enteroglucagon concentration and postnatal age. Figure 14.4 illustrates that a mean of only 15 ml of human milk per kg body weight is associated with a threefold rise from the 'unfed' enteroglucagon level. This would correspond, in a very low birthweight infant, to an intake of 1 ml of milk per hour for less than 24 hours. After a mean of 125 ml/kg has been consumed, a maximal enteroglucagon response is seen. These results indicate that subnutritional quantities of food may exert a potent effect on gastrointestinal hormone release. The quantity and quality of enteral feeding needed to ameliorate the hypotrophic effects of parenteral nutrition in newborn infants requires detailed investigation. Animal studies (reviewed by Hughes 1984) indicate, for instance, that intraluminal long chain triglycerides may have a potent effect in partially preventing TPN-induced changes in the gut, and this observation is of interest in view of the major effect of these lipids in stimulating enteroglucagon release. Thus, the possibility is raised that enteral nutrients may be used as a 'drug' in neonatal intensive care to achieve a biological rather than a nutritional effect.

REFERENCES

Abbas T M, Tovey J E 1960 Proteins of the Liquor Amnii. British Medical Journal
  i: 476–479
Aynsley Green A 1985 Metabolic and endocrine interrelations in the human fetus and
  neonate. Am J Clin Nutr 41: 399–418
Aynsley Green A, Bloom S R, Williamson D H, Turner R C 1977 Endocrine and metabolic
  response in the human newborn to the first feed on breast milk. Archives of Disease in
  Childhood 52: 291–295
Aynsley Green A, Lucas A, Bloom S R 1979 The effect of feeds of differing composition
  on entero-insular hormone secretion in the first hours of life in human neonates. Acta
  Paediatrica Scandinavica 68: 265–270
Aynsley Green A, Adrian T E, Bloom S R 1982 Feeding and the development of
  enteroinsular hormone release in the preterm infant: effects of continuous gastric infusion
  of human milk compared with intermittent boluses. Acta Paediatrica Scandinavica
  71: 379–383
Bernbaum J C, Pereira G R, Watkins J B, Peckham G J 1983 Non-nutritive sucking during

gavage feeding enhances growth and maturation in premature infants. Pediatrics
71: 41–45

Besterman H S, Bloom S R, Adrian T E, Cristofides N D, Sarson D L, Mallinson C N,
Pero A, Modigliani R 1978a Gut hormone profile after gut resection. Gut 19:A972

Besterman H S, Sarson D L, Blackburn A M, Cleary J, Pilkington T R, Bloom S R 1978b
The gut hormone profile in morbid obesity and following jejuno-ileal bypass.
Scandinavian Journal of Gastroenterology 13 Supplement 49:15

Bloom S R, Polak J M 1981 Gut Hormones. Churchill Livingstone, Edinburgh

Buchan A M J, Bryant M G, Polak J M, Gregor M, Ghatei M A, Bloom S R 1981
Development of regulatory peptides in the human fetal intestine. In: Bloom S R, Polak
J M (eds) Gut Hormones. Churchill Livingstone, London. pp 119–126

Chayvialle J A, Paulin C, Dubois P M, Descos F 1979 Immunoreactive somatostatin in the
digestive tract of the human fetus. Gastroenterology 76:1112

Creutzfeldt W 1979 The incretin concept today. Diabetologia. 16: 75–85

Dembinski A, Gregory M, Konturek S J, Polanski M 1982 Trophic action of epidermal
growth factor on the pancreas and gastroduodenal mucosa in rats. In: Robinson J W L,
Dowling R H, Reiken E O (eds) Mechanisms of Intestinal Adaptation. MTP Press,
Lancaster. pp 281–284

Dupre J, Ross S A, Watson D, Brown J C 1973 Stimulation of insulin secretion by gastric
inhibitory polypeptide in man. Journal of Clinical Endocrinology and Metabolism
37: 826–828

Euler A R, Bryne W J, Cousins L M, Ament M E, Leake R D, Walsh J D 1977 Increased
serum gastrin concentrations and gastric acid hyposecretion in the immediate newborn
period. Gastroenterology 72: 1271–1273

Feldman E J, Aures D, Grossman R I 1978 Epidermal growth factor stimulates ornithine
decarboxylase activity in the digestive tract of the mouse. Proceedings of the Society for
Experimental Biology and Medicine 159: 400–402

Friis-Hansen B 1982 Body water metabolism in early infancy. Acta Paediatrica Scandinavica.
Supplement 296: 44–48

Giuraldes E 1981 The effect of cortisone on postnatal development of ion transport in
rabbit small intestine. Pediatric Research 16: 1530–1532

Gleeson M H, Bloom S R, Polak J M, Henry K, Dowling R M 1971 An endocrine tumour
in kidney affecting small bowel structure, motility and absorptive function. Gut
12: 773–782

Greenberg G R, Mitznegg P, Bloom S R 1977 Effect of pancreatic polypeptide on DNA
synthesis in the pancreas. Experientia 33: 1332–1333

Hughes C A 1984 Intestinal adaptation. In: Tanner M S, Stocks R J (eds) Neonatal
Gastroenterology. Intercept Ltd, Newcastle upon Tyne. pp 69–91

Johnson L R 1976 The trophic action of gastrointestinal hormones. Gastroenterology
70: 278–288

Johnson L R 1977 New aspects of the trophic action of gastrointestinal hormones.
Gastroenterology 72: 788–792

King K C, Schwartz R, Yamaguchi K, Adam P J 1977 Lack of gastrointestinal
enhancement of the insulin response to glucose in newborn infants. Journal of Pediatrics
91:783

Koldovsky O, Vaucher Y, Gasparo M, Auteri A, Tenore A, Parks J, Orth D 1980 TSH
and ACTH are present in rats milk: they retain physiological activity when given
perorally to sucking rats. Pediatric Research 14:502, A.462

Kramer M S 1981 Do breast feeding and delayed introduction of solid foods protect against
subsequent obesity? Journal of Pediatrics 98: 883–887

Larsson L-I, Jorgensen L M 1978 Ultrastructural and cytochemical studies on the
cytodifferentiation of duodenal endocrine cells. Cell and Tissue Research 194: 79–102

Lebenthal E, Lee P C 1983 Interaction of determinants in the ontogeny of the
gastrointestinal tract: a unified concept. Pediatric Research 17: 19–24

Lehy T, Christina M L 1979 Ontogeny and distribution of certain cells in the human
fetal large intestine. Cell and Tissue Research. 203: 415–426

Lichtenberger L, Johnson L R 1977 Gastrin in the ontogenic development of the small
intestine. American Journal of Physiology 227(2): 390–395

Lowy C, Schiff D 1968 Urinary excretion of insulin in the healthy newborn. Lancet
i: 225–227

Lucas A, Mitchell M D 1980 Prostaglandins in human milk. Archives of Disease in Childhood 55: 950–952

Lucas A, Adrian T E, Aynsley Green A, Bloom S R 1979 Gut hormones in fetal distress. Lancet ii:968

Lucas A, Adrian T E, Bloom S R, Aynsley Green A 1980a Plasma pancreatic polypeptide in the human neonate. Acta Paediatrica Scandinavica 69: 211–214

Lucas A, Adrian T E, Christofides N D, Bloom S R, Aynsley Green A 1980b Plasma motilin, gastrin and enteroglucagon and feeding in the human newborn. Archives of Disease in Childhood 55: 673–677

Lucas A, Adrian T E, Bloom S R, Aynsley Green A 1980c Plasma secretin in neonates. Acta Paediatrica Scandinavica 69: 205–210

Lucas A, Sarson D L, Bloom S R, Aynsley Green A 1980d Developmental aspects of gastric inhibitory polypeptide and its possible role in the enteroinsular axis in neonates. Acta Paediatrica Scandinavica 69: 321–325

Lucas A, Blackburn A M, Aynsley Green A, Sarson D L, Adrian T E, Bloom S R 1980e Breast vs bottle: endocrine responses are different with formula feeding. Lancet i: 1267–1269

Lucas A, Bloom S R, Aynsley Green A 1980f The development of gut hormone response to feeding in neonates. Archives of Disease in Childhood 55: 678–682

Lucas A, Bloom S R, Aynsley Green A 1982a Postnatal surges in plasma gut hormones in term and preterm infants. Biology of the Neonate 41: 63–67

Lucas A, Bloom S R, Aynsley Green A 1982b Vasoactive intestinal peptide (VIP) in preterm and term neonates. Acta Paediatrica Scandinavica 71: 71–74

Lucas A, Bloom S R, Aynsley Green A 1983 Metabolic and endocrine consequences of depriving preterm infants of enteral nutrition. Acta Paediatrica Scandinavica 72: 245–249

Mainz D L, Black O, Webster P D 1973 Hormonal control of pancreatic growth. Journal of Clinical Investigation 52:2300

Mayston P D, Barrowman J A 1971 The influence of chronic administration of pentagastrin on the rat pancreas. American Journal of Experimental Physiology 56: 113–122

Nakai T, Hayashi M, Kanazawa T, Sakamoto S 1976 Alterations of insulin-secreting response to glucose in human infants during the early postnatal period. Endocrinology Japan 23: 61–64

Neu J 1982 Prostaglandins alter growth and small intestinal development in the rat. Pediatric Research 16: 172A

Rogers I M, Davidson D C, Lawrence J, Ardill J, Buchanan K D 1974 Neonatal secretion of gastrin and glucagon. Archives of Disease in Childhood 49: 796–801

Ruppin H, Sturm G, Westhoff D, Domschke S, Domschke W, Wiinsch E, Demling L 1976 Effect of 13NLe motilin on small intestinal transit time healthy subjects. Scandinavian Journal of Gastroenterology (Supplement) 11(39): 85–88

Sack J 1980 Hormones in milk. In: A I Eidelman, S Frier (eds) Human Milk, its Biological and Social Value. Excerpta Medica, Amsterdam. pp 56–61

Smith C A 1976 Physiology of digestion.In: N M Nelson, C A Smith (eds) The Physiology of the Newborn Infant, Thomas, Springfield, Illinois. pp 259–279

Sperling M A 1982 Integration of fuel homeostasis by insulin and glucagon in the newborn. Monographs in Pediatrics 16: 39–58

Starkey R H, Orth D N 1977 Radioimmunoassay of human epidermal growth factor (urogastrone). Journal of Clinical Endocrinology and Metabolism 45: 1144–1153

Stoddart R W, Widdowson E M 1976 Changes in the organs of pigs in response to feeding for the first 24 hours after birth. III. Fluorescence histochemistry of carbohydrates of the intestine. Biology of the Neonate 29: 18–27

Vaucher Y, Anna J, Lindberg R, Bustamante S, Jorgensen E, Krulich L, Koldovsky O 1982 Maturational effect of tri-iodothyronine and its analogue on sucrase activity in the small intestine of the developing rat. Pediatric Research 16:181A

Von Berger L, Henrichs I, Raptis S et al 1976 Gastrin concentration in plasma of the neonate at birth and after the first feeding. Pediatrics 58: 264–267

Werner S, Widstro A-M, Wahlberg V, Eneroth P, Winberg J 1982 Immunoreactive calcitonin in maternal milk and serum in relation to prolactin and neurotensin. Early Human Development 6: 77–82

Acute infective diarrhoea and vomiting

PREDISPOSING FACTORS

Diarrhoeal disease, with or without vomiting, remains a major world health problem. The magnitude of the problem of acute infective diarrhoea and vomiting has been emphasized recently (Snyder & Merson 1982). An estimated 700–1000 million episodes of diarrhoea and 5 million deaths occurred in children under 5 years of age in the developing countries (excluding China) in 1980. This group of diarrhoeal diseases is therefore the leading cause of death in childhood. While deaths due to diarrhoea are uncommon in developed countries it ranks second only to respiratory diseases as an indication for admission to paediatric medical wards. In developing countries the highest incidence of diarrhoeal disease is during the second year of life when it coincides with the peak incidence of malnutrition. Thus both occur together and are related to the age of weaning; if weaning occurs earlier then the peak incidence of diarrhoea occurs earlier too. In contrast, in the developed world the peak incidence for diarrhoeal disease occurs during the first year of life. Mortality rates in European countries for children aged 0–5 years with acute diarrhoea range from 17 deaths per 100 000 live births in Denmark, and 56 per 100 000 in England and Wales, to 150 per 100 000 in Italy (Tripp et al 1977). The problem in underdeveloped countries is of such magnitude as to overwhelm the already overstretched health services. It is clear that overcrowding and contaminated drinking water play a major role in maintaining the enormity of this problem, however removal of these factors in developing countries is unlikely in the foreseeable future. Experience from developed countries shows that elimination of these factors alone will not eradicate the problem of diarrhoea, and other preventative strategies including campaigns to encourage breast feeding, infant welfare clinics, family planning advice and improved management, are required.

No satisfactory definition of diarrhoea is available. A frequently used definition of a diarrhoeal stool is one 'taking the shape of the container' but the normal stools of breast fed babies also fulfil this criterion. Accordingly, parental perception of increasing looseness and frequency of stool in the child may be taken to mean diarrhoea.

Appreciable morbidity occurs in children following the acute effects of the fluid and electrolyte losses associated with a diarrhoeal episode. The nutritional impact on the child may be measured by longitudinal studies of subsequent growth. Mata et al (1977) first highlighted the significant association between diarrhoeal episodes and growth failure compared to other infective illnesses. This association has recently been reaffirmed, and in particular linked with bacterial rather than viral diarrhoea (Black et al 1984). Since children in developing countries may expect to experience an attack of acute diarrhoea every four to six weeks, it becomes apparent that repeated bouts of acute diarrhoea will initiate a downward spiral of malnutrition, secondary immunodeficiency, repeated infections and death. This process will be accelerated by inappropriate nutritional management, or by protraction of the diarrhoea (see Ch. 16).

AETIOLOGY AND PATHOGENESIS

Recent advances in identification of bacteria and viruses allow for the identification of potential pathogens in the stools of up to 80% of children with diarrhoea, thus strongly supporting an infective aetiology. Development of specific treatment and preventative measures will depend on precise identification of the microorganism causing the acute gastrointestinal upset. Problems still remain, compounded by the simultaneous presence of more than one potential pathogen in the gastrointestinal tract of a particular child during an episode of diarrhoea. The importance of controlled studies was emphasized by Wadström et al (1976) who found potentially pathogenic bacteria and parasites in the stools of Ethiopian children with or without diarrhoea. A further potential difficulty with currently available data on microbial aetiology is that most are derived from hospital-based studies and few have included techniques to identify all known pathogens. Extensive community-based studies are urgently required in centres throughout the world to identify the seasonality, frequency and effects of the various agents capable of causing diarrhoeal disease.

Infecting agents

Table 15.1 lists the bacteria and viruses which have been implicated in acute diarrhoea in humans. The epidemiological data linking certain species of bacteria and virus with acute diarrhoea is variable and stool cultures need

Table 15.1 Bacteria and viruses implicated in acute infective diarrhoea and vomiting

Bacteria	Viruses
Vibrio cholerae	Parvovirus-like agents:
Escherichia coli	Norwalk agent
Salmonella sp.	Montgomery County agent
Shigella sp.	Hawaii agent
Campylobacter sp.	W agent
Clostridium perfringens	Ditchling agent
Clostridium difficile	Cockle agent
Staphylococcus aureus	Parramatta agent
Yersinia enterocolitica	
Aeromonas hydrophila	Reoviridiae:
Klebsiella sp.	Rotavirus
Enterobacter sp.	Astrovirus
Proteus sp.	
Citrobacter sp.	Picornaviruses:
Edwardsiella tarda	Calicivirus
Vibrio parahaemolyticus	Adenovirus
Bacillus cereus	
Pseudomonas aeruginosa	Coronaviruses
Plesiomonas shigelloides	

to be interpreted with caution: bacteria including *Klebsiella* sp, *Enterobacter* sp., *Proteus* sp., and *Pseudomonas* may be increased in diarrhoeal stools irrespective of aetiology (Gorbach et al 1971).

Amongst the protozoa capable of colonizing the gastrointestinal tract, *Giardia lamblia* can cause acute diarrhoea. It is generally acknowledged that extraintestinal infections, e.g. urinary tract infections, can also cause diarrhoea (so-called parenteral diarrhoea; Nelson 1979).

Pathogenesis of infective diarrhoea

The pathogenesis of infective diarrhoea is summarized in Figure 15.1. It is self-evident that increased frequency of ingestion of potential pathogens will lead to an increased attack rate. Provision of an abundant water supply free from pollution with faecal microorganisms would be likely to decrease diarrhoea in developing countries to the level of disease in developed countries. Breastfeeding is an important mechanism for the provision of passive immunization against enteric infection in small infants; the protective factors are listed in Table 15.2. By contrast, foods prepared under conditions of poor hygiene and left at ambient temperatures for prolonged periods before consumption are a fertile breeding ground for diarrhoeagenic bacteria.

The gastric acid barrier

Hydrochloric acid secreted by the normal stomach presents a formidable barrier to most microorganisms. A gastric pH of less than 4 is lethal to the

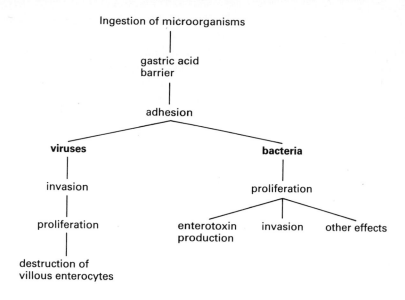

Fig. 15.1 Pathogenesis of infective diarrhoea

majority of microorganims ingested. The invasive bacteria, particularly *Shigella* and *Campylobacter* are relatively resistant to this defence mechanism, the infective dose being as low as 5 and 500 organisms respectively, compared with 10^9 and 10^{10} *Escherichia coli* or *Vibrio cholerae*. If gastric acidity is reduced by H_2-receptor blocking drugs, malnutrition or previous gastric surgical resection, for example, then this predisposes to gastrointestinal infection.

Bacterial colonization of the small intestine

Many pathogenic and nonpathogenic gram negative bacteria which survive transit through the stomach may avoid expulsion into the distal intestine by binding to the brush border of the mucosa using hairlike protein strands on the surface of bacteria, originally called fimbriae ('fringe') (Duguid et al 1955) and subsequently pili ('hair') (Brinton 1959). Those fimbriae whose adhesion phenomena are inhibited specifically by D-mannose are termed common, or type 1 fimbriae. The genetic information necessary for common fimbrial adhesion resides in the bacterial chromosome. By contrast, diarrhoeagen *Esch. coli* of humans and herd animals produce fimbriae whose species-specific adhesion to jejunal brush borders and erythrocytes is unaffected by D-mannose. These fimbriae are coded on extrachromosomal DNA called plasmids which are transmissible to other bacteria. Specific colonization fimbriae are essential virulence factors since loss of the ability to elaborate them, plasmid loss for example, results in complete loss of the ability to cause diarrhoea.

Whilst in the pig, lamb and calf only a few surface proteins are involved in binding strains of the organism to the brushborder, the situation in humans may be more complex. Two colonization factors (CFA/I and CFA/II) have been isolated in *Esch. coli* from humans with diarrhoea. CFA/I from serogroups 078, 025 and 063, and CFA/II with serogroups 06, 08 and 015 (Gaastra & De Graaf 1982). GFA/II exists as three antigenic variants, while the mechanisms by which human *Esch. coli* of other serogroups adhere to human brush borders remains to be elucidated.

One of the most important gut-associated immunological defence mechanisms is the ability to secrete IgA specifically directed against colonization factors. Once the IgA binds to colonization factors and the bacteria are inhibited from brush border adhesion, they can be expelled, without stimulation of an inflammatory reaction characterized by IgG and IgM responses. Hence colonization factors represent potential vaccines against bacterial diarrhoea (Levine et al 1983). Such protection may be passive, as in the vaccination of pregnant herd animals, with colonization factors, so that their sucklings receive breast milk containing specific anti-colonization factor antibodies. This confers a high degree of protection against diarrhoea induced by *Esch. coli* which produce colonization factors contained in the vaccine.

Protective effects of breast-feeding

Breast-feeding provides an extremely effective system of passive immunization against infectious diarrhoea by a variety of mechanisms (Table 15.2).

Table 15.2   Protective factors in breast milk against infective diarrhoea

Low bacterial count
IgA
Lactoferrin
Phagocytes
Lymphocytes
Enterotoxin receptor analogues
Antiviral factors

Breast milk contains IgA, specifically directed against maternal bowel flora, to which the nursing infant is likely to be exposed. The lactoferrin content of breast milk may limit growth of bacteria in the upper small intestine by competing for iron in the gut lumen with iron-binding proteins associated with bacteria. The macrophage, neutrophil and lymphocyte content of breast milk may also contribute. Antiviral factors have been described in breastmilk, while the predominance of bifidobacteria in the stools of breastfed infants may inhibit intestinal colonization with enteropathogens.

Enterotoxins. Having overcome the intestinal defence mechanism outlined above, certain genera of bacteria can cause diarrhoea by synthesizing proteins or peptides called enterotoxins which are capable of inhibiting

Table 15.3   Enterotoxins of *Vibrio cholerae* and *Escherichia coli* (After Sack 1980)

	Cholera toxin	LT	ST
Molecular weight (Mr)	84 000	73 000	5000
Subunits	5B (binding) A (active toxin)	5B A	None
Genetic control	Chromosomal	Plasmid	Plasmid
Brush border receptor	GM$_1$ ganglioside	GM$_1$ ganglioside	?
Biochemical action	Activation adenylate cylase	Activation adenylate cyclase	Activation guanylate cyclase
Effect on electrolyte secretion by small intestine	Delayed onset prolonged	Delayed onset prolonged	Rapid onset
Immunological properties	Related to LT	Related to cholera toxin	Weakly immunogenic
Assays	Animal models Cell culture Immunological Radiolabelled gene probe	Animal models Cell culture Immunological Radiolabelled gene probe	Animal models Radioimmunoassay Radiolabelled gene probe

LT = heat-labile enterotoxin of *Esch. coli*; ST = heat-stable enterotoxin of *Esch. coli*

small intestinal ion absorption or inducing ion secretion. The enterotoxins of *V. cholerae* and *Esch. coli* are the best characterized (Table 15.3). Cholera toxin and the heat-labile enterotoxin of *Esch. coli* (LT) are thought to induce intestinal secretion via elevation of mucosal cyclic adenosine monophosphate (cAMP) while the heat-stable enterotoxin (ST) of Esch. coli exploits cyclic guanosine monophosphate (cGMP) as its intracellular messenger (Guerrant 1985). Until recently, the detection of such enterotoxigenic bacteria has relied upon cumbersome bioassays, chinese hamster ovary for LT and the infant mouse assay for ST. Recently, simple Elisa assays for LT and radiolabelled gene hybridization for ST have been developed.

Pathophysiology of infecting agents

Bacteria

Enterotoxigenic bacteria. Enterotoxins from organisms other than *V. cholerae* and *Esch. coli* have been less extensively studied, but enterotoxins from staphylococci (O'Brien & Kapral 1976), *Bacillus cereus* (Stephen & Pietrowski 1981), salmonella (Stephen et al 1985) and *Campylobacter jejuni* (Ruiz-Palacios et al 1983) may elevate intestinal cAMP while a heat-stable enterotoxin of *Yersinia enterocolitica* and *Klebsiella* elevates cGMP (Rao et al 1979).

Enteropathogenic Esch. coli. Until recently enteropathogenic *Esch. coli* were implicated in infantile diarrhoea on epidemiological grounds. Specific lipoprotein somatic antigens (O serogroups) were isolated in diarrhoeal outbreaks but the mechanism of the intestinal secretion was unknown until recently. Enteropathogenic *Esch. coli* have been shown to induce a pathognomonic lesion of this intestinal brush border in humans and experimental animals. Ultrastructural studies have shown brush border destruction (effacement) and formation of 'pedestals' of bare plasma membrane to which the enteropathogenic *Esch. coli* become attached (Rothbaum et al 1982). The changes are seen throughout the gastrointestinal tract of colonized infants. The microbial determinants mediating this specific mode of attachment and enterocyte/colonocyte damage are not known, but it is likely that a plasmid is involved (Baldini et al 1983). More recently, enteropathogenic *Esch. coli* have been shown to synthesize the toxin of *Shigella dysenteriae* type 1 (see below) but the role of this toxin in diarrhoeal disease remains to be determined (O'Brien et al 1982).

Enteroinvasive Esch. coli and Shigella spp. Certain specific O serogroups of *Esch. coli* (especially 0124 and 0164) behave biochemically and induce an identical clinical syndrome to *Shigella* (Rowe 1979); thus these organisms can be considered together. There are four *Shigella* species (*S. dysenteriae, S. flexneri, S. boydii* and *S. sonnei*) which together with enteroinvasive *Esch. coli* cause watery diarrhoea, often followed by dysentery. *S. dysenteriae* is the most virulent, *S. sonnei* produces a less severe illnesses, while *S. flexneri* and *S. boydii* can be severe or mild (Keusch et al 1982). *Shigella* which have lost the ability to penetrate colonic epithelial cells are avirulent, nevertheless in rhesus monkeys, watery diarrhoea follows jejunal colonization with shigellae when secretion occurs without bacterial invasion or mucosal damage.

Dysentery follows invasion of colonic epithelium, intracellular multiplication and cell death leading to an acute infective colitis. *Shigella* produce a toxin (Shiga toxin), MW 72 000, which has a variety of biological effects, including inhibition of ribosomal protein synthesis in cultured cells, paralysis and death in mice, and induction of fluid secretion in closed loops of rabbit ileum. It is possible to speculate that Shiga toxin released in the jejunal lumen induces the fluid secretion which leads to watery diarrhoea, while in the colon intracellular release of toxin results in colonic mucosal cell death via inhibition of protein synthesis (Keusch et al 1982).

Non-typhoid Salmonellae. The occurrence of dysenteric symptoms in a proportion of patients with *Salmonella* attests to the ability of nontyphoid salmonellae to invade the distal bowel. The diarrhoea may not however be due entirely to the damage produced by mucosal invasion, for although all invasive strains of *S. typhimurium* cause mucosal damage, it has been shown experimentally that not all invasive strains induce fluid secretion (Giannella et al 1973). Thus a bacterial factor may be present in addition to the essential prerequisite of intestinal invasion to cause intestinal secretion. Both cholera-like toxin and Shiga toxin are produced in vitro by non-typhoid salmonellae (Stephen et al 1985).

Campylobacter jejuni. The invasive potential of *Campylobacter* has been demonstrated by isolation of the organism from blood cultures in humans and by animal studies in which *Campylobacter* have been demonstrated in the caecal wall of chicks (Butzler & Skirrow 1979). A cholera-like toxin has been reported (Ruiz-Palcios et al 1983).

Yersinia enterocolitica. Y. enterocolitica causes gastroenteritis in children which may be dysenteric. In adults, acute terminal ileitis with mesenteric adenitis and reactive athritis occur (O'Morain 1981).

A guanylate-cyclase activating stable toxin is produced but the role of this toxin has not been established (Rao et al 1979).

Viruses

Viruses are the commonest cause of diarrhoea in infants. Two major clinical syndromes are recognized, sporadic infantile gastroenteritis, a severe diarrhoeal disease mainly associated with rotavirus infection, and a milder epidemic illness which affects older children and adults, commonly associated with parvovirus-like agents.

Rotavirus. Rotavirus is the commonest cause of diarrhoea in children under the age of 2 years. Our knowledge of the pathophysiology of rotavirus infection is based largely on challenge studies of human rotavirus administered to conventional piglets (Davidson et al 1977).

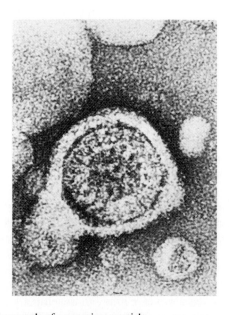

Fig. 15.2 Electron micrograph of a rotavirus particle

Rotavirus selectively infects the mature absorptive cells of the tips of small intestinal villi. The cells are thereby killed and are shed into the gut lumen with the viruses (Fig. 15.2). At the height of the diarrhoeal episode, there is no detectable viral antigen in the small intestinal mucosa. As a result of the loss of mature enterocytes which are replaced by immature crypt-type cells, there is villous atrophy, loss of surface area and decreased disaccharidase activity. The immature surface cells are ill-equipped to absorb luminal fluid, electrolytes and nutrients; thus diarrhoea appears to result from failure of small bowel absorptive ability rather than secretion. Once the virus is shed, normal epithelial cell kinetics are restored and the mucosal damage is repaired.

Other viruses. Epidemics of nonbacterial gastroenteritis have been associated with the presence of 27 nm viral particles called parvovirus-like agents. They are often named after the site of the outbreak (e.g. Norwalk, Hawaii, Montgomery County agents) and the syndrome produced is called 'Winter Vomiting Disease' (Greenberg et al 1979). Adult volunteers show similar histological appearances to those produced by rotavirus infection; thus similar pathophysiological mechanisms may be operating.

Adenoviruses which are detected in diarrhoeal stools but cannot be cultivated in tissue culture have been linked with diarrhoea in children which may be fatal (Vesikari et al 1981); as yet there have been no published studies on pathogenesis.

A number of other viruses have been implicated and these include calicivirus, astrovirus, coronavirus and small round viruses.

Epidemiology

The epidemiological features of the various diarrhoeal pathogens discussed above are summarized in Table 15.4.

CLINICAL FEATURES

Acute infection of the gastrointestinal tract by any of the organisms discussed above produces a clinical syndrome that is characterized by varying combinations of nausea, vomiting, abdominal cramps and diarrhoea.

Careful clinical appraisal of the individual case begins by excluding, on clinical grounds, other diseases that can produce acute diarrhoea, vomiting or abdominal pain. These are listed in Table 15.5 and will be considered in detail later.

Infants under the age of 1 year, and less than 6 months in particular, are especially liable to develop dehydration and other metabolic complications (Finberg 1973b), and are also more likely to develop a septicaemia following infection with invasive pathogens.

Infectious agent	Distribution	Seasonality	Age group	Main route of transmission[1]	Asymptomatic excretion
Vibrio cholerae	West Coast Africa, India, Far East	Variable but definite	Uncommon under 1 year	Water, Shellfish	Man–man	Uncommon
Enterotoxigenic *Escherichia coli*	West Africa, India, Far East, South America, Mexico	March–September (Bangladesh)	6 months–2 years in endemic areas	Water, Food	Man–man[2]	Common (especially LT strains)
Enteropathogenic *Escherichia coli*	Worldwide	Summer	Infants, especially at weaning, Nursery outbreaks	Water, Food	Man–man[3]	Common
Enteroinvasive *Escherichia coli*	Common in Brazil, Eastern Europe	?	Adults and young children	Food	Man–man	Common
Shigellae	Worldwide	Summer	Young children	Water, Food	Man–man[4]	Uncommon
Salmonellae	Developed countries	Summer	Infants and young children, Food-born outbreaks in adults	Meat	Animals–man	Very common
Campylobacter jejuni	Worldwide	Summer	Older children, Young adults	Poultry, Milk, Puppies, Birds	Animals–man	Uncommon
Yersinia enterocolitica	France, Scandinavia, Canada	Winter	Children	Uncertain	Man–man, Animals–man	Common
Rotavirus	Worldwide	Winter	6 months–1 year	?Airborne	Man–man	Occurs in neonates
Parvovirus-like agents	Developed countries	Winter	Family outbreaks	Shellfish, ?Airborne	Man–man	Uncommon

[1] All pathogens listed are transmitted by the faecal-oral route. Man–man or animal–man signifies principle reservoirs of infection. Where other routes of transmission are listed, this indicates that infection may be transferred indirectly via the named route.

[2] May be imported into temperate countries as Travellers' diarrhoea.

[3] ?Upper respiratory tract carriage in adults (Bois et al 1964)

[4] Infective dose as small as 10 organisms — hence direct faecal-oral spread very likely.

Table 15.5   Differential diagnosis of acute diarrhoea and vomiting

Gastroenteritis
Food poisoning
Acute food protein (e.g. cow's milk) intolerance
Systemic infections
    Septicaemia
    Meningitis
    Urinary tract infection
    Respiratory tract infection
Surgical disorders
    Appendicitis
    Intussusception
    Pyloric stenosis
    Necrotizing enterocolitis
    Incomplete intestinal obstruction including Hirschprung's disease
Metabolic disorders
    Diabetic precoma
    Haemolytic-uraemic syndrome
    Congenital adrenal insufficiency
Miscellaneous
    Coeliac disease
    Inflammatory bowel disease
    Immune deficiency states
    Selective inborn errors of metabolism
    Poisoning

If the patient is known to have an underlying gastrointestinal disorder such as inflammatory bowel disease or recently treated coeliac disease, an acute intestinal infection may produce relapse of the underlying condition and a severe illness.

Underlying renal or other metabolic disease may exaggerate the fluid and electrolyte disturbance caused by the present infective episode. Recurring episodes of acute infective diarrhoea may be a manifestation of an immuno-deficiency state.

Malnutrition

In world-wide terms the vicious cycle that links malnutrition to diarrhoea is the most important health challenge of today (Puffer & Serrano 1973). At the level of the individual infant or child, preexisting malnutrition probably increases susceptibility to all infections, including gastrointestinal infection, and certainly increases the likelihood of dehydration, acidosis, hypoglycaemia and hypothermia during an acute diarrhoeal episode (Mata et al 1972, Ortiz 1978).

Dehydration

The success of regimes of oral rehydration (see Management, oral rehydration) in reducing mortality from acute gastroenteritis (Lancet 1983) have

Table 15.6 Features of (extracellular) dehydration

2–3%	Thirst, mild oliguria.
5%	Thirst, oliguria. Slightly sunken eyes and fontanelle. Discernible alteration in skin turgor.
6–9%	Very obvious sunken eyes with loss of eyeball tension. Sunken fontanelle, loss of skin turgor. Marked thirst and oliguria. Increasing apathy.
10%+	All the above, plus shock. Anuric.

Remember: in hypernatraemic states, classical signs of dehydration are less obvious, but CNS signs (lethargy, irritability) are prominent early.

confirmed that dehydration is *the* essential clinical feature that must be accurately measured and treated.

The clinical assessment of dehydration (water loss) is made with reference to the estimated deficit in lean body mass expressed as a percentage and referred to inaccurately as 'percentage dehydration'. Most of the clinical features that are used to assess the state of hydration (Table 15.6) reflect the state of the extracellular fluid (ECF) compartment of the body. Thus thirst, oliguria, dry mucous membranes, sunken fontanelle, loss of skin turgor and eyeball tension, hypotension and tachycardia are all signs of depletion of ECF volume. In broad terms, depletion of ECF volume can be taken as a mirror for the volume depletion of total body water. However, for reasons discussed below this general statement has to be modified under two circumstances; namely when there is hypernatraemia or hyponatraemia.

In hypernatraemic dehydration, the ECF volume is relatively well maintained at the expense of intracellular dehydration. The 'classical' signs of dehydration listed above will underestimate the true loss of total body water (Finberg 1973a). The skin feels doughy and the fontanelle may actually bulge. Peripheral circulation remains adequate until late in the illness. Lethargy and hyper-irritability may give the vital clue to the diagnosis.

Conversely, in dehydration with hyponatraemia the ECF volume will be depleted to a relatively greater extent, and formal signs of dehydration will be obvious. There is more shock per degree of water loss than in normonatraemic states.

It is easy to underestimate the degree of dehydration in obese infants because of the small amount of water present in adipose tissue. Information about recent weight loss is particularly helpful and emphasis on examination should be placed on signs not affected by obesity, such as thirst, oliguria fontanelle and eyeball tension, tachycardia and hypotension.

In recent years there has been a changing trend in the UK in the type of dehydration seen in infants. A decade ago about 20% of all infants admitted to hospital with gastroenteritis had hypernatraemia (Ironside et al 1970) and similar figures were reported in the USA (Finberg 1970). Since then the proportion of cases with hypernatraemia has fallen steadily to only 1 to 2%. The beginning of this trend coincided with the introduction of low-solute formulae for young infants, and with a year-by-year increase in breast-feeding (Davies et al 1977). Hypernatraemia remains common in such countries as Nigeria where high-solute milks are fed to a relatively well nourished infant population (Ahmed & Agusto-Odutola 1970). In contrast hyponatraemia which is seen rarely in the UK is common in malnourished breastfed infants with gastroenteritis (Kingston 1973).

Metabolic disturbances

Acidosis

The metabolic acidosis that accompanies severe gastroenteritis is a result of bicarbonate losses in the stool compounded by poor renal perfusion and fasting ketosis. From a clinical standpoint the tachypnoea that is produced can be misinterpreted by the inexperienced clinician as evidence of pneumonia.

Hypokalaemia

In severe diarrhoea body losses of K^+ can be as much as 10–12 mmol/kg/d. Serum levels of K^+ are a poor guide to body K^+ status and may remain normal or even elevated (in the presence of a metabolic acidosis with displacement of intracellular K^+ by H^+ ions). Hypokalaemia with abdominal distension, absent bowel sounds, bradycardia and ECG changes, occurs clinically under two cases: first in association with hyponatraemic dehydration in the malnourished; and second in the post-emergency treatment of severe dehydration with acidosis.

Abnormal blood glucose concentrations

Hyperglycaemia of uncertain cause can be found in hypernatraemic states with acidosis. Hypoglycaemia is seen in malnourished infants with prolonged diarrhoea.

Hypocalcaemia

This is seen in hypernatraemia, particularly where there has been concomitant K^+ loss, and is the result of equilibration of body fluids with the skeleton (Finberg 1957). Tetany is rare but can occur in cases where there is failure to replace K^+ deficits.

Fever

Dehydration itself can produce fever in the very young infant and is particularly common in hypernatraemic states. Fever is more common in certain nonviral diarrhoeas but the rule is not absolute.

Renal failure

Anuria is a common feature of severe dehydration because of reduced renal perfusion. Restoration of urine flow is to be expected within a few hours of the successful introduction of an anti-shock and rehydration regime. If anuria still persists the possibility of structural renal damage should be considered. Further management is outlined below.

CNS signs

Lethargy is of course a feature of any severely ill child. Marked lethargy combined with extreme hyper-irritability on handling is the hallmark of hypernatraemic dehydration, and results from shrinkage of the brain. Haemorrhage and the production of intracellular 'idiogenic osmols' may contribute to the pathogenesis (McDowell et al 1955).

Convulsions can occur when there are sudden shifts of water across the blood-brain barrier in either direction. Thus erroneous administration of appreciable quantities of glucose-water to a dehydrated child can produce brain swelling, as will an attempt to correct hypernatraemia too rapidly.

Convulsions can also occur as a result of fever and are particularly common during the acute phase of *Shigella* infection (Donald et al 1956).

Differential diagnosis

Table 15.5 lists conditions which could present with diarrhoea and vomiting and be mistakenly diagnosed as acute gastroenteritis. Some are more important than others.

The clinician must exclude infections at another site which can be associated with concomitant diarrhoea and/or vomiting. Respiratory tract infections, including otitis media, are most frequent though it should be remembered that rotavirus and perhaps adenovirus enteritis may have prodromal upper respiratory symptoms. Meningitis may mimic hypernatraemia closely with fever, lethargy, irritability, full fontanelle, neck stiffness and tachypnoea. Urinary tract infections can only be excluded by appropriate urinary microscopy and culture, and these tests are essential.

There is the ever present fear of misdiagnosing a surgical disorder as gastroenteritis, and only a high index of suspicion will serve as insurance. Abdominal distension and tenderness and 'toxicity' out of proportion to the degree of dehydration are warning signs. A straight X-ray of the abdomen is mandatory as is a rectal examination (specifically for acute appendicitis and intussusception). In practice, it may be very difficult to distinguish the radiological features of 'functional' obstruction associated with gastroenteritis and its metabolic consequences from anatomical obstruction. A combined medical and surgical team should be involved and frequent review in the early hours after admission is required.

Investigation

The above paragraphs outline a diagnostic approach to exclude other disorders. If the diagnosis is considered to be acute infective gastroenteritis, are any investigations needed? At one end of the scale it can be argued that none is necessary. In the developing world with its overwhelming numbers of cases, the pragmatic approach — acute diarrhoea, assume gastroenteritis, institute oral rehydration — has proved practical, safe and effective. A similar approach can be, and is, adopted in the UK by many family doctors treating mild cases of diarrhoea and vomiting.

In the severely ill dehydrated child who is admitted to hospital, regular measurement of body weight, urine output, fluid balance, serum electrolytes and acid-base status, plus monitoring of vital signs, allow fine control of management.

Is there a need in the individual case to try to identify the aetiological agent? Again in most cases, pragmatism says no. But stool culture may be indicated under special epidemiological circumstances or to identify (invasive) pathogens for which antibiotic therapy may be required; for example: hospital in-patients, nursery outbreaks, severe diarrhoea, delayed resolution, blood and mucus in stools, systemic illness, fever or foreign travel.

MANAGEMENT

Dehydration, and its complications, are usually the cause of death in acute infective diarrhoea and its correction is the fundamental aim of treatment. Infants are particularly at risk as a result of their high basal fluid requirement, immature renal concentration of solute and an inability to increase fluid intake when thirsty.

The indications for hospital admission are summarized in Table 15.7. None is absolute and they should be considered in the light of the availability of local hospital facilities, the capabilities of the parents and the degree of trained supervision available in the home.

Table 15.7   Indications for hospital referral of patients with acute diarrhoea and vomiting

Clinically dehydrated
Less than 6 months of age
Short history of profuse diarrhoea
Parents unable to comply with oral rehydration advice, for whatever reason
Poor social circumstances
Pre-existing medical condition present which may worsen dehydration (e.g. diabetes mellitus, adrenogenital syndrome)
Suspected surgical condition (e.g. intussusception, appendicitis)
Frequent supervision in the home by adequately trained personnel unavailable

Investigations

Many patients require no investigation, particularly those with mild symptoms of abrupt onset, who are seen in the home or as outpatients. In some patients, however, fresh stool microscopy and culture is helpful, either for the purpose of tracing/preventing cross-infection in hospital or nurseries, or because an antimicrobial agent may be indicated as discussed above. If the patient is dehydrated, plasma electrolytes and urea should be measured as the results may have a major influence on subsequent fluid replacement.

Prevention and Correction of Dehydration

Dehydration absent or mild

In this group of patients, the prime aim is the *prevention* of dehydration. Older children with mild symptoms often require no more than a modest increase in their fluid intake. However, the younger the patient, the more important it is to provide not only clear instructions to the parents about management, but also to observe the patient at frequent intervals in order to check that he or she is not becoming dehydrated.

In the well nourished child, the withdrawal of normal feeds for 24 hours and their replacement by a sugar-electrolyte solution or dilute milk feeds is traditionally performed. Fluids should be administered in small amounts, initially by teaspoon if necessary. After 24 hours the infant is regraded onto a normal diet by stepwise increases in the strength of milk offered, usually over 3–4 days. In the malnourished patient with mild diarrhoea, feeding is not interrupted and a sugar-electrolyte solution is given to replace stool losses.

Table 15.8 Composition of some oral solutions used in the management of acute diarrhoea (mmol/l)

	Sodium	Chloride	Potassium	Bicarbonate	Glucose	Sucrose
Dextrolyte	35	30	13	18[1]	200	—
Dioralyte	35	37	20	18	200	—
Rehidrat	50	50	20	20[2]	91	94
WHO-UNICEF	90	80	20	30[3]	110	—

[1] as lactate
[2] also contains 8 mmol/l citric acid
[3] now replaced with 10 mmol/l citric acid

When a sugar-electrolyte solution is given with the aim of preventing dehydration, it is appropriate to administer one containing 30–60 mmol/l sodium (Table 15.8); higher concentrations of sodium are unnecessary and may be harmful in nondehydrated children in whom the net sodium deficit is small. It seems likely that the sugar content of many commercially available oral rehydration solutions (ORS) is at the upper limits of acceptability (Kjellman & Ronge 1982). Certainly, the high sugar content and osmolarity, and negligible electrolyte content of most carbonated soft drinks make them entirely unsuitable as ORS (Head et al 1983) and their use often results in an osmotic diarrhoea with the passage of large amounts of watery stools, low in sodium, with the consequent risk of hypernatraemia (Hirschhorn 1980).

Although the use of home-made rehydration solutions prepared from sucrose and salt represents a reasonable alternative to prepackaged solutions when these are unavailable, they are not without some risk as a result of incorrect formulation or administration (Whitelaw et al 1975, Levine et al 1980). Furthermore, sucrose-salt solutions contain no added bicarbonate or potassium and their use is associated with prolonged hypokalaemia (Clements et al 1981). If prepackaged mixtures are readily available, there seems little justification in risking the use of home-made solutions.

Moderate to severe dehydration

More severe diarrhoea is associated with the emergence of clinically detectable dehydration which is usually overt when 5% or more of the total body weight has been lost. In obese infants, tissue turgor may be maintained until dehydration is severe and undue reliance should not, therefore, be placed on this sign in fat patients. As fluid losses progress and the signs of dehydration become more obvious (see Table 15.6), urine output diminishes and the pulse becomes rapid and low in volume; postural hypotension may be present.

Patient management closely reflects the economic climate in which their disease occurs. In developed countries, most dehydrated patients are admitted to hospital and rehydrated intravenously, whereas in developing countries oral rehydration, often as an outpatient, is the usual practice. The concept that intravenous rehydration is of necessity better than oral, is an outmoded one.

Intravenous rehydration

The regimen is based upon the nature of the fluid, electrolyte and acid-base disturbance present on admission. Blood for electrolytes, urea and bicarbonate are therefore sent to the laboratory as soon as possible. While these investigations are being performed, an infusion of 40–80 ml/kg of half-normal saline (sodium 75 mmol/l with 2.5% dextrose is given over four hours. Potassium is not added to the infusion until the plasma potassium concentration is known and urine flow has been established. Subsequent rehydration is planned according to the results of plasma electrolyte determinations. Examples of the necessary calculations are given in Appendix 1, and daily requirements of water, sodium and potassium in Table 15.9.

Hyponatraemic dehydration. Hyponatraemic dehydration occurs most commonly in developing countries, characteristically in breastfed infants (Kingston 1973), those who have had repeated episodes of diarrhoea, are

Table 15.9 Maintenance requirements of water, sodium and potassium (Requirements/kg/24 h)

Age(months)	Water(ml)	Sodium(mmol/l)	Potassium(mmol/l)
0–6	120–150	1.0–2.5	1.0–2.5
6–12	100–120	2.5	2.5
12–24	80–100	2.5	2.5
> 24	70–90	1.5–2.5	1.5–2.5

malnourished and who receive salt-poor fluid replacements. Fluid and electrolyte losses result in an initial contraction of the extracellular fluid compartment and a compensatory increase in aldosterone and antidiuretic hormone secretion (Hirschhorn 1980). As a result, urinary potassium losses are increased. Potassium depletion is further enhanced by the displacement of potassium from the intracellular compartment by retained hydrogen ions. Sodium and water move intracellularly, thereby enhancing the initial contraction of the extracellular fluid. The administration of hypotonic solutions, and a greater retention of water than sodium exaggerate this phenomenon. Thus, in hyponatraemic dehydration, the intracellular compartment is maintained at the expense of the extracellular space and plasma volume, resulting in relatively early circulatory collapse. Fluid replacement with solutions containing a sodium concentration approximating to that of extracellular rather than intracellular fluid is therefore appropriate.

Although potassium depletion may be severe and prolonged, it is important not to exceed the maximum safe concentration in the infusion fluid of 40 mmol/l. When calculating the intravenous dose of potassium, it may be assumed to be half the sodium requirement for the first 24 hours, as the potassium concentration in diarrhoeal stools is approximately half that of sodium. Following the initial period of intravenous rehydration, oral potassium supplements may be required.

Normonatraemic dehydration. Most dehydrated patients with acute diarrhoea are normonatraemic. Although large deficits of fluid and electrolytes may be present, the absence of preceding malnutrition and potassium depletion, and a freedom from the administration of salt-poor fluids to excess, mitigates the development of frank hyponatraemia. The deficit of water may be calculated, as in hyponatraemic dehydration, from the percentage dehydration at the start of treatment. Sodium deficit may be approximately assessed if it is assumed that the fluid loss has a sodium concentration equal to half that of normal saline (see Appendix 1).

Hypernatraemic dehydration. Hypernatraemic dehydration (plasma sodium > 150 mmol/l) results from a disproportionately large loss of body water compared with sodium. Excess body losses of water result in desiccation of the intracellular compartment; because sodium is retained within the extracellular space, the volume of this compartment and hence plasma volume are relatively well maintained. Consequently, for a given degree of dehydration there is less circulatory disturbance in this form than in hyponatraemic dehydration. However, intracellular water depletion within the central nervous system results in a marked neurological disturbance (Finberg 1973b).

Patients at greatest risk of developing hypernatraemic dehydration are those under 1 year of age receiving high-solute feeds, whose diarrhoea is accompanied by high fever and who are nursed in a hot, dry environment; renal immaturity also impairs the patient's ability to excrete a sodium load (Spitzer 1978). The oral administration of hyperosmolar fluids induces additional water loss in excess of sodium, by the induction of an osmotic diarrhoea and the ensuing passage of large volumes of stool low in sodium (Hirschorn 1980). In the United Kingdom, the recent widespread administration of low-solute milk formulae during infancy has coincided with a fall in the incidence of hypernatraemic dehydration (Walker-Smith et al 1981).

The intravenous correction of hypernatraemic dehydration poses a considerable dilemma. The rapid administration of excess free water may rapidly correct dehydration but may also result in a rapid lowering of extracellular osmolality so that water enters the intracellular compartment down an osmotic gradient. The ensuing intracellular 'water intoxication' leads to brain swelling which may result in convulsions. Thus, after the initial four hour period during which half-normal saline is administered, subsequent fluid replacement should take place slowly over a total of 48 hours (Finberg 1973b). When calculating the sodium requirement, it is assumed that the sodium content is derived solely from the estimated fluid deficit and that this is between 100 and 130 mmol/l of deficit. To this requirement is added 48 hours sodium-free maintenance fluid requirement, so that the required sodium concentration of the given infusion is reduced to between 25 and 40 mmol/l. Thus, following an initial infusion of half-normal saline over 4 hours, an infusion of fifth normal saline with 4% dextrose (sodium 30 mmol/l) is infused over the remaining 44 hours of the 48 hour period (see Appendix 1). Once urine has been passed, potassium is added to the infusion (40 mmol/l). This addition not only increases the solute content of the infusion and corrects potassium depletion which may be considerable, but also facilitates the passage of water into cells by providing an ion which moves intracellularly. The further addition of calcium (10 ml of 10% calcium gluconate per 500 ml) guards against the rare occurrence of tetany during rehydration. Additional volumes of the solution may be given to replace any ongoing stool losses, since, with the exception of toxigenic diarrhoea, the electrolyte concentrations in this solution are approximately those in stool water (Pizarro et al 1984).

Acidosis. A metabolic acidosis usually accompanies diarrhoea, mainly because a reduced renal hydrogen ion excretion follows a reduction in glomerular filtration rate; but faecal bicarbonate losses and ketosis are important contributory reasons. The most important factor in the correction of acidosis is rehydration and the re-establishment of urine flow. Infusion of bicarbonate is reserved for severe acidosis with an arterial pH of less than 7.0. The administration of bicarbonate leads to the formation of CO_2:

$$HCO_3^- + H^+ \longleftrightarrow H_2CO_3 \longleftrightarrow H_2O + CO_2$$

The permeability of cell membranes and of the blood-brain barrier is greater to CO_2 than to bicarbonate, and consequently bicarbonate given intravenously causes an initial, paradoxical fall in intracellular and cerebro-spinal fluid pH. It is only when pH falls below 7.0 that the depressant effect of acidosis on the myocardium becomes sufficient to justify slow bicar-bonate administration.

Bicarbonate requirements are calculated as follows: deficit = weight (kg) × 0.3 × base deficit. The bicarbonate should be diluted with other infusion fluids. The addition to calcium-containing fluids results in a precipitate.

Oral rehydration

The observation that sodium transport is enhanced by concurrent glucose transport in the small intestine (Riklis & Quastel 1958, Schultz & Zalusky 1964, Crane 1965) and that this co-transport is intact during most acute enteric infections, provided a rational basis for using glucose-electrolyte solutions in the management of acute diarrhoea. More recently, sucrose (Palmer et al 1977) and rice-powder (Molla et al 1982), both of which release luminal glucose following intestinal hydrolysis, have been shown to be satisfactory alternatives to glucose. Although rotavirus infection is as-sociated with impaired glucose-coupled sodium co-transport (Davidson et al, 1977, Telch et al 1981), oral rehydration therapy (ORT) is equally as effective in rotavirus infection as in toxigenic diarrhoea (Nalin et al 1979).

The widespread use of ORT in the management of moderate to severe diarrhoeal dehydration in develping countries arose from its spectacular efficiency in the management of cholera in children (Anon 1981). Subse-quent studies have confirmed ORT to be effective as a rehydrating agent in children (Anon 1983), and neonates (Pizarro et al 1983a), and also as a means of reducing diarrhoea-associated mortality (Rahaman et al 1979). The efficacy, cheapness and simplicity of ORT has led the World Health Organ-isation to promote the worldwide use of an oral rehydration solution (WHO ORS) containing sodium 90 mmol/l (see Table 15:8) and to publish guide-lines concerning its use (WHO 1980).

In the management of moderate and moderately severe dehydration in developing countries, WHO ORS is currently administered to infants in a volume of 100 ml/kg body weight over 4 hours followed by 50 ml/kg of water (or breast milk *ad lib*) over the next two hours. After this six-hour course of therapy, the infant is re-examined (clinically and by weight gain).

If complete rehydration has been achieved, the infant enters a maintenance phase of therapy. If dehydration is now mild (about 5%), WHO ORS is continued for six more hours with half the volume being offered (50 ml/kg), as for the moderately dehydrated state. The above regime is successful in over 95% of patients and is the treatment of choice in all but the shocked child, when intravenous fluids should be administered. Successful rehydration occurs in 50% of children by 6 hours, in 65% by 12 hours and in 95% by 18–24 hours. Following rehydration, ORS is given in maintenance amounts; 100 ml/kg over 24 hours. In addition, oral nutrients are now recommended in the form of breast milk *ad lib*, or a half-strength cow's milk formula feed (120 ml/kg per 24 h), both of which provide free water with which to handle the sodium load given during the maintenance period of rehydration. Plain water or an alternative low solute fluid is also offered during this phase, to provide more free water if necessary. The child is regraded onto a normal diet; in the malnourished child this should be supplemented with locally available high calorie feeds wherever possible.

In developed countries, oral rehydration with the WHO ORS is used much less frequently than intravenous rehydration. This is largely as a result of experience obtained in developed countries during the 1950's and early 1960's when hypernatraemic dehydration was relatively common and many paediatricians have been concerned about the use of a single high sodium solution (90 mmol/l) particularly when used as a maintenance solution, or for the replacement of ongoing loses in nondehydrated infants. In this age-group an immature renal concentrating capacity, increased insensible water losses and an impaired natriuretic response may all predispose to the development of hypernatraemia.

Recently however, the safety of 90 mmol/l sodium ORS has been examined in well nourished in-patients and well supervised out-patients in the United States and Latin America (Santosham et al 1982, 1983; Pizarro et al 1983b). Dehydrated children with a wide range of electrolyte disturbance, including specifically those with hypernatraemia, were safely and effectively rehydrated orally. Thus, current evidence, which is still limited, suggests that a 90 mmol/l sodium ORS is suitable for the initial rehydration of overtly dehydrated, well nourished, bottlefed children, irrespective of the initial plasma sodium concentration and may, in fact be safer than intravenous rehydration (Santosham 1982). In patients who are hypernatraemic on admission, administration of a 90 mmol/l sodium rehydration solution over twelve, rather than six, hours may lead to fewer convulsions during rehydration (Pizarro et al 1984). Oral rehydration is contraindicated in those patients who are shocked on admission, have an impaired level of conciousness or absent bowel sounds, and such patients should be resuscitated intravenously (vide infra).

With correct administration, significant hypernatraemia does not occur with 90 mmol/l. However, gross errors by poorly instructed parents who dissolve the mixture in insufficient water lead to a high incidence of subsequent hypernatraemia (Cleary et al 1981). Probably an even more important determinant of hypernatraemia complicating ORT is an inappropriately high sugar concentration in the solution, leading to an osmotic diarrhoea and an excess loss of water over electrolytes (Meeuwisse 1983).

When using a 90 mmol/l sodium solution for rehydration, water should be administered in addition to ORS in a ratio of 2:1 (ORS : water) unless the patient is known to be severely hyponatraemic. It is important to differentiate between rehydration and the use of an ORS in either the prevention of dehydration, or in the maintenance phase after rehydration; in the latter circumstance, considerable free water should be administered with a 90 mmol/l sodium solution (1:1). Alternatively, a separate solution should be used when economically feasible for prevention/maintenance purposes. Ideally this would contain (mmol/l): sodium 50–60, potassium 20–30, chloride 30–50, bicarbonate or citrate 30, glucose 110 (Finberg et al 1982). Although such a solution contains adequate free water for excretion of any excess electrolytes, additional fluids such as breast milk or plain water should be offered as an additional precaution. Guidelines for the use of ORT are given in Appendix 2.

Severe dehydration with shock

Restoration of the circulating volume is an emergency and this may be achieved by the intravenous administration of i) plasma or purified protein fraction (20 ml/kg body weight over 10–15 minutes) or ii) normal saline or Ringer's lactate (30–40 ml/kg body weight over 30–40 minutes). Following this emergency phase of resuscitation, rehydration may be continued intravenously with half-normal saline with 2.5% dextrose, as outlined in 'Moderate to severe dehydration': alternatively ORT may be commenced (see Appendices 1 and 2).

Management after rehydration

Once rehydration has been achieved and vomiting has ceased, the decisions regarding subsequent management are strongly influenced by the nutritional status of the child and also by local medical and cultural traditions.

In the *developing* world, diarrhoea and malnutrition commonly go together (Morley 1973). Acute diarrhoea is a potent contributory factor in the pathogenesis of protein-energy malnutrition (Rowland et al 1977, Martorell et al 1980), probably as a result of stress-induced catabolism, carbohydrate and other dietary intolerances (Hirschorn et al 1969) and maternal withdrawal of foods. Anorexia is another important factor. Children with acute diarrhoea eat 30% less food than usual, mainly because of a diminished intake of weaning foods; breast milk intake tends to be well maintained (Molla et al 1983).

Following diarrhoea, particularly after the weaning period, a vicious cycle may be readily established, leading to protracted diarrhoea and progressively worsening malnutrition (see Chapter 16). Thus, the more malnourished the patient, the greater the necessity for feeds early in the illness. Breast feeding or a half-strength cow's milk formula may be started as soon as the patient is rehydrated, and ORS given concurrently to replace any continuing losses. Subsequently, the child is regraded rapidly onto a normal diet, supplemented by locally available high-calorie feeds whenever possible.

It has long been recognized that early refeeding after rehydration does not affect the mean duration of diarrhoea (Chung & Viscorova 1948) and it has recently been shown that it may actually shorten it (Isolauri & Vesikari 1985). Furthermore, the absorption of substantial amounts of nitrogen, fat and carbohydrate takes place during early refeeding, even during acute diarrhoea. In general, stool volume does not seem to increase, although continued absorption of macronutrients still occurs in those patients in whom it does increase (Chung 1948, Chung & Viscorova 1948, Molla et al 1983). Clearly these observations, together with those that suggest that the use of ORT is related to improved subsequent nutrition (International Study Group 1981, Barzgar et al 1980), have important implications for the management of the malnourished child with acute diarrhoea. It is becoming increasingly clear that the prolonged withdrawal of adequate nutrients during and after acute diarrhoea is an important cause of iatrogenic malnutrition. (Mahalanabis 1983).

In *developed* countries, the vast majority of children presenting with acute diarrhoea are well nourished and the reintroduction of oral nutrients is less urgent than in a previously malnourished patient. The optimal way in which to introduce milk feeds is not known, but following rehydration, milk feeds are usually introduced on a graded basis over the following four days. A low sodium (e.g. 30 mmol/l) ORS is used to dilute the milk feed during the period of regrading. Breast milk is usually well tolerated following acute diarrhoea, so that the early reintroduction of breast-feeding is to be encouraged. Whether gradual reintroduction of cow's milk formula feeds is strictly necessary after *mild* diarrhoea is uncertain. In nonbreastfed patients with mild diarrhoea the rapid reintroduction of milk feeds is associated with less weight loss and is not associated with a longer stay in hospital than in those managed conventionally (Rees & Brook 1979, Dugdale et al 1982). However, delayed recovery is more common in infants under six months of age (Edmeades et al 1981), and Placzek & Walker-Smith (1984) have recently shown that the rapid reintroduction of milk feeds to infants under nine months of age is associated with a return of watery diarrhoea or vomiting in 30%. Therefore, in children under nine months of age, a gradual reintroduction of milk feeds seems to be a wise precaution. In even younger babies of less than three months of age, the use of a lactose-free, hydrolysed protein formula should be considered, particularly after moderate to severe diarrhoea. The indications for such feedings in this group of patients do, however, require more precise definition.

Treatment with drugs

The indications for the use of drugs in the management of acute diarrhoea in children are extremely limited (Anon 1983), although they continue to be widely prescribed (Catford 1980). All classes of anti-diarrhoeal agents are associated with considerable disadvantages. The drugs currently used in the management of acute diarrhoea may be classified into four main groups:

Anti-motility agents

The anti-diarrhoeal effect of opioids in adults has long been recognized, and drugs such as diphenoxylate (Lomotil®), codeine, morphine (with kaolin) and loperamide (Imodium®) are currently widely used to treat the social distress associated with mild, acute diarrhoea. However, there is no evidence that agents which affect intestinal motility and prolong transit time are beneficial in younger age groups. Diphenoxylate, for example, does not reduce stool output or the volume of rehydration fluid required by infants with acute diarrhoea (Portnoy et al 1976). These drugs may even be harmful when administered to patients affected with an enteroinvasive organism like *Shigella*. In human subjects with shigellosis, diphenoxylate prolongs both fever and the period of faecal excretion of the pathogen (Du Pont & Hornick 1973), while guinea pigs pretreated with opioids are converted from a state of shigella resistance to one of extreme susceptibility (Formal et al 1963). In children the use of these agents may predispose to post-enteritis diarrhoea (Halliday et al 1982). The presence of opioid-containing anti-diarrhoeals in the home represents a serious health hazard for children, even when the drug is prescribed for adult use. Diphenoxylate is a potent respiratory depressant when taken in accidental overdose and is one of the commonest causes of fatal poisoning in childhood.

Anti-secretory agents

The pathophysiological mechanisms underlying intestinal secretion have been intensively studied over recent years and many of the biochemical events underlying the secretory processes which take place are now understood. This work has led to the identification of a galaxy of agents which modify experimentally-induced intestinal secretion in the experimental animal in vivo and in vitro (Powell & Field 1980). Currently no anti-secretory agent (e.g. loperamide, chlorpromazine, aspirin) has been shown to be an unequivocally useful adjunct to rehydration therapy in acute diarrhoea in children and none can be currently recommended, despite claims to the contrary (Diarrhoeal Diseases Study Group 1984).

Adsorbents

The rationale of administering adsorbents like kaolin or activated charcoal is the luminal binding of bacterial enterotoxins. Kaolin does not, however, reduce stool output in acute diarrhoea, but does make the stools appear more formed (Portnoy et al 1976). The use of this agent may therefore lead to a dangerous underestimation of the severity of diarrhoea. Pectin actually increases faecal sodium output in control subjects (Sandberg et al 1983).

Antibiotics

The vast majority of children with acute diarrhoea of both a viral and bacterial aetiology, have a self-limiting illness which responds to oral rehydration without antibiotics (Lambert 1979). Oral neomycin is contraindicated as it may cause diarrhoea and a reversible malabsorptive state associated with marked changes in villous architecture (Jacobson & Faloon 1961, Jacobson et al 1960). Antibiotics in *Salmonella* gastroenteritis, uncomplicated by systemic spread, do not favourably affect the clinical course of the illness, and may lead to prolonged faecal excretion of the pathogen and the promotion of antibiotic-resistant strains.

Table 15.10   Indications for antibiotics in acute diarrhoea in childhood

Indication	Suggested first line antimicrobial agent (until sensitivities known)[1]
Shigella dysentery	Co-trimoxazole
Typhoid/paratyphoid fever	Co-trimoxazole or chloramphenicol
Systemic salmonellosis	Co-trimoxazole or chloramphenicol
Cholera	Tetracycline
Campylobacter enteritis when severe and diagnosed early, or prolonged	Erythromycin
Pseudomembranous colitis (*Clostridium difficile*)	Vancomycin or metronidazole
Giardiasis	Metronidazole
Amoebic dysentery	Metronidazole
Severe persistent diarrhoea in travellers	Co-trimoxazole
Diagnostic doubt between gastroenteritis and septicaemia	As indicated by full clinical assessment of the child

[1] The sensitivities of certain organisms, particularly *Shigella*, frequently change, and an up-to-date knowledge of the sensitivities of the organisms in the affected community is essential.

There are, however, circumstances in which antibiotics are indicated and these are summarized in Table 15.10. The need for an antimicrobial agent will usually only be recognized following fresh stool microscopy and culture, but when faced with a sick infant with bloody diarrhoea and fever it is safer to begin treatment with an anti-*Shigella* agent rather than await the results of stool culture.

Anti-emetics

Although vomiting is frequently seen as an early symptom of acute enteric infection, the volumes are generally small and do not preclude the successful use of ORT. Anti-emetics such as metoclopramide or prochlorperazine are therefore rarely, if ever, indicated, particularly as the extrapyramidal side effects of the dystonic type occur more frequently in children. Instead, persistent vomiting requires a re-evaluation of the working diagnosis.

Complications

Extraintestinal spread of infection

Infection beyond the intestine may occur during infection with Salmonellae, Shigellae and enteroinvasive *Esch. coli*, as a result of the ability of these organisms to penetrate the intestinal epithelium, and is an indication for chemotherapy. Rigors, high fevers and a marked leucocytosis in a child with diarrhoea, indicate the need for regular blood cultures and repeated observation for localized extraintestinal infection. Salmonellae may cause metastatic infection in any tissue, particularly the meninges, joints and bones (especially in patients with sickle cell disease), renal parenchyma and lungs; an endocarditis may occur. Generalized convulsions are a relatively frequent complication of shigellosis in children (Barrett-Connor & Connor 1970); pneumonia may occur in some patients and a sterile effusion into large joints may occur several weeks after the initial symptoms have resolved. Extraintestinal infection is more common in neonates and in the immuno-deficient.

Anuria

Following the restoration of the circulation in shocked patients, the passage of small amounts of highly concentrated urine may be expected within 4–8 hours. Typically, urinary sodium concentration will be low (less than 10 mmol/l) and the urine/plasma osmolarity ratio greater than 1.3. If no urine has been passed despite adequate rehydration (adequate weight gain, markedly improved tissue turgor and increased blood pressure and pulse volume), the administration of large doses of frusemide may induce urine flow and protect against the development of tubular necrosis. An intravenous dose of frusemide (1–2 mg/kg body weight) may be repeated 4–6 hourly if a response is seen. Frusemide should be given slowly, as ototoxicity may infrequently follow rapid intravenous infusion. When diuresis begins, the state of hydration must be checked frequently and plasma sodium and potassium concentrations monitored every 4–6 hours, as urinary water and electrolyte losses may be large.

Anuria persisting after rehydration and the administration of frusemide, suggests that intrinsic renal damage may have occurred and referral to a centre equipped to perform dialysis if necessary, is indicated. Fluids are restricted to an amount equal to insensible water loss (30 ml/m²/day) plus any urinary output. Hyperkalaemia (>7.5 mmol/l) in the presence of ECG changes is a dangerous complication and emergency treatment is required. Calcium gluconate (0.5 ml/kg of a 10% solution) injected intravenously over several minutes with ECG monitoring, antagonizes the cardiac effects of hyperkalaemia. Correction of acidosis with intravenous sodium bicarbonate also lowers plasma potassium, but the extra sodium may exacerbate any preexisting sodium overload.

Hyperglycaemia

Hyperglycaemia of uncertain aetiology is commonly seen in patients with hypernatraemic dehydration. Often the blood glucose is 11–14 mmol/l but may occasionally be as high as 30 mmol/l. Almost always, rehydration with consequent correction of acidosis results in a fall in blood glucose concentration. Insulin, even in small amounts, may cause a precipitous fall in blood glucose which may contribute to an over-rapid lowering of plasma osmolality, and is to be avoided.

Convulsions

Convulsions may occur as a result of fever, hypernatraemia, infection with an enteroinvasive organism, or a rapid reduction in raised plasma osmolality. Management comprises maintenance of an airway and oxygenation, and the administration of diazepam intravenously. Subsequently, phenobarbitone (5 mg/kg IM) may be helpful in controlling fits. Lumbar puncture should be performed as soon as the clinical state of the patient permits.

Chronic faecal excretion of pathogens

Up to one-third of patients excrete salmonellae eight weeks after an infection (Association for the Study of Infectious Disease 1970); excretion is prolonged by antibiotic administration (Aserkoff & Bennett 1969) and in patients under one year of age (Anon 1978). Following shigellosis, less than 10% of patients excrete Shigellae three months post infection and only a small minority for longer; prolonged excretion, sometimes intermittent, may be associated with episodes of diarrhoea and abdominal pain. Following *Campylobacter* enteritis, faecal excretion usually continues for 2–5 weeks in the absence of chemotherapy. Prolonged excretion of rotavirus or other enteroviruses is uncommon, but when associated with protracted diarrhoea, raises the possibility of an underlying immunodeficiency state.

IMMUNIZATION

The development of effective vaccines for acute diarrhoeal diseases is a high priority for the control of such diseases worldwide. Promising vaccines for cholera, enterotoxigenic *Esch. coli* (ETEC) and rotavirus have been developed.

Cholera vaccines have been based on manipulating cholera organisms so that their virulence is attenuated and either the binding subunit of the toxin alone is produced (Texas Star SR) or no enterotoxin is produced (JBK70). In volunteer trials mild diarrhoea was produced in vaccinees.

Successful trials of ETEC vaccines in piglets and calves administered to lactating mother animals providing protection by specific anti-fimbrial antibodies in colostrum have stimulated the development of CFA/I and CFA/II vaccines for man (Levine et al) 1983. The potential effectiveness of these vaccines is however somewhat limited as a proportion of ETEC are negative for both CFA/I and CFA/II.

Attenuated human rotavirus strains are being developed. A bovine-derived rotavirus (RIT4237) vaccine has been used with considerable success. Interestingly, the incidence of all diarrhoeal episodes was reduced in three quarter of the vaccinees.

APPENDIX 1
CALCULATION OF THE INTRAVENOUS REQUIREMENTS IN THE MANAGEMENT OF DEHYDRATION (from Tripp & Harries 1977)

The maintenance requirements for water, sodium and potassium for different age groups are listed in Table 15.9.

In the examples below a hypothetical patient will be considered. The infant weighed 3.72 kg on admission, was estimated to be 7% dehydrated (7% dry) and received half normal saline at a rate of 60 ml/h for the first four hours.

Example 1 — **Hyponatraemia (plasma sodium = 115 mmol/l)**

(1) Estimated rehydrated weight (WR)
   WR = Admission weight × 100 ÷ (100 − % dry)
      = 3.72 × 100 ÷ 93 = 4 kg

(2) Water required (ml)

Deficit $= WR \times 1000 \times \% \text{ dry} \div 100$

$\qquad = 4 \times 1000 \times 7 \div 100$ $\qquad\qquad = + 280$

24 hours maintenance $= 4 \times 150$ $\qquad\qquad = + 600$

Less $\frac{1}{2}$ normal saline given $= 4 \times 60$ $\qquad\qquad = - 240$

$\qquad\qquad\qquad\qquad\qquad$ Total $\qquad = + 640$

(3) Sodium required (mmol)

Deficit $= WR \times 0.6 \times (140 - \text{plasma sodium})$

$\qquad = 4 \times 0.6 \times (140 - 115)$ $\qquad\qquad = + 60$

24 hours maintenance $= 4 \times 2.5$ $\qquad\qquad = + 10$

Less $\frac{1}{2}$ normal saline given (0.24×75) $\qquad = - 18$

$\qquad\qquad\qquad\qquad\qquad$ Total $\qquad = + 52$

(4) Potassium required (mmol/l)

Deficit $= \text{sodium deficit} \div 2$

$\qquad = 60 \div 2$ $\qquad\qquad\qquad = + 30$

24 hours maintenance $= 4 \times 2.5$ $\qquad\qquad = + 10$

$\qquad\qquad\qquad\qquad\qquad$ Total $\qquad = + 40$

An intravenous infusion of half normal saline with 2.5% dextrose and potassium chloride (40 mmol/l) at a rate of 32 ml/h for 20 hours would provide:

		Amounts provided	Require- ments	Differences to requirements
Water (ml)	$= 20 \times 32$	$= 640$	640	0
Sodium (mmol/l)	$= 0.64 \times 75$	$= 48$	52	$- 4$
Potassium (mmol/l)	$= 0.64 \times 40$	$= 25$	40	$- 15$

Note that though water and sodium requirements are met, only just over half the potassium requirements are given.

Example 2 — **Normonatraemia** (plasma sodium $= 135$ mmol/l)

Rehydrated weight and water requirements as for Example 1 and equal 4 kg and 640 ml, respectively,

(1) Sodium required

Deficit $= \text{fluid deficit as } \frac{1}{2} \text{ normal saline}$

$\qquad = 0.28 \times 75$ $\qquad\qquad\qquad = + 21$

24 hours maintenance $= 4 \times 2.5$ $\qquad\qquad = + 10$

Less $\frac{1}{2}$ normal saline given $\qquad\qquad\qquad = - 18$

$\qquad\qquad\qquad\qquad\qquad$ Total $\qquad = + 13$

(2) Potassium required

Deficit = sodium deficit ÷ 2

$\qquad$ = 21 ÷ 2   = + 10.5

24 hours maintenance = 4 × 2.5   = + 10

$\qquad\qquad\qquad\qquad\qquad$ Total   = + 20.5

An intravenous infusion of one-fifth normal saline with 4% dextrose and potassium chloride (30 mmol/l) at a rate of 32 ml/h for 20 hours would provide:

		Amounts provided	Requirements	Difference to requirements
Water	= 20 × 32 = 640	640	640	0
Sodium	= 0.64 × 30 = 19	19	13	+ 6
Potassium	= 0.64 × 30 = 19	19	21	− 2

Example 3 — **Hypernatraemia** (plasma sodium 164 mmol/l)

Water required

Deficit   = + 280 ml

48 hours maintenance requirement (4 × 150 × 2)   = + 1200 ml

Less ½ normal saline given (4 × 60)   = − 240 ml

Total requirement over remaining 44 hours   = +1240 ml

An infusion of one-fifth normal saline with 4% dextrose plus potassium chloride (40 mmol/l) and 10% calcium gluconate (10 ml/500 ml) is therefore infused at 28 ml/h for 44 hours.

APPENDIX 2
GUIDELINES FOR ORAL REHYDRATION THERAPY

It is important to differentiate between the three aims of treatment: prevention, rehydration and maintenance:

Prevention (dehydration absent or mild)

a) 35–60 mmol/l sodium solution (150 ml/kg/24 h) plus additional plain water or human milk to satisfy thirst,

$\qquad$ or:

b) 90 mmol/l sodium solution (e.g. WHO) given in a ratio ORS 1: water/breast milk 1.

Rehydration (moderate to severe dehydration, but not shocked)

a) Administer *twice* estimated total fluid deficit over six hours, with two thirds of calculated deficit given as 90 mmol/l sodium ORS over the first four hours and remaining one-third as water over the next two hours.

b) Patient reviewed clinically and by weighing at 6 hours:

i) successfully rehydrated: enter maintenance phase

ii) still dehydrated: further 6 hours course of ORS and water as in (a), with the volume based on the re-estimated deficit

iii) more dehydrated: intravenous therapy

Maintenance

Once rehydration has been achieved, solutions are used as outlined under 'Prevention'. Breast feeding may now be continued.

Note

Vomiting is common during the first few hours administration of ORT, but volumes are usually small and it does not prevent a successful outcome. To reduce vomiting, ORS can initially be offered by teaspoon or as sips.

REFERENCES

Ahmed I, Agusto-Odutola T B 1970 Hypernatraemia in diarrhoeal infants in Lagos. Archives of Disease in Childhood 45: 97–103

Anon 1978 Persistent excretion of salmonellas. British Medical Journal ii:509

Anon 1981 Oral therapy for acute diarrhoea. Lancet ii: 615–617

Anon 1983 Management of acute diarrhoea. Lancet i: 623–625

Aserkoff B, Bennet J V 1969 Effect of antibiotic therapy in acute salmonellosis on the fecal excretion of salmonellae. New England Journal of Medicine 281: 636–640

Association for the Study of Infectious Disease 1970 Effect of neomycin in non-invasive salmonella infections of the gastrointestinal tract. Lancet ii: 1159–1161

Baldini M M, Kaper J B, Levine M M, Candy D C A, Moon H W 1983 Plasmid-mediated adhesion in enteropathogenic Escherichia coli. Journal of Paediatric Gastroenterology and Nutrition 2: 534–538

Barrett-Connor E, Connor J D 1970 Extraintestinal manifestations of shigellosis. American Journal of Gastroenterology 53: 234–245

Barzgar M A, Ourshano S, Nasser Amin J 1980 The evaluation of the effectiveness of oral rehydration in acute diarrhoea in children under three years of age in West Azerbaijan. Journal of Tropical Paediatrics 26: 217–222

Black R E, Brown K H, Becker S 1984 Effects of diarrhoea associated with specific enteropathogens on the growth of children in rural Bangladesh. Pediatrics 73: 799–805

Booth I W, Levine M M, Harries J T 1984 Oral rehydration in acute diarrhoea in childhood. Journal of Pediatric Gastroenterology and Nutrition 3: 491–499

Boris M, Thomason B M, Hines V D, Montague T S, Sellers T F 1964 A community epidemic of enteropathogenic Escherichia coli 0126:B16:NM gastroenteritis associated with asymptomatic respiratory infection. Pediatrics 33: 18–29

Brinton C C 1959 Non-flagellar appendages of bacteria. Nature 183:782

Butzler J P, Skirrow M B 1979 Campylobacter enteritis. Clinics in Gastroenterology 8: 737–741

Catford J C 1980 Quality of prescribing for children in general practice. British Medical Journal 280: 1435–1437

Chung A N 1948 The effect of oral feeding at different levels on the absorption of foodstuffs in infantile diarrhea. Journal of Pediatrics 33: 1–13

Chung A N, Viscorova B 1948 Effect of oral feeding versus oral starvation on course of infantile diarrhea. Journal of Pediatrics 33: 14–22

Clearly T G, Clearly K R, Du Pont H L et al 1981 The relationship of oral rehydration solution of hypernatraemia in infantile diarrhoea. Pediatrics. 99: 739–741

Clements M L, Levine M M, Cleaves F et al 1981 Comparison of simple sugar/salt versus glucose/electrolyte oral rehydration solutions in infant diarrhoea. Journal of Tropical Medicine and Hygiene 84: 189–94

Crane R K 1965 Na⁺-dependent transport in the intestine and other animal tissues. Federation Proceedings 24: 1000–1006

Davies D P, Ansari B M, Mandal B K 1977 Hypernatraemia and gastroenteritis. Lancet i:252

Davidson G P, Gall D G, Petric M, Butler D G, Hamilton J R 1977 Human rotavirus enteritis induced in conventional piglets. Intestinal structure and transport. Journal of Clinical Investigation 60: 1402–1409

Diarrhoeal Diseases Study Group (UK) 1984 Loperamide in acute diarrhoea in childhood: results of a double blind, placebo controlled multicentre clinical trial. British Medical Journal 289: 1263–1267

Donald W D, Winkler C H, Bargeron L M 1956 The occurrence of convulsions in children with *Shigella* gastroenteritis. Journal of Pediatrics 48: 323–329

Dugdale A, Lovell S, Gibbs V, Ball D 1982 Refeeding after acute gastroenteritis: a controlled study. Archives of Disease in Childhood 57: 76–78

Duguid J P, Smith I W, Dempster G, Edmunds P N 1955 Non-flagellar filamentous appendages ('fimbriae') and haemaglutinating activity in *Bacterium coli*. Journal of Pathology and Bacteriology 7: 335–345

Dupont H L, Hornick R B 1973 Adverse effect of Lomotil therapy in shigellosis. Journal of the American Medical Association. 225: 1525–1528

Edmeades R, Halliday K, Shepherd R 1981 Infantile gastroenteritis relationship between cause, clinical course and outcome. Medical Journal of Australia 2: 29–32

Finberg L 1957 Experimental studies of the mechanisms producing hypocalcaemia in hypernatremic states. Journal of Clinical Investigation 36: 434–439

Finberg L 1970 The management of the critically ill child with dehydration secondary to diarrhea. Pediatrics 45: 1029–1036

Finberg L 1973a Hypernatraemic (hypertonic) dehydration in infants. New England Journal of Medicine 289: 196–198

Finberg L 1973b Diarrhoeal dehydration. In: Winters R W (ed) The Body Fluids in Pediatrics. Littler Brown & Co, Boston. Ch. 18, pp 349–371

Finberg L, Harper P A, Harrison H E, Sack R B 1982 Oral rehydration for diarrhea. Journal of Paediatrics 101: 497–499

Formal S B, Abrams G D, Schneider H, Sprinz H 1963 Experimental shigella infections. VI Role of the small intestine in an experimental infection in guinea pigs. Journal of Bacteriology 85: 119–125

Gaastra W, De Graaf F K 1982 Host-specific fimbrial adhesins of non-invasive enterotoxigenic *Escherichia coli* strains. Microbiological Reviews, 46, 129–161

Giannella R A, Formal S B, Dammin G J, Collins H 1973 Pathogenesis of salmonellosis. Studies of fluid secretion, mucosal invasion, and morphological reaction in the rabbit ileum. Journal of Clinical Investigation 52: 441–453

Gorbach S L, Banwell J G, Chatterjee B D, Jacobs B, Sack R B 1971 Acute undifferentiated diarrhea in the tropics. I: Alterations in intestinal microflora. Journal of Clinical Investigation 50: 881–889

Greenberg H B, Valdesuso J, Yolken R H, Gangaroso E, Gary W, Wyatt R G, Konno T, Suzuki H, Chanock R M 1979 Role of Norwalk virus in outbreaks of nonbacterial gastroenteritis. Journal of Infectious Diseases 139: 564–568

Guerrant R L 1985 Microbial toxins and diarrhoeal diseases: introduction and overview. In: D Evered, J Whelan (eds) Microbial toxins and diarrhoeal disease. Ciba Symposium 112, Pitman, London. 1–13

Halliday K, Edmeades R, Shepherd R 1982 Persistent post-enteritis diarrhoea in childhood. Medical Journal of Australia 1: 18–20

Head J, Hogarth M, Parsloe J, Broomhall J 1983 Soft drinks, electrolytes and sick children. Lancet i:1450

Hirschhorn N 1980 The treatment of acute diarrhea in children. An historical and physiological perspective. American Journal of Clinical Nutrition 33: 637–663

Hirschhorn N, Molla A, Molla A M 1969 Reversible jejunal disaccharidase deficiency in cholera and other acute diarrhoeal diseases. Johns Hopkins Medical Journal 125: 291–300

International Study Group 1981 Beneficial effects of oral electrolyte-sugar solutions in the treatment of children's diarrhoea. Journal of Tropical Pediatrics 27: 62–67

Ironside A G, Tuxford A F, Heyworth B 1970 A survey of infantile gastroenteritis. British Medical Journal 3: 20–24

Isolauri E, Vesikari T 1985 Oral rehydration, rapid feeding and cholestyramine for treatment of acute diarrhoea. Journal of Pediatric Gastroenterology and Nutrition 4: 366–374

Jacobson E D, Faloon W W 1961 Malabsorptive effects of neomycin in commonly used doses. Journal of the American Medical Association 175: 181–190

Jacobson E D, Prior J T, Faloon W W 1960 Malabsorption syndrome induced by neomycin; morphologic alterations in the jejunal mucosa. Journal of Laboratory and Clinical Medicine 55: 245–250

Keusch G T, Donohue-Rolfe A, Jacewicz M 1982 *Shigella* toxin(s): description and role in diarrhea and dysentery. Pharmacology and Therapeutics 15: 403–438

Kingston M E 1973 Biochemical disturbances in breastfed infants with gastroenteritis and dehydration. Journal of Pediatrics 82: 1073–1079

Kjellman B, Ronge E 1982 Oral solutions for gastroenteritis — optimal glucose concentration. Archives of Disease in Childhood 57: 313–315

Lambert H P 1979 Antimicrobial agents in diarrhoeal disease. Clinics in Gastroenterology 8: 827–833

Lancet Editorial 1983 Management of acute diarrhoea i: 623–625

Levine M M, Edelman R 1984 Enteropathogenic *Escherichia coli* of classic serotypes associated with infant diarrhea: epidemiology and pathogensis. Epidemiologic Reviews 6: 31–35

Levine M M, Hughes T P, Black R E 1980 Variability of sodium and sucrose levels of simple sugar/salt oral rehydration solutions prepared under optimal and field conditions. Journal of Pediatrics 97: 324–327

Levine M M, Kaper J P, Black R E, Clements M L 1983 New knowledge on pathogenesis of bacterial enteric infections as applied to vaccine development. Microbiological Reviews 47: 510–550

McDowell M E, Wolf A V, Steer A 1955 Osmotic volumes of distribution. Idiogenic changes in osmotic pressure associated with administration of hypertonic solutions. American Journal of Physiology 180: 545–558

Mahalanabis D 1983 Feeding practices in relation to childhood diarrhoea and malnutrition. In: Chen L C, Scrimshaw N S (eds) Diarrhoea and Malnutrition: Interacting Mechanisms and Interventions. Plenum Press, New York. Ch. 14 pp 223–234

Martorell R, Yarborough C, Yarborough S, Klein R F 1980 The impact of ordinary illnesses on the dietary intakes of malnourished children. American Journal of Clinical Nutrition 33: 345–350

Mata L J, Urrutia J J, Albertazzi C, Pellecer O, Arellano E 1972 Influence of recurring infections on nutrition and growth of children in Guatemala. American Journal of Clinical Nutrition 25: 1267–1275

Mata L J, Kromal R A, Urrutia L J, Garcia B 1977 Effect of infection on food intake and the nutritional state: perspectives as viewed from the village. American Journal of Clinical Nutrition 30: 1215–1227

Meeuwisse 1983 High sugar worse than high sodium in oral rehydration solutions. Acta Paediatrica Scandinavica 72: 161–166

Molla A M, Hossain M, Sanker S A, Molla A, Greenough W B 1982 Rice-powder electrolyte solutions as oral therapy in diarrhoea due to *Vibrio cholerae* and *Escherichia coli*. Lancet i: 1317–1319

Molla A M, Molla A, Sarker S A, Rahaman M M 1983a Food intake during and after recovery from diarrhoea in children. In: Chen L C, Scrimshaw N S (eds) Diarrhea and Malnutrition: Interactions, Mechanisms and Interventions. Plenum Press, New York. Ch. 7 p 113–123

Molla A, Molla A M, Sarker S A, Khatoon M, Rahaman M M 1983b Effects of acute diarrhea on absorption of macronutrients during disease and after recovery. In: Chen L C, Scrimshaw N S (eds) Diarrhoea and Malnutrition: Interactions, Mechanisms and Interventions. Plenum Press, New York. Ch. 9 pp 143–154

Morley D 1973 Paediatric Priorities in the Developing World. Butterworths, London pp 180–184

Nalin D R, Levine M M, Mata L et al 1979 Oral rehydration and maintenance of children with rotavirus and bacterial diarrheas. Bulletin of WHO 57: 453–459

Nelson J D 1979 Diarrhea. In: V C Vaughan, R J McKay Jr, R E Behman (eds) Nelson Textbook of Pediatrics, 11th Ed. Saunders, Philadelphia. pp 710–712

Oakley J R, McWeeney P M, Hayes-Allen M, Emery J L 1976 Possibly avoidable deaths in hospital in the age group one week to two years. Lancet i: 770–772

O'Brien A D, Kapral F A 1976 Increased cyclic adenosin 3', 5'-monophosphate content in guinea pig ileum after exposure to *Staphylococcus aureus* delta toxin. Infection and Immunity 13: 152–162

O'Brien A D, LaVeck G D, Thompson M R, Formal S B 1982 Production of *Shigella dysenteriae* Type 1-like cytotoxin by *Escherichia coli*. Journal of Infectious Diseases 146: 763–769

O'Morain C 1981 Acute ileitis. British Medical Journal 283: 1075–1976

Ortiz A 1978 Acute diarrhoea in young children. In: Jellife D, Stanfield J P (eds) Diseases of Children in the Subtropics and Tropics, 3rd edn. Edward Arnold, London. Ch. 19, pp 474–492

Palmer D L, Koster F T, Islam A F, Rahman A S, Sack R B 1977 A comparison of sucrose and glucose in oral electrolyte therapy of cholera and other severe diarrheas. New England Journal of Medicine 297: 1107–1110

Pizarro D, Posada G, Mata L 1983a Treatment of 242 neonates with dehydrating diarrhoea with an oral glucose-electrolyte solution. Journal of Pediatrics 102: 153–156

Pizarro D, Posado G, Villavicencio N, Mohs E, Levine M M 1983b Oral rehydration in hyper- and hyponatraemic diarrheal dehydration. American Journal of Diseases of Children 137: 730–734

Pizarro D, Posada G, Levine M M 1984 Hypernatraemic diarrheal dehydration treated with 'slow' (12-hour) oral rehydration therapy: A preliminary report. Journal of Pediatrics 104: 316–319

Placzek M, Walker-Smith J A 1984 Comparison of two feeding regimens following acute gastroenteritis in infancy. Journal of Pediatric Gastroenterology and Nutrition 3: 245–248

Portnoy B L, Dupont H L, Pruitt D, Abdo J A, Rodriquez J T 1976 Antidiarrhoeal agents in the treatment of acute diarrhea in children. Journal of the American Medical Association 236: 844–846

Powell D W, Field M 1980 Pharmacological approaches to the treatment of secretory diarrhea. In: Field M, Fordtran J S, Schultz S G (eds) Secretory Diarrhea. American Physiological Society, Bethesda, USA. Ch. 15: pp 187–209

Puffer R R, Serrano C V 1973 Patterns of mortality in childhood. Pan American Health Organisation Science Publication No. 262

Rahaman M M, Aziz K M S, Patwani Y, Munshi M H 1979 Diarrhoeal mortality in two Bangladeshi villages with and without community-based oral rehydration therapy. Lancet ii: 809–812

Rao M C, Guandalini S, Laird W J, Field M 1979 Effects of a heat stable enterotoxin of *Yersinia enterocolitica* on ion transport and cyclic guanosine 3', 5'-monophosphate metabolism in rabbit ileum. Infection and Immunity 26: 875–878

Rees L, Brooke C G D 1979 Gradual reintroduction of full-strength milk after acute gastroenteritis in children. Lancet i: 770–771

Riklis E, Quastel J H 1958 Effects of cations on sugar absorption by isolated surviving guinea pig intestine. Canadian Journal of Biochemistry and Physiology 36: 347–362

Rothbaum R, McAdams A J, Giannella R, Partin J C 1982 A clinicopathologic study of enterocyte-adherent *Escherichia coli*: a cause of protracted diarrhea in infants. Gastroenterology 83: 441–454

Rowe B 1979 The role of *Escherichia coli* in gastroenteritis. Clinics in Gastroenterology 8: 625–651

Rowland M G, Cole T J, Whitehead R G 1977 A quantitative study into the role of infection in determining the nutritional status of Gambian village children. British Journal of Nutrition 37: 441–450

Ruiz-Palacios G M, Torres J, Torres N I, Escamilla E, Ruiz-Palacios B R, Tamayo J 1983 Cholera-like enterotoxin produced by *Campylobacter jejuni*. Characterisation and clinical significance. Lancet ii: 250–253

Sack R B 1980 Enterotoxigenic *Escherichia coli*: identification and characterization. Journal of Infectious Diseases 142: 279–286

Sandberg A S, Ahderinne R, Andersson H, Hallgreen B, Hulten L 1983 The effect of citrus pectin on the absorption of nutrients in the small intestine. Human Nutrition: Clinical Nutrition 37: 171–183

Santosham M, Daum R S, Dillman L et al 1982 Oral rehydration therapy in infantile diarrhoea: a controlled study of well-nourished children hospitalised in the United States and Panama. New England Journal of Medicine 306: 1070–1076

Santosham M, Carrera E, Sack R B 1983 Oral rehydration therapy in well-nourished ambulatory patients. American Journal of Tropical Medicine and Hygiene 32: 804–808

Schultz S G, Zalusky R 1964 Ion transport in isolated rabbit ileum. II The interaction between active sodium and active sugar transport. Journal of General Physiology 47: 1043–1059

Snyder J D, Merson M H 1982 The magnitude of the global problem of acute diarrhoeal disease: a review of active surveillance data. Bulletin of the World Health Organisation 60:605

Spitzer A 1978 Renal Physiology and Functional Development. In: Edelmann C M (ed) Pediatric Kidney Disease, Little, Brown and Co., Boston. pp 25–128

Stephen J, Pietrowski R A 1981 *Bacillus cereus* enterotoxins. In: Bacterial Toxins, Nelson, Walton-on-Thames. Ch. 4, p 65

Stephen J, Wallis T S, Starkey W G, Candy D C A, Osborne M P, Haddon S 1985 Salmonnellosis: retrospect and prospect. In: Microbial Toxins and Diarrhoeal Disease. Ciba Foundation Symposium 112. Pitman, Tunbridge Wells. pp 175–192

Telch J, Shepherd R W, Butler D G, Perdue M, Hamilton J R, Gall D G 1981 Intestinal glucose transport in acute viral enteritis in piglets. Clinical Science 61: 29–34

Tripp J H, Harries J T 1977 Infective diarrhoea and vomiting. In: Harries J T (ed) Essentials of Paediatric Gastroenterology. Churchill Livingstone, Edinburgh. pp 192–194

Tripp J H, Wilmers M J, Wharton B A 1977 Gastroenteritis: a continuing problem of child health in Britain. Lancet, ii: 233–236

Vesikari T, Maki M, Sarkkinen H K, Arstila P P, Halonen P E 1981 Rotavirus, adenovirus and non-viral enteropathogens in diarrhoea. Archives of Disease in Childhood 56: 264–270

Wadstrom T, Aust-Kettis A, Habte D, Holmgren J, Meeuwisse G, Mollby R, Soderling O 1976 Enterotoxin-producing bacteria and parasites in stools of Ethiopian children with diarrhoeal disease. Archives of Disease in Childhood 51: 865–870

Walker-Smith J A, Manuel P D, Placzek M 1981 The decline in the incidence of hypernatraemic dehydration in the United Kingdom. American Journal of Clinical Nutrition 34: 1975–1976

Whitelaw A G L, Dillon M J, Tripp J H 1975 Hypertension, oedema and suppressed renin-aldosterone system due to unsupervised salt administration. Archives of Disease in Childhood 50: 400–401

WHO 1980 World Health Organisation. A manual for the treatment of acute diarrhoea. WHO/CDD/SER/80.2 Geneva

Protracted diarrhoea

Protracted diarrhoea is defined as the passage of four or more watery stools per day persisting for longer than two weeks in a child whose body weight either remains static or declines. The condition can present major problems both in diagnosis and management and may carry an appreciable mortality. Unless the disease process is arrested at an early stage, severe malnutrition may ensue, with all the clinical features of protein-energy deficiency as seen in the developing parts of the world (see Ch. 7).

AETIOLOGY OF PROTRACTED DIARRHOEA

Protracted diarrhoea may result from a wide variety of conditions (Table 16.1) but in only 60–70% of cases will a specific entity be recognizable (Avery et al 1968, Larcher et al 1977). In the remaining 30%, a diagnosis cannot be made despite extensive investigations. Larcher et al (1977) were able to identify the cause in 57 (72%) of 82 infants presenting with severe protracted diarrhoea of infancy (SPDI); the commonest diagnosis being coeliac disease (33.2%), disaccharide intolerance (12.2%) and cow's milk protein intolerance (11.3%). Other conditions included primary sucrase-isomaltase deficiency, Shwachman's syndrome, ulcerative colitis, ganglioneuroma, defective opsonization, staphylococcal pneumonia and Hirschsprung's disease. The overall mortality for the whole series was 5%, all four deaths being among infants with 'idiopathic protracted diarrhoea'.

PATHOPHYSIOLOGY OF PROTRACTED DIARRHOEA

The condition commonly appears to complicate an episode of acute gastroenteritis in infants under the age of 6 months in which the acute illness is assumed to be infective.

353

Table 16.1   Differential diagnosis of protracted diarrhoea in infancy

Causes	Example
Idiopathic	
Acquired sugar intolerance	Lactose intolerance
Acquired protein intolerance	Cow's milk, soya, egg, fish and rice
Coeliac disease	
Pancreatic insufficiency	Cystic fibrosis, Shwachman-Diamond syndrome, isolated pancreatic enzyme deficiency
Extraintestinal infections	Otomastoiditis, urinary tract infections, respiratory tract infections
Intrauterine infection	Cytomegalovirus
Surgical anomalies	Hirschsprung's disease, mid-gut malrotation
Following abdominal surgery	Short-gut syndrome
Selective inborn errors of metabolism	Congenital chloridorrhoea, glucose-galactose, malabsorption, Acrodermatitis enteropathica
Immune deficiency states	Defective opsonization, severe combined immunodeficiency, x-linked hypogammaglobulinaemia
Inflammatory bowel disease	Ulcerative colitis
Tumours	Neuroblastoma, histiocytosis
Nonaccidental injury	Laxatives
Endocrine	Adrenogenital syndrome, Addison's disease, thyrotoxicosis
Enterocolitis	
Miscellaneous	Intestinal lymphangiectasis, abetalipo-proteinaemia, renal tubular acidosis, autoimmune disease, congenital idiopathic intestinal pseudo-obstruction

Table 16.2   Pathophysiology of protracted diarrhoea

Protein intolerance	Cow's milk
	Eggs
	Fish
	Chicken
	Soya
	Rice
Carbohydrate intolerance	Disaccharides
	Monosaccharides
Gluten intolerance	See Chapter 8
Bacterial overgrowth of the small intestine	
Intraluminal metabolism of substrates	Bile acids
	Hydroxy fatty acids
	Short chain organic acids
Extraintestinal infections	
Autoimmunity	
Nonaccidental injury	
Idiopathic	? Defective enterocyte differentiation
? Defects of intestinal motility, gastrointestinal polypeptide metabolism, and changes in permeability	

"THE VICIOUS CYCLE"

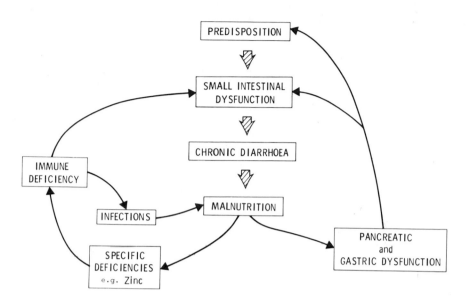

Fig. 16.1 The perpetuation of diarrhoea as a result of a vicious cycle of interacting events which have their basis in malabsorption and/or malnutrition.

A variety of pathophysiological mechanisms (listed in Table 16.2) acting singly or in concert, result in a diarrhoeal illness which may be trivial at its onset, and progress to a severe life-threatening disease. The concerted action of a number of events and the consequence of these is shown in Figure 16.1 and illustrates the vicious cycle of malabsorption-malnutrition that is in many cases associated with the perpetuation of the diarrhoea.

The intestinal dysfunction is perpetuated by a series of secondary events; malabsorption leads to malnutrition with consequent impairment of gastric and pancreatic function (Barbezat & Hansen 1968). In addition to maldigestion, we now know that pancreatic insufficiency may also result in impaired amino acid absorption (Milla et al 1983) thus perpetuating malnutrition. It is well established that malnutrition is also associated with reduced immune competence and loss of gastric acidity, which is in turn associated with increased bacterial contamination of the small intestine.

Acquired protein intolerance

Intolerance is not necessarily synonymous with the capacity of a dietary protein to induce morphological abnormalities of the small intestinal mucosa; it is this latter phenomenon which will be considered first. A wide variety of dietary proteins including cow's milk, eggs, wheat or gluten, soya, fish, rice and chicken (Kuitunen et al 1975, Iyngkaran et al 1982,

Victoria et al 1982) have now been shown to be capable of inducing an enteropathy. It has been suggested that an acute infective insult may be the prime event in sensitizing the small intestine to foreign proteins (Harrison et al 1976). The presence of relatively minor immunodeficiency by virtue of age, malnutrition or as a specific inherited defect (Harrison et al 1976, Candy et al 1980, Booth et al 1982) seems important in the pathogenesis of the enteropathy. The immunological mechanisms involved are discussed in detail in Chapter 8.

The diagnosis of protein intolerance is difficult at present because of the lack of adequate simple tests. Currently, response to food elimination and challenge is central to diagnosis. These aspects are discussed in more detail in Chapter 8.

Carbohydrate intolerance

Disaccharide intolerance may accompany a protein intolerance and since the disaccharidase enzymes are located at the brush border of the absorptive cells, reduced activity can be anticipated to accompany any factor which induces mucosal damage. Lactase is the last enzyme to reach maturity during fetal development, and for this reason premature babies who develop enteric infection are particularly at risk of becoming lactose-intolerant. Of the three disaccharides lactose, sucrose and maltose, clinical intolerance to lactose is by far the most important entity. Following mucosal damage lactase is the last enzyme to recover; this may take several months and be preceded by complete recovery of mucosal morphology (Gray et al 1968). The development of clinical symptoms of disaccharide intolerance will depend not only on the magnitude of the decreased enzyme activity, but also on its extent along the small intestine. For example, proximal small intestinal lesions are usually not accompanied by intolerance because the unabsorbed disaccharides can be hydrolysed and absorbed by the remaining normal mucosa. Similarly, where there is a severe enteropathy, monosaccharide intolerance might be expected as the mucosa will be populated with immature or damaged cells whose ability to actively absorb glucose/galactose is markedly reduced. Transient secondary intolerance to one or all of the three monosaccharides, (glucose, galactose and fructose) is now recognized as a clinical entity (Harries & Francis 1968, Lifshitz et al 1970a, 1970b). The clinical features and diagnosis are similar to those for disaccharide intolerance.

Symptoms include vomiting, abdominal distension and pain, and watery acid stools which are often frothy and result in perianal excoriation. The pathophysiology of these symptoms is discussed in detail in Chapter 9.

Disaccharide intolerance can be diagnosed relatively simply. The diagnosis may be suspected on the basis of a historical relationship between symptomatology and intake of dietary sugars, and should be confirmed by appropriate tests. The Clinitest® method (Kerry & Anderson 1964) is simple and determines the amount of reducing substances in the stool. The method can be applied to immediate testing of stools in the ward or even in field conditions. The test must be performed on the fluid component of the stool and must be done promptly to avoid bacterial degradation of sugars. A value of greater than 0.5% of stool-reducing sugars suggests sugar intolerance. Sucrose is a non-reducing sugar, and prior hydrolysis of the stool fluid with hydrochloric acid is necessary for its detection. Paper chromatography of stool water provides a semiquantitative method for determining the individual sugars. Oral sugar tolerance tests involve the determination of serial blood glucose levels following the administration of the suspected sugar (1 to 2 g/kg). If intolerant of the sugar, the patient develops gastrointestinal symptoms as described above, a rise of blood glucose of less than 1.6 mmol/l (30 mg/100 ml) and loose acid stools containing excessive amounts of reducing substances. It should be stressed that sugar loading tests may precipitate severe gastrointestinal symptoms and dehydration in susceptible children, particularly if they are sick infants with protracted diarrhoea. In most instances a confident diagnosis of sugar intolerance can be made on the basis of the history, examination of the stools and the response to withdrawal of the offending sugar from the diet. Stool pH is an unreliable test and merely creates additional work for the ward staff.

Determination of mucosal enzyme activities is unnecessary since it does not influence clinical management.

Bacterial overgrowth of the small intestine

Bacterial overgrowth of the small intestine in infants with protracted diarrhoea is common in both the developing (Coello-Ramirez & Lifshitz 1972, Heyworth & Brown 1975) and developed (Challacombe et al 1974a, Gracey et al 1969) parts of the world. The relationship between the bacterial overgrowth and the persistent diarrhoea is not at present clear. It is known however that bacterial toxins may have a direct effect on mucosal function (see Ch. 15), or an indirect effect secondary to the metabolism of certain intraluminal substrates as discussed below. More recently a cytopathic effect directed primarily against the brush border of the enterocyte has been described in young infants (Ulshen & Rollo 1980).

A variety of bacteria have been commonly found in the duodenum of infants with protracted diarrhoea, especially those that are malnourished (*Escherichia coli*, Clostridia, *Klebsiella pneumoniae*). Toxins elaborated by such bacteria have been shown to cause active secretion and inhibition of water and electrolyte absorption in the experimental animal (Field 1974, Klipstein et al 1976, McDonel 1974). The ability of the bacteria to adhere to a mucosal surface is probably essential for their colonization of the small intestine and their ability to produce disease. Candy et al (1983) found increased adhesion of *Esch. coli* (O1-K1-H7) to mucosal cells from infants with protracted diarrhoea compared to children with acute diarrhoea, and healthy infants and adults. In addition, bacteria isolated from the jejunum or stools of patients with protracted diarrhoea adhered to far greater numbers of their own buccal epithelial cells than those from healthy adults.

Intraluminal metabolism of substrates

A number of intraluminal substrates may be metabolized by bacteria to produce products of pathophysiological importance such as deconjugated bile acids and hydroxy fatty acids. Anaerobic bacteria contain enzymes which catalyse the deconjugation and 7-α-dehydroxylation of conjugated bile salts leading to the production of free dihydroxy bile acids such as deoxycholate and chenodeoxycholate. Deoxycholate has been shown to inhibit absorption of fluid and electrolytes in both the small and large bowel, and to inhibit monosaccharide absorption and mucosal (Na^+-K^+)-ATPase activity in the jejunum. At high concentrations the bile acid produces gross structural abnormalities of the jejunal mucosa (Harries & Sladen 1972, Sladen & Harries 1972, Guiraldes et al 1975). Deoxycholate and other free bile acids have been shown to be present in the duodenal contents of some infants with protracted diarrhoea (Gracey et al 1969, Challacombe et al 1974b, Schneider & Viteri 1974); the three infants reported by Gracey et al (1969) were also intolerant of monosaccharides.

Morphological abnormalities of the ileal mucosa have been reported in infants dying during the acute phase of gastroenteritis (Walker-Smith 1972) and it is likely that similar lesions may be present in some patients with protracted diarrhoea. This could result in bile salt malabsorption followed by bacterial degradation in the colon, with the free bile acids inducing colonic secretion of fluid and electrolytes. Cholestyramine is a nonabsorbable anion-exchange resin which is capable of binding bile acids and bacterial endotoxins. In this context it is of some interest that successful treatment with this resin of infants with intractable diarrhoea has been reported in an uncontrolled study (Tamer et al 1974).

In addition to free bile acids, bacterial production of hydroxy fatty acids and short chain organic acids may also result in inhibition of fluid absorption and the production of secretion particularly in the colon (Binder et al 1975).

Extraintestinal infections

Whilst the role of intraluminal enteric infection seems clear in the production of diarrhoeal states, the role of extraintestinal infection is not clear (De Sousa et al 1980). It is, however, the experience of all paediatricians that extraintestinal infections such as those of the urinary tract, lungs and meninges may be accompanied by diarrhoea in infants. The mechanisms involved are likely to be multifactorial and include underlying immunodeficiency, the production of toxins which, at least theoretically, may affect the serosal surface of the enterocyte, and enteric colonization with organisms such as *Esch. coli* and *Klebsiella* that are known to produce enterotoxins; this latter factor may be particularly true for urinary tract infection.

Autoimmunity

A recent communication raises the important concept that autoimmune processes may play a role in the pathogenesis of protracted diarrhoea in some infants. Mirakian et al (1986) reported cases of protracted diarrhoea in which autoantibodies to intestinal enterocytes were present as part of a polyendocrinopathy syndrome. The antibody to intestinal enterocytes was a complement-fixing IgG and reacted preferentially with a cytoplasmic antigen in villous tip enterocytes and also with colonic epithelium, but not with the stomach, oesophagus, rectum or skin. In addition, the patients produced a variety of other autoantibodies including pancreatic exocrine and islet cell, thyroid and smooth muscle antibodies. These patients bear some resemblance to a 14-year-old boy with isolated IgA deficiency reported by McCarthy et al (1978) who, following a febrile diarrhoeal illness, developed subtotal villous atrophy and IgG small intestinal antibodies. This patient failed to respond to a gluten-free diet but did respond to cyclophosphamide, the other cases responded variably to diet, steroids, azathioprine and cyclophosphamide.

Nonaccidental injury

Self-administered laxatives are a well recognized cause of chronic diarrhoea in adults (Cummings et al 1974) and sadly this possibility must now be considered in children with unexplained protracted diarrhoeal states. Ackerman & Strobel (1981) reported a 34-month-old girl who had been admitted on 12 occasions because of diarrhoea and dehydration for no apparent cause. The condition ultimately proved to result from phenolphthalein administered by the mother.

We have encountered similar episodes in infants with severe life-threatening diarrhoea, one following maternal administration of common table salt and another where the mother consistently fed her child cow's milk-containing formulae despite the firm diagnosis of a cow's milk-induced enteropathy.

The administration of a noxious agent to a child by a parent has now been firmly recognized and designated the 'Munchausen by proxy syndrome'. The presence of laxatives in the stool may be suspected by high concentrations of magnesium sulphate or anthrane derivatives in stool water (Read et al 1980) and other specific laxatives can be confirmed by appropriate tests.

Idiopathic protracted diarrhoea

In approximately 30% of patients with SPDI (Avery et al 1968, Candy et al 1981, Larcher et al 1977, Stankler et al 1982), particularly in those presenting at birth or soon after, a specific diagnosis will not be established and there is often a strong familial tendency. Candy et al (1981) reported 24 children with protracted 'cholera like' diarrhoea from 10 families, in which at least one sibling was affected. In two families the siblings were from first cousin marriages. In addition, extraintestinal anomalies were common. The mortality was high, 21 (87.5%) infants died after an illness that lasted between 12 days and 6 years, despite periods of prolonged intravenous feeding and the administration of a wide variety of pharmacological agents. Candy et al (1981) termed this condition 'lethal familial protracted diarrhoea'. Two other reports have described familial protracted diarrhoea also with a high mortality rate (Davidson et al 1978, Stankler et al 1982). The family histories were compatible with an autosomal recessive mode of inheritance, but studies by Davidson et al (1978), Milla et al (1981) and Heath & Milla (1983) suggested that this was a heterogenous group of conditions. Using a steady state perfusion technique Milla et al (1981) studied transport of water, electrolytes and hexoses in the proximal jejunum and colon of six infants with lethal familial protracted diarrhoea. In five of the six infants the jejunum was in a marked secretory state; in the sixth, water absorption was markedly reduced. Absorption of glucose and fructose was markedly impaired in all the infants as was the glucose-evoked transmural potential. In the proximal jejunum, glucose failed to induce an increase in Na^+ and water absorption in three of the patients. Estimation of the activity of the two transport enzymes $Na^+K^+ATPase$ and adenylate cyclase showed a marked reduction of the $N^+K^+ATPase$ activity in the five infants with marked secretion. The adenylate cyclase activity was variable. Colonic transport in these infants appeared normal suggesting that the diarrhoea was due to small intestinal secretion overwhelming the reabsorptive capacity of the colon.

All the families studied by Davidson et al (1978) suffered from a crypt hypoplastic villous atrophy. Transport studies in the proximal jejunum showed glucose absorption to be reduced and the response of Na^+ absorption to both glucose and phenylalanine impaired. In two of the three patients studied there was net secretion of water and sodium in the basal state; the clinical course of the third patient was milder and clearly different. In addition to the active secretory process, the defect in glucose absorption in both studies could be accounted for by either abnormal Na^+ coupled organic solute translocation at the apical cell membrane or by a defect in Na^+ extrusion at the baso-lateral cell membrane. In the infants studied by Milla et al (1981) at least the latter was playing a role. However, the findings of both studies could be accounted for if the enterocytes populating the villus were immature and retained their 'crypt-like' characteristics. Thus a defect in cell differentiation and replication may also play a role and this may be either an acquired or inherited defect.

In at least one of the families studied by Davidson et al (1978) a defect of the microvillus membrane has since become apparent. The condition has been termed congenital microvillus atrophy (Schmitz et al 1982, Phillips et al 1985) and is described in detail in Chapter 8.

Nonfamilial cases of idiopathic SPDI may have a better outlook. In those reported by Larcher et al (1977), 74% presented about one month after birth and the prognosis was good. Few pathophysiological studies have been made in this group of children. Rossi et al (1980) studied the extent and duration of small intestinal mucosal damage in 30 infants, 18 of whom suffered from idiopathic SPDI. Various degrees of villous atrophy persisting for an average period of six months were present in all patients. One might expect, therefore, that the small intestine would be in a secretory state with respect to water and electrolytes and that there would be malabsorption of a variety of organic solutes.

In summary, the information currently available suggests that whilst in many situations only one major factor such as altered cell turnover and the consequent enteropathy may be the prime cause of the diarrhoea, in others, most of the factors discussed above, toxin-induced secretion, toxic luminal metabolites, altered cell turnover, and increased prostaglandin production, may all be playing a part in the pathogenesis of the diarrhoeal state. Other factors such as gastrointestinal polypeptide metabolism, changes in motility and permeability, alterations in cell replication and differentiation may clearly be involved but are as yet poorly understood.

MANAGEMENT

The management of infants with protracted diarrhoea depends on the cause and the general condition of the infant when first seen. It can pose major therapeutic problems. If the infant's condition is reasonable, appropriate investigations can be performed to provide a logical basis for treatment. Often, however, the child's condition limits the time available for diagnostic investigations, and empirical treatment based on theoretical assumptions is necessary.

Dietetic

The basis of management is dietetic, to which most patients respond. A skilled dietitian is a key member of any team involved in the care of infants with protracted diarrhoea.

Cause determined

If investigation reveals that the infant is intolerant to one or more of the dietary constituents listed in Table 16.2, then a rational approach is possible. A wide variety of commercial food products are available for the treatment of various sugar and protein intolerances, and for detailed information the reader is referred to the excellent monography by Francis (1987). Generally speaking, preparations containing fat in the form of medium chain triglycerides (MCT) and nitrogen as amino acids or peptides are unnecessary, and most infants respond to more physiological preparations. Moreover, the high osmolality of many preparations containing MCT may in itself exacerbate the diarrhoea. The management of infants who are unable to tolerate all three monosaccharides deserves special mention. Successful treatment depends on the complete elimination of all carbohydrates from the diet and such therapy makes these infants extremely susceptible to development of severe hypoglycaemia, which may be fatal (Lifshitz et al 1970a, 1970b). Limited hepatic glycogen stores may be a predisposing factor, particularly if the infant is malnourished. Whilst receiving carbohydrate-free feeds, frequent determination of blood glucose levels is essential, and hypothermia may be a sign of severe hypoglycaemia. Preventive measures include daily infusions of glucose, and ephedrine and epinephrine have also been successful in some patients. Details of the diets for such patients can be obtained from Francis (1987). Intravenous feeding may be required to support the patient prior to recovery of monosaccharide tolerance.

Cause undetermined

When the cause of the protracted diarrhoea cannot be established or when the infant's condition precludes detailed investigation, we have found that a diet which is free of disaccharides, cow's milk protein and gluten gives excellent results. Protein is provided as comminuted chicken (which contains some long chain triglycerides), carbohydrate as Caloreen® (a

Table 16.3 Constituents of the initial full-strength feed for the treatment of protracted infantile diarrhoea of undetermined cause

Constituents	Amount in 100 ml
Protein (contained in comminuted chicken[1])	2.25 g
Fat (contained in chicken)	1.65 g
Caloreen®[2]	5.0 g
Sodium[3]	1.85 mmol
Potassium[3]	2.32 mmol
Calcium[3]	1.75 mmol
Other minerals[3]	—
Total energy provided:	approximately 200 kJ

[1] See Table 16.4 for further details of composition.
[2] Caloreen® is a glucose polymer; (Roussel Laboratories).
[3] Sodium, potassium, calcium and other minerals derived from the comminuted chicken and the metabolic mineral mixture; further details in Table 16.4 and Table 16.6.

Table 16.4 Composition of comminuted chicken[1] (Cow & Gate Baby Foods, England)

Constituents	Amount in 100 g
Protein	7–8 g
Fat	2.5–4 g
Carbohydrate	Nil
Sodium	0.4 mmol
Potassium	1.3 mmol
Calcium	0.2 mmol
Magnesium	0.3 mmol
Iron	0.1 mmol
Phosphorus	1.5 mmol

[1] Minced chicken can also be simply prepared in the home (see Francis 1987); sterility is extremely important because of the not infrequent endogenous bacterial contamination of poultry (e.g. Salmonellae).

glucose polymer) and fat as Calogen® (an emulsion of long chain triglycerides). Carbohydrate can also be given solely as glucose or as a mixture of glucose and fructose, up to a maximum concentration of 8 to 10%. The basic constituents of 100 ml of the initial full strength feed are shown in Table 16.3. Caloreen® (5 g) and the metabolic mineral mixture (10 g) are made up to 100 ml with water. Initially this formula is given as a quarter-strength feed with added sugar (5% Caloreen®) in a suitable volume every one to two hours, together with disaccharide-free complete vitamin and mineral supplements, e.g. three Ketovite® tablets and 5 ml Ketovite® liquid per 24 hours and a metabolic mineral mixture 1.5 g/kg/24 h to a total of 8 g/24 h. (See Tables 16.5, 16.6 and 16.7).

Any orally administered drugs must be free of disaccharides. The feeds are then slowly built up over a period of 10 to 30 days. This is achieved

Table 16.5 Composition of Ketovite® (Paines & Byrne Ltd, England)

Tablets	Content per tablet (mg)
Aneurine hydrochloride	1.0
Riboflavin	1.0
Pyridoxine hydrochloride	0.33
Nicotinamide	3.3
Calcium pantothenate	1.16
Ascorbic acid (C)	16.6
α-tocopheryl acetate (E)	5.0
Inositol	50.0
Biotin	0.17
Folic acid	0.25
Acetomenaphthone (K)	0.5

Liquid	Contents per 5 ml
Vitamin A	2500 units
Vitamin D	400 units
Choline chloride	150 mg
Cyanocobalamin (B_{12})	12.5 μg

Table 16.6 Composition of metabolic mineral mixture (Scientific Hospital Supplies, England)

Constituents	Amount (mg) in 1 g
Calcium	82
Potassium	83
Phosphorus	59
Sodium	39.6
Magnesium	9.7
Iron	0.63
Copper	0.13
Zinc	0.48
Manganese	0.057
Iodine	0.007
Aluminium	0.0002
Molybdenum	0.0015

by first increasing the feeds to full strength and then by adding Caloreen® (1% increments per day) until the child is on 10% Caloreen®.

Calogen® is next added to 1 ml/100 ml of feed per 24 hours to a total of 8 ml/100 ml to provide the requirements shown in Table 16.4. If this feeding regime is tolerated and the patient begins to thrive, then the following modifications are implemented prior to discharge home: (1) the intervals between feeds are increased (e.g. four hourly × 5); (2) introduction of suitable weaning solids (e.g. Robinson®'s baby rice mixed with 5% dextrose; milk-free mashed potato and puree meat). The dietitian then spends two to three sessions with the mother teaching her the diet. Following a period of protracted diarrhoea infants often become ravenously hungry and there is a real danger of them becoming overweight. This should be discussed with the mother during the dietary teaching sessions.

Table 16.7 Details of the full-feeding regime in the treatment of protracted infantile diarrhoea of undetermined cause

Constituents	Amounts in feeds
Comminuted chicken	30 g/100 ml of feed
Gastrocaloreen	10 g/100 ml of feed
Fat (from Calogen®[1] and comminuted chicken)	4 g/100 ml of feed
Metabolic mineral mixture	1.5 g/kg/24 h[2] (provided quantities do not exceed 1 g/100 ml of feed, or a total of 8 g/24 h)
Calcium (from comminuted chicken, metabolic mineral mixture and added calcium gluconate)	200 ml/kg/24 h
Total energy provided:	750 or more kJ/kg/24 h

[1] Calogen® is a 50% arachis oil emulsion of long chain triglycerides; Scientific Hospital Supplies Ltd., Liverpool
[2] Units of weight refer to actual not expected body weight. Vitamin supplements are given as Ketovite® tablet × 3/24 h) and liquid (5 ml/24 h) − see Table 16.5 for composition for Ketovite®

We have used this feeding regime for many years at The Hospital for Sick Children, Great Ormond Street, London, in infants with protracted diarrhoea who have failed to respond to other dietary manipulations and have been impressed by the excellent response which has been achieved in the majority of patients (Larcher et al 1977).

Intravenous feeding

In patients who are severely malnourished or who fail to respond to dietetic management, a period of intravenous feeding may be life-saving (Booth & Harries 1982); details are discussed in Chapter 24.

Other approaches

Where diarrhoea continues to pose a major problem, a number of therapeutic agents may be tried in addition to intravenous feeding or oral oligoantigenic feeds. On occasions they may be life-saving and in severe situations have a place in the management of the diarrhoeal state. If there is evidence of bacterial overgrowth and bile salt degradation, cholestyramine and antimicrobial agents are worth trying. Where *Clostridia difficile* toxin is found, vancomycin is the drug of choice, otherwise septrin and metronidazole. A number of agents enhance intestinal absorption directly, such as corticosteroids, or indirectly by interfering with prostaglandin synthesis such as salicylates and indomethacin.

Some agents are truly antisecretory in nature and these include phenothiazines and opioids. Both are effective in secretory states; chlorpromazine has been shown to reduce intestinal secretion in cholera (Rabbani et al 1982) although at the expense of some sedation, and it is currently thought to act by inhibiting calmodulin (Levin & Weiss 1977). Loperamide may also be extremely effective in modifying a secretory state (Sandhu et al 1983).

Duration of treatment

After a period of 2–3 months the patient is readmitted and reintroduction of disaccharides and cow's milk protein is attempted according to the following scheme:

Day 1: Lactose replaces the feed carbohydrate, initially in a concentration of 1%. If this is tolerated the concentration of lactose is increased on days 2, 3 and 4, to 3, 5 and 7% respectively.

Day 5: If lactose is tolerated, a challenge (5 ml) of fresh pasteurized cow's milk is given.

Day 6: If the milk challenge does not precipitate any symptoms, the volume of a suitable low solute cow's milk formula is slowly increased over the next four days so as to completely replace the chicken feeds. Sucrose is added to the diet (e.g. a fruit puree) prior to discharge. If lactose is tolerated then almost invariably sucrose will also be tolerated, since lactose intolerance usually persists for longer periods of time than sucrose intolerance.

Day 10: The patient is discharged home on a temporary gluten-free diet. After 2–3 months of treatment the majority of infants are able to tolerate disaccharides and cow's milk protein, but occasionally this is not the case. In those circumstances a further period of dietetic treatment is indicated, and one of the many commercially available disaccharide-free milk formulae containing soy protein or hydrolysed protein should be considered.

Assuming disaccharides and cow's milk protein are tolerated, the patient is followed up and growth and development checked at regular intervals. Failure to thrive may indicate persistent cow's milk protein intolerance, and a peroral intestinal biopsy may be helpful in confirming the diagnosis (see Ch. 8). If the infant continues to thrive, a gluten-free diet is continued for approximately six months. Following the reintroduction of a gluten-containing diet, follow up is continued for a year or more; the development of any biochemical or clinical abnormalities suggestive of gluten intolerance is an indication for biopsy. If there is a family history of coeliac disease or a clinical suspicion that the initial cause of the protracted diarrhoea was due to coeliac disease, a gluten-free diet is continued for at least two years when a formal gluten challenge is performed as outlined in Chapter 8.

PROGNOSIS

In those patients that present some time after birth the prognosis is excellent (Larcher et al 1977). However, in those that present from birth, unless the cause can be found, the prognosis is extremely poor with a mortality rate in the region of 80% (Larcher et al 1977). In this latter group there is a high familial incidence (Candy et al 1981).

REFERENCES

Ackerman N B, Strobel C T 1981 Polle syndrome: Chronic diarrhoea in Munchausen's child. Gastroenterology 81: 1140–1142
Avery G B, Villavicencio O, Lilly J R, Randolph J G 1968 Intractable diarrhoea in early infancy. Pediatrics 41: 712–722
Barbezat G O, Hansen J D L 1968 The exocrine pancreas and protein calorie malnutrition. Pediatrics 42: 77–92
Binder H J C, Filburn C, Volpe B T 1975 Bile salt alteration of colonic electrolyte transport: role of cyclic adenosine monophosphate. Gastroenterology 68: 503–508
Booth I W, Harries J T 1982 Parenteral nutrition in young children. British Journal of Intravenous Nutrition 3: 31–40
Booth I W, Christie I L, Levinsky R J, Marshall W C, Pincott J, Harries J T 1982 Protracted diarrhoea, immunodeficiency and viruses. European Journal of Paediatrics 138: 271–272
Candy D, Larcher V F, Tripp J H, Harries J T, Harvey B A M, Soothill J F 1980 Yeast opsonisation in children with chronic diarrhoeal states. Archives of Disease in Childhood 55: 189–193

Candy D, Larcher V F, Cameron D J S et al 1981 Lethal familial protracted diarrhoea. Archives of Disease in Childhood 56: 15–23

Candy D, Leung T S M, Marshall W C, Harries J T 1983 Increased adhesion of *Escherichia coli* to mucosal cells from infants with protracted diarrhoea: A possible factor in pathogenesis of bacterial overgrowth and diarrhoea. Gut 24: 538–541

Challacombe D N, Richardson J M, Rowe B, Anderson C M 1974a Bacterial microflora of upper gastrointestinal tract in infants with protracted diarrhoea. Archives of Disease in Childhood 49: 270–277

Challacombe D N, Richardson J M, Edkins S 1974b Anaerobic bacteria and deconjugated bile salts in the upper small intestine of infants with gastrointestinal disorders. Acta Paediatrics Scandinavica 63: 581–587

Coello-Ramirex P, Lifshitz F 1972 Enteric microflora and carbohydrate intolerance in infants with diarrhea. Pediatrics 49: 233–242

Cummings J H, Sladen G E, James O F W, Samer M, Misiewicz J J 1974 Laxative induced diarrhoea: A continuing clinical problem. British Medical Journal I: 537–541

Davidson G P, Cutz E, Hamilton J R, Gall D G 1978 Familial enteropathy: a syndrome of protracted diarrhoea from birth, failure to thrive, and hypoplastic villous atrophy. Gastroenterology 75: 783–790

De Sousa J S, De Silva A, De Costa Ribeiro V 1980 Intractable diarrhoea of infancy and latent otomastoiditis. Archives of Disease in Childhood 55: 937–940

Field M 1971 Intestinal secretion. Gastroenterology 66: 1063–1084

Francis D E M 1987 Diets for Sick Children, 4th edn. Blackwell, Oxford

Gracey M, Burke V, Anderson C M 1969 Association of monosaccharide malabsorption with abnormal small intestinal flora. Lancet ii: 384–385

Gray G M, Walter W M, Colver E H 1968 Persistent deficiency of intestinal lactase in apparently cured tropical sprue. Gastroenterology 54: 552–558

Guiraldes E, Lamabadusuriya S P, Oyesiku J E J, Whitfield A E, Harries J T 1975 A comparative study on the effects of different bile salts on mucosal ATPase and transport in the rat jejunum in vivo. Biochimica et Biophysica Acta 389: 495–505

Harries J T, Francis D E M 1968 Temporary monosaccharide intolerance. Acta Paediatrica Scandinavica 57: 505–511

Harries J T, Sladen G E 1972 The effects of different bile salts on the absorption of fluid, electrolytes, and monosaccharides in the small intestine of the rat in vivo. Gut 13: 596–603

Harrison M, Kilby A, Walker-Smith J A, France N E, Wood C B S 1976 Cow's milk protein intolerance: a possible association with gastroenteritis, lactose intolerance and IgA deficiency. British Medical Journal 1: 1501–1504

Heath A, Milla P J 1983 Development of colonic transport in early childhood: implications for diarrhoeal disease. Gut, 24:A977

Heyworth B, Brown J 1975 Jejunal microflora in malnourished Gambian children. Archives of Disease in Childhood 50: 27–33

Iyngkaran N, Abidin Z, Meng L L, Yadav M 1982 Egg protein induced villous atrophy. Journal of Pediatric Gastroenterology and Nutrition 1: 29–33

Kerry K R, Anderson C M 1964 A ward test for sugar in faeces.Lancet i: 981–982

Klipstein F A, Horowitz I R, Engert R F, Schenk E A 1976 Effect of *Klebsiella pneumoniae* enterotoxin on intestinal transport in the rat. Journal of Clinical Investigation 56: 799–807

Kuitunen P, Visakorpi J K, Savilahti E, Pelkonon P 1975 Malabsorption syndrome with cow's milk intolerance. Clinical findings and course in 54 cases. Archives of Disease in Childhood 50: 351–356

Larcher V F, Shepherd R, Francis D E M, Harries J T 1977 Protracted diarrhoea in infancy. Archives of Disease in Childhood 52: 597–605

Levin R M, Weiss B 1977 Binding of trifluoperazine to the calcium-dependent activation of cyclic nucleotide phosphodiesterase. Molecular Pharmacology 13: 690–697

Lifshitz F, Coello-Ramirez P, Gutierrez-Topete G 1970a Monosaccharide intolerance and hypoglycemia in infants with diarrhea. I. Clinical course of 23 infants. Journal of Pediatrics 77: 595–603

Lifshitz F, Coello-Ramirez P, Gutierrez-Topete G 1970b Monosaccharide intolerance and hypoglycemia in infants with diarrhea. II. Metabolic studies in 23 infants. Journal of Pediatrics 77: 604–612

McCarthy D M, Katy S I, Gayzi L, Waldman T A, Nelson D L, Strober W 1978 Selective IgA deficiency associated with total villous atrophy of the small intestine and organ specific anti-epithelial cell antibody. Journal of Immunology 120: 932–938

McDonel J L 1974 In vivo effects of *Clostridium perfringens* enteropathogenic factors on the rat ileum. Infection and Immunity 10: 1156–1162

Milla P J, Ogilvie D A, Harries J T 1981 Studies on the pathophysiology of severe protracted diarrhoea of infancy (SPDI). Pediatric Research 15:1194

Milla P J, Kilby A, Rassam U B, Ersser R, Harries J T 1983 Small intestinal absorption of amino acids and a dipeptide in pancreatic insufficiency. Gut 24: 818–824

Mirakian R, Richardson A, Milla P J 1986 Protracted diarrhoea of infancy: evidence in support of an autoimmune variant. British Medical Journal 293: 1132–1136

Phillips A D, Jenkins P, Raafat F, Walker-Smith J A 1985 Congenital microvillus atrophy: specific diagnostic features. Archives of Disease in Childhood 60: 135–140

Rabbani G H, Greenough III W B, Holmgren J, Kirkwood B 1982 Controlled trial of chlorpromazine as antisecretory agent in patients with cholera hydrated intravenously. British Medical Journal 284: 1361–1364

Read N W, Krejs G J, Read M G, Santa Ana C A, Morawski S G, Fordtran J S 1980 Chronic diarrhoea of unknown origin. Gastroenterology 78: 264–271

Rossi T M, Lebenthal E, Nord K S, Faizili R R 1980 Extent and duration of small intestinal mucosal injury in intractable diarrhoea of infancy. Pediatrics 66: 730–735

Sandhu B K, Tripp J H, Milla P J, Harries J T 1983 Loperamide in severe protracted diarrhoea. Archives of Disease in Childhood 58: 39–45

Schneider R E, Viteri F E 1974 Luminal events of lipid absorption in protein-calorie of the duodenal content to achieve micellar solubilizatiton of lipids. American Journal of Clinical Nutrition 27: 777–787

Sladen G E, Harries J T 1972 Studies on the effects of unconjugated dihydroxy bile salts on rat small intestinal function in vivo. Biochimica et Biophysica Acta 288: 443–456

Schmitz J, Ginies J L, Arnaud-Battandier F et al 1982 Congenital microvillus atrophy, a rare case of neonatal intractable diarrhoea. Pediatric Research 16:1041

Stankler L, Lloyd D, Pollitt R J, Gray E, Thom H, Russell G 1982 Unexplained diarrhoea and failure to thrive in 2 siblings with unusual facies and abnormal scalp hair shafts: a new syndrome. Archives of Disease in Childhood 57: 212–216

Tamer M A, Santora T R, Sandberg D H 1974 Cholestyramine therapy for intractable diarrhoea. Pediatrics 53: 217–220

Ulshen M M, Rollo J L 1980 Pathogenesis of *Escherichia coli* gastroenteritis in man — another mechanism. New England Journal of Medicine 302: 99–101

Vitoria J C, Camarero C, Sojo A, Ruiz A, Rodriguez-Soriano J 1982 Enteropathy related to fish, rice and chicken. Archives of Disease in Childhood 57: 44–48

Walker-Smith J A 1972 Uniformity of dissecting microscope appearances in proximal small intestine. Gut 13: 17–20

Diseases of the exocrine pancreas during childhood

Pancreatic disease during childhood is a relatively uncommon occurrence. This fact, however, makes recognition of pancreatic disease, evaluation, and treatment more difficult. In this review acute and chronic pancreatitis and exocrine pancreatic insufficiency are discussed. For reference purposes, the laboratory evaluation of pancreatic function is considered separately.

ACUTE AND CHRONIC PANCREATITIS

Pancreatitis is not common during childhood but reliable figures for incidence are not available. Evidence of acute pancreatitis is seen in 0.01% of all autopsies in children (Eichelberger et al 1981). With increasing awareness and improved diagnostic methods, the incidence of pancreatitis may, however be higher.

Aetiology and pathophysiology

The various factors thought to cause acute and chronic pancreatitis are listed in Table 17.1. The mechanisms by which these factors produce pancreatitis are not fully known, although a combination of duct obstruction, loss of vascular integrity, or primary insult to the pancreatic parenchyma is likely. Unfortunately, an aetiological agent frequently cannot be identified.

Trauma is one of the commonest causes (13–42% cases) of acute pancreatitis during childhood (Jordan & Ament 1977, Buntain et al 1978, Eichelberger et al 1982) and unfortunately many episodes of trauma are secondary to abuse (Pena & Medovy 1973). Symptoms usually appear soon after injury, although occasionally they occur much later.

Table 17.1   Causes of acute pancreatitis during childhood

Acute pancreatitis	Chronic pancreatitis
Trauma	Hereditary

Drugs
   valproic acid
   prednisone
   azathioprine
   cytosine arabinoside
   L-asparaginase
   tetracycline
   thiazides
   nitrofurantoin
	Metabolic
	   hyperlipidaemia
	   hyperparathyroidism
	   cystic fibrosis
	   (Wilson's disease) (alpha$_1$-antitrypsin
	   deficiency)

Infections
virus
   coxsackie
   echo
   mumps
   Epstein–Barr
bacteria
   leptospira
   mycoplasma
   typhoid
fungus
   candida
parasite
   ascaris
   malaria
   rickettsia
	Duct anomalies/obstruction
	   choledochal cyst
	   duodenal duplicatiton
	   duodenal diverticulum
	   anomalous duct insertion
	   pancreas divisum
	   (ectopic pancreas)
	   (annular pancreas)
	
	Idiopathic

Gallstones	

Vasculitis
   Henoch–Schonlein purpura
   systemic lupus erythematosus	

Inflammatory bowel disease	

Metabolic
   refeeding malnutrition
   parenteral alimentation
   Reye's syndrome
   diabetic ketoacidosis	

Ulcer disease	
Miscellaneous	
Idiopathic	

Drugs are frequently incriminated in pancreatitis (Jordan & Ament 1977, Buntain et al 1978, Mallory and Kern 1980, Eichelberger et al 1982), although the children are often being treated for an illness which itself might lead to pancreatic disease (see below). Such drugs include valproic acid (Allen & Coulter 1980), azathioprine (Isenberg 1978), prednisone (Jordan & Ament 1977, Eichelberger et al 1982), L-asparaginase (Land et al 1972), tetracycline (Elmore & Rogge 1981), thiazides (Weaver et al 1982), cystosine arabinoside (Altman et al 1982), and nitrofurantoin (Nelis 1983). In general, the development of signs and symptoms suggestive of pancreatitis in any child taking medication should raise the possibility of drug-induced disease.

Infection (commonly viral) is probably a frequent cause of childhood pancreatitis, although confirmation of this relationship is difficult. Various agents are listed in Table 17.1, the most notable being mumps. However, surprisingly few rigorous studies exist which establish that the amylase elevation seen during mumps-like illness is truly pancreatic in origin (Naficy et al 1973, Jordan & Ament 1977, Buntain et al 1978). Other viruses include Epstein-Barr virus (Werbitt & Mohsenifar 1980), echo and Coxsackie viruses (Ursing 1973). A variety of other agents including bacteria (Mardh & Ursing 1974), fungus (Richter et al 1982), parasites (Gilbert & Carbonnell 1964), and rickettsia (Mansueto et al 1983) have been reported to cause pancreatitis.

Gallstone pancreatitis is seen in children as well as in adults (Auldist 1972, Jordan & Ament 1977, Eichelberger et al 1982). Although the relative infrequency of cholelithiasis would suggest this to be an uncommon cause of the disease, between 10 and 20% of instances of acute pancreatitis during childhood seem to be related to the passage of gallstones.

Vasculitic diseases may also cause pancreatitis, including Schönlein–Henoch purpura (Garner 1977), and systemic lupus erythematosus (Buntain et al 1978, Reynolds et al 1982). Pancreatitis has also been reported in association with inflammatory bowel disease (Seidman et al 1983).

Several metabolic diseases have been postulated to cause pancreatitis. These include pancreatitis that develops during refeeding of patients with severe malnutrition (Barbezat & Hansen 1968, Gryboski et al 1980, Cox et al 1983), parenteral alimentation (Ellis et al 1979, Izsak et al 1980), Reye's syndrome (Reye et al 1963, Ellis et al 1979), diabetic ketoacidosis (Jordan & Ament 1977), cystic fibrosis, Wilson's disease, alpha$_1$-antitrypsin deficiency, severe hyperlipidaemia and hyperparathyroidism. Caution is necessary before assuming that hypercalcaemia or hypertriglyceridaemia are the causative agents of acute pancreatitis. Serum lipids are often elevated during the course of acute pancreatitis of any cause. In addition, serum calcium levels may drop from previously elevated levels to normal during acute pancreatitis.

The various causes of chronic pancreatitis are listed in Table 17.1. Perhaps the most common of these is hereditary pancreatitis. This illness was first reported by Comfort & Steinberg in 1952, and subsequently many other kindreds have been identified (e.g. Gross et al 1961, Kattwinkel et al 1973, Riccardi et al 1975, Perrault et al 1976, Sibert 1978). The condition is inherited as an autosomal dominant trait with penetrance that varies between 40 and 80%. The underlying defect is not known, although much attention has been placed recently on structural abnormalities of the pancreatic duct or possibly abnormal pancreatic stone protein (Sarles 1984). The onset of symptoms is usually under the age of 20, and most frequently between 10 and 12 years. As with other forms of pancreatitis, pain is usually the first manifestation. Episodes of pancreatitis may be severe and lead to debilitating disease. An aid in diagnosis is the relatively high frequency of characteristic calcifications of the pancreas seen on plain films of the abdomen. Aminoaciduria is not a necessary factor in the diagnosis. The diagnosis should be suspected in any situation where more than one family member has developed pancreatitis, especially at an early age, in the absence of other causative factors.

Several duct anomalies and obstructions have been implicated in chronic pancreatic disease during childhood. Annular pancreas (Johnston 1978, Kiernan & ReMine 1980) may cause symptoms, but does not usually lead to pancreatic inflammation. Duodenal duplications and diverticulae (Williams & Hendren 1971, Scully et al 1982), midgut malrotation and volvulus (Jordan & Ament 1977), choledochal cysts (Agrawal & Brodmerkel 1979), pancreatic duct diverticulae (Hatfield et al 1982), and congenital strictures of the pancreatic duct (Turner 1983) have also been reported to lead to pancreatitis.

The occurrence of these structural defects supports the need for rigorous evaluation of duct anatomy in otherwise unexplained chronic pancreatitis during childhood. Pancreas divisum is a congenital lesion found quite frequently, in which the drainage system of the pancreas does not fuse during development. Increasing recognition of this anomaly as a causative agent for pancreatitis is accumulating (Cotton 1980, Richter et al 1981). Although not necessarily an 'illness' leading to development of pancreatitis, the ectopic tissue itself occasionally becomes inflamed and presents problems with differential diagnosis (Dolan et al 1974, Thoeni & Gedgaudas 1980, Fam et al 1982). The ectopic tissue is found most commonly in the stomach, duodenum, or jejunum, but is responsible for disease in <10%. It is, however, as susceptible to the development of acute and chronic pancreatitis as is the proper gland.

Clinical presentation

The symptoms of acute pancreatitis and chronic relapsing pancreatitis are quite similar and will be discussed together. For simplicity, the differences between chronic relapsing and chronic recurrent pancreatitis will not be stressed. Clearly, children with chronic relapsing pancreatitis have repeated episodes of clinical similarity, and can develop pancreatic insufficiency, as opposed to those with chronic recurrent pancreatitis in whom the inflammation of the gland supposedly resolves between episodes.

In general, except for children with traumatic pancreatitis who may develop symptoms rapidly after injury, children with pancreatitis present with an illness of less than two months duration. The pain of pancreatitis is usually located in the epigastrium to periumbilical regions, with occasional radiation to the shoulder, back or lower abdomen. Inflammation in an ectopic focus of pancreatic tissue may present significant confusion. The pain is often precipitated or exacerbated by eating, although not necessarily by a fatty meal as is commonly supposed. Few alleviating factors are to be found. The pain tends to be rather constant in nature and can be measured in terms of hours and perhaps days, rather than minutes. Associated symptoms frequently include nausea, vomiting and anorexia.

Icterus is a less common manifestation and deep jaundice should raise suspicions of complicated disease. Unless pancreatitis is particularly severe, high fever is not present and evidence of vascular compromise is absent. Children with pancreatitis tend to lie rather still with some flexion at the hips. The abdomen is often mildly distended but visible loops of bowel are usually not seen. Other signs noted at inspection may include the Grey–Turner sign (bluish-grey colouration of the flanks) and Cullen's sign discolouration of the umbilical region. These are uncommon in children but suggest haemorrhagic pancreatitis. Auscultation of the abdomen usually reveals diminished bowel sounds and percussion reveals some degree of tympany. Tenderness may be elicited if early peritoneal signs are present. The retroperitoneal location of the gland may, however, change the localization of the pain; tenderness may be epigastric, but more commonly it is difficult to localize. A mass is not usually palpated unless a pseudocyst is present. Cutaneous manifestations include subcutaneous fat necrosis, which may occur during the acute disease or up to months later.

Differential diagnosis

Several other illnesses may mimic the signs and symptoms seen in acute and chronic pancreatitis and these are listed in Table 17.2. They include both diseases of the gastrointestinal tract and of other organ systems. Ulcer disease, especially in younger children, is at times quite difficult to differentiate from pancreatitis. A classic history of burning epigastric pain

Table 17.2 Differential diagnosis — pancreatitis

Gastrointestinal	Systemic
Ulcer disease	Pneumonia
Gastritis	Urinary tract disease
Oesophagitis	Gynaecological disease
Cholecystitis	
Inflammatory bowel disease	
Appendicitis	
Bowel obstruction	

relieved by antacids or eating is unusual in childhood. Ulcer disease in children is often accompanied by nausea and abdominal tenderness. Differentiation from pancreatitis, however, is usually possible on the basis of laboratory tests. An elevated serum amylase may be seen with ulcer disease, but penetration of the ulcer into the pancreas does not usually cause severe pancreatitis. Gastritis and oesophagitis are usually accompanied by pain which is more fleeting in nature and will not usually be confused with pancreatitis. Hepatitis may cause persistent abdominal pain but enlargement of the liver, more pronounced icterus, and simple laboratory testing allows the correct diagnosis to be made.

Cholecystitis may present more difficulty. A mild elevation in the serum amylase is not uncommon in cholecystitis and conversely mildly abnormal liver tests are often seen in pancreatitis. Laboratory testing, discussed below, and the clinical course allow appropriate diagnosis. Inflammatory bowel disease is usually associated with more persistent symptoms of gastrointestinal disease, including diarrhoea and pain lower in the abdomen and ponderal or linear growth delay. Appendicitis may at times be extremely difficult to differentiate from pancreatitis but generally, even the youngest child with appendicitis demonstrates more localized tenderness in the lower abdomen. Laparotomy is at times the only way to resolve this diagnostic dilemma. Small bowel obstruction may be associated with a mildly elevated serum amylase. Vomiting is usually more significant when obstruction is complete and abdominal distension is more pronounced than in pancreatitis. Bowel sounds also tend to be more active with bowel obstruction. Other non-gastrointestinal causes of abdominal pain need to be considered in the differential diagnosis of pancreatitis. These include pulmonary disease, urinary tract infection and obstruction, and gynaecological abnormalities.

Treatment

The treatment of acute pancreatitis differs little from that of adults and is aimed at resuscitative measures, 'rest of the gland,' and expectation of complications. Most important is awareness of the presence of the disease and prompt initiation of therapy. This usually consists of prohibiting all intake by mouth and placing an intravenous cannula for administration of fluids. Maintenance of adequate systemic circulation should be a primary aim of therapy. Passage of a nasogastric tube is not mandatory unless significant pain, vomiting, or complications exist. Provision of adequate analgesia is important. Pethidine in doses of 1–2 mg/kg intravenously or intramuscularly usually suffices and does little to exacerbate the disease through spasm of the sphincter of Oddi. The patient should be monitored frequently for evidence of severe disease, including circulatory collapse, peritoneal signs, hyperglycaemia and hypocalcaemia. Other complications of pancreatitis should be anticipated, including pulmonary disease (pleural effusions, respiratory failure, and intrathoracic pseudocyst formation), pseudocyst formation, and abscess formation. The latter two complications are suggested by a particularly prolonged course, either clinically or biochemically. The usual course of uncomplicated acute pancreatitis is measured in days. The diet should be advanced only when signs are abating and the serun amylase level is approaching normal. A prolonged course may require parenteral alimentation, which seems to pose no threat to the inflamed gland (Silberman et al 1982). Patients with chronic pancreatitis often suffer from severe and refractory abdominal pain. Analgesics are indeed necessary, although the risk is significant for development of dependencies. Many techniques have been employed in efforts to reduce this dependency, including a variety of biofeedback techniques. Recent attention has focused on the provision of supplemental exogenous pancreatic enzymes, even when exocrine function is good. Only in rare instances is surgery indicated during childhood either in the acute or chronic phase. Results, however, tend to be better in children than in adults.

EXOCRINE PANCREATIC INSUFFICIENCY

Cystic fibrosis

Cystic fibrosis is the commonest cause of pancreatic exocrine insufficiency during childhood. The disease affects approximately one in every 2000 live Caucasian births. Since almost 80% of these patients now live into adulthood (Shwachman et al 1977) and the diagnosis is, at times, first established in adulthood (Scully et al 1982), awareness of the disease is important to physicians of all subspecialties. Monographs and textbooks devoted to fibrosis are available (Shwachman 1978, Lloyd-Still 1983, Taussig 1985), therefore the current discussion will be limited to gastrointestinal involvement (Park & Grand 1981).

Cystic fibrosis is inherited in an autosomal recessive manner, with an estimated gene frequency of 4–5% among Caucasian populations (Wood et al 1976). The disease is much less common in other racial groups. Pathogenetic mechanisms leading to disease are not well understood at present, although factors leading to inhibition of electrolyte transport in ductular epithelium and to abnormal mucus composition, are most often implicated.

Histologically, the pancreatic lesion appears to be initiated by obstruction of small ductules with eosinophilic concretions (Andersen 1958). The pancreas may be nearly normal in neonates (Oppenheimer & Esterly 1973), although the characteristic lesions of cystic fibrosis may even then be present with luminal concretions, distension of ducts and acini, mild inflammation and fibrosis, and cysts lined by a single layer of epithelial cells. Older children with established disease usually demonstrate this lesion. Cysts may occasionally be relatively large, up to 3 mm in diameter, and calcifications are sometimes present. The main pancreatic ducts and islet cells are normal. Late in the course of the disease, the characteristic lesions may be lost and the gland entirely replaced by fat and fibrous tissue. At this stage, differentiation between cystic fibrosis and other forms of chronic pancreatic injury may be difficult.

Exocrine pancreatic insufficiency occurs in approximately 85% of patients with cystic fibrosis (Shwachman 1975). Pancreatic secretions in these patients are of small volume, thick, and deficient in both enzymes and bicarbonate (Hadorn et al 1968a, Lapey et al 1974), although variations in severity exist. Those without clinical pancreatic insufficiency usually show near-normal enzyme concentrations, but abnormal volume and bicarbonate responses to pancreatic stimulation (Hadorn et al 1968, Kopelman et al 1985). A few patients without pancreatic insufficiency develop recurrent acute pancreatitis (Shwachman 1975). The resulting malabsorption, steatorrhea, and azotorrhea are the most frequent gastrointestinal manifestations of cystic fibrosis and usually present by the age of 2 years and often by 2 months of age. It has often been stated that children with a voracious appetite are much more likely to have cystic fibrosis than other malabsorptive diseases, such as coeliac sprue, where anorexia seems more frequent. This concept has not been supported when examined carefully. Usually, only young infants have increased appetites, while older infants and children have diminished appetites (Chase et al 1979). Watery diarrhoea without a particularly foul odour is often seen in the first six months, progressing only later to characteristic foul, bulky, pale stools. Malabsorption, anorexia, and increased energy demands worsen as adolescence is approached.

At times, however, the severity of the disease is less and normal growth and development may persist into adulthood. Older patients often choose to discontinue enzyme replacement with little change in symptoms, although significant steatorrhoea persists (Lapey et al 1974). This may reflect compensation for the greatly dminished pancreatic lipase activity by lingual lipase which is still secreted in patients with cystic fibrosis (Abrams et al 1984, Roulet et al 1980). Other manifestations of fat malabsorption include deficiencies of fat soluble vitamins (Chase et al 1979), abnormal fatty acid profiles and occasionally overt essential fatty acid deficiency (Chase et al 979). Water soluble vitamin deficiency is less of a problem.

As suggested above, 15–20% of patients with cystic fibrosis do not manifest clinical exocrine pancreatic insufficiency. An interesting subset of these has been identified who suffer from recurrent acute pancreatitis. This is discussed in the section dealing with pancreatitis.

Meconium ileus is the earliest manifestation of cystic fibrosis in 15% of patients (Donnison et al 1966). These children present with abdominal distension, delayed passage of meconium, and evidence of gastrointestinal obstruction such as bilious emesis. This occurs within the first day or two of life. An occasional history of polyhydramnios is present and physical examination may reveal visible loops of bowel. Volvulus, atresia, or peritonitis may also occur. Abdominal X-ray often shows small air bubbles trapped within obstructing meconium in the distal small bowel with more proximal distension and a lack of air in the colon, which is normally present at 3 to 6 hours of age. Intraabdominal calcifications suggest bowel perforation in utero. Barium enema supports the diagnosis when a microcolon and distal left ileal mass are demonstrated. A similar illness occurs in as many as 10% of older children with cystic fibrosis (Matseshe et al 1977), the so-called meconium ileus equivalent. In practice, this syndrome includes almost any condition due to partial or complete bowel obstruction in a patient with cystic fibrosis. Symptoms include abdominal pain, and a palpable mass in the right lower quadrant, or obstruction. Rectal prolapse occurs in up to 22% of patients with cystic fibrosis and may be a presenting and recurring complaint particularly between 1 and 2 years of age (Kulczycki & Schwachman 1958). Intussusception is less common, being seen in approximately 1% of patients with cystic fibrosis (Holsclaw et al 1971).

A mucosal defect in small bowel function has been suggested by findings of poor uptake of some amino acids (Morin et al 1976, Milla et al 1980). Although previously thought to be prominent, the incidence of lactase insufficiency is no higher than that seen in age-matched controls (Antonowicz et al 1978, Shwachman 1978). Radiographic changes in the bowel are frequently seen and include thickening and distortion of small bowel loops (Taussig et al 1973) and pneumatosis intestinalis (Wood et al 1976). These X-ray findings are not fully explained by local histologic changes, although abnormalities have been reported in the small bowel and rectum. Small bowel crypts may contain increased mucus, and villous structure is usually normal (Thomaidis & Arey 1963), although mild to moderate villous shortening has been described (Cox et al 1979). More severe abnormalities in villous structures suggest concomitant disease, including coeliac disease (Katz et al 1976).

Many patients with cystic fibrosis show evidence of liver disease, although this is of clinical significance in less than 5% of patients (Oppenheimer & Esterly 1975, Stern et al 1976). Oppenheimer & Esterly (1975) identified three types of hepatic lesions. An early lesion, probably peculiar to cystic fibrosis is seen in infants and is characterized by focal accumulation of mucus in the biliary tree. This is most marked in the porta hepatis and is rarely found in extrahepatic ducts. Periportal changes include mild inflammation and fibrosis and often bile duct proliferation and cholestasis. The second lesion although similar, was considered nonspecific because of a lack of mucus collections. The third and most characteristic hepatic lesion of cystic fibrosis is 'focal biliary cirrhosis'. It consists of inspissated eosinophilic material within bile ducts, increased periportal inflammation and fibrosis, and bile duct proliferation. These changes are focal and are more frequent in older patients. In 5% of patients with cystic fibrosis, these lesions progress with the development of regenerative nodules, increased fibrosis, and collapse of lobules representing severe post-necrotic cirrhosis (Stern et al 1976, Schuster et al 1977). Other histologic lesions include nutritionally-induced fatty changes and central lobular necrosis from right heart failure. Corresponding clinical entities are usually limited to neonatal jaundice, hypersplenism, variceal bleeding, and hepato-cellular failure, plus nonspecific abnormalities of liver tests, especially alkaline phosphatase. Prolonged obstructive jaundice in infants with cystic fibrosis has also been associated with 'giant cell hepatitis' in the absence of other characteristic changes (Rosenstein & Oppenheimer 1977).

Abnormalities in the biliary tree are found in approximately one-third of patients on autopsy analysis and in over 40% by cholecystography (L'Heureux et al 1977). The gallbladder is often small, containing thick colourless bile within its lumen and mucus-filled cysts within its epithelial lining (Oppenheimer and Esterly 1975). An oral cholecystogram is abnormal in 40–50% of patients, although malabsorption of contrast material is often the explanation. In a significant number of patients, however, the gall bladder is not visualized at intravenous cholangiogram. Gallstones are detected in approximately 12% of patients (L'Heureux et al 1977). Not unexpectedly, the presence of stones does not necessarily correlate with symptoms.

The bile salt pool is depleted in cystic fibrosis with an increased fractional turnover rate secondary to faecal losses (Watkins et al 1977, Harries et al 1979). Analysis of relative lipid composition of gallbladder bile may reveal supersaturation with cholesterol (Roy et al 1977).

The diagnosis of cystic fibrosis begins with awareness of the disease. More than 95% of children with pancreatic insufficiency, most with meconium ileus, 30% with meconium peritonitis and 15% with small bowel atresia (Noblett 1979) will have cystic fibrosis. Other indications for evaluation include unexplained chronic pulmonary disease, chronic hepatobiliary disease, hypoproteinaemia and oedema, and failure to thrive. Siblings of an affected family member should also be screened. The diagnosis of cystic fibrosis depends at present on analysing the sweat sodium and/or chloride concentrations, and chloride concentrations are elevated in 99% of patients with cystic fibrosis. The test, however, must be performed carefully. Classically, quantitative pilocarpine iontophoresis (Shwachman 1978) has been the method of choice for sweat testing. False negative results occur with improper testing techniques. False positive results have been reported in a variety of conditions including adrenal insufficiency, nephrogenic diabetes insipidus, congestive heart failure and other oedematous states, fever, dehydration, ectodermal dysplasia and malnutrition, for a variety of causes. In these situations, however, abnormalities in sweat chloride are usually transient. Medications, including diuretics, and high or low sodium diets may also affect results. Other methods of detecting sweat chloride concentrations have recently been introduced. Most useful among these seems to be the Medtronics® apparatus. Other methods include Orion® and Medtherm® probes. A positive result should be confirmed at least once at a major cystic fibrosis centre before diagnosis is made. Results must then be correlated with clinical findings, family history, and clinical course. 99% of patients with cystic fibrosis with a confidence level of 99% will have sweat chloride and sodium concentrations above 77 mmol/l and 74 mmol/l respectively. In addition the concentration of chloride will be slightly greater than that of sodium which is the reverse of normal. Borderline values between 45 and 75 are difficult clinical problems and require repeat testing and clinical correlation.

Screening tests have been suggested to establish a neonatal diagnosis of cystic fibrosis. These have included determination of serum immunoreactive trypsin levels as discussed later. Most neonates with cystic fibrosis have highly elevated serum levels of immunoreactive trypsin. Whether this will prove to be a useful screening test remains to be determined.

The prognosis of cystic fibrosis is improving, although it is still far from acceptable. Currently, between 80 and 90% of patients which cystic fibrosis survive into early adulthood. Male patients tend to live longer than females by about four years. Most of the significant morbidity and mortality are related to lung disease. The relative influence of nutritional support, pancreatic enzyme replacement, and aggressive treatment of pulmonary disease on improving the quality of life is uncertain.

Schwachman's syndrome

In 1964, Schwachman's syndrome became a distinct clinical entity (Bodian et al 1964, Schwachman et al 1964). The combination of exocrine pancreatic insufficiency, bone marrow and haematological abnormalities, and normal sweat electrolytes typified the syndrome which has been expanded in the last few years to include abnormalities in many other organ systems. It is currently thought to be the second most frequently diagnosed cause of pancreatic insufficiency in children.

The disease seems to be inherited in an autosomal recessive manner (Aggett et al 1980, Schwachman et al 1964). The pathogenetic mechanisms, however, are unclear. Some sort of fetal injury may occur, since pancreatic exocrine tissue and the myeloid portion of the bone marrow both develop at around the fifth month of gestation. This alone would not, however, explain the familial incidence.

At laparotomy, the pancreas varies in size from normal to small, and usually has a fatty appearance. The main pancreatic ducts are normal. Histologically, acinar tissue is replaced by fat with preservation of islet cells (Figs 17.1 and 17.2) (Bodian et al 1964) Schwachman et al 1964, Caselitz et al 1979, Aggett et al 1980).

There is no sex preponderance, and children almost always develop

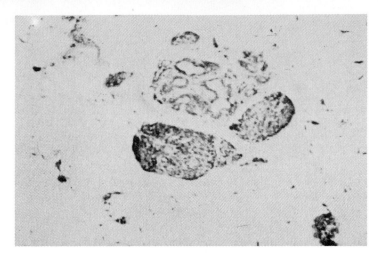

Fig. 17.1 Histological appearances of the pancreas in Schwachman's syndrome. Acinar tissue is very sparse with preservation of the islets of Langerhans and the ducts. The acinar cells are almost completely replaced by fat, and there is an absence of fibrosis and inflammatory cells.

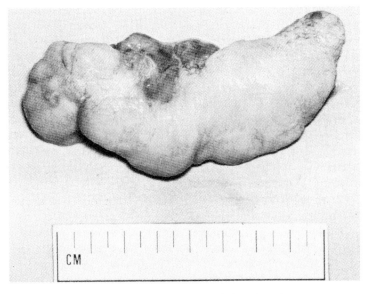

Fig. 17.2 Macroscopic appearances of the pancreas in Schwachman's syndrome. The gland appears as a lobulated, fat-laden structure

malabsorption by four to six months of age (Schwachman et al 1964, Shmerling et al 1969, Aggett et al 1980). Failure to thrive, feeding difficulties and impaired growth present from an early age.

Pancreatic exocrine function is impaired with diminished secretion of lipase, amylase, and trypsin (Schwachman et al 1964, Shmerling et al 1969,

Aggett et al 1980). Volume and bicarbonate content, however are variable but tend not to be as low as in cystic fibrosis. Values range from low (Shmerling et al 1969, Liebman et al 1979) to normal (Saunders et al 1979). Serum enzyme activities have been low, including pancreatic isoamylase (Levitt et al 1977). Symptomatic response to pancreatic enzyme replacement is good, although growth failure does not abate despite intensive therapy (Aggett et al 1980). Endocrine pancreatic function is usually maintained. By definition, the sweat electrolytes are normal.

Infection is a frequent problem and is related in part to both quantitative and qualitative defects of neutrophils.

Neutropenia is almost always present at some time during the course of the disease. This may be cyclical in nature, fluctuating over intervals as frequent as days. Patients usually respond with a normal or elevated white count when infection is present (Schwachman et al 1964, Saunders et al 1979, Aggett et al 1980). The cause of the neutropenia is not known. Neutrophil function is also defective in over 90% of patients (Aggett et al 1980) with impaired mobility in response to a standard bacterial stimulus. Improved mobility may result from treatment with cimetidine or large doses (0.5 g) of ascorbic acid. Thrombocytopenia is seen in approximately two-thirds of patients and may also be a cyclic event (Aggett et al 1980). Severe bleeding, however, is unusual (Aggett et al 1979, Saunders et al 1979). Anaemia seems to be the least common haematological abnormality, occurring in 50% of patients at most. Malignancies have been reported in patients with Schwachman's syndrome, including chronic myeloid leukaemia (Caselitz et al 1979), acute lymphoblastic leukaemia (Strevens et al 1978), acute monocytic leukaemia (Nezelof & Watchi 1961), acute myeloblastic leukaemia (Huijgens et al 1977) and erythroleukaemia (Aggett et al 1980). Bone marrow aspiration may be entirely normal (Aggett et al 1980) or show arrest of the myeloid series with occasionally marrow replacement by fibrous tissue and fat (Schwachman et al 1964, Shmerling et al 1969).

Bony changes have been frequently reported (Shmerling et al 1969, Aggett et al 1980). Metaphyseal chondrodysplasia is usually the most frequent lesion, involving the femoral neck. The lesion tends to be symmetrical and may be progressive, at times leading to clincial disease. Other osseous lesions have included abnormally short ribs with anterior flaring, vertebral wedging, clinodactyly, and long bone changes (Aggett et al 1980).

Abnormalities in liver structure and function have also been reported (Schwachman et al 1964, Liebman et al 1979, Aggett et al 1980). Hepatomegaly is seen in about two-thirds of patients when young, and less frequently in older individuals. Serum amino-transferase levels are elevated in half to three quarters of patients, again most frequently in the young. Bilirubin levels are usually normal, with minimal elevation of alkaline phosphatase. Chronic liver disease has been documented, although infrequently (Liebman et al 1979).

Other lesions, including endocardial fibrosis, right-sided hypertrophy due to lung disease (Graham et al 1980), icthyosis (Aggett et al 1980), testicular fibrosis (Graham et al 1980), pubertal delay (Aggett et al 1980), renal tubular dysfunction (Schwachman et al 1964, Aggett et al 1980) have been reported.

The diagnosis of Schwachman's syndrome should be suspected in any child with exocrine pancreatic insufficiency who on careful testing has normal sweat electrolytes, particularly if haematological abnormalities are present. Repeat blood counts may be necessary, as may radiographs of the hips in older children.

In the past, between 15 and 20% of patients died because of severe infections, but improved care has substantially reduced the prognosis.

Treatment of exocrine pancreatic insufficiency in this illness is discussed below. Growth deficiency, however, persists despite enzyme replacement.

Other causes of pancreatic insufficiency

Other causes of pancreatic insufficiency during childhood are rare although several isolated enzyme defects have been reported. These include isolated lipase deficiency which was first reported by Sheldon (1964) and subsequently confirmed by other observers (e.g. Rey et al 1966, Muller et al 1975, Figarella et al 1972). The origin of this deficiency is not clearly established. An unusual manifestation of this disease is the passage of oil rectally, separate from stools. Interestingly failure to thrive and other systemic manifestations have not been associated. Treatment of this condition is orientated towards reduction in the distressing discharge of faecal oil. Isolated trypsin deficiency was first reported by Townes (Townes 1965, Townes et al 1967), and presents with severe growth failure, hypoproteinaemia, and oedema. In addition to absent tryptic activity, chymotrypsin and carboxypeptidase activity was also diminished in the children reported. This disorder has not been clearly differentiated from enterokinase deficiency. Children with enterokinase deficiency present similarly with malabsorption, hypoproteinaemia and growth failure (Hardon et al 1969). As expected, amylase and lipase activities are normal, while trypsin activity is low. Intraluminal trypsinogen can be activated by the addition of exogenous enterokinase.

Other rare selected deficiencies have included absent amylase (Lowe & May 1951) and absent lipase and proteolytic activity (Townes 1969).

Treatment of exocrine pancreatic insufficiency

The treatment of exocrine pancreatic insufficiency in children is similar to that of adults. Special attention, however, must be paid to adequate nutrition to ensure proper growth and development.

Treatment of exocrine pancreatic insufficiency would seem at first to be a simple matter. Exogenous enzyme should easily replace deficient pancreatic secretions once the product is delivered to the duodenum. It is estimated, in fact, that only 10% of normal lipase activity is needed to prevent steatorrhoea and as little as 2–3% to prevent severe symptoms (DiMagno et al 1973). In practice however, this minimum level seems difficult to reach. As little as one-quarter of ingested trypsin and 10% of ingested lipase actually arrives active within the duodenal lumen (DiMagno et al 1977). This has been thought to result from inactivation of enzyme by either intragastric or intraduodenal acidity. Initial therapy of exocrine pancreatic insufficiency in children consists of the administration of exogenous pancreatic enzymes. The dose of exogenous lipase seems to be most critical in alleviating clinical problems. Usually, a total dose of between 3000 and 15 000 units of lipase given just before each meal and a lesser amount with snacks is appropriate. A precise dosing regimen is variable and depends upon patient age and clinical response. In general, infants can be started on a quarter teaspoon of porcine pancreatic enzyme extract before each feed and the amount adjusted according to response. The powder can be mixed with a small amount of apple sauce or other appropriate vehicle.

To protect the enzyme during gastric transit, acid-resistant coatings and pH sensitive microsphere preparations have been developed. These products must also be mixed in an appropriate vehicle before administration as there can be a problem with spherules becoming stuck between the buccal mucosa and gingiva, creating superficial ulcerations and bleeding. For unexplained reasons, some neonates do not respond as well to coated preparations, whereas older children and adults usually prefer capsules (with or without an acid-resistant coating) to powder. Therapy usually begins with one or two capsules of enzyme at each meal or snack. An insufficient dose will of course, lead to inadequate relief of steatorrhoea and malnutrition. Excessive administration produces few symptoms other than a perianal rash at times, or, more importantly, constipation, and possible bowel obstruction. In certain patients, between 10 and 20 capsules are needed with meals and approximately half that amount with snacks to obtain an adequate response. In situations where replacement therapy is unsuccessful and there is confirmation that appropriate medication is being taken, additional medications can be of benefit. This has generally included agents which are able to eradicate the acid milieu. Antacids and H_2 histamine receptor blockers (Regan et al 1977, Saunders et al 1977, Durie et al 1980a) have been tried alone or in combination, with variable response.

Vitamin supplementation is usually recommended in patients with exocrine pancreatic insufficiency, particularly the fat soluble vitamins A, D, E and K. One to 5 mg of vitamin K, 10 mg/kg/24 h of vitamin E, and vitamin A in a dose of 5 to 10 000 international units/24 h are also appropriate. Vitamin D deficiency seems to be less common; 5000 international units/24 h is appropriate therapy for documented deficiency, while 500 to 1000 international units daily is suggested as maintenance.

Other therapies including the use of medium chain triglycerides have been recommended but they still do not eliminate the need for adequate intraluminal enzyme activity (Durie et al 1980b). Essential fatty acid deficiency is unusual. Elemental diets have also been recommended, but these diets, as well as the use of total parenteral alimentation (Chase et al 1979) are reserved for those patients with problems maintaining adequate nutrition by food alone.

MISCELLANEOUS PANCREATIC DISEASE

Congenital structural abnormalities of the pancreas such as annular pancreas may be associated with pancreatitis or pancreatic insufficiency as well as with bowel obstruction (Kiernan et al 1980). Ectopic pancreas is found at autopsy in between 0.5 and 14% of studies (Dolan et al 1974, Thoeni & Gedgaudas 1980) and is found most frequently in the stomach, duodenum, and then jejunum. It appears on X-ray as a small hemispherical mass usually 2–3 cm diameter with a central umbilication. At endoscopy, the lesion appears as a submucosal tumour. A great debate exists concerning the contribution of this anomaly to clinical disease. Most agree that unless evidence of an obstruction exists or a clearly inflamed gland is seen at endoscopy, correlation between the presence of ectopic pancreatic tissue and symptoms is poor.

Pancreas divisum is found at autopsy in 4–11% of patients and at endoscopic retrograde cholangiopancreatography in approximately half that number (Cotton 1980, Richter et al 1981). This developmental anomaly occurs when fusion of the dorsal and ventral pancreas fails to occur. Symptoms are thought to occur because of poor drainage of the body and tail of the pancreas by a relatively insufficient accessory pancreatic duct.

Other anomalies, including duodenal duplication, choledochal cysts, duodenal diverticulae, and anomalous insertion of the common bile duct may also contribute to the development of pancreatitis (Williams & Hendren 1971, Agrawal & Brodmerkel 1979, Griffin et al 1981, Jordan & Ament, 1977).

Pancreatic tumours are unusual during childhood but have been reported in families with hereditary pancreatitis (Kattwinkel et al 1973), von Hippel-Landau disease (Fishman & Bartholomew 1979) and ataxia telangiectasia (Swift et al 1976).

INVESTIGATION OF PANCREATIC DISEASE

The available laboratory and radiological tests for the investigation of pancreatic disease are listed in Table 17.3. Details and critical assessment of these investigations can be found in Chapter 3.

In summary, in searching for evidence of inflammation of the pancreas, serum amylase determinations should be performed first. If these levels are

Table 17.3 Laboratory evaluation

Blood tests
  Amylase
  Isoamylase
  Amylase/creatinine clearance ratio
  Lipase
  Serum immunoreactive trypsin/trypsinogen

Faecal tests
  Enzymes
  Fat

Duodenal intubation

Tubeless function tests
  N-benzoyl-L tyrosyl-p-aminobenzoic acid (BTP)
  Fluorescein dilaurate
  Breath tests

Radiography
  Plain X-ray
  Contrast studies
  Ultrasound
  CT
  NMR
  ERCP

elevated, then a search should be made to clarify whether the amylase truly originated from the pancreas. In the appropriate clinical situation, either a concomitant elevation of the amylase to creatinine clearance ratio or of the serum lipase is of most use. Other tests, including serum immunoreactive trypsin, ultrasound and CT may occasionally be necessary to establish a diagnosis of pancreatitis. In searching for evidence of pancreatic insufficiency the investigation of choice is pancreatic stimulation and duodenal intubation. The findings of low to absent serum immunoreactive trypsinogen or pancreatic isoamylase levels would suggest exocrine pancreatic insufficiency. These tests are however not very sensitive. The 'tubeless' tests using either N-benzoyl-L-tyrosyl-p-aminobenzoic acid (BTP) or fluorescein dilaurate give false positive and negative values which limit their usefulness. The use of radiolabelled substrate in breath tests is not desirable in children and the cost of the instrumentation for the quantitative measurement of stable isotopes is very high. All these methods are also dependent on normal gastric emptying and intermediary metabolism. If the availability of the required investigations is limited, referral should be made to a centre experienced in the investigation of pancreatic disorders.

REFERENCES

Abrams C K, Hamosh M, Hubbard V S, Dutla S K, Hamosh P 1984 Lingual lipase in cystic fibrosis. Journal of Clinical Investigation 73: 374–382

Aggett P F, Harries J T, Harvey B A M, Soothill J F 1979 An inherited defect of neutrophil mobility in Schwachman's syndrome. Journal of Pediatrics 94: 391–394

Aggett P J, Cavanagh N P C, Matthew D J, Pincott J R, Sutcliffe J, Harries J T 1980 Schwachman's syndrome. Archives of Disease in Childhood 55: 331–347

Agrawal R M, Brodmerkel J G 1979 Choledochal cysts presenting as pancreatitis. American Journal of Gastroenterology 71: 408–413

Allen R J, Coulter D L 1980 Valproic acid induced pancreatitis in children. Pediatrics 65:1194

Altman A J, Dinndorf P, Quinn J, 1982 Acute pancreatitis in association with cytosine arabinoside therapy. Cancer 49: 1384–1387

Andersen K D 1958 Cystic fibrosis of the pancreas. Journal of Chronic Disease 7: 58–90

Antonowicz I, Lebenthal E, Shwachman H 1978 Disaccharidase activities in small intestinal mucosa in patients with cystic fibrosis. Journal of Pediatrics 92: 214–219

Auldist A W 1972 Pancreatitis and choledocholithiasis in childhood. Journal of Pediatric Surgery 7: 78–83

Barbezat G O, Hansen J D L 1968 The exocrine pancreas and protein-calorie malnutrition. Pediatrics 42: 77–84

Bodian M, Sheldon W, Lightwood R 1964 Congenital hypoplasia of the exocrine pancreas. Acta Paediatrica 53: 282–293

Buntain W L, Wood J B, Wooley M M 1978 Pancreatitis in childhood. Journal of Pediatric Surgery 13: 143–145

Caselitz J, Kloppel G, Delling G, Grattner R, Holdhoff U, Stern M 1979 Schwachman's syndrome and leukemia. Virchows Archiva 385: 109–116

Chase H P, Long M A, Lavin M H 1979 Cystic fibrosis and malnutrition. Journal of Pediatrics 95: 337–347

Comfort M W, Steinberg A G 1952 Pedigree of a family with hereditary chronic relapsing pancreatitis. Gastroenterology 21: 554–559

Cotton P B, 1980 Congenital anomaly of pancreas divisum as cause of obstructive pain and pancreatitis. Gut 21: 105–114

Cox K L, Cannon R A, Ament M E, Phillips H E, Schaffer C B 1983 Biochemical and ultrasonic abnormalities of the pancreas in anorexia nervosa. Digestive Diseases and Sciences 28: 225–229

DiMagno E P, Go V L W, Summerskill H J 1973 Relations between pancreatic enzyme outputs in malabsorption and severe pancreatic insufficiency. New England Journal of Medicine 288: 813–815

DiMagno E P, Malagelada J R, Go B L W, Moertel C G 1977 Fate of orally ingested enzymes in pancreatic insufficiency. New England ·Journal of Medicine 296: 1318–1322

Dolan R V, ReMine W H, Dockerty M B 1974 The fate of heterotopic pancreatic tissue. Archives of Surgery 109:762

Donnison A, Shwachman H, Gross R 1966 A review of 164 children with meconium ileus seen at Children's Hospital Medical Center, Boston. Pediatrics 37: 833–850

Durie P R, Bel L W, Corey M L, Forstner G G 1980 Effect of cimetidine and sodium bicarbonate on pancreatic replacement therapy in cystic fibrosis. Gut 21: 778–786

Durie P R, Newgh C J, Forstner G G, Gall D G 1980b Malabsorption of medium-chain triglycerides in infants with pancreatic insufficiency and cystic fibrosis: Correction with pancreatic enzyme supplements. Journal of Pediatrics 96: 862–864

Eichelberger M R, Chattin J, Bruce D A, Garcia Z F, Goldman M, Koop C E 1980 Acute pancreatitis and increased intracranial pressure. Journal of Pediatric Surgery 16: 562–564

Eichelberger M R, Hoelzer D J, Koop C E 1982 Acute pancreatitis: the difficulties of diagnosis and therapy. Journal of Pediatric Surgery, 17:244

Ellis G H, Mirkin L D, Mills M C 1979 Pancreatitis and Reye's syndrome. American Journal of Diseases of Children 133: 1014–1017

Elmore M F, Rogge J S 1981 Tetracycline-induced pancreatitis. Gastroenterology. 81: 1134–1137

Fam S, O'Briain D S, Borger J A 1982 Ectopic pancreas with acute inflammation. Journal of Pediatric Surgery 17: 86–87

Figarella C, Negri G A, Sarles H 1972 Presence of colipase in congenital pancreatic lipase deficiency. Biochimica Biophysica Acta. 280: 205–210

Fishman R S, Bartholomew L G, 1979 Severe pancreatic involvement in three generations in von Hippel-Lindau disease. Mayo Clinic Proceedings 54: 329–331

Garner J A 1977 Acute pancreatitis as a complication of anaphylactoid purpura. Archives of Disease in Childhood 52: 971–972

Gilbert M G, Carbonnell M L 1964 Pancreatitis in childhood associated with ascariasis. Pediatrics 33: 589–591

Graham A R, Walson P D, Paplanus S H, and Payne C M 1980 Testicular fibrosis and cardiomegaly in Schwachman's syndrome. Archives of Pathology and Laboratory Medicine 104: 242–244

Griffin M, Carey W D, Hermann R, Buonocore E 1981 Recurrent acute pancreatitis and intussusception complicating an intraluminal duodenal diverticulum. Gastroenterology 81: 345–348

Gross J B, Gambill E E, Ulrich J A 1961 Hereditary pancreatitis. American Journal of Medicine 33:358

Gryboski J, Hillemeier C, Kocoshis S, Anyan W, Seachore J S 1980 Refeeding pancreatitis in malnourished children. Journal of Pediatrics 97: 441–446

Hadorn B, Zoppi G, Shmerling D H, Prader A, McIntyre I, Anderson C M 1968 Quantitative assessment of exocrine pancreatic function in infants and children. Journal of Pediatrics 73: 39–50

Hadorn B, Tarlow M J, Lloyd J K, Wolff O H 1969 Intestinal enterokinase deficiency. Lancet, i: 812–813

Harries J T, Muller D P R, McCollum J P K, Lipson A, Roma E, Norman A P 1979 Intestinal bile salts in cystic fibrosis. Archives of Disease in Childhood 54: 19–24

Hatfield A R W, Dent D M, Marks I N 1982 An intrapapillary pancreatic duct diverticulum: A rare, but surgically correctable cause of juvenile pancreatitis. British Journal of Surgery 69: 430–432

Holsclaw D, Rocmans C, Shwachman H 1971 Intussusception in patients with cystic fibrosis. Pediatrics 48: 51–58

Huijgens P C, van der Veen E A, Meijer S, Muntinghe O G 1977 Syndrome of Schwachman and leukemia. Scandinavian Journal of Haematology 18: 20–24

Isenberg J N 1978 Pancreatitis, amylase clarance and azathioprine. Jonrnal of Pediatrics 93: 1043–1045

Izsak E M, Shike M, Roulet M, Jeejeebhoy K N 1980 Pancreatitis in association with hypercalcemia in patients receiving total parenteral nutrition. Gastroenterology 79: 555–559

Johnston D W B 1978 Annular pancreas: A new classification and clinical observation. Canadian Journal of Surgery 21:241

Jordan S C, Ament M E 1977 Pancreatitis in children and adolescents. Journal of Pediatrics 91: 211–215

Katz A, Falchuk M, Shwachman H 1976 The co-existence of cystic fibrosis in celiac disease. Pediatrics 57: 715–721

Kattwinkel J, Lapey A, di Sant'agnese P A, Edwards W A, Hufty M P 1973 Hereditary pancreatitis: Three new kindreds and a critical review in the literature. Pediatrics 51:55–69

Kiernan P C, ReMine W H 1980 Annular pancreas. Archives of Surgery 115: 56–50

Kopelman H, Durie P, Gaskin K, Weizman Z, Forstner G 1985 Pancreatic fluid secretion and protein hyperconcentration in cystic fibrosis. New England Journal of Medicine 312: 329–334

Kulczycki L, Shwachman H 1958 Studies of cystic fibrosis of the pancreas: Occurrence of rectal prolapse. New England Journal of Medicine 259: 409–412

Land V J, Sutow W W, Fernback D J, Lane D M, Williams T E 1972 Toxicity of L-asparaginase in children with advanced leukemia. Cancer 30: 339–345

Lapey A, Kattwinkel J, Di Sant'agnese P, Laster L, 1974 Steatorrhea and azotorrhea and their relation to growth and nutrition in adolescents and young adults with cystic fibrosis. Journal of Pediatrics 84: 328–334

Levitt M D, Ellis C, Engel R R 1977 Isoelectric focusing studies of human serum and tissue amylase. Journal of Laboratory and Clinical Medicine 90: 141–152

L'Heureux P, Isenberg J N, Sharp H, Warwick W 1977 Gallbladder disease in cystic fibrosis. American Journal of Roentgenology 128: 953–956

Liebman W M, Rosenthal E, Hirschberger M, Thaler M M 1979 Schwachman-Diamond syndrome and chronic liver disease. Clinical Pediatrics. 18: 694–698

Lloyd-Still et al 1983 Textbook of cystic fibrosis. John Wright P G Inc, Boston

Lowe C U, May C D 1951 Selective pancreatic deficiency. American Journal of Diseases of Children 82: 459–464

Mallory A, Kern F 1980 Drug-induced pancreatitis: A critical review. Gastroenterology 78:813

Mansueto S, Di Leo R, Tringali G 1983 Unusual abdominal involvement in rickettsial diseases. JAMA, 249:1709

Mardh P, Ursing B 1974 The occurrence of acute pancreatitis in mycoplasma pneumonia infection. Scandinavian Journal of Infectious Disease 6: 167

Matseshe J, Go V, DiMagno E 1977 Meconium ileus equivalent complicating cystic fibrosis in post and neonatal children and young adults. Gastroenterology. 72: 732–736

Milla P J, Rassam U B, Kilby A, Ersser R, Harries J T 1980 Small intestinal absorption of amino acids and dipeptide in pancreatic insufficiency. In: Sturgess J M (ed) Perspectives in Cystic Fibrosis. Canadian Cystic Fibrosis Foundation, Toronto, Canada. pp 177–180

Morin C L, Roy C C, LaSalle R, Bonin A 1976 Small bowel mucosal dysfunction in patients with cystic fibrosis. Journal of Pediatrics 88: 213–216

Muller D P R, McCollum J P K, Trompeter R S and Harries J T 1975 Studies on the mechanism of fat absorption in congenital isolated lipase deficiency. Gut 16:838

Naficy K, Nategh R, Ghadimi H 1973 Mumps pancreatitis without parotitis. British Medical Journal 1:529

Nelis G F 1983 Nitrofurantoin-induced pancreatitis: Report of a case. Gastroenterology 84: 1032

Neutra M R, Trier J S 1978 Rectal mucosa in cystic fibrosis. Gastroenterology 75: 701–710

Nezelof C, Watchi M 1961 L'hypoplasie congenitale lipomateuse du pancreas exocrine chez l'enfant. Archives Francaises de Pediatrie 18: 1135–1172

Noblett H 1979 Meconium ileus. In: Ravitch M, Welch K, Benson C, Aberdeen E, Randolph J (eds) Pediatric Surgery. Yearbook Medical Publishers, Chicago. pp 943–953

Oppenheimer E, Esterly J 1973 Cystic fibrosis of the pancreas: Morphologic findings in infants with and without pancreatic lesions. Archives of Pathology 96: 149–154

Oppenheimer E, Esterley J 1975 Hepatic changes in young infants with cystic fibrosis: Possible relation to focal biliary cirrhosis. Journal of Pediatrics 86: 683–689

Park R, Grand R J 1981 Gastrointestinal manifestations of cystic fibrosis. Gastroenterology 8: 1143–1161

Pena S D J, Medovy H 1973 Child abuse and traumatic pseudocyst of the pancreas. Journal of Pediatrics 83:1026

Perrault J, Gross J B, Kanya J E, 1976 Endoscopic retrograde cholangiopancreatography in familial pancreatitis. Gastroenterology 71: 138

Regan B T, Malagelada J R, DiMagno E P, Glanzeman S L, Go V L W 1977 Comparative effects of antacids, cimetidine, and enteric coating on the therapeutic response to oral enzymes in secure pancreatic insufficiency. New England Journal of Medicine 297: 854–858

Rey J, Frezal J, Royer P, Lamy M 1966 Absence congenitale de lipase pancreatique. Archives Françaises de Pédiatrie 23: 5–14

Reye R D K, Morgan G, Boral J 1963 Encephalopathy and fatty degeneration of the viscera: A disease entity in childhood. Lancet ii:749

Reynolds J C, Inman R D, Kimberly R P, Chuong J H, Kovacks J E, Walsh M B 1982 Acute pancreatitis in systemic lupus erythematosus, report of 20 cases and a review of the literature. Medicine 61: 25–31

Riccardi, B M, Shih V E, Holmes L B, Nardi G L 1975 Hereditary pancreatitis. Archives of Internal Medicine 135: 822–825

Richter J M, Jacoby G A, Schapiro R H, Warshaw A L 1982 Pancreatic abscess due to Candida albicans. Annals of Internal Medicine 97: 221–224

Richter J M, Schapiro R H, Mulley A G, Warshaw A L 1981 Association of pancreas divisum and pancreatitis, and its treatment by sphincteroplasty of the accessory ampulla. Gastroenterology 81: 1104–1109

Rosenstein B J, Oppenheimer E H 1977 Prolonged obstructive jaundice and giant cell hepatitis in an infant with cystic fibrosis. Journal of Pediatrics 91: 1022–1023

Roulet M, Weber A, Roy C 1980 Increased gastric lipolytic activity in cystic fibrosis. In: Sturgess J M (ed) Perspective in Cystic Fibrosis. Canadian Cystic Fibrosis Foundation Toronto, Canada. pp 172–176

Roy C C, Weber A M, Morin C L, Combes J C, Nussle D, Megevand A, Lasalle R 1977 Abnormal biliary lipid composition and cystic fibrosis. New England Journal of Medicine 297: 1301–1305

Sarles H 1984 Epidemiology and pathophysiology of chronic pancreatitis and the role of the pancreatic stone protein. Clinical Gastroenterology 3: 895–912

Saunders J H B, Drummond S, Wormsley K G 1977 Inhibition of gastric secretion in treatment of pancreatic insufficiency. British Medical Journal 1: 418–419

Saunders E F, Gall G, Freedman M H 1979 Granulopoiesis in Shwachman's syndrome. Pediatrics 64: 515–519

Schuster S, Shwachman H, Toyama W, Rubino A, Khaw K 1977 The management of portal hypertension in cystic fibrosis. Journal of Pediatric Surgery 12: 201–206

Schwachman H 1975 Gastrointestinal manifestations of cystic fibrosis. Pediatric Clinics of North America 22: 787–805

Schwachman H 1978 Cystic fibrosis. Current Problems in Pediatrics, 8: 1–72

Schwachman H, Diamond L K, Oski F A, Khaw K T 1964 The syndrome of pancreatic insufficiency and bone marrow dysfunction. Journal of Pediatrics 65: 645–663

Schwachman H, Kowalski M, Khaw K 1977 Cystic fibrosis: A new outlook, 70 patients above 25 years of age. Medicine 56: 24–49

Scully R E, Mark E J, McNealy B U, 1982 Case Records of the Massachusetts General Hospital. New England Journal of Medicine 307: 1438–1443

Seidman E G, Deckelbaum R J, Owen H, de Chadarevian J, Weber A M, Morin C L, Roy C C 1983 Case report: Relapsing pancreatitis in association with Crohn's disease. Journal of Pediatric Gastroenterology and Nutrition 2: 178–182

Sheldon W 1964 Congenital pancreatic lipase deficiency. Archives of Disease in Childhood 39: 268–271

Shmerling D H, Prader A, Hitzig W H, Giedion A, Hadorn B, Kuhni M 1969 The syndrome of exocrine pancreatic insufficiency, neutropenia, metaphyseal dysostosis, and dwarfism. Helvetica Paediatrica Acta 24: 547–575

Sibert J R 1978 Hereditary pancreatitis in England and Wales. Journal of Medical Genetics 15:189

Silberman H, Dixon N P, Eisenberg D 1982 The safety and efficacy of a lipid based system of parenteral nutrition in acute pancreatitis. American Journal of Gastroenterology 77: 494–497

Stern R, Stevens D, Boat T, Doershuk C, Izant B, Matthews L 1976 Symptomatic hepatic disease in cystic fibrosis. Incidence, course and outcome of portal systemic shunting. Gastroenterology 70: 645–649

Strevens M J, Lilleyman J S, Williams R B 1978 Shwachman's syndrome and acute lymphoblastic leukemia. British Medical Journal 2: 18–20

Swift M, Sholman L, Perry M, Chase C 1976 Malignant neoplasms in the families of patients with ataxia-telangiectasia. Cancer Research 36: 209–215

Taussig L 1985 Cystic Fibrosis. Thienne-Stratton, New York

Taussig L, Saldino R, di Sant'Agnese P 1973 Radiographic abnormalities of the duodenum and small bowel in cystic fibrosis of the pancreas. Radiology 196: 369–376

Thoeni R F, Gedgaudas R K 1980 Ectopic pancreas: Usual and unusual features. Gastrointestinal Radiology 5:37

Thomaidis D S, Arey J B 1963 The intestinal lesions in cystic fibrosis of the pancreas. Jornal of Pediatrics 63: 444–453

Townes P L 1965 Trypsinogen deficiency disease. Journal of Pediatrics 66: 275–279

Townes P L 1969 Proteolytic and lipolytic deficiency of the exocrine pancreas. Journal of Pediatrics 75: 221–228

Townes P L, Bryson M F Miller G 1967 Further observations on trypsinogen deficiency disease: Report of a second case. Journal of Pediatrics 71: 220–224

Turner L J 1983 Chronic pancreatitis and congenital strictures of the pancreatic duct. American Journal of surgery 145: 582–584

Ursing B 1973 Acute pancreatitis in Coxsackie B infections. British Medical Journal 3:524

Watkins J B, Tercyak A M, Szcepanik P, Klein P D 1977 Bile salt kinetics in cystic fibrosis: Influence of pancreatic enzyme replacement. Gastroenterology 73: 1023–1028

Weaver G A, Bordley K, Guiney W B, D'Accurzio A 1982 Chronic pancreatitis with cyst formation after prednisone and thiazide treatment. American Journal of Gastroenterology 77:164

Werbit W, Mohsenifar Z 1980 Mononucleosis pancreatitis. South Medical Journal 73: 1094–1096

Williams W H, Hendren W H 1971 Intrapancreatic duodenal duplication causing pancreatitis in a child. Surgery 60: 708–710

Wood R, Boat I, Doershuk C 1976 Cystic fibrosis. American Review of Respiratory Disease 113: 833–877

Inborn errors of hepatic metabolism

The liver has a central role in many metabolic processes. It produces substrates for the generation of energy, synthesizes both structural and enzymatic proteins, and is the site of catabolism of numerous substances. Inborn errors involving many of these pathways have been identified and, although most of the disorders are rare, recognition is important in order that treatment can be given at an early stage before irreversible harm has occured. Even in those conditions for which treatment is not currently available, accurate identification is needed for genetic counselling.

The clinical manifestation of inborn errors of hepatic metabolism are very variable. In some there is evidence of acute or chronic liver dysfunction with jaundice, hepatomegaly or signs of hepatic failure, but in others there maybe little to indicate that the basic defect is within the liver. The disorders discussed in this chapter have been selected because they have overt hepatic and/or gastrointestinal symptoms or signs. No attempt is made to review all inborn errors involving the liver.

All the disorders described are inherited as autosomal recessives except where this is stated. Certain inherited disorders which also cause liver disease, notably alpha$_1$-antitrypsin deficiency and cystic fibrosis are discussed elsewhere (Chapter 21 and 19).

DISORDERS OF CARBOHYDRATE METABOLISM

After a meal there is net uptake of glucose and other monosaccharides by the liver followed by synthesis and storage of glycogen. The enzymes responsible are glycogen synthetase and the brancher enzyme (Fig. 18.1).

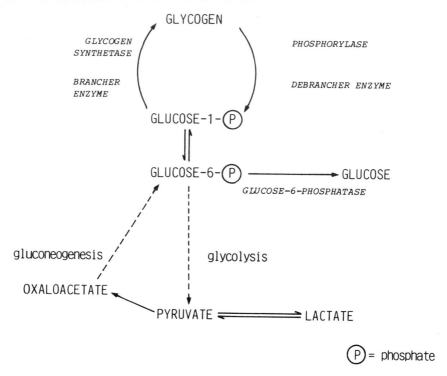

Fig. 18.1 Glucose and glycogen metabolism in the liver.

Glucose is also synthesized from other substrates (glycerol, lactate, alanine, etc.) by gluconeogenesis. During fasting, glycogen is broken down by phosphorylase and the debrancher enzyme to form glucose 1-phosphate. Release of glucose from the liver requires hydrolysis of glucose 6-phosphate to form free glucose (Fig. 18.1)

Glycogen storage disease (GSD)

Although many inborn errors of the synthesis and of the breakdown of glycogen in liver and muscle have been described, not all involve the liver (Howell & Williams 1983, Hug 1980). Only the hepatic forms will be described here and a classification with details of the alternative names is given in Table 18.1

Glucose 6-phosphatase deficiency

Clinical features

As patients with glucose 6-phosphatase deficiency (type Ia GSD) cannot release glucose from the liver, fasting hypoglycaemia is a common

Table 18.1   Classification of hepatic glycogen storage disease

Enzyme deficiency	Type	Inheritance
Glycogen synthetase deficiency	0	AR
Glucose 6-phosphatase deficiency	Ia	AR
Glucose 6-phosphate translocase deficiency	Ib	AR
Debrancher deficiency	III	AR
Brancher deficiency	IV	AR
Phosphorylase deficiency	VI	AR
Phosphorylase kinase deficiency	VI/IX (both numbers are used and may be subdivided into a, b, c)	AR and X-linked inheritance

AR = autosomal recessive.
  The original classification of glycogen storage disease by Roman numerals was proposed before the enzymology was understood. It is preferable to refer to the enzymes, pariculary as there is confusion about the numbering of enzymes in the phosphorylase cascade.

presenting feature. It may be evident in the neonatal period (Hufton & Wharton 1982) but because feeds are usually given frequently in the early weeks of life, symptoms often do not develop until later in the first year. The liver progressively enlarges and abdominal distension may be the initial manifestation. Failure to thrive and diarrhoea are also frequent symptoms so that gastrointestinal disease may be suspected initially. Occasionally patients present with tachypnoea (often attributed to a chest infection) as a result of lactic acidosis; this develops because glucose 6-phosphate accumulates in the liver cell and is metabolized via the glycolytic pathway to form pyruvate and lactate which are then released into the blood stream (Fig. 18.1).

In type Ib GSD clinical features are similar to glucose 6-phosphatase deficiency (Senior & Loridan 1968) but the children also have recurrent infections and oral ulceration because of immune deficiency and neutropenia (Schaub and Heyne 1983).

Diagnosis

A combination of short stature, hepatomegaly and fasting hypoglycaemia with lactic acidosis is strongly suggestive of glucose 6-phosphatase deficiency. Other biochemical abnormalities include hypertriglyceridaemia and elevated plasma urate concentrations. A glucagon test will usually show a blood glucose increase of less than 2 mmol/l after glucagon with a rise in blood lactate (Dunger & Leonard 1982). Confirmation of the diagnosis should be obtained by assaying glucose 6-phosphatase activity in a liver biopsy sample. It is important to carry out the assay in both fresh and frozen samples, as in the variant glucose 6-phosphate translocase deficiency (type Ib — see table 18.1) the enzyme deficiency is only apparent in fresh liver (Igarashi et al 1979).

Treatment

Because glucose release from the liver is impaired treatment necessitates the administration of glucose to maintain the plasma glucose within normal limits throughout the 24 hours. By day this can be achieved with frequent drinks of glucose or a soluble glucose polymer. At night regular drinks are rarely satisfactory and it is preferable to give the glucose by a nasogastric infusion (Greene et al 1976, Fernandes et al 1979). In infants under the age of 2 years a rate of 0.4–0.5 g/kg/h is usually sufficient. For older children the dose should be reduced to about 0.15–0.2 g/kg/h. It is very important not to overtreat; giving too much glucose may cause excessive insulin secretion resulting in rapid swings in blood glucose with severe and potentially fatal hypoglycaemia (Leonard & Dunger 1978). Considerable care is needed to ensure that the patients get their glucose regularly and that nothing interrupts this, particularly at night.

When treatment with glucose is properly controlled, children can be expected to do well with reduction in liver size, normal growth and development and improvement of the secondary biochemical changes. For older patients uncooked corn starch (which is hydrolysed slowly in the gut) given regularly as a suspension, may maintain satisfactory blood glucose concentrations (Smit et al 1984).

Debrancher deficiency (Type III GSD)

Clinical features

These are similar to those of glucose 6-phosphatase deficiency though they tend to be less severe. As the branch points of glycogen cannot be hydrolysed, there is no accumulation of glucose 6-phosphate and hence no lactic acidosis.

Hypoglycaemia, which is common in the first year of life improves with age. Hepatomegaly and short stature are often presenting features. Cardiac and skeletal muscle metabolism is also affected and a mild myopathy may be detectable.

Diagnosis

Short stature, hepatomegaly and fasting hypoglycaemia are suggestive of glycogen storage disease but unlike glucose 6-phosphatase deficiency blood lactate is not raised but transaminases and creatine kinase are markedly elevated. Hypercholesterolaemia and mild hypertriglyceridaemia are also usual. The rise in blood glucose after glucagon is usually less than 2 mmol/l. Although there may be a greater rise if the test is repeated after a carbohydrate meal, this finding is neither invariable nor diagnostic (Dunger & Leonard 1982). The diagnosis should be confirmed by measuring debrancher activity in white blood cells. The glycogen content of the red blood cells is also markedly elevated. Only in a few complex cases is it necessary to proceed to a liver biopsy.

Treatment

Because glucose synthesized via gluconeogenesis can be released from the liver the mainstay of treatment is a high protein diet to provide aminoacids that form substrates for the synthesis of glucose (Fernandes & Van der Kamer 1968). Such a regime will usually prevent hypoglycaemia and promote better growth. Although patients often remain short during childhood and puberty is usually delayed, catch-up growth during adolescence generally results in a normal final height (Dunger et al 1984).

Disorders of the phosphorylase system (Type VI/IX GSD)

Phosphorylase exists in two interconvertible forms, one active and the other inactive. Interconversion is initiated by glucagon and catecholamines through a series of enzymes. Inborn errors involving several of these enzymes have been described, the commonest being phosphorylase kinase deficiency (de Barsy & Lederer 1980).

Clinical features, diagnosis and treatment

Clinical manifestations are usually mild; hypoglycaemia is rare and the presentation is generally with hepatomegaly and/or short stature. The glucagon test is almost always normal and the diagnosis is established by measuring phosphorylase kinase activity in red blood cells (Lederer et al 1975). The prognosis is good. Hepatomegaly gradually becomes less apparent. Children with short stature will catch up during childhood, pass through puberty normally and achieve a normal final height (Dunger et al 1984). Specific treatment is not usually necessary but, if required, is a high protein diet.

Other forms of glycogen storage disease (Glycogen synthetase deficiency, Brancher deficiency)

Inborn errors involving the synthesis of glycogen are very rare. Glycogen synthetase deficiency is characterized by fasting hypoglycaemia without hepatomegaly (Aynsley-Green et al 1977a). The hypoglycaemia can be prevented by a high protein diet (Aynsley-Green et al 1977b).

Deficiency of the brancher enzyme results in the synthesis of an abnormally structured glycogen molecule (Howell & Williams 1983). This causes progressive liver cirrhosis and is the only form of glycogen storage disease in which the spleen is enlarged in addition to the liver. Histochemical studies of the liver show glycogen with abnormal staining and characteristics. The diagnosis is confirmed by measuring brancher activity in liver or white blood cells. Liver transplantation offers the only hope of effective treatment.

Galactosaemia

Galactose is converted to glucose by the reactions shown in Figure 18.2. Patients with galactosaemia lack galactose 1-phosphate, uridyl transferase and as a result, galactose 1-phosphate accumulates within cells (Segal 1983).

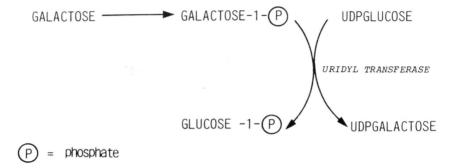

P = phosphate

Fig. 18.2 Galactose metabolism.

Clinical features

Symptoms occur only after the ingestion of galactose and in most milkfed babies these develop during the neonatal period. The earliest manifestations are usually poor feeding, vomiting and sometimes diarrhoea. Signs of liver disease soon develop with jaundice, hepatomegaly and a bleeding diathesis. Cataracts may appear at a very early age and should be specifically sought if the diagnosis is suspected. Infection is common and septicaemia due to *Escherichia coli* may cause death before the underlying diagnosis has even been suspected (Levy et al 1977).

Occasionally infants have a milder neonatal course and are not diagnosed at this stage, presenting later with failure to thrive, signs of liver disease, cataracts and developmental retardation.

Diagnosis

A provisional diagnosis may be made by the finding of reducing substances in the urine. However, if the child is not receiving milk at the time of urine collection (because, for instance, intravenous fluid therapy has already been started) reducing substances may not be present. If the diagnosis is suspected, lactose (and hence galactose) should immediately be removed from the diet and the diagnosis confirmed by measuring the uridyl transferase activity in red blood cells. This test should be done on cord blood if a previous sibling has been affected and milk feeding delayed until the result is known.

Treatment

All feeds must be free of lactose. The immediate response is usually excellent with resolution of all acute symptoms. During the early months of life there are usually few problems with treatment as a lactose-free formula can provide all nutritional needs. With the introduction of weaning foods the help of a skilled dietitian is essential as many processed foods contain milk or milk-based products. The diet should be monitored by regular measurements of galactose 1-phosphate in the red cells.

Long-term studies of the outcome have been disappointing (Anon 1983). Children have tended to have a lower IQ than expected and school problems have been common (Donnel et al 1980). Many of the girls have been shown to have hypergonadotrophic hypogonadism (Kaufman et al 1981). Although it is not certain that these problems are related to dietary relaxation it is now thought advisable for lactose to be excluded for life.

Fructosaemia

The metabolism of fructose is shown in Figure 18.3. Patients with fructosaemia lack fructose 1-phosphate aldolase so that fructose 1-phosphate accumulates within cells (Gitzelmann et al 1983).

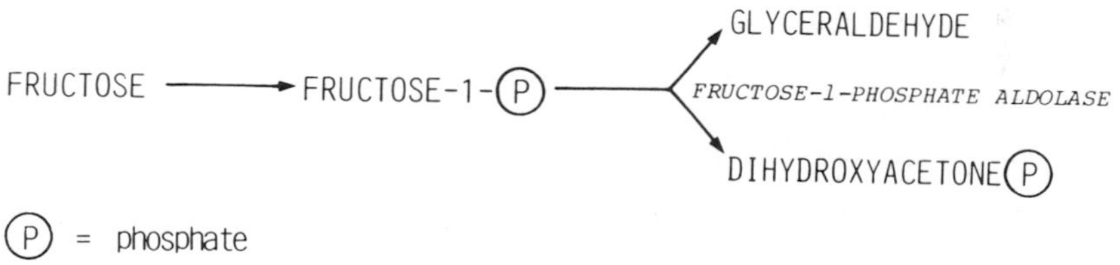

Fig. 18.3 Fructose metabolism.

Clinical features

Patients remain well until fructose is ingested. As feeds in early infancy seldom include sucrose or fructose, symptoms are rare in the neonatal period but occur when fruit juices, sweetened pureed foods or medicines containing sucrose or sorbitol are given. The most common early symptoms are vomiting and refusal to feed. Later the child fails to thrive, becomes irritable, develops hepatomegaly and a variety of other nonspecific symptoms. If the condition is not recognized, infants who continue to ingest sucrose and fructose deteriorate relentlessly with signs of severe liver disease and renal tubular dysfunction culminating in death. Some families, however, notice that sweet foods make the child unwell and evolve a diet low in fructose so that symptoms are minimized and the child survives. Older children usually develop a marked aversion to food containing fructose and thereby effectively treat themselves.

Diagnosis

The diagnosis should be suspected from the history and all sucrose and fructose-containing foods should be immediately stopped. Confirmation is possible by intravenous fructose loading and measuring the changes in the plasma glucose, phosphate and urate, or by direct estimation of the fructose 1-phosphate aldolase activity in either a liver or jejunal mucosal biopsy specimen.

Treatment

A strict sucrose and fructose-free diet usually produces a dramatic improvement and provided the diagnosis is made early the outcome is excellent. The diet needs to be continued for life.

DISORDERS OF AMINO ACID METABOLISM

Disorders of the urea cycle

Nitrogen which is not used for biosynthetic purposes has to be excreted and the major waste product is urea, formed as shown in Figure 18.4. One nitrogen atom of urea is derived from ammonia; thus any block within the urea cycle results in accumulation of ammonia which is highly toxic, particularly to the central nervous system. Inborn errors of each step of the urea cycle have now been described (Fig. 18.4) (Walser 1983). With the exception of arginase deficiency (defect 5 of Figure 18.4), the clinical manifestations have close similarities so that they will be considered together.

Clinical features

There is a broad spectrum of clinical presentation with the most severe forms developing symptoms in the neonatal period and milder variants presenting in later infancy and childhood.

In the neonatal form babies usually present after the first 24 hours of life with lethargy, vomiting, changes in tone, fits and finally coma. Terminally there may be evidence of liver failure with bleeding.

Less severely affected patients may present in infancy with a history of vomiting and failure to thrive so that a gastrointestinal disorder is often suspected. However, periods of lethargy and more specific neurological

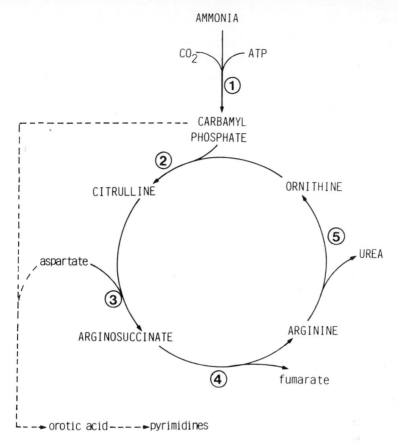

Fig. 18.4 The urea cycle. Inborn errors of each step have been described.

Enzyme	Inborn error
1 Carbamyl phosphate synthetase	CPS deficiency
2 Ornithine carbamoyl transferase	OCT deficiency
3 Arginosuccinate synthetase	Citrullinaemia
4 Arginosuccinate lyase	Arginosuccinic aciduria
5 Arginase	Argininaemia

features such as extreme irritability and developmental delay almost always develop. Seizures and focal neurological signs such as hemiplegia may occur. In older children symptoms are commonly intermittent or episodic with lethargy, confusion, behaviour problems, convulsions and sometimes focal neurological signs. Cerebral oedema may supervene with irreversible damage or a fatal outcome.

Arginase deficiency causing hyperarginaemia is rare. Symptoms due to hyperammonaemia are less prominent and patients usually present with progressive spastic diplegia and retardation beginning around the age of 3 years.

Diagnosis

Patients presenting in the neonatal period and older children who are ill have raised plasma ammonia levels but few other abnormalities on routine biochemical tests; transaminases may be raised; blood urea is normal. The normal concentration of ammonia in the plasma is usually less than 40 μmol/l and is dependent on the age of the patient and the protein intake. Symptomatic children with urea cycle disorders generally have values well in excess of this and concentrations in comatose patients usually exceed 250 μmol/l. Plasma aminoacid analysis shows raised concentrations of glutamine and alanine. In citrullinaemia (defect 3 of Fig. 18.4), arginosuccinic aciduria (defect 4) and arginase deficiency (defect 5), measurement of the blood and urine aminoacids is diagnostic. However in carbamyl phosphate synthetase deficiency (defect 4) and ornithine carbamoyl transferase deficiency (defect 2) the abnormalities in the plasma aminoacids are more easily overlooked. Alanine and glutamine are raised and the citrulline often low; although these are often helpful, they are not diagnostic. In these children the estimation of urinary orotic acid is useful. This compound is a pyrimidine precursor which is synthesized from carbamyl phosphate, an intermediate in the urea cycle. Excess urinary orotate may be present even with only minimal hyperammonaemia and is virtually diagnostic of a urea cycle disorder (Bachmann & Columbo 1980).

Treatment

Reduction in dietary protein plays a major role in the management of the urea cycle disorders. The intake is adjusted according to the age, the severity of the disorder, and the child's growth rate, and is usually between 0.7–2.0 g/kg/24 h. For some children diet alone may be sufficient to control hyperammonaemia, but for more severely affected individuals other forms of treatment are necessary. Some of the natural protein can be replaced with an essential aminoacid mixture (Snyderman et al 1975). This enables total nitrogen intake to be reduced whilst still meeting the essential aminoacid requirements for growth. The major advance in therapy, however, has been the exploitation of other pathways of nitrogen excretion (Batshaw & Brusilow 1980, Batshaw et al 1982). Sodium benzoate and sodium phenylacetate are conjugated in the liver with glycine and glutamine to form hippurate and phenylacetylglutamine respectively, which are then rapidly excreted by the kidney. Hyperammonaemia is reduced because of the removal of glycine and glutamine from the waste nitrogen pool in the liver, thus reducing the load on the urea cycle. Both sodium benzoate and sodium phenylacetate are well tolerated in dosages of 250 mg/kg/24 h and can be used in acute as well as chronic hyperammonaemia.

Arginine is normally synthesized in the urea cycle and is therefore not an essential aminoacid. However, in patients with urea cycle disorders (except for argininaemia) the synthesis of arginine may be insufficient because of the metabolic block (Fig. 18.4). Arginine then becomes an essential (or semiessential) aminoacid and supplements need to be given (Kline et al 1981, Brusilow 1984) Indeed the administration of arginine, to patients with citrullinaemia and arginosuccinic aciduria is important in order to replenish the supply of ornithine. Patients with arginosuccinic-acidaemia can in fact be maintained on moderate restriction of dietary protein (between 1.2–2.0 g/kg/24 h) and arginine supplements (350–700 mg/kg/24 h) alone.

When children with urea cycle disorders have an intercurrent illness their plasma ammonium concentrations may rise rapidly due to breakdown of muscle protein. An emergency dietary regime is therefore required. All protein intake is stopped and a high carbohydrate intake given to inhibit the protein catabolism. Additional sodium benzoate and arginine is given. If there is depression of consciousness urgent admission to hospital is essential for review and more intensive therapy is necessary.

Prognosis

The outlook for babies who present early in the neonatal period is not good (Msall et al 1984) but for older children, provided that the diagnosis is made before neurological damage has occured, the prognosis is much better and normal growth and development can be achieved.

Genetic advice is important. With the exception of ornithine carbamoyl transferase deficiency these disorders have an autosomal recessive mode of inheritance. Prenatal diagnosis is posssible although sophisticated techniques may be required. Ornithine carbamyl transferase has X-linked inheritance. Most affected boys but not all, will have severe neonatal disease. Expression in females is very variable, some having no symptoms at all. Detection of these asymptomatic carriers is important for genetic counselling and may require a protein challenge. Recombinant DNA techniques may also be helpful (Rozen et al 1985).

Disorders of tyrosine metabolism

Plasma tyrosine concentrations may be raised as a secondary consequence of generalized liver disease as well as resulting from inborn errors of the metabolic pathway (Goldsmith 1983) (Fig. 18.5). Detailed investigation is necessary to determine the cause of raised tyrosine concentrations.

Hereditary tyrosinaemia (Type I)

This disorder is characterized by severe liver dysfunction. It may present with acute liver failure in the early months of life or later in infancy with failure to thrive and rickets with evidence of renal tubular abnormalities.

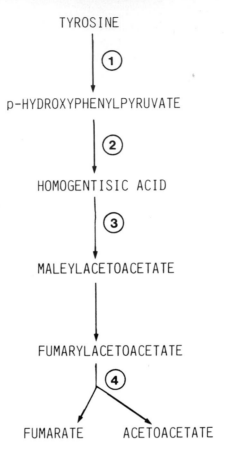

Fig. 18.5 Pathway of the catabolism of tyrosine.

Enzyme	Inborn error
1 Tyrosine aminotransferase	TAT deficiency (Hereditary tyrosinaemia type II)
2 p-hydroxyphenylpyruvate oxidase	
3 Homogentisic acid oxidase	Alkaptonuria
4 Fumarylacetoacetate lyase	Hereditary tyrosinaemia type I

The primary defect is a deficiency of fumarylacetoacetate, the last step in the pathway of the tyrosine catabolism (Lindblad et al 1977) (Fig. 18.5), resulting in the accumulation of toxic metabolites in the liver. Plasma concentrations of tyrosine, phenylalanine and methionine are raised and other liver function tests are abnormal with a severe clotting disorder, unresponsive to vitamin K. Renal involvement causes generalized tubular dysfunction with glycosuria and in particular phosphaturia that is responsible for the rickets.

The patients excrete a marked excess of succinylacetone in plasma and urine which appears to be specific for the disorder. Further confirmation can be obtained by measuring the activity of fumarylacetoacetate in liver or cultured fibroblasts.

Treatment is difficult and unsatisfactory. Whilst it is possible to correct the aminoacid abnormalities by dietary means, hepatic and renal tubular function only partially improve and the urinary excretion of succinyl-acetone persists. Liver damage progresses relentlessly with the development of cirrhosis; a high proportion of patients subsequently develop a hepatoma. Liver transplantation appears to offer the only hope of long-term cure. (Starzl et al 1985).

Tyrosine aminotransferase deficiency (Hereditary tyrosinaemia Type II)

The clinical presentation is varied and seldom points to the liver. Symptoms include photophobia, keratitis that does not respond to conventional treatment, painful hyperkeratosis of palms and soles, and occasionally developmental delay and other neurological abnormalities. Plasma tyrosine concentrations are greater than 2 mmol/litre without other evidence of liver disease. The skin and corneal abnormalities improve with a low tyrosine diet.

Transient neonatal tyrosinaemia

In newborn babies, particularly those who are preterm, the activity of the enzyme p-hydroxyphenylpyruvate oxidase (defect 2, Fig. 18.5) is low, and, because a relatively high protein intake provides considerably more tyrosine than required, not all the tyrosine can be catabolized and plasma concentrations rise. The infants may appear lethargic and unwell and often have prolonged jaundice; these symptoms, however, may be more related to their immaturity than the tyrosinaemia. Some patients will improve rapidly when given vitamin C, the co-factor of p-phdroxyphenylpyruvate oxidase; for others the protein intake should be reduced. The condition is self-limiting, usually resolving within a few weeks. The increased frequency of breast-feeding and the introduction of infant formulas with a low protein content have greatly reduced the incidence of this disorder.

WILSON'S DISEASE

In Wilson's disease copper accumulates particularly within the liver, brain, kidney and cornea. The basic defect is not known; although rare it is an important and treatable cause of liver disease in childhood (Danks 1983).

Clinical features

The presentation is very varied and the disorder may mimic many other diseases (Walshe 1962).

It is, however, rare for symptoms to develop before the age of 4 years. During the first decade liver disease predominates but in adolescence neurological abnormalities are often more prominent.

The presentation may be acute, mimicking acute hepatitis or even fulminating acute liver failure. In other patients the hepatic disorder is more chronic and may even present with haematemesis due to varices. Thus the possibility of Wilson's disease must be considered in all patients with undiagnosed liver disease over the age of 4 years, especially in those with chronic or recurrent illness.

Many neurological symptoms have been described but as the copper accumulation in the brain particularly involves the basal ganglia, movement and speech disorders are common. Initial manifestations may be very subtle such as school difficulties, speech problems, clumsiness, or an odd gait. Psychiatric problems, such as depression and emotional lability may also occur. Deposition of copper in the cornea causes the Kayser–Fleischer ring. This is always present in patients with neurological disease but may not be found in younger patients with liver disease. Nevertheless in any patient in whom Wilson's disease in suspected the eyes should be examined with a slit lamp.

Diagnosis

To establish the diagnosis can be difficult because the simpler tests are not wholly reliable. Plasma copper and caeruloplasmin concentrations are usually reduced and urinary copper excretion increased. The copper content of the liver is increased and this is a more reliable test especially in younger children with liver disease. Occasionally more complex tests using copper isotopes are necessary.

Treatment

Treatment should be started immediately the condition is diagnosed and has to be life-long. Penicillamine is currently the drug of choice, though if the patient is intolerant of penicillamine an alternative such as trientine may be used. Treatment is monitored by measurement of urinary copper excretion. The outcome depends on the stage at which the diagnosis is made; when treatment is started early the outlook is good. Unfortunately delay in diagnosis is common and since improvement with treatment is only gradual, patients may still die or have serious residual problems.

LYSOSOMAL STORAGE DISORDERS

Many lysosomal storage disorders, for example the mucopolysaccharidoses, cause hepatosplenomegaly but other features usually provide clues to the diagnosis and liver function is generally not impaired. A few conditions, however, may present with cholestatic jaundice in infancy (e.g.

Niemann–Pick type C, GM_1 gangliosidosis and β-glucuronidase deficiency) and in Wolman's disease (acid esterase deficiency) failure to thrive, vomiting and diarrhoea are prominent symptoms (Assman & Fredrickson 1983). Liver disease is common in older patients with Gaucher's disease (James et al 1982).

It is beyond the scope of this chapter to discuss individual lysosomal storage disorders but if such as a condition is suspected a peripheral blood film should be examined for vacuolation in white blood cells and bone marrow aspiration may show storage cells. A specific diagnosis may be possible by enzyme assay on white blood cells. Liver biopsy is rarely necessary.

DISORDERS OF BILIRUBIN METABOLISM

Bilirubin is formed by the breakdown of the haemproteins particularly haemoglobin. Unconjugated bilirubin is virtually insoluble in water and is transported to the liver bound to albumin. In the liver it is conjugated by uridine diphosphate (UDP) glucuronyl transferase to form bilirubin diglucuronide which is water-soluble and is excreted in the bile. Several inherited defects in the metabolism of bilirubin have been described, all of which cause chronic jaundice (Wolkoff et al 1983).

Crigler–Najjar syndrome

This disorder is caused by a deficiency of UDP glucuronyl transferase activity and is therefore characterized by unconjugated hyperbilirubinaemia. Two types are described which appear to be genetically distinct.

Type I

Severe jaundice develops shortly after birth and, if untreated, levels of unconjugated bilirubin rise rapidly to much as 850 μmol/l causing kernicterus. There is no other evidence of liver dysfunction, nor are there signs of haemolysis. The bile does not contain pigment.

Treatment is difficult and even early exchange transfusion may fail to prevent kernicterus. For chronic therapy, plasmapheresis is currently the best option. Phototherapy may have a slight effect but there is no response to phenobarbitone.

Type II

Although the activity of UDP glucuronyl transferase is usually very low in vitro, type II Crigler–Najjar is a milder disease than type I as levels of unconjugated bilirubin seldom exceed 350μmol/l. Patients do not develop kernicterus. The bile contains some pigment but the ratio of monoglucuronide to diglucuronide is greatly increased.

The mode of inheritance is not clear, both autosomal dominant with incomplete penetrance and autosomal recessive have been postulated. It has been suggested that it may represent the homozygous form of Gilbert's disease.

Treatment with phenobarbitone induces enzyme activity with a fall in plasma bilirubin concentrations. The condition is, however, benign and treatment is largely cosmetic.

Gilbert's syndrome

It is now clear that the term Gilbert's syndrome encompasses a heterogeneous group of disorders characterized by mild fluctuating unconjugated hyper-bilirubinaemia which seldom exceeds 85 μmol/l and is entirely benign. The jaundice is increased by calorie restriction. All other tests of liver function and liver histology are normal.

At least some patients with Gilbert's syndrome have reduced levels of UDP glucuronyl transferase and produce bile with an increased ratio of mono- to diglucuronide as in type II Crigler–Najjar. They also respond to phenobarbitone with a reduction in plasma bilirubin but such treatment is seldom necessary.

Although these disorders are clearly familial the mode of inheritance is unclear.

Dubin–Johnson and Rotor syndrome

In these disorders the secretion of bilirubin diglucorinide by the liver into the bile is impaired with consequent conjugated hyperbilirubinaemia. Jaundice is usually mild and often fluctuating. There is no specific treatment and the prognosis for both disorders is good.

Whereas it used to be thought that Dubin–Johnson and Rotor syndrome were variants of the same disorder it is now clear that they are different and can be distinguished by the appearance of the liver, with accumulation of a dark pigment in Dubin–Johnson disease, a gross delay in the excretion of bromsulphthalein in Rotor syndrome, and the ratio of coproporphyrins I and III in the urine (Wolkoff et al 1983).

GENERAL REFERENCES

Stanbury J B, Wyngaarden J B, Fredrickson D B, Goldstein J L, Brown M S (eds) 1983. The metabolic basis of inherited disease, 5th edn. McGraw-Hill, New York.
Newsholme E A, Leech A R 1983 Biochemistry for the medical sciences. John Wiley and Sons, Chichester.
Francis D E M 1987 Diets for Sick Children, 4th edn. Blackwell, Oxford.

REFERENCES

Anonymous 1983 Clouds over galactosaemia (Editorial). Lancet ii: 1379–1380
Assmann G, Fredrickson D B 1983 Acid lipase deficiency: Wolman's disease and cholesteryl ester storage disease. In: Stanbury J B, Wyngaarden J B, Fredrickson D B,

Goldstein J L, Brown M S (eds) The metabolic basis of inherited disease, 5th edn.
McGraw-Hill, New York. Ch. 39, pp 803–819

Aynsley-Green A, Williamson D H, Gitzelmann R 1977a Hepatic glycogen synthetase
deficiency. Archives of Disease in Childhood 52: 573–579

Aynsley-Green A, Williamson D H, Gitzelmann R 1977b The dietary treatment of hepatic
glycogen synthetase deficiency. Helvetica Paediatrica Acta 32: 71–75

Bachmann C, Columbo J P 1980 Diagnostic value of orotic acid excretion in heritable
disorders of the urea cycle and in hyperammonaemia due to organic acidurias. European
Journal of Paediatrics 134: 109–113

Batshaw M L, Brusilow S W 1980 Treatment of hyperammonaemic coma caused by inborn
errors of urea synthesis. Journal of Pediatrics 97: 893–900

Batshaw M L, Brusilow S, Waber L et al 1982 Treatment of inborn errors of urea
synthesis. New England Journal of Medicine 306: 1387–1392

Brusilow S W 1984 Arginine, an indispensible amino acid for patients with inborn errors
of urea synthesis. Journal of Clinical Investigation 74: 2144–2148

Danks D M 1983 Hereditary disorders of copper metabolism in Wilson's disease and
Menke's disease. In: Stanbury J B, Wyngaarden J B, Fredrickson D B, Goldstein J L,
Brown M S (eds) The metabolic basis of inherited disease, 5th edn. McGraw-Hill, New
York. Ch. 58 pp 1251–1268

de Barsy T, Lederer B 1980 Type VI glycogenosis: identification of subgroups. In: Burman
D, Holton J B, Pennock C A (eds) Inherited disorders of carbohydrate metabolism. MTP
Press, Lancaster. Ch 19, pp 369–380

Donnell G N, Koch R, Fishler K, Ng W G 1980 Clinical aspects of galactosaemia. In:
Burman D, Holton J B, Pennock C A (eds) Inherited disorders of carbohydrate
metabolism. MTP Press, Lancaster. Ch 5, pp 103–115

Dunger D B, Leonard J V 1982 The value of the glucagon test in screening for hepatic
glycogen storage disease. Archives of Disease in Childhood 57: 384–389

Dunger D B, Leonard J V, Preece M A 1984 Patterns of growth in hepatic glycogenoses.
Achives of Disease in Childhood 59: 657–660

Fernandes J, van der Kamer J H 1968 Hexose and protein tolerance tests in children with
liver glycogenosis caused by a deficiency of the debranching enzyme system. Pediatrics
41: 935–44

Fernandes J, Jansen H, Jansen T C 1979 Nocturnal gastric drip feeding in glucose-6-
phosphate deficient children. Pediatric Research 13: 225–229

Gitzelmann R, Steinmann B, Van den Berghe G 1983 Essential fructosuria, hereditary
fructose intolerance, and fructose-1, 6-diphosphatase deficiency. In: Stanbury J B,
Wyngaarden J B, Fredrickson D B, Goldstein J L, Brown M S (eds) The metabolic
basis of inherited disease, 5th edn. McGraw-Hill, New York. Ch 5 pp 118–140

Goldsmith L A 1983 Tyrosinaemia and related disorders. In: Stanbury J B,
Wyngaarden J B, Fredrickson D B, Goldstein J L, Brown M S (eds) The metabolic basis
of inherited disease, 5th edn. McGraw-Hill, New York. Ch 13 pp 287–299

Greene H L, Slonim A E, O'Neill J A, Burr I M 1976 Continuous nocturnal intragastric
feeding for management of type I glycogen storage disease. New England Journal of
Medicine 294: 423–425

Howell R R, Williams J C 1983 The glycogen storage diseases. In: Stanbury J B,
Wyngaarden J B, Fredrickson D B, Goldstein J L, Brown M S (eds) The metabolic
basis of inherited disease, 5th edn. McGraw-Hill, New York. Ch 6 pp 141–166

Hufton B R, Wharton B A 1982 Glycogen storage disease type I presenting in the neonatal
period. Archives of Disease in Childhood 57: 309–311

Hug G 1980 Pre- and post natal diagnosis of glycogen storage disease In: Burman D,
Holton J B, Pennock (eds) Inherited disorders of carbohydrate metabolism. MTP
Press, Lancaster. Ch 18 pp 327–367

Igarrashi Y, Otomo H, Narisawa K, Tada K 1979 A new variant of glycogen storage
disease type I: probably due to a defect in the glucose-6-phophate transport system.
Journal of Inherited Metabolic Disease 2: 45–49

Kaufman F R, Kogut M D, Donnel G N, Goebelsmann U, March C, Koch R 1981
Hypergonadotrophic hypogonadism in female patients with galactosaemia. New England
Journal of Medicine 304: 994–998

Kline J J, Hug G, Schubert W K, Berry H 1981 Arginine deficiency syndrome. American
Journal of Disease of Children 135: 437–442

James S R, Stromeyer F W, Stowens D W, Barranger J A 1982 Gaucher disease: Hepatic abnormalities in 25 patients. In: Desnick R J, Gatt S, Grabowski G A (eds) Gaucher disease: A century of delineation and research. Alan Liss, New York. pp 131–142

Lederer B, van Hoof F, Van den Berghe G, Hers H G 1975 Glycogen phosphasates of normal human subjects and patients with type VI glycogen storage diseasee. Biochemical Journal 147: 23–35

Leonard J V, Dunger D B 1978 Hypoglycaemia complicating feeding regimens for glycogen storage disease (letter). Lancet ii: 1203–1204

Levy H L, Sepe S J, Shih V E, Vawter G F, Klein J O 1977 Sepsis due to *Escherichia coli* in neonates with galactosaemia. New England Journal of Medicine 297: 823–825

Lindblad B, Lindstedt S, Steen G11977 On the enzyme defects of hereditary tyrosinaemia. Proceedings of National Academy of Sciences (USA) 74: 4641–4645

Msall M, Batshaw M L, Suss R, et al 1984 Neurologic outcome in children with inborn errors of urea synthesis. New England Journal of Medicine 310: 1500–1505

Rozen R, Fox J, Fenton W A, Horwich A L, Rosenberg L E 1985 Gene deletion and restriction length polymorphisms at the human ornithine transcarbamylase locus. Nature 313: 815–817

Schaub J, Heyne K 1983 Glycogen Storage Disease type Ib. European Journal of Paediatrics 140: 283–288

Segal S 1983 Disorders of galactose metabolism. In: Stanbury J B, Wyngaarden J B, Fredrickson D B, Goldstein J L, Brown M S (eds) The metabolic basis of inherited disease 5th edn. McGraw-Hill, New York. Ch 7 pp 167–191

Senior B, Loridan L 1968 Studies of liver glycogenoses, with particular reference to the metabolism of intravenously administered glycerol. New England Journal of Medicine 279: 958–965

Smit G P A, Berger R, Potasnick R, Moses S W, Fernandes J 1984 The dietary treatment of children with type I Glycogen Storage Disease with slow release carbohydrate. Paediatric Research 18: 879–881

Snyderman S E, Sansaricq C, Phansalkar S V, Schacht R G, Norton P M 1975 The therapy of hyperammonaemia due to ornithine transcarbamylase deficiency in a male neonate. Pediatrics 56: 65–73

Starzl T E, Zitelli B J, Shaw B W, et al 1985 Changing concepts: Liver replacement for hereditary tyrosinaemia and hepatoma. Journal of Pediatrics 106: 604–606

Walser M 1983 Urea cycle disorders and other hereditary hyperammonaemic syndromes. In: Stanbury J B, Wyngaarden J B, Fredrickson D B, Goldstein J L, Brown M S (eds) The metabolic basis of inherited disease. 5th edn. McGraw-Hill, New York. Ch 20 pp 402–438

Walshe J M 1962 Wilson's disease: the presenting symptoms. Archives of Disease in Childhood 37: 253–256

Wolkoff A W, Chowdury J R, Arias I M 1983 Hereditary jaundice and disorders of bilirubin metabolism In: Stanbury J B, Wyngaarden J B, Fredrickson D B, Goldstein J L, Brown M S (eds) The metabolic basis of inherited disease. 5th edn. McGraw-Hill, New York. Ch 61 pp 1385–1420

Persistent jaundice in infancy

Persistent jaundice in the first months of life has many causes (for a recent review see Balistreri 1985) and may be classified according to whether the raised serum concentrations of bilirubin are conjugated or unconjugated. In unconjugated hyperbilirubinaemia the concentration of conjugated bilirubin is not raised, whereas in conjugated hyperbilirubinaemia the concentration of conjugated bilirubin is raised to usually more than 20% of the total. In both types of jaundice the intensity and duration is accentuated by the temporarily increased production and ineffective hepatic excretion of bilirubin commonly called physiological jaundice. Since nearly all newborn infants have some degree of jaundice, the term 'hyperbilirubinaemia' in this age-group is used to indicate a degree of jaundice which should alert the physician to further investigate the infant so that treatable causes of jaundice can be detected and kernicterus prevented. 'Hyperbilirubinaemia' is defined as serum concentrations of greater than 255 μmol/l (15 mg/100 ml) in the full-term infant, and greater than 204 μmol/l (12 mg/100 ml) in the preterm infant.

UNCONJUGATED HYPERBILIRUBINAEMIA

The unconjugated hyperbilirubinaemia can be classified according to the pathophysiological mechanisms which contribute to the increased serum concentrations of bilirubin (Table 19.1).

Physiological jaundice

Serum unconjugated bilirubin exceeds 34 μmol/l (2 mg/100 ml) in the first week of life in over 90% of normal full term infants: maximum levels occur on the second to fourth day of life and rarely exceed 102 μmol/l (6 mg/100 ml). In preterm infants, levels of 204 to 238 μmol/l (12 to

Table 19.1   Pathophysiological mechanisms and causes of unconjugated hyperbilirubinaemia

Pathophysiological mechanism	Examples of causes
1 Increased haemolysis	
Blood group incompatibility	Rhesus and ABO incompatibility
Defects of RBC membrane	Hereditary spherocytosis
RBC enzyme deficiencies	Glucose-6-phosphate dehydrogenase deficiency
Haemolytic agents	Vitamin K
Infections	Septicaemia
Extravasated blood	Cephalhaematoma
2 Increased red cells mass	Placental transfusion
	Twin-to-twin transfusion
3 Defective hepatic uptake and/or conjugation of bilirubin	Prematurity
	Hypoxia
	Hypoglycaemia
	Dehydration
	Drugs sharing metabolic pathways of bilirubin
	Hypothyroidism
	Breast-milk jaundice
	Transient familial neonatal hyperbilirubinaemia
	Gilbert's syndrome
	Crigler–Najjer syndrome
4 Increased enteric absorption	Meconium retention
5 Ill-understood; possibly involving some or all of above mechanisms	Hypothyroidism
	Pyloric stenosis and high intestinal obstruction
	Infants of diabetic mothers
	Down's syndrome
	Galactosaemia

14 mg/100 ml) are commonly reached by the fifth to seventh day. Jaundice may persist until the tenth day of life. The diagnosis may be established by excluding known cases of jaundice.

The physiology of bilirubin formation and excretion is briefly referred to in chapter 18. The pathophysiology of self-limiting jaundice of early infancy is imperfectly understood. Contributory temporary defects include increased bilirubin production, impaired hepatic uptake of bilirubin from plasma into the hepatocytes, impaired conjugation of bilirubin and an increased enterohepatic circulation of bilirubin (Odell 1980, Maisels 1981).

In the newborn infant bilirubin production may be twice that of the adult as a result of shortened red blood cell survival, increased turnover of haem-containing enzymes and from ineffective erythropoiesis. There is impaired hepatic uptake of bilirubin due to a variety of factors, such as ineffective hepatic perfusion associated with the complex vascular changes occurring after birth, including persistent patency of the ductus venosus and inequality of the hepatic sinusoidal perfusion. In addition, it has been postulated that there may be inefficiency of hepatocyte uptake of bilirubin secondary to defective transport across the hepatocyte membrane, or lack of anion binding transport proteins such as ligandin in the hepatic cyto-plasm. There is impaired ability to form bilirubin conjugates. Although xylose and glucose conjugates of bilirubin are formed in man, the major conjugate is thought to be glucuronide (Heirwegh et al 1973). The reasons for the deficient glucuronidation are not clear; there may be transient deficiency of glucuronide donors such as uridine diphosphate glucuronic acid (UDPGA), which is derived exclusively from hepatic glycogen via glucose 1-phosphate; equally, deficiency of the enzyme UDP glucuronyl-transferase may be rate-limiting. It is also postulated that hepatic excretion of bilirubin glucuronide may be transiently impaired, although there is no information on this in the human neonate. In primates bilirubin clearance may be inhibited by saturation of the excretion process between day two and day four after birth.

A major factor in physiological jaundice can probably be attributed to the intestinal reabsorption of unconjugated bilirubin; meconium contains 40 mg of bilirubin per 100 g and thus presents a total load of 200 mg of bilirubin to be excreted by the gut. To this must be added absorption of bilirubin released from bilirubin glucuronide by the action of the enzyme β glucu-ronidase which is present in high concentration in the intestine of the neonate. There is also little bacterial degradation of bilirubin due to limited bacteriological colonization.

Persistent jaundice with hyperbilirubinaemia in the first 4 days of life

The many factors which cause neonatal hyperbilirubinaemia must be briefly considered since they are commonly followed by jaundice which persists beyond the tenth day of life. The most important are those which cause increased erythrocyte destruction. Blood group incompatibility between the infant and mother (isoimmunization) must always be considered when jaun-dice occurs in the first 24 hours of life and is associated with features of erythroblastosis. Rhesus isoimmunization remains the most frequent cause in Western Europe, but this is falling with the successful use of anti-D-gammaglobulin which, when given in the puerperium following the birth of a Rhesus positive infant to a Rhesus negative mother, prevents sensitiz-ation to the Rhesus factor. In other areas, incompatibility of the ABO blood groups and minor blood groups may be more important. Structural abnormalities of red cells such as hereditary spherocytosis and red cell enzyme deficiencies, such as glucose-6-phosphate dehydrogenase deficiency or pyruvate kinase deficiency, are rarer causes but in some parts of the world are important.

Bacterial infections and intrauterine viral infections are also important causes of hyperbilirubinaemia since they promote bilirubin production by haemolysis; they may, however, also impair bilirubin excretion. Bilirubin formation is also excessive where marked bruising has occurred. There are also many factors which singly or in combination add to the functional inefficiency of the liver in the newborn period and cause hyperbilirubin-aemia and persistence of jaundice. These include prematurity, hypoxia, hypoglycaemia, dehydration, drugs which compete with bilirubin for the same excretory pathways and any circumstance which leads to meconium retention.

Transient familial hyperbilirubinaemia

Jaundice in this condition starts in the first few days of life and persists into the second or third week. It is thought to be associated with an unidentified in vitro inhibitor of glucuronide formation which can be recovered from the serum of mothers and their children. All infants born to such mothers develop jaundice of this nature.

Crigler–Najjar syndrome

Type I Crigler–Najjar syndrome must be considered in any infant who has a persistent severe, unconjugated hyperbilirubinaemia requiring continuous phototherapy to prevent kernicterus.

Persistent jaundice without hyperbilirubinaemia

Breast-milk jaundice syndrome

During the first week of life, jaundice is more commonly observed in breast-fed than in bottle-fed infants (Seigal et al 1982). The reasons for this are not clear, but possibly result from the combination of handicaps causing physiological jaundice aggravated by steroids in breast milk, possibly inhibition of bilirubin excretion by fatty acids, increased betaglucosonidase activity and contentiously by some action of prostaglandins. In most instances jaundice disappears within two weeks of birth.

A rarer form of jaundice associated with breast-feeding is that in which serum bilirubin concentrations of 255–360 μmol/l (15–20 mgm/100 ml) occur in the second or third week of life in infants who are entirely well. The jaundice may persist for as long as 10 weeks. If breast-feeding is discontinued, however, the jaundice usually resolves within six days and may not recur if breast-feeding is recommenced.

The aetiology of this syndrome is not known; 75% of the siblings of such infants are similarly affected. Breast milk from the mothers of affected infants competitively inhibits glucuronide formation in vitro; pregnane 3α–20β pregnanediol, a powerful inhibitor of glucuronide formation has been isolated from such milk in a few instances, but it is likely that this steroid is not the sole cause of the jaundice. Free unsaturated fatty acids in milk have also been implicated but the evidence is far from conclusive (Odievre & Luzeau 1978) and hence bilirubin reabsorption from the intestine due to lack of an inhibitory factor has also been postulated (Gartner

& Lee 1979). An inhibitor of glucuronyl transferase activity has been identified in colostrum and breast milk in the first 3 days of life in mothers of Navajo American Indians whose infants have exaggerated unconjugated hyperbilirubinaemia. (Sal and et al 1974).

Although kernicterus has not been described, breast-feeding should be discontinued for 24 to 48 hours if serum bilirubin levels are greater than 290 μmol/l (17 mg/100 ml).

Hypothyroidism

Hypothyroidism may be associated with prolonged jaundice lasting 3–4 weeks and should be considered in any infant in whom jaundice lasts more than two weeks; the precise cause of the jaundice is not certain.

High intestinal obstruction

Jaundice may complicate any high intestinal obstruction such as pyloric stenosis; again the reasons are not certain, but the jaundice resolves when the obstruction is removed (Bleicher et al 1979).

Kernicterus

Kernicterus is a disorder in which death or permanent neurological damage follows the deposition of unconjugated bilirubin in the brain, and occurs when the serum concentration of unconjugated bilirubin exceeds the capacity of serum proteins to bind bilirubin.

There is no clinically valid technique for measuring free or unbound bilirubin, the reserve capacity of serum proteins to bind more bilirubin or the measurement of bilirubin bound to albumin (Odell 1980). At present there is no published evidence that such measurements lead to more appropriate intervention and better outcome for the infant than treatment based on measurement of the total unconjugated bilirubin concentration (Gitzelmann-Cumarasamy & Kuenzle 1979). The accurate estimation of the reserve capacity of serum proteins to bind bilirubin may provide a more precise indication of the risk of kernicterus than serum bilirubin concentrations, but this has only been demonstrated for the salicylate saturation index method, which is technically difficult and available only in a limited number of laboratories (Odell et al 1970)

In full term infants, a serum bilirubin of 340 μmol/l (20 mg/100 ml) or more is associated with a significant risk of kernicterus. There are several conditions in which kernicterus may occur at lower serum bilirubin concentrations because of diminished capacity of the serum proteins to bind bilirubin. These include prematurity, hypoalbuminaemia, asphyxia, acidosis and the administration of drugs which compete with bilirubin for albumin binding (Pearlman et al 1980).

Do elevations of serum bilirubin concentration which are not sufficiently marked to cause kernicterus cause intellectual impairment? Although studies have been reported which do show such an association, others have not demonstrated this and even if such an association is established, it does not necessarily confirm a direct relationship (Scheidt et al 1977). The effects of hypoxia and prematurity become very difficult to unravel from the effects of hyperbilirubinaemia.

Management of unconjugated hyperbilirubinaemia

Identification and treatment of the cause of hyperbilirubinaemia and the prevention of kernicterus are dual objectives in management. Diagnosis will be established by careful history, together with scrutiny of the obstetrical case record, physical examination of the infant and appropriate laboratory investigations (See tables 19.1 and 19.2).

Table 19.2   Laboratory investigation of unconjugated hyperbilirubinaemia

Serial determination of total and direct serum bilirubin
Haemoglobin
Red blood cell morphology, reticulocyte and normoblast count
Blood group in mother and child
Direct Coomb's test in saline and albumin
Maternal antibodies and haemolysins
Urine microscopy and culture
Urine-reducing substances
Blood culture and other appropriate bacteriological studies
Specific tests for abnormalities of red blood cells, e.g. G-6-PD deficiency
Serum T4 concentration
Breast-milk inhibitors of bilirubin conjugation in vitro

General measures

In controlling unconjugated hyperbilirubinaemia and preventing kernicterus, the factors which cause aggravation of physiological jaundice must be identified and minimized. It is particularly important to prevent hypoxia and hypothermia and to maintain an appropriate intake of fluid and calories.

Exchange transfusion

Exchange transfusion is a most effective means of removing bilirubin when the risk of kernicterus is high and must be undertaken when the serum level of unconjugated bilirubin exceeds 340 μmol/l (20 mg/100 ml). In may be indicated at lower levels, e.g. 255 μmol/l (15 mg/100 ml), in premature infants particularly if they are acidotic or if serum albumin levels are low. In infants with haemolytic disorders a rise of serum bilirubin of greater than 8.5 μmol/l/h (0.5 mg/100 ml/h) usually indicates that bilirubin will accumulate more rapidly than it can be excreted, and exchange transfusion usually proves necessary.

Phototherapy

In the last two decades it has been unequivocally shown that exposing the jaundiced infant to artificial light of moderate intensity is effective in preventing hyperbilirubinaemia and in lowering elevated serum bilirubin except in the presence of severe haemolysis. Light of a wavelength near 450 nm is perhaps most effective, but white light is to be preferred since observation of the patient is easier. A radiant flux of 4–6 micro-watts/m²/min is most effective (Modi & Keay 1983).

The precise mechanism by which phototherapy reduces serum bilirubin concentrations in infants is unclear. It certainly changes bilirubin to a more polar diazo negative water-soluble product and causes the enhanced excretion of unconjugated bilirubin in the bile. Photobilirubin is produced by rotation of the terminal ring of bilirubin through 180° to give a product which is rapidly excreted in the bile. Much of the action of phototherapy takes place in the skin but shielding the liver in experimental animals decreases efficiency of phototherapy, suggesting a direct hepatic effect. Photochemical derivatives of bilirubin are less toxic to microsomal functions in vitro than bilirubin itself.

A number of side-effects have been recognized as complicating phototherapy. The most frequent is an increased insensible water loss which may lead to dehydration and aggravate hyperbilirubinaemia. Diarrhoea has been reported but where detailed observations have been made with appropriate controls the incidence of loose stools has not in fact increased. Skin reactions such as maculopapular rashes, tanning of Negro infants and bronzing of the skin with acute haemolysis in infants with liver disease occur rarely. Other possible biological effects of phototherapy must be considered. These include neuroendocrine functions mediated through the pineal gland and photoreceptors in the retina, which may possibly affect growth, diurnal rhythms, sexual maturation and direct photochemical reactions on other body tissues including the retina itself; with appropriate protection of the eye this last side-effect can be avoided.

Elevated levels of leutinizing hormone have been observed 3–4 weeks after phototherapy in preterm infants (Lemaitre et al 1977) and increased FSH production has also been documented (Dacou-Voutetakis et al 1978). Phototherapy to the retina of newborn, stumped-tailed monkeys produced changes similar to those of premature ageing (Messner et al 1978). Follow-up of infants whose eyes have been adequately shielded have yielded normal visual function as assessed clinically or by electroretinography.

Perhaps the most damaging effect of phototherapy arises from its injudicious use prior to precise diagnosis and the disturbance it causes to the mother/child relationship.

To date, no permanent abnormalities have been detected in human infants treated with phototherapy. Nevertheless this type of treatment should be limited to those infants who strictly need it and therapy should not be given for longer than is absolutely necessary.

Phototherapy is primarily used to prevent the serum bilirubin level reaching values at which exchange transfusion is indicated. Since it is easy to use and the side-effects are not as life-threatening or immediately damaging as those due to exchange transfusion or kernicterus, it tends to be employed at relatively low serum bilirubin concentrations. Although increased phototherapy together with other measures, has reduced kernicterus in premature nurseries (Pearlman et al 1980), it has yet to be shown that the widespread use of phototherapy in the management of non-haemolytic anaemia in low birthweight infants is in the patient's best interests.

Phenobarbitone

Phenobarbitone, particularly if given to the mother for some days before delivery of the infant, is effective in both premature and full term infants in controlling neonatal hyperbilirubinaemia, even when caused by haemolysis due to ABO or Rhesus incompatibility. The mechanism of action of phenobarbitone is not clear. Animal studies suggest that the drug stimulates hepatic uptake, conjugation and excretion of bilirubin, as well as stimulating the bile salt-independent component of bile flow. If treatment is instituted at birth (8 mg/kg/24 h), the frequency of exchange transfusion in infants with Rhesus isoimmunization and glucose-6-phosphate dehydrogenase deficiency is significantly reduced. Since the effect of phenobarbitone is not apparent until at least 48 hours after the drug is commenced, it is of no value in treating established hyperbilirubinaemia. In addition to its effects on bilirubin, phenobarbitone influences other metabolic systems. It stimulates haem synthesis and may therefore aggravate jaundice. It modifies the activity of many microsomal enzymes which are involved in the metabolism of drugs, vitamins, clotting factors and hormones; also, it influences the intracellular ratios of the reduced and oxidized forms of NAD(H) (nicotinamide-adenine dinucleotide, reduced form) and NADP(H) nicotinamide-adenine dinucleotide phosphate, reduced form. The routine use of phenobarbitone in the management of hyperbilirubinaemia is thus to be discouraged. In circumstances, however, where optimal perinatal care cannot be achieved the small risks of phenobarbitone and phototherapy may be discounted if they increase the chance of survival with an intact neurological system.

CONJUGATED HYPERBILIRUBINAEMIA

The causes of the conjugated hyperbilirubinaemias are listed in Table 19.3.

Table 19.3 Classification and aetiological factors associated with intrahepatic disorders of conjugated hyperbilirubinaemia in infancy

Infective	Bacterial:
	   Urinary tract infection
	   Syphilis
	   Listeriosis
	
	Protozoal:
	   Toxoplasmosis
	
	Viral:
	   Cytomegalovirus
	   Rubella
	   Herpes simplex
	   Coxsackie B
	   Herpes zoster
	   Adenovirus
	   Non-A non-B hepatitis

Genetic-Metabolic disorder	Alpha$_1$-antitrypsin deficiency Cystic fibrosis Galactosaemia Fructosaemia Tyrosinosis Neimann–Pick disease type III Wolman's disease Neonatal iron storage disease Mucopolysaccharidosis Abnormal bile salt metabolism Zellweger's syndrome Byler's syndrome Dubin–Johnson syndrome Rotor syndrome
Endocrine	Hypothyroidism Hypopituitarism Hypoadrenalism
Parenteral Nutrition	
Rare familial syndromes	e.g. with cardiac lesions, lymphoedema, mental retardation and abnormal facies, and skeletal abnormalities Familial neonatal hepatic steatosis
Chromosomal abnormalities	Trisomy 13, 18, 21, Turner's Syndrome
Posthaemolytic disorders	
Microcystic disease of the liver and kidney	
Toxins, drugs etc., e.g. Halothane	
Fulminant hepatic failure	
Intrahepatic cholestasis	
Vascular lesions	Haemangiomata Poor perfusion syndrome Veno-occlusive disease
Idiopathic hepatitis of infancy	

Hepatitic syndrome of infancy

The clinical features of this syndrome are jaundice with raised conjugated bilirubin, dark bile-containing urine and stools with absent or reduced yellow or green pigment. Such infants usually show hepatomegaly and frequently splenomegaly and failure to thrive. Irrespective of the cause of such disease, these infants have a marked propensity to spontaneous bleeding usually from the umbilicus but occasionally intracranially. This is due to impaired blood clotting caused by vitamin K malabsorption. Rarely, patients present with features of hypoalbuminaemia or hypoglycaemia. Investigation often reveals a mild, haemolytic anaemia and standard biochemical tests of liver function are abnormal with raised serum transaminase, alkaline phosphatase, and gammaglutamyl transpeptidase activities as well as increased bilirubin concentrations. The prothrombin time is the most urgent investigation in such infants.

The onset of the liver disease usually dates from birth, with the jaundice continuing from what has been considered physiological jaundice. Such infants, however, frequently have yellow urine from birth. A small percentage of cases start after the first four weeks of life and few as late as 4–5 months. Rarely, a history is obtained of the mother having had an infectious illness during the pregnancy, e.g. rubella or hepatitis type B, rhesus isoimmunization, or of a genetic disorder which affects the liver, such as cystic fibrosis. Clinical examination shows the features mentioned above. Infants with biliary atresia are frequently very well nourished and typically have no stigmata of chronic liver disease other than a firm or hard liver. Rarely, there are clinical signs of diagnostic importance (Alagille 1972, Mowat et al 1976, Henricksen et al 1981) (Table 19.4).

Investigations

Priorities in management are the recognition of those causes which are amenable to specific therapy, those patients who require surgical intervention, and the genetically determined disorders (see Ch. 18 and 21). Careful consideration should be given to ascertain before laparotomy, whether or not there is bile duct obstruction. This is important since laparotomy findings may be misleading in up to 20% of cases (Hays et al 1967). Even with operative cholangiography the operator may be unable to demonstrate a lumen in very narrow but patent bile ducts in infants with severe intrahepatic disease and marked reduction in bile flow. Experienced surgeons have removed such bile ducts in the mistaken belief that the patient was suffering from biliary atresia (Markowitz et al 1983).

The difficulty in determining the presence of biliary obstruction is compounded by the evidence that extrahepatic biliary atresia is a progressive disease and the longer corrective surgery is delayed, the less likelihood there is that it will be successful (Kasai 1983a). It is essential

Table 19.4 Infectious causes of the hepatitis syndrome of infancy

Infecting agents	Screening investigations	Definitive investigations	Principal extrahepatic clinical manifestations
Cytomegalovirus	CF antibody in serum	Isolation from urine and liver with demonstration of virus in liver by IF	Small for dates; microcephaly; meningoencephalitis; intracranial calcification; neonatal thrombocytopaenic purpura; splenomegaly; retinitis, deafness
Rubella virus	CF and HAI antibodies in serum	Specific IgM antibody, virus isolation from nasopharynx and liver	Small for dates; cataracts; retinitis; congenital heart defects; microphthalmia, buphthalmos and corneal oedema; myocarditis; neonatal thrombocytopaenic purpura; splenomegaly; osteopathy; lymphadenopathy
Hepatitis B virus	HBs antigen in mother	Hepatitis Bs antigen in infant Demonstration of Hepatitis B antigen in liver by IF and EM	None described
Herpes simplex virus	Perinatal herpes in mother	Isolation and demonstration of virus from superficial lesions and liver	Splenomegaly; heart failure, pneumonitis; skin vesicles; meningoencephalitis
Coxsackie B virus	Isolation from respiratory tract and faeces	Isolation from liver	Myocarditis; meningoencephalitis pneumonitis
Varicella zoster virus	Demonstration of virus from superficial lesions	Demostration of virus in the liver	Disseminated infection as in herpes simplex; skin lesions more obvious
Bacterial infection		Blood culture, urine culture, CSF	Anaemia; any other system may be involved
Listeria		Isolation of organisms from blood culture, CSF or liver	Septicaemia; meningitis; pneumonitis; purpura
Trepomema pallidum	VDRL or TPI, particularly in mother	Demonstration of Trepomema by dark ground illumination	Rhinitis; skin rash; bone lesions; anaemia; lymphadenopathy; meningoencephalitis
Toxoplasma gondii	CF antibody in serum	Rising antibody titre in infant; specific IgM antibody; isolation of organisms from liver and CSF; visualization of organism from liver and CSF	Microcephaly; macrocephaly; meningoencephalitis; intracranial calcification; choreoretinitis; thrombocytopaenia; purpura

CF = Complement fixing; HAI = Haem. agglutination inhibition; IF = Immunofluorescence microscopy; EM = Electron microscopy;
CSF = Cerebrospinal fluid

therefore that infants with acholic stools should be referred to units with experience in interpreting the diagnostic investigations as outlined above and in the assessment of laparotomy findings in such patients.

Erythroblastosis

Transient conjugated hyperbilirubinaemia occurs during the recovery stage of erythroblastosis in which it appears that bilirubin is conjugated more rapidly than it can be excreted. When the unconjugated hyperbilirubinaemia has been protracted and severe or when there has been marked anaemia at birth, elevated serum amino transferase levels, hepatocellular necrosis and giant transformation of hepatocytes may occur (Walker 1971). The prognosis is good.

Acute neonatal hepatic necrosis

Neonatal hepatic necrosis is a rare condition presenting in the first four weeks of life with a haemorrhagic diathesis which usually precedes jaundice. There is a rapid downhill course, and at autopsy the liver is small with indistinct greyish-yellow streaks. Microscopically there is massive necrosis, collapse of liver reticulum, marked haemosiderin deposition and scanty giant cells are present. The aetiology is unknown. Vigorous supportive therapy with fresh blood transfusions, vitamin K and steroids is indicated (Reubner et al 1969, Philip & Larson 1973, Dupuy et al 1975).

Intrahepatic cholestasis of the newborn

This disorder is characterized pathologically by cholestasis without hepatocellular necrosis (Hass 1968). The liver architecture is preserved, and variable inflammatory cell changes occur in the portal tracts. These findings may represent a resolving hepatitis, and the prognosis is considered to be good.

Cryptogenic disease

In most series the aetiology of the disease remains obscure in a large percentage of cases (Alagille 1972, Henriksen et al 1981, Mowat et al 1976). The frequency with which genetic, infectious, environmental causes, or structural abnormalities are identified depends not only on the prevalance of these in the community but also on the referral patterns and sophistication of investigative facilities. In a study of infants with jaundice lasting for two weeks identified by paediatricians in South-east England, idiopathic intrahepatic disorders were approximately three times more common than biliary atresia and four times as frequent as liver disease associated with alpha$_1$-antitrypsin deficiency or the combined incidence of all other specific diagnoses (Mowat et al 1976).

Acute liver failure in infancy

Acute liver failure in infancy differs from that in the older child or adult in that bleeding complications predominate over neurological ones, and the severity of the bleeding diathesis frequently seems to be out of proportion to other manifestations of liver involvement. It must be assumed to be due to galactosaemia, fructosaemia or hereditary tyrosinosis until proved otherwise, as there is specific therapy for these conditions which in the first two is very effective. Bacterial infections presenting with septicaemia and if complicated, by septic shock, may initiate massive hepatic necrosis. Viral diseases, however, are more frequently implicated and usually occur without any of the congenital viral syndromes familiar to paediatricians and probably result from infection occurring in the perinatal period. In the first ten days of life the herpes virus and echo virus are commonly responsible. In the third week of life Epstein–Barr virus may be implicated and from six weeks of age, hepatitis B if the infection has been blood-borne but rather later if infection has been acquired by the gastrointestinal route (Delaplane et al 1983). In many infants the illness suggests a viral cause but no virus is isolated. Shock and vascular collapse due to cardiac lesions may occasionally cause liver damage, particularly in left ventricular hypoplasia (Alagille & Odievre 1979).

Clinical features. The first sign of hepatic involvement is frequently a bleeding diathesis. Jaundice with pale stools and dark urine may be another early feature, ofter occurring with a background of anorexia, vomiting and occasionally diarrhoea. The cardinal clinical feature is however a decrease in liver size. Neurological signs are absent or appear late in the course of the disease. They include meningeal irritation and features of hypoglycaemia. Many proceed to seizures followed by respiratory and cardiovascular complications which may require assisted ventilation.

Infections

Generalized infection acquired in utero, during delivery, or early in the newborn period by agents such as *Toxoplasma gondii*, *Treponema pallidum*, *Listeria*, *Mycobacterium tuberculosis*, rubella, cytomegalovirus, herpes simplex virus, coxsackie B and adenovirus, may be associated with a hepatitis. The infective agents, screening and definitive investigations and the principal extrahepatic clinical manifestations are listed in Table 19.4. It is particularly important to exclude those agents for which specific therapy is available. In addition to these generalized perinatal infections, liver damage in infancy may be caused by hepatotrophic viruses, particularly hepatitis B (HBV). The incidence of this in any community will depend on the frequency of the carrier-state for hepatitis B in the community. HBV infection appears to be acquired perinatally. The mode of infection is conjectural. Transplacental maternal/fetal blood transfusion, skin exposure to infected maternal blood at delivery, swallowing of maternal blood at delivery and postnatal infection by blood, e.g. from cracked nipples, are suggested modes of infection. All infants born to HBsAg (hepatitis B surface antigen) positive mothers are at risk. Infection occurs in 80–90% of infants whose mother has had an acute hepatitis in the last trimester of the pregnancy or early in the puerperium, with a 10–30% chance of infection if hepatitis has occurred in the early pregnancy. If the mother is an asymptomatic carrier the risk of infection depends on the Hepatitis Be antigen status of the mother. If her serum is HBe antigen positive there is a 90% chance of the infant being affected, while if the serum contains antibody to HBe antigen, infection occurs in less than 10%. When an infant is born to a mother whose serum contains neither HBe antigen or antibody, there is an intermediate risk of infection.

The onset of clinically evident liver disease is usually between 4 weeks and 5 months after birth. Infected infants show a wide range of severity of hepatitis ranging from asymptomatic acquisition of anti-HBs status through all grades of acute hepatitis to fulminant hepatic failure, or they develop a chronic hepatitis which may lead to the chronic persistent variety or chronic aggressive, passing on to cirrhosis (Mowat 1980, Delaplane et al 1983).

Vigorous supportive therapy with fresh blood transfusions and exchange transfusions may be required. Carbohydrates should be given as glucose as part of the intravenous therapy regimen. Oral feeding should be recommenced after 48 hours but should be low in protein; glucose polymers are useful to halt catabolism. Patients with disease due to a metabolic cause may rapidly improve but viral illnesses frequently lead to death, either acutely, or over a course of 3–4 months.

Genetic or familial causes of liver disease in infancy

Liver disease associated with alpha₁-antitrypsin deficiency. Genetic deficiency of the serum protein alpha₁-antitrypsin has in the last decade been shown to be an important factor in liver disease in infancy and childhood, and this condition is discussed in Chapter 21.

Other genetic, chromosomal and familial disorders. Liver disease presenting with conjugated hyperbilirubinaemia may be the first manifestation of a number of inherited metabolic disorders including galactosaemia, fructosaemia, tyrosinosis and more unusual disorders such as Nieman–Pick type C, Zellweger's syndrome or trihydroxy coprostanic acidaemia (see Chapter 18), cystic fibrosis, Gaucher's disease, and the mucopolysaccharidoses are disorders which may sometimes be associated with conjugated hyperbilirubinaemia with abnormal biochemical tests of liver function, but such liver manifestations are not present in all subjects (Mowat 1982). The Dubin–Johnson syndrome and Rotor syndrome may cause hyperbilirubinaemia but other aspects of liver function are normal. Liver disease may also occur in a number of major chromosomal abnormalities including trisomy 13, 18, and 21, and 45 X Turner's syndrome (Gardner 1974). Other recessively inherited disorders, but with an as yet unknown genetic or metabolic basis include Byler's disease and familial cholestasis with lymphoedema (Aagenaes 1974). Byler's disease, first described in an Amish family of that name, is characterized by vomiting, diarrhoea and recurrent episodes of cholestasis with persistently abnormal biochemical tests of liver function, going on to cirrhosis with death by ten years of age. The term 'Byler's syndrome' tends to be applied to any familial cholestatic syndrome leading to cirrhosis and early death. There is no diagnostic test or characteristic pathology that allows this diagnosis to be made with certainty.

In familial cholestasis with lymphoedema there are recurrent attacks of cholestatic jaundice throughout life, occasionally progressing to cirrhosis. Lymphoedema starts at puberty. The mechanism of the liver disease is unknown. There are deficient lymphatics in the peripheries.

A syndrome with intrahepatic biliary hypoplasia and a range of non-hepatic features has been increasingly recognized in the last decade (Alagille et al 1975) (see p. 432). This disorder is thought to be inherited as an autosomal dominant with variable penetrance.

Idiopathic

In most cases none of the above can be cited as causes (Silverman et al 1971). In a recent analysis of an on-going study in South-east England which included 103 patients with intact extraphepatic bile ducts, we found that 57 cases were without an identifiable cause, and in a further 14 the association of liver disease with a possible cause could not be firmly established. In some instances parenchymal damage or intrahepatic cholestasis may be associated with exposure to agents such as halothane, or drugs, but their association is tenuous and the frequency rare.

Other causes

Other rare causes of the hepatitis syndrome of infancy include choledocal cysts which may be responsible for 1–2% of such cases; spontaneous perforation of the bile ducts, in which bile-stained ascites may occur, may add to the usual clinical features of the syndrome (Howard et al 1976). In both cases surgical correction is necessary. Other causes are gallstones, microcystic disease of the liver and kidney and Rotor syndrome (Sass-Kortsak 1974).

Prognosis for infants with intrahepatic disease

The prognosis for infants with known genetic abnormalities, chromosomal lesions or infections, is usually determined by the overall effects of these, rather than purely hepatic damage. In liver disease associated with alpha$_1$-antitrypsin deficiency and in some forms of biliary hypoplasia the prognosis is poor. For infants with jaundice due to hepatic disease of unknown cause the prognosis is unknown. Danks et al (1977) gave a poor prognosis with 15 deaths and 6 with chronic liver disease amongst 52 such infants. This poor prognosis was confirmed by Deutsch et al in 1985. Henriksen et al (1981) also gave a poor prognosis with 15 out of 27 dying and 4 of 7 survivors studied having biochemical evidence of continuing liver disease. In contrast, Odievre et al (1981) reported only 4 deaths in 64 infants with 85% of the survivors making a good recovery. In another study 2 of 29 cases with cryptogenic hepatitis died but only 2 of the survivors followed up for 10 years had any hepatic abnormality (Dick & Mowat 1985). A similarly favourable prognosis was reported from Japan (Shiraki et al 1966). Infants with the worst prognosis appear to be those who have stools that are acholic for more than 4 weeks, hard livers, a positive family history for similar liver disease or histological features suggesting mechanical bile duct obstruction mimicking extrahepatic biliary atresia (Danks et al 1977, Odievre et al 1981).

Management of conjugated hyperbilirubinaemia

Rational management requires an accurate diagnosis. For infants who develop jaundice associated with bacterial infection, antibiotic therapy, generally in the form of intravenous gentamycin and a cephalosporin, is indicated. *Listeria*, syphilis and toxoplasmosis require specific therapy. Glucose should be the only dietary carbohydrate source used until galactosaemia and fructosaemia have been excluded as causes of the liver damage by specific tests. There is no effective treatment for idiopathic hepatitis of infancy or hepatitis associated with viral infections. Prolongation of the prothrombin time frequently occurs, usually due to vitamin K malabsorption rather than failure of synthesis of vitamin K-dependent coagulation proteins. If parenteral vitamin K fails to correct clotting abnormalities, fresh frozen plasma, whole fresh blood transfusion, platelet transfusion and even exchange transfusion may be required. When weight gain is poor or linear growth is subnormal, nutrition may be improved by supplementing the diet with glucose polymers or medium chain triglycerides. Proprietary milk preparations with long chain fat replaced by medium chain triglycerides may help weight gain in infants with marked cholestasis. Parenteral fat-soluble vitamins A and D are given to all patients. Vitamin D requirements are very variable and close biochemical and radiological monitoring is required. Vitamin E is particularly dependent on bile salts for solubilization and absorption and a number of reports have now appeared relating a neurological syndrome to a severe deficiency of vitamin E in children with cholestatic liver disease (Muller 1986). In general, patients with inadequate intestinal bile salt concentrations are unable to absorb oral supplements of vitamin E and require intramuscular preparations. There have been reports of neurological improvement following such treatment (Guggenheim et al 1982, Sokol et al 1985).

Liver damage associated with parenteral nutrition

In the last decade liver damage has emerged as a sporadic problem in infants receiving intravenous alimentation. The incidence is inversely proportional to gestation and increases with increased duration of intra-venous feeding or lack of oral feeding (Beal et al 1979, Pereira et al 1981, Whittington 1985). Affected infants usually have other disorders which may adversely affect hepatic function or bile flow, e.g. intra-abdominal sepsis, intractable diarrhoea, and disorders causing either acute or chronic hypoxia; very frequently, infants are receiving other forms of drug therapy. Liver damage or abnormal liver function tests have been reported with feeding regimens containing solutions of aminoacids, lipids, dextrose, vitamins and electrolytes but have also been reported in the absence of each of these constituents. (Mowat 1981). The pathogenesis of the liver injury is unknown. Lack of essential nutrients including trace elements, an imbalanced supply of aminoacids and lack of intestinal stimulation to bile secretion or gall-bladder contraction have all been postulated as possible contributory factors. If intravenous feeding can be stopped, liver function tests usually return to normal over a period of 1–5 months unless severe hepatic fibrosis or cirrhosis has already developed. If intravenous feeding has to be continued in spite of evidence of liver disease these irreversible complications may occur in those most severely affected.

Microscopically there is canalicular and hepatocellular cholestasis with hepatocyte distension and an increased number of nuclei. The Kupffer cells are distended with large amounts of para-aminosalicylic acid (PAS)-positive pigment and often bile. There may be lobular disarray with distension of portal tracts. A fine panlobular perisinusoidal or pericellular fibrosis is present in up to 50% of cases. Severe cases show portal-to-portal tract bridging necrosis or cirrhosis. Ultrastructural studies of liver biopsies show giant mitochondria of various shapes and sizes and abnormalities in the endoplasmic reticulum, and the cell sac frequently contains a glassy, homo-geneous, faintly electron-dense material. Follow-up biopsies 5–9 months after regression of the hepatitis still show mild hepatocellular cholestasis, ballooning of hepatocytes, lobular disarray and increased fibrosis (Dahms & Halpin 1981). There are no reported long-term follow-up studies. It is clearly important, therefore, to closely monitor liver function tests in infants who receive intravenous nutrition, particularly if they are premature. A rise in lipoprotein X concentration is usually followed later by a rise in trans-aminases. These tests should be carried out at weekly intervals during intravenous feeding. Intravenous feeding should be curtailed as much as possible in those patients whose tests become markedly abnormal.

Extrahepatic biliary atresia (see Daum & Fischer 1983)

Extrahepatic biliary atresia, a disorder unique to infancy, is characterized by a complete inability to excrete bile and by obstruction, destruction or absence of the bile duct(s) anywhere between the duodenum and the first or second order of branches of the right and left hepatic ducts. The condition is the end result of a destructive, inflammatory process. The extent and site of the obstruction, destruction or absence of the bile ducts is extremely variable (Hays & Kimura 1981). In terms of management and prognosis, three types, Type I, Type II, and Type III of the Classification of the Japanese Association of Surgeons should be identified. Atresia is limited to the common bile duct in Type I, the hepatic duct in Type II, with both the proximal extrahepatic bile ducts being patent to the porta-hepatis, while in Type III, atresia extends to the portahepatis. In Types I and II, bile duct to bowel anastomosis may be possible. It is in Type III that the radical surgical treatment introduced by Kasai can given effective bile drainage. In 80–85% of cases Kasai showed that excision of all remnants of the obliterated extrahepatic bile ducts up to the level of the portahepatis could result in bile drainage from minute residual channels which communicated with intrahepatic bile ducts. A roux-en-Y loop of jejunum is anastomosed to the cut surface of the residual bile duct tissue. A large number of cases with effective bile drainage after portoenterostomy have now been reported, the oldest survivors being over 23 years of age (Kasai 1983a). The results of surgical treatment in the UK improve with the experience of the unit in which the surgery is performed (McClement et al 1985).

In the first 2–3 months after birth the main intrahepatic bile ducts are patent. Three-dimensional reconstruction of the bile ducts in the vicinity of the portahepatis show that at this level the major intrahepatic bile ducts divide into many small branches which terminate in the fibrous tissue at the portahepatis. After two months of age the destructive process progressively destroys the main intralobular bile ducts (Kasai et al 1980). The more distal bile ducts or bile ductules in the peripheral portal tracts show proliferation of small ductule structures which starts in the first month of life and reaches its peak between six and ten months of age, and then starts to decline (Kasai 1983b). For surgery of extrahepatic biliary atresia to be effective it must be carried out at a time when it interrupts the progression of events that leads to these intrahepatic changes.

Portal tracts at the periphery of the liver show distension with oedema, inflammatory cell infiltrate, increasing fibroblastic activity and fibrous tissue accumulation. Portal hypertension is established by 6–10 weeks of age (Kasai et al 1978). The rate of biliary fibrosis varies widely with cirrhosis being established at any age between 6 weeks and three years.

Aetiology

The aetiology of biliary atresia is unknown. Familial cases are extremely rare. Up 25% of infants have minor or major abnormalities outside the biliary system with a particularly high frequency of abnormalities of a vascular nature below the diaphragm. Polysplenia and splenic hypoplasia with or without situs inversus is a rare association. It has been suggested that the precarious blood supply to the biliary tree may be further jeopardized by such abnormalities (Gautier & Elliot 1981), although experimental evidence does not suggest that ischaemic injury is a likely cause (Pickett & Briggs 1969 Okamoto et al 1980).

Miyano and his colleagues (1979) have reported an abnormally long common channel at the junction of the bile duct and the pancreatic duct in post mortem studies of infants with atresia, and suggest that pancreatic juice may enter the biliary system and initiate mucosal damage and a subsequent inflammatory response. There have been many suggestions that perinatal infection might be a possible cause for biliary atresia, the most recent candidate being the Reo virus Type III (Banjura et al 1980). Ultrastructural examination of tissue resected at surgery has failed to identify any infective agent. In experimental animals the Reo virus produces lesions of the bile ducts but without atresia.

Clinical and laboratory features

Yellow urine is usually present from birth with jaundice persisting from the second or third day of life and associated with stools that contain no bile pigment. The jaundice may be exaggerated by coexistent physiological jaundice. In up to 25% of cases stools with green or yellow pigment are reported but they eventually become quite acholic. Clinical examination shows a hard, enlarged liver and a degree of splenomegaly which increases with increased intrahepatic fibrosis. The infant is frequently very well nourished without any features of complications of cirrhosis until after two months of age.

Biochemical tests of liver function show a conjugated hyperbilirubinaemia with raised serum aspartate aminotransferase, alkaline phosphatase and gamma glutamyltranspeptidase activities. The serum albumin and prothrombin time are normal if the infant has received parenteral vitamin K.

Table 19.5 Histological features of the hepatitis syndrome of infancy and biliary atresia

Hepatitis	Biliary atresia
Hepatocellular necrosis	Widened portal tracts with prominent,
Giant cell transformation	distorted, elongated and angulated bile
Disorganization of liver cords	ducts; increased fibrosis; inflammatory cell
Inflammatory cell infiltrate in parenchyma	infiltrate
and portal tracts	Normal hepatic architecture
Cholestasis	Cholestasis with bile lakes
Focal portal bile duct proliferation	Giant cell transformation

The essential steps in prelaparotomy diagnosis have been considered earlier. The diagnostic features on percutaneous liver biopsy are given in Table 19.5. It is noteworthy that no single histological feature distinguishes biliary atresia from hepatitis. The principal difficulty occurs in infants who go on to develop the histological features of biliary hypoplasia but at this stage the condition still has bile duct reduplication in the portal tracts. The importance of excluding alpha$_1$-antitrypsin deficiency has already been stressed.

Many blood tests have been advocated for the distinction of extrahepatic biliary atresia from hepatitis but sadly their value has not been confirmed in prospective clinical trials. Such tests include alpha-fetoprotein (Johnson et al 1976), lipoprotein X (Manolaki & Mowat, unpublished observations), gamma glutamyltranspeptidase (Manolaki et al 1983), and bile acid ratios (Manthorpe & Mowat 1976).

Management (see Ohi et al 1985)

In up to 10% of cases it is possible to establish bile drainage by anastomosing the gallbladder or distended proximal bile duct to a Roux-en-Y loop from the small bowel. If the gallbladder or bile duct contains bile, biliary drainage should be established, but even with such a procedure long-term survival is infrequent (Berenson et al 1974). For the remaining patients, hepatic portoenterostomy or one of its variants is required. After hepatic portoenterostomy bile drainage may occur as evidenced by pigment in the stool and a fall in serum bilirubin. A deterioration in liver function and a fall in biliary excretion after operation has been correlated in many series with the onset of febrile illnesses and positive cultures of a large variety of organisms from liver and blood. Such infections are thought to be the result of ascending bacterial cholangitis (Lilley & Hitch 1978) and are followed by an increase in hepatic fibrosis and more severe portal hypertension. A large number of operations with variation in the construction and anastomosis of the intestinal conduit have been designed to try to prevent this serious complication. There is as yet no evidence that such complicated procedures decrease the incidence of serious or sustained cholangitis (Sawaguchi et al 1980).

Complications after portoenterostomy

Cholangitis. Ascending cholangitis is a major hazard and has been discussed above. Patients with suspected cholangitis require very prompt treatment with broad spectrum antibiotics, usually in the form of intravenous gentamicin and cephalosporin pending the result of bacteriological investigation. Prophylatic antibiotics have not been shown to reduce the incidence of cholangitis.

Portal hypertension. Portal hypertension is present in the majority of infants at the initial operation. In patients in whom the serum bilirubin falls to normal following surgery, endoscopic study may reveal disappearance of varices (Odievre 1978). Episodes of ascending cholangitis increase portal pressure. These patients should be advised to avoid aspirin. If bleeding occurs, injection sclerotherapy would appear to be the treatment of choice at this time (Stamatakis et al 1982).

Malabsorption. Malabsorption from lack of bile leads to poor growth and a deficiency of the fat-soluble vitamins. Natural bile flow is not achieved until one year after operation and even then, bile salts tend to be excreted preferentially to cholesterol and phospholipids.

Prognosis

The short-term results of portoenterostomy have gradually improved since its introduction by Kasai. The outcome of surgery appears to be related to the age at which surgery is performed, the severity of hepatic parenchymal damage at the time of the surgery, the frequency of ascending cholangitis and the experience of the surgeon (Hays & Kimura 1980). The best results are obtained in patients operated on before 8 weeks of age by a surgeon experienced in this work (McClement et al 1985). In such patients, up to 80% may be expected to be jaundice-free. With increasing age, effective bile drainage becomes less common.

The long-term results of portoenterostomy are encouraging (Ohio et al 1985). Hays & Kimura in Japan (1980) reported 85 patients over 5 years of age, 95% of whom were asymptomatic. In 1983 Kasai reported 41 jaundice-free survivors ranging in age from 5–28 years. 21 were more than ten years of age, all were well-grown and normally active. Only one was jaundiced. Approximately 50% of these long-term survivors had persistently abnormal liver function tests. Kitamura and co-workers (1980) have shown that satisfactory long-term survival, over 20 years, is compatible with a histological diagnosis of cirrhosis as the abnormal liver histology may be very irregularly distributed.

These results are extremely encouraging when one considers that the mean age of death in uncorrected biliary atresia is 11 months (Adelman 1978) and survival beyond 2 years of age is exceptional (Mowat et al 1976). It remains very disappointing that so many patients with biliary atresia are suspected of having serious disease after 6–8 weeks of life. It cannot be stressed too strongly that infants with jaundice associated with yellow urine and pale stools require urgent investigation.

Intrahepatic biliary hypoplasia

This disorder is characterized by complete absence or reduction in the number of bile ducts in the hepatic portal tracts. The diagnosis rests on the microscopic appearance of a number of portal tracks which contain normal portal vein and hepatic artery branches, but no accompanying bile ducts. This abnormality is seen in three circumstances; firstly, in patients with extrahepatic biliary atresia who have survived beyond the age of 12 months; secondly, in association with genetic disorders such as alpha$_1$-antitrypsin deficiency, and in infants with trihydroxy coprostanic acidaemia (Hanson et al 1975) and an isolated, ill-understood syndrome in which the extrahepatic bile ducts are intact.

The latter condition commonly presents as a hepatitis syndrome in the newborn period, and the early pathological picture is dominated by cholestasis with variable changes in the portal tract; there is usually minimal fibrosis. Bile ducts may be absent or initially may proliferate, and there is a minimal to moderate polymorphonuclear inflammatory response; the extrahepatic ducts are patent but small. In some instances, severe fibrosis develops in the portal tracts to give the pathological features of so-called 'biliary cirrhosis', and portal hypertension and varices eventually develop. Pruritus and xanthoma are prominent, and may be presenting features in some patients. Thirdly, a syndromic form of illness highlighted by Alagille et al in 1975 has been increasingly reported in the last decade. These children, in addition to biliary hypoplasia, have a range of extrahepatic features. The most constant features are systolic murmurs due to a range of cardiac anomalies, but particularly pulmonary stenosis which may be peripheral, embryotoxon seen by slit-lamp examination on the posterior aspects of the cornea overlying the iris, and abnormalities of formation or fusion of the anterior vertebral bodies, particularly in the thoracolumbar spine. In Alagille's original description, a distinct facial appearance was highlighted but subsequent observations suggest that this facial appearance is rather that of any form of persistent hepatic cholestasis of childhood (Sokol et al 1983).

Clinically, the majority of these cases have persisting jaundice with abnormal liver function tests starting in early infancy. By 5–9 months of age they develop severe pruritus followed by xanthelasma and very high serum cholesterol concentrations. In 10–20% of cases there is no jaundice, the disease presenting with pruritus, sometimes followed by xanthomata. Liver function tests in such cases are abnormal. Severe failure to thrive with malabsorption are major problems in early childhood, but in some cases the cholestasis gradually clears and the patient may make a complete recovery. Others seem to develop progressive, intrahepatic disease with increasing fibrosis. Although for the majority the prognosis in this syndrome is better than that for biliary hypoplasia as an isolated abnormality, cardiovascular difficulties, delayed development, growth failure and the effects of malabsorption cause much morbidity in childhood.

REFERENCES

Aagenaes Ø 1974 Hereditary recurrent cholestasis with lymphoedema. Acta Paediatrica Scandinavica 63: 465–469

Adelman S 1978 Prognosis of uncorrected biliary atresia: an update. Journal of Pediatric Surgery 13: 389–391

Alagille D 1972 Clinical aspects of neonatal hepatitis. American Journal of Diseases of Children 123: 287–293

Alagille D, Odievre M 1979 Acute liver failure in infants. In: Liver and Biliary Tract Disease in Children. John Willoughby & Sons Inc. New York, Ch. 5, pp 94–101

Alagille D, Odievre M, Gautier M, Domergues J P 1975 Hepatic ductular hypoplasia associated with characteristic facies, vertebral malformations, retarded physical, mental and sexual development and cardiac murmur. Journal of Pediatrics 86: 63–71

Balistreri W F 1985 Neonatal cholestasis. Journal of Pediatrics 106: 171–184

Banjura B, Morecki R, Glaser H, Gartner L M, Horwitz H S 1980 Comparative studies of biliary atresia in the human newborn and Reo virus-induced cholangitis in weaning mice. Laboratary Investigation 43: 456–461

Beal E F, Nelson R N, Bucciarelli R L 1979 Intrahepatic cholestasis associated with parenteral nutrition in premature infants. Pediatrics 64: 342–349

Berenson M M, Garde A R, Moody F G 1974 Twenty five year survival after surgery for complete extrahepatic biliary atresia. A case report. Gastroenterology 66: 260–263

Bleicher M A, Reiner M A, Rappoart S, Track N S 1979 Extraordinary hyperbilirubinaemia in a neonate with idiopathic hypertrophic pyloric stenosis. Journal of Pediatric Surgery 40: 427–431

Dacou-Voutetakis C, Anagnostakis D, Matsoniotis N 1978 Effect of prolonged illumination (phototherapy) on concentration of lutinising hormone in human infants. Science 199: 1299–1230

Dahms B B, Halpin T C 1981 Serial liver biopsies in parenteral nutrition — associated cholestasis of early infancy. Gastroenterology 81: 136–144

Danks D M, Campbell P E, Smith A L, Rogers J 1977 Prognosis of babies with neonatal hepatitis. Archives of Disease in Childhood 52: 368–372

Daum F, Fischer S E 1983 Extrahepatic biliary atresia. Marcel Dekker, New York

Delaplane D, Yogev R, Crussi F, Shulman S T 1983 Fatal hepatitis B in early infancy: importance of identifying HBsAg positive pregnant women and providing immuno-prophylaxis to the newborn. Pediatrics 72: 176–180

Deutsch J, Smith A L, Danks D M, Campbell P E 1985 Long-term prognosis in babies with neonatal liver disease. Archives of Disease in Childhood 60: 447–451

Dick M C, Mowat A P 1985 Hepatitis syndrome in infancy — an epidemiological study with 10-year follow up. Archives of Disease in Childhood 60: 512–516

Dupuy J M, Frommel D, Alagille D 1975 Severe viral hepatitis type B in infancy. Lancet i:191–194

Gardner L I 1974 Intrahepatic bile stasis in 45X Turners Syndrome. New England Journal of Medicine 290: 406–407

Gartner L M, Lee K S 1979 The effect of starvation and milk feeding on intestinal lumen absorption. Gastroenterology 77:A13

Gautier M, Elliot N 1981 Extrahepatic biliary atresia: morphological study of 94 biliary remnants. Archives of Pathology and Laboratory Medicine 105: 397–402

Gitzelmann-Cumarasamy N, Kuenzle C C 1979 Bilirubin-binding tests: living up to expectations? Pediatrics 64: 375–378

Guggenheim N A, Ringel S B, Silverman A, Grabert P E 1982 Progressive neuro-muscular disease in children with chronic cholestasis and Vitamin E deficiency: diagnosis and treatment with alpha-tocopherol. Journal of Pediatrics 100: 51–58

Hanson R F, Eisenberg J N, Williams G G, Hachey D, Szczepanic P, Kline P D, Sharp H L 1975 Metabolism of 3,7,12-trihydroxy-5 beta cholestan-26-oic acid in two siblings with cholestasis due to intrahepatic bile duct abnormalities. Journal of Clinical Investigation 56: 577–581

Hass L 1968 Intrahepatic cholestasis in the newborn. Archives of Disease in Childhood 48: 438–442

Hays D M, Kimura K 1980 Biliary Atresia — The Japanese Experience. Harvard University Press, Cambridge, Mass.

Hays D M, Wooley M, Snyder W H, Reid G, Gwinn J L, Landing B H 1967 Diagnosis of biliary atresia — relative accuracy of percutaneous liver biopsy, open liver biopsy and operative cholangiography. Journal of Paediatrics 71: 598–607

Heirwegh K P M, Meuwissen G A T P, Fevery G 1973 Critique of the assay and significance of bilirubin conjugation. Advances in Clinical Chemistry 16: 239–244

Henriksen N T, Drablos P A, Aagenaes Ø 1981 Cholestatic jaundice in infancy. The importance of familial and genetic factors in the aetiology and prognosis. Archives of Disease in Childhood 56: 622–627

Howard E R, Johnson D I, Mowat A P 1976 Spontaneous perforation of the common bile duct in infants. Archives of Disease in Childhood 51: 883–886

Johnson D I, Mowat A P, Orr H, Kohn J 1976 Serum alpha-fetoprotein levels in extrahepatic biliary atresia, idiopathic neonatal hepatitis, and alpha[1] antitrypsin deficiency (PiZ). Acta Paediatrica Scandinavica 65: 623–629

Kasai M 1983a Advances in treatment of biliary atresia. Japanese Journal of Surgery 13: 265–76

Kasai M 1983b Biliary atresia and its disorders. Excerpta Medica — Amsterdam, Oxford and Princeton (International Congress Series 627)

Kasai M, Suzuki H, Ohashi E, Ohi R, Chiva T, Okamoto A 1978 Technique & results of operative management of biliary atresia. World Journal of Surgery 2: 571–580

Kasai M, Ohi R, Kiba T 1980 Intrahepatic bile ducts in biliary atresia. Intrahepatic bile ducts. In: Kasai M, Shirake A (eds) Cholestasis in Infancy. Japan Medical Research Foundation, University of Tokyo press, Tokyo, pp 181–188

Kitamura K, Sawaguchi S, Akiyama H, Nakajo T 1980 Long-term results of the operation for extrahepatic biliary atresia in 144 infants. Zeitschrift fur Kinderchirurgie 31: 239–262

Lemaitre B, Toubas P L, Guillo T M, Drew N C, Relier J P 1977 Changes of serum gonadotrophin concentrations in premature infants admitted to phototherapy. Biology of the Neonate 32: 113–117

Lilly J R, Hitch D C 1978 Post-operative ascending cholangitis following portoenterostomy for biliary atresia. Measures for control. World Journal of Surgery 2: 581–585

McClement J W, Howard E R, Mowat A P 1985 Results of surgical treatment for extrahepatic biliary atresia in the United Kingdom 1980–82. British Medical Journal 290: 345–347

Maisels M J 1981 Neonatal Jaundice. In: Avery G B (ed) Neonatology, pathophysiology and management of the newborn, 2nd Edition. Lippencot Company, Philadelphia. pp 473–543

Manolaki A G, Larcher V F, Mowat A P, Barrett J J, Portmann B, Howard E R 1983 The pre-laparotomy diagnosis of extrahepatic biliary atresia. Archives of Disease in Childhood 58: 591–594

Manthorpe D J, Mowat A P 1976 Serum bile acids in the neonatal hepatitis syndrome. In: Alagille D (ed) Liver Diseases in Children. INSERM, Paris. pp 57–61

Markowitz J, Daum M, Kahn E I et al 1983 Arterio-hepatic dysplasia. 1. Pitfalls in diagnosis and management. Hepatology 3: 74–76

Messner K H, Maisels M J, Leure du Pree A E 1978 Phototoxicity to a newborn primate retina. Investigative Ophthalmology 17: 178–188

Miyano T, Suruga K, Suda K 1979 Abnormal choledocho-pancreaticoductal junction related to the aetiology of infantile obstructive jaundice. Journal of Pediatric Surgery 14: 16–26

Modi N, Keay A J 1983 Patotherapy for neonatal hyperbilirubinaemia: the importance of dose. Archives of Disease in Childhood 58: 406–409

Mowat A P 1980 Viral hepatitis in infancy and childhood. Clinics in Gastroenterology 9: 191–212

Mowat A P 1981 Paediatric Liver Disease. In: Arias I M, Frankel M, Wilson J H B (eds) Liver Annual. Vol. 1. Excerpta Medica, Amsterdam, pp 210–203

Mowat A P 1982 Familial inherited hepatic disorders. In: Clinics in Gastroenterology 11:(1) 171–205

Mowat A P, Psacharopoulos H T, Williams R 1976 Extrahepatic biliary atresia versus neonatal hepatitis. Review of 137 prospectively investigated infants. Archives of Disease in Childhood 51: 763–770

Muller D P R 1986 Vitamin E — its role in neurological function. Postgraduate Medical Journal 62: 107–112

Odell G B 1980 Neonatal hyperbilirubinemia (Monographs in Neonatology Series). Grune & Stratton, New York

Odell G B, Storey G N B, Rosenberg L A 1970 Studies in kernicterus. 3. Saturation of serum proteins with bilirubin during neonatal life and its relationship to brain damage at 5 years of age. Journal of Pediatrics 76: 12–23

Odievre M 1978 Long term results of surgical treatment of biliary atresia. World Journal of Surgery 2: 589–593

Odievre M, Luzeau R 1978 Lipolytic activity in milk from mothers of unjaundiced infants. Acta Paediatrica Scandinavica 67: 49–54

Odievre M, Hadchouel M, Landrieu Alagille D, Elliot N 1981 Long-term prognosis for infants with intrahepatic cholestasis and patent extrahepatic biliary tract. Archives of Disease in Childhood 56: 373–376

Ohi R, Hanamatsu M, Mochizuki I, Chiba T, Kasai M 1985 Progress in the treatment of biliary atresia. World Journal of Surgery 9: 285–293

Okamoto P, Okasora T, Toyosaka A 1980 An experimental study in the aetiology of congenital biliary atresia. In: Kasai M, Shiraki K (eds) Cholestasis in Infancy. Japan Medical Research Foundation, University of Tokyo Press, pp 217–224

Pearlman M A, Gartner L M, Lee K-S, Eidehman A I, Morecki R, Houroupian D S 1980 The association of kernicterus with bacterial infection in the newborn. Pediatrics 65: 26–32

Pereira G R, Sherman M S, Digiacimo J 1981 Hyper-alimentation-induced cholestasis. American Journal of Diseases of Childhood 135: 842–845

Philip A, Larson E 1973 Overwhelming neonatal infection with ECHO 19 virus. Journal of Pediatrics 82: 391–397

Pickett L K, Briggs H C 1969 Biliary obstruction secondary to hepatic vascular ligation in fetal sheep. Journal of Pediatric Surgery 4: 95–101

Psacharopoulos H T, Howard E R, Portmann B, Mowat A P 1980 Extrahepatic biliary atresia, pre-operative assessment and surgical results in 47 consecutive cases. Archives of Disease in Childhood 55: 851–856

Ruebner B H, Bhagavan B S, Greenfield A J, Campbell P, Danks D M 1969 Neonatal hepatic necrosis. Pediatrics 43: 963–970

Saland J, McNamara H, Cohen M I 1974 Navajo jaundice: A variant of neonatal hyperbilirubinemia associated with breast feeding. Journal of Pediatrics 85: 271–277

Sass-Kortsak A, 1974 Management of young infants presenting with direct reacting hyperbilirubinaemia. Pediatric Clinics of North America 21: 777–799

Sawaguchi S, Ikiyama H, Nakajo T 1980 Long-term follow up after radical operation for biliary atresia. In: Kasai M, Shiraki K (eds) Cholestasis in Infancy. University of Tokyo Press, Tokyo. pp 371–379

Scheidt P C, Mellits A D, Hardy J B, Draga J S, Boggs T R 1977 Toxicity to bilirubin in neonates. Infant development during first year in relation to maximum neonatal serum bilirubin concentration. Journal of Pediatrics 91: 292–297

Seigal S, Lunyk O, Bennett K J, Patterson M C 1982 Serum bilirubin levels in breast and formula-fed infants in the first 5 days of life. Canadian Medical Association Journal 127: 985–989

Shiraki K, Okamoto Y, Takatsu T 1966 A follow-up study of prolonged obstructive jaundice in infancy. Paediatrie Universitatas, Tokyo, 12: 41–49

Silverman A, Roy C C, Cozzetto F J 1971 In Pediatric Clinical Gastroenterology, p. 299. St. Louis: Moseby

Sokol R J, Heubi J E, Balistreri W F 1983 Intrahepatic cholestasis facies: is it specific for Alagilles syndrome. Journal of Pediatrics 103: 205–208

Sokol R J, Guggenheim M A, Iannaccone S T et al 1985 Improved neurological function after long-term correction of vitamin E deficiency in children with chronic cholestasis. New England Journal of Medicine 313: 1580–1586

Stamatakis J D, Howard E R, Psacharopoulos H T, Mowal A P 1982 Injection sclerotherapy for oesophageal varices in children. British Journal of Surgery 69: 74–75

Walker W 1971 Haemolytic disease in the newborn. In: Gairdner G, Hull D (eds) Recent Advances in Paediatrics. 4th edition. Churchill, London. pp 119–170

Whittington P F 1985 Cholestasis associated with total parenteral nutrition in infants. Hepatology 5:693

Infectious and drug-induced acute liver damage

This chapter will concentrate on infections in which the main or major clinical manifestation is hepatic. A wide range of viruses, Rickettsia, bacteria, fungi, protozoa and helminths may cause an infectious process within the liver. With many infections hepatic involvement is part of a widespread infection in which the major involvement may be of other organs. In these infections liver disease is usually asymptomatic unless there is already chronic liver damage. A brief mention is also made of non-microbial causes of liver damage and in particular that caused by drugs and poisons.

VIRAL INFECTIONS

Two distinct hepatotropic viruses, hepatitis A virus (HAV) and hepatitis B virus (HBV) have been identified and their laboratory and clinical features extensively studied. HAV and HBV account for much of the symptomatic hepatitis in man. A third hepatotropic virus, the Delta virus causes hepatitis in patients already infected by HBV. Sensitive, specific serological tests are available for the detection of both IgM and IgG antibodies to all three viruses. Epidemiological and laboratory evidence indicates that there are at least four other distinct hepatotropic viruses which are as yet, poorly characterized and without reliable serological markers. These are termed 'non-A, non-B hepatitis' (Deinhardt & Gust 1982, Zuckerman 1984.)

Hepatitis A

HAV is a cubic ribonucleic acid (RNA)-containing virus classified toxonomically on the basis of its physical and biochemical properties as a picorna

virus of the enterovirus genus with the designation enterovirus type 72
(Melnick 1982). It is however still referred to as the hepatitis A virus. HAV
is transmitted from person to person primarily by the faecal/oral route but
blood may carry the infection during the short period of viraemia. (Noble
et al 1984)

Hepatitis A virology

The incubation period is usually 2–4 weeks but may be as short as one
week. Viraemia, viral accumulation in hepatocytes and viral shedding in the
stools, become detectable 1–2 weeks after exposure and are maximal at
20–25 days just as nonspecific symptoms start and before biochemical
evidence of hepatitis. By this time, IgM antibodies which become detectable
after 7–10 days of exposure, are present in high concentrations. The
concentration of virus in the stool falls rapidly thereafter but virus may be
recovered for up to 8 weeks after the onset of jaundice. IgM antibodies are
usually undetectable after 60 days. IgG antibodies become detectable
20–40 days after exposure and persist for up to 30 years (Fig. 20.1). The
virus is cytopathogenic. There is no chronic 'carrier-state' (Siegal &
Frosner 1978a, 1978b, Duermayer & Van den Veen 1978).

Epidemiology

Close contact in a crowded environment and poor hygienic conditions
predispose to spread of infection. In countries in which drinking water is

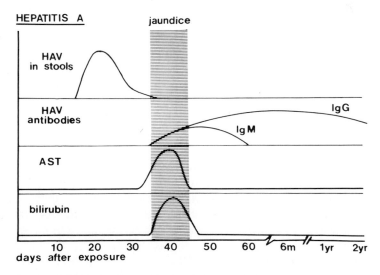

Fig. 20.1 Sequential appearance of hepatitis A virus (HAV) in the stool, the appearance of
hepatitis A antibodies, biochemical and clinical evidence of hepatitis in course of acute
hepatitis A.

contaminated by sewage, infection in early childhood is almost universal. Epidemics have been caused by stool contamination of water and food. Shellfish may carry the virus. Blood transfusion is a rare cause (Noble et al 1984).

Clinical features

The illness is frequently mild. It ranges in severity from asymptomatic infection to fulminant hepatic failure. Asymptomatic or anicteric infection is particularly frequent in young children. Jaundice is rare in those of less than 3 years of age (Capps et al 1952). In symptomatic patients anorexia, nausea, vomiting, abdominal pain, diarrhoea and fever may precede jaundice by 3–5 days. Occasionally pre-icteric symptoms are absent or mild and the first evidence of infection is the appearance of bile in the urine followed by jaundice, sometimes complicated by pruritus. With the appearance of the jaundice there is frequently considerable improvement in other symptoms.

On examination the liver is usually enlarged and tender. 20–30% of cases have splenomegaly and occasionally there will be generalized lymph gland enlargement. Stools may be pale. The icteric phase usually lasts from 3–7 days, but rarely it may persist for months. Complete recovery is the rule unless subacute hepatic necrosis or fulminant hepatic failure develops. Clinically this becomes evident by a recurrence of initial symptoms, deepening of jaundice, development of ascites or the appearance of features of hepatic encephalopathy. In children this frequently takes the form of unusual, aggressive behaviour as well as drowsiness. Other cardinal signs are a reduction in liver size, the liver frequently becoming impalpable and the development of spontaneous bleeding. Prompt recognition of these rare complications is essential so that appropriate treatment measures may be undertaken. Aplastic anaemia, pancreatitis and myocarditis are very rare complications. Chronic liver disease has not been shown to follow a serologically proven HAV infection.

Laboratory findings

A rise in serum aspartate aminotransferase or alanine aminotransferase occurs as symptoms begin. Concentrations rise progressively over the course of three or four days to values as high as 20–25 times the upper limit of normal. When, the serum bilirubin rises, the transaminase concentration falls and frequently returns to normal values within four weeks but occasionally remains abnormal for as long as three months. Serum alkaline phosphatase concentrations are rarely elevated more than fifty % above the upper limit of normal for the patient's age. The prothrombin time is normal. Elongation by more than three seconds suggests the presence of some other liver disorder or the development of subacute or fulminant hepatic failure. A mild leucocytosis, sometimes followed by lymphopaenia with a few atypical lymphocytes is frequently seen.

The diagnosis is confirmed by the demonstration of IgM antibodies to HAV. If this test is not available, the diagnosis is based on the exclusion of other causes of acute hepatitis, perhaps supported by an elevation of serum immunoglobulin IgM.

In atypical or isolated cases, particularly where specific serological tests are not available, consideration has to be given to excluding other treatable causes of liver damage which may present in a similar fashion. This includes chronic active hepatitis, Wilson's disease, and choledochal cysts.

Management

There is no specific treatment. The child should be encouraged to choose his own diet, trying to maintain a protein intake of 1 g/kg/24 h and a carbohydrate intake of 4 g/kg/ 24 h. Fats aggravate nausea but do not cause other difficulties. Enforced bed-rest is unnecessary (Repsher & Freebern 1969). Corticosteroids have no place in management.

Prevention

With the high incidence of asymptomatic cases and with maximum infectivity preceding the onset of recognized disease, the essential step in prevention is the provision of facilities which will allow a safe disposal of sewage and guarantee drinking water uncontaminated by faecal pathogens. Person-to-person spread may be minimized by scrupulous handwashing after defaecation and before handling food.

Normal immunoglobulin prepared from pools of at least 1000 donations of human plasma contain sufficient antibodies to HAV to give immunological protection for three months when given in a dose of 0.02–0.04 ml/kg. This dose should be used to control infection in closed institutions and for school and home contacts. Larger doses of 0.06–0.12 m/kg should be given to travellers going to highly endemic areas. The dose should be repeated every 4–6 months if exposure continues.

Hepatitis A virus has been successfully propagated in several primary tissue culture media, and with serial passages it has been possible to produce an attenuated, nonpathogenic virus capable of producing antibody in the chimpanzee which protects against virulent hepatitis type A (Provost et al 1983). It should therefore be possible to develop a live attenuated HAV. Since the genome for hepatitis A has been cloned it may also be possible to produce a vaccine virus synthetically or to synthesize an antigenic oligopeptide (Zuckerman 1984).

Hepatitis B

HBV is a member of a family of deoxyribonucleic acid (DNA) viruses termed Hepadna viruses with unique molecular, ultrastructural and biochemical properties (Melnick 1982). Using recombinant DNA and molecular hybridization techniques HBV has been found in the genome of liver cells of infected patients, (Shafritz et al, 1981). Unlike HAV the host immunological response is variable; it is occasionally excessive causing fulminant hepatic failure but more frequently it is ineffective leading to a longlasting infective carrier-state. The carrier may have normal liver structure and function or a range of pathological changes with up to 10% of those infected developing chronic liver disease, including cirrhosis or hepatocellular carcinoma. The host or environmental factors causing the variable immune and cytopathological effects are the subject of intensive research but remain to be fully elucidated (Bianchi 1982). Lack of a convenient laboratory model hampers progress.

Biology of hepatitis B virus

The complete and presumed infective form of HBV is a 42 nm spherical particle known as the Dane particle. It consists of an inner nucleocapsid core 27 nm in diameter termed the 'hepatitis B core' (HBc) and an outer lipoprotein coat comprising the hepatitis B surface antigen (HBsAg). Three different morphological forms of HBs may be detected in the sera of individuals acutely or chronically infected with HBV; i.e. Dane particles, spherical 22 nm HBsAg particles or filamentous HBsAg particles 22 nm in diameter. In most sera the ratio of 22 nm HBsAg to Dane particles exceeds 1 000:1. Four major virus-determined subtypes of HBsAg termed adw, ayw, ayr and adr, which breed true in infected people and experimental animals, have also been identified. No clinicopathological correlates of these viral subtypes have been identified but they are useful markers in epidemiological studies. It is disputed whether infection with one subtype confers immunity to the others. The respective antibodies to the two components of HBV are anti-HBc and anti-HBs. The antibody to the complete viron is termed the 'anti-Dane' antibody.

In sera two additional indicators of HBV infection are HBV specific DNA polymerase and the e antigen which are present in sera containing Dane particles. Although HBe antigen is clearly coded for by the viral genome as are the major polypeptides of HBsAg and HBcAg, the exact nature of HBeAg remains to be determined. Since it may be detected by serological techniques it remains a very useful marker of high infectivity of the HBV carrier.

Serological response in HBV infection. The serological response is variable in time and intensity and is summarized in Figure 20.2 and Table 20.1. Viral components may never be detected or may persist in high concentrations for up to 30 years. Antibodies to viral components may be detected

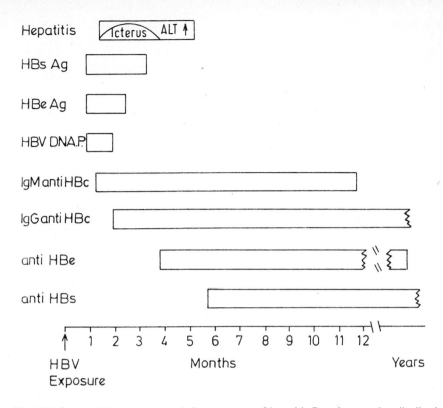

Fig. 20.2 Sequential appearance and disappearance of hepatitis B antigens and antibodies in an uncomplicated course of acute hepatitis type B with transient hepatitis B surface antigenaemia. In a small percentage of individuals with type B hepatitis, hepatitis B antigens may not be detected in spite of weekly blood sampling and the primary antibody response is detected.

In contrast, in the carrier state antibodies to surface and e antigen do not develop. An end to the carrier state is heralded by the appearance of antibody to the e antigen, the subsequent clearance of the e antigen and eventually clearance of the surface antigen.

HBV = hepatitis B virus; Ag = antigen; p = polymerase.

when the patient presents within a few weeks of exposure or may never appear. Commonly there is a time interval during which the viral antigens disappear from the serum and antibodies are undetectable. When antigens or antibodies are present the range of concentration may be wide.

Carriers. In the carrier state HBsAg, HBeAg and HBV DNA polymerase activity persists in the serum. Although HBc antibody (Ab) is present there is failure to develop HBeAb and HBsAb. High titres of anti-HBc suggests viral replication and persisting liver damage. After years of the carrier-state antigens may disappear and antibodies develop in the same pattern as in acute hepatitis. The time scale is protracted.

Evidence of HBc in the liver may be found in the absence of serological markers (Vergani et al 1982).

Table 20.1   Serological markers of hepatitis B infection and their significance

Marker	Antigen	Antibody
HBs	Acute infection, chronic infection, 'healthy' carriers	Past infection, passive or active immunization
HBe	Highly infectious state, acute infection, chronic infection	Past infection, healthy carrier (less infective than antigen positive status)
Dane particle	Highly infectious state, acute infection, chronic infection	Past infection
Hepatitis B core		IgM Very recent or ongoing infection IgG Past infection
HBV DNA polymerase HBV DNA (direct molecular hybridization technique)	)))))	Active viral replication and infective state in acute or chronic infections

HBV = hepatitis B virus; DNA = deoxyribonucleic acid

Hepatocellular damage in HBV infection. The pathogenesis of hepatocellular injury in HBV infection is unclear. Current evidence suggests that viral products or the virus enters the hepatocytes via Kupffer cells. The viral genome becomes encoded in host DNA (deoxyribonucleic acid) producing changes in the cell surface membrane and antibodies to surface antigens are produced. An antibody-dependent cellular autoimmune response to these hepatocyte membrane autoantigens and T-lymphocyte cytotoxicity against HBc expressed on the liver cell surface, are thought to cause hepatocellular injury. (Mondelli et al 1982). Defects in suppressor cell numbers and function involved in the maintenance of normal immune tolerance have been identified in chronic HBV infections. The humoral and/or non-circulating substances which cause immunoregulatory dysfunction are as yet unknown. The introduction of viral DNA fragments containing the HBcAg polypeptide coding sequence into a human hepatoma cell line already producing HBsAg without impairment of cell growth or function, led to a significant cytopathic effect when HBcAg was expressed. Thus, a direct cytotoxic effect of HBV remains a possibility (Yoakum et al 1983).

A wide range of pathological changes occur (Table 20.2). Asymptomatic subjects without abnormal clinical features and with normal biochemical tests of liver function may have advanced liver disease.

HBV within the liver. Using immunofluorescent and immunoperoxidase techniques, HBc can be detected within the nucleus of the hepatocyte as granular deposits, while in the endoplasmic reticulum HBsAg accumulates. It is believed that HBc is extruded from the nucleus and surrounded by

Table 20.2   The expression of hepatitis B virus infection in childhood

Asymptomatic development of HBsAb
Acute hepatitis, icteric or anicteric
Papular acrodermatitis
Acute hepatitis proceeding to chronic hepatitis and cirrhosis
Disorders associated with 'circulating immune complexes'
    glomerulonephritis, periarteritis, pericarditis, arthritis
Chronic liver disease
Hepatocellular carcinoma
Carrier state with immune deficiency,
    Down's syndrome, malignant disease, renal failure

HBsAb = Hepatitis B surface antibody

its protein code in the cytoplasm. How it gets into the blood stream of the host is unknown. In 'healthy' carriers without liver disease, few nuclei show HBc but there is abundant HBs in the cytoplasm of some hepatocytes, frequently clumped together. In contrast, in those with persisting hepatitis, intranuclear HBc is detected in many nuclei but little HBsAg is detected in the cytoplasm. Cytoplasmic HBsAg may be identified by its ground-glass appearance with haematoxylin and eosin or Masson's trichrome stains, or as brown material with orcein staining.

Epidemiology

As well as being present in the blood and serum, HBV may be detected in urine, saliva, tears, impetigenous lesions, semen and breast milk. Sources of infection in childhood are given in Table 20.3

It is now clear that therapeutic transfusions or injection of blood products is a relatively uncommon mode of transmission, particularly in childhood. In North-west Europe and North America infection in infancy and childhood is very uncommon. When it does occur it is usually in the setting of a family epidemic where an adult relative has HBV infection with HBe

Table 20.3   Sources of hepatitis B infection in childhood

HBsAg positive Mother	Maximum risk of infection in the perinatal period
HBsAg positive family member	50% of cases subclinical, drug addict, renal dialysis subject
Close contact	Infection via fomites, arthropod-borne or via abrasions
Blood products, particularly clotting factor concentrates	e.g. antihaemophilic globulin

HBsAg = Hepatitis B surface antigen

antigen in serum. It also occurs in up to 40% of institutionalized handicapped children, particularly those with Down's syndrome. It is more common in patients with leukaemia and other disorders with impaired immunity, particularly if much hospitalization is required or if multiple transfusions of blood products or coagulation factors are given. Patients with haemophilia receiving infusions of cryoprecipitate are at a particularly high risk.

In much of Asia and Africa and to a lesser extent, the Mediterranean countries and South America, HBV infection is predominantly a disease of infancy and childhood. The higher the adult carrier rate, particularly carriers who are HBeAg positive, the higher the rate of acquisition in childhood. Close contact with an HBsAg HBeAg positive mother or other family members is a particularly important predisposing factor.

In South-East Asia up to 30% of children become infected in the first year of life predominantly in the perinatal period. In contrast, in parts of Africa, only 5% may be infected in the first year of life (Botha et al 1984). Thereafter however, evidence of HBV infection appears in a gradually increasing percentage of children so that in some communities up to 90% may be infected in the first decade (Mowat 1984b). There is some evidence that the earlier in life infection is acquired, the longer the carrier state will last.

Clinical and laboratory features

In acute hepatitis the clinical and laboratory features are similar to those of Type A hepatitis except that fever and other systemic upset is less marked. The course is often more protracted. 50% of patients are asymptomatic and anicteric infection is frequent. In general the more acute the onset, the more marked the clinical or laboratory evidence of hepatocellular necrosis, and the greater the likelihood of affective antibody production and the early clearance of infection.

In chronic infections there may be clinical and laboratory features of chronic liver disease, cirrhosis or hepatocellular carcinoma, but frequently the clinical and laboratory features are no guide to the underlying liver pathology. Liver biopsy is the only means of assessing this. Patients with the histological features of chronic persistent or lobular hepatitis have a low risk of developing cirrhosis but the risk is high in those with chronic aggressive hepatitis. Because serological markers of HBV infection may be present without symptoms for years, their presence in acute hepatitis does not confirm that HBV infection is the cause of the acute hepatitis.

The specific accurate laboratory diagnosis of acute HBV infection is made by the detection of IgM HBcAb in high concentration.

Papular acrodermatitis. This disorder first described by Gianotti in 1973 appears to be a peculiarly paediatric manifestation of HBV infection. It takes the form of a non-itching erythematous, papular rash on the face and limbs which spreads rapidly initially and then clears spontaneously within a month. Lymphadenopathy, hepatomegaly and serological evidence of HBV infection is always present. The hepatitis is frequently anicteric but may progress to chronic liver disease. HBsAg is present in the serum during the acute phase of the dermatitis. The maximum incidence appears to be between 2 and 8 years of age.

Membranous glomerulonephritis. Glomerulonephritis appears to be more common in children with HBV infection than in adults (Dienstag 1982). It is thought to be mediated by immune complexes involving HBV virus antigens. Hepatitis Be antigen-antibody complexes have been identified in glomerular deposits in such children. The clinical outcome of the glomerulonephritis does not appear to differ from that observed in children who do not have HBV infection (Cadrobbi et al 1985).

The Delta agent. In 1977 Rizzetto and co-workers identified a new antigen antibody system closely related to HBV infection. This is the Delta agent which is identified in the liver by immunofluorescence, and in serum, IgM and IgG antibodies can be detected by radioimmunoassay. Subsequent studies have shown that the Delta agent is related to a small RNA-containing infectious agent, smaller than the genome of known animal RNA viruses, which requires the presence of HBV for its replication. Simultaneous infection with Delta agent and HBV results in an acute hepatitis of duration and course similar to acute HBV hepatitis. In contrast, Delta infection in individuals persistently infected with HBV results in an acute hepatitis which may have a fulminant course or progress to chronic disease. Up to 60% may develop chronic progressive disease which is unresponsive to immunosuppression (Hadler et al 1984).

Delta infection is world-wide but the incidence is relatively low in Asia. Patients with evidence of Delta infection are usually HBsAg positive with only 4 of 148 HBsAg negative HBsAb positive patients having Delta antibodies (Rizetto et al 1982). Infection may be acquired in the perinatal period (Zanetti et al 1982), and children and adults in areas with a high incidence of HBV infection are at risk of this super infection. Infection rates in drug addicts in Western Europe range from 30–60%, while up to 25% of haemophilic children in Italy have evidence of Delta infection.

Management

Hepatitis B viral infection is usually a self-limiting disorder. There is no specific treatment. The measures advised for Hepatitis A are also appropriate for HBV infection. In chronic infections antiviral drugs and human and synthetic interferon are being evaluated but their role in therapy has not yet been defined.

Prevention. All blood for transfusions or to provide products such as antihaemophilic globulin must be screened by the most sensitive methods and rejected where positive.

HBsAg positive patients, particularly if HBeAg positive, are potential sources of infection because of the presence of HBV in secretions and at high concentrations in blood. HBV persists on fomites. HBV appears to gain entrance via injured or infected skin and mucosa or orally. If attendants are advised of the modes of infection and take appropriate precautions, the risks of infection are small. If contaminated by blood or secretions, vigorous washing is advised. If there is skin or mucosal damage, immunoglobulin with high HBsAb titres may prevent infection.

Active immunization. Highly effective vaccines prepared from HBsAg persistent carriers are commercially available. Although expensive they are recommended for staff caring for many infective HBV patients. As yet no adverse long-term effects have been reported.

To prevent the development of a persistent HBsAg carrier state and thereby subsequent sequelae, vaccination of newborn infants and young children at risk is essential. All infants born to HBsAg positive mothers whether they are HBe antigen positive or have antibody to the e antigen, require immunization, as do infants born into communities with a high incidence of HBV infection. Hyperimmune gammaglobulin with hepatitis B vaccine given immediately after birth and with the vaccine repeated at 1, 2 and 6 months is of confirmed efficacy in preventing postnatal HBV infection in two double-blind randomized placebo control studies (Beasley et al 1983, Manzel et al 1984).

Synthetic vaccines should be commercially available in the near future and hopefully they will be freely available where they are most needed (Skellie et al 1981, Yong et al 1984).

Non-A, Non-B Hepatitis

The diagnosis of non-A, non-B hepatitis is made clinically by serological exclusion of HAV, HBV, Epstein–Barr, cytomegalovirus, herpes and echovirus infection in patients without other causes of acute liver injury such as drugs. There are no specific diagnostic tests.

Epidemiological, virological and clinical features

Non-A, non-B hepatitis accounts for 80–95% of post-transfusion hepatitis in North America and Northern Europe (Locasciulli et al 1983). There is an increased incidence in drug abusers and homosexuals. Family contacts are rarely affected. These observations suggest direct serum or blood spread. Two distinct incubation periods are seen, less than 5 weeks and from 2–26 weeks. The occurrence of sporadic cases is unexplained. Animal transmission studies suggest at least two distinct agents are responsible. Infection may be asymptomatic, anicteric or icteric and the hepatitis fulminant. Liver function tests remain abnormal in two-thirds of cases for up to six months with 60% of these developing chronic liver disease.

At least three common source epidemics of non-A, non-B hepatitis have been reported and these were presumed to have been water-borne. Immuno-electronmicroscopy of faecal samples and transmission experiments suggested that the cause was a virus similar to HAV with an incubation period of approximately 40 days. The clinical course was similar to that of HAV infection without progression to chronic liver disease. The disorder is frequently fatal in pregnancy (Zuckerman 1982). There is no known specific treatment.

Infectious mononucleosis (Epstein–Barr virus): EBV

This is an acute, usually benign, self-limiting infectious illness in which there is a generalized reticuloendothelial reaction with fever, lymphadenopathy, sore throat, rash, hepatosplenomegaly and a lymphocytosis with atypical lymphocytes (Christie 1980). Diagnosis is established by the presence of heterophil antibodies (Paul-Bunnell test) with a rising IgM antibody titre to EBV. Classical clinical features are seen in young adults. Young children frequently have asymptomatic infection or a less generalized reaction. The virus may be recovered from the pharynx for up to three months during an acute illness. Infection is life-long and may be periodically reactivated. Fatal abberations of immune function are rare complications.

Hepatic features

The spectrum of liver disease extends from hepatomegaly with or without tenderness to a picture resembling an acute type A hepatitis, but with features of a generalized disease. 5–15% have overt jaundice and 50% will have mild hyperbilirubinaemia. Raised serum transaminase levels are almost universal with over 80% having values more than 20 times the upper limit of normal (Kirkpatrick 1966). Histologically there is dense accumulation of large mononuclear cells in and around the portal tracts and within the hepatic parenchyma. The Kupffer cells are large and numerous. There are foci of liver cell necrosis but these are usually less diffuse than in viral hepatitis. The viral particles have not been identified in the liver. Histological recovery takes up to 8 months. Prolonged, severe jaundice and even fatal hepatocellular necrosis, has been recorded (Allen & Bass 1963, Harries & Fergusson 1968).

There is no specific treatment but in severely ill patients a dramatic improvement may be produced by corticosteroids.

Cytomegalovirus (CMV)

Cytomegalovirus has the physical and biological characteristics of a herpes virus. It causes a persistent, generalized infection with three main clinical syndromes: a multisystem infection acquired in utero, a variable illness in infants, young children and adults, and an opportunistic infection in immunosuppressed patients. Whether the latter category is due to reinfection or reactivation or both is unclear. In all syndromes the majority of infections are asymptomatic. The virus is excreted in the urine, in almost all secretions and is present in circulating leucocytes. Persistent excretion may follow intrauterine infection (Weller 1971).

Hepatic Features

Hepatomegaly and mildly abnormal liver function tests are frequently found in asymptomatic individuals excreting CMV in the urine and in patients with CMV mononucleosis. In those with jaundice the features are those of a viral hepatitis with transaminases as high as 20 times normal. The jaundice may persist for up to three months. Rarely, fatal massive hepatic necrosis develops (Schusterman et al 1978). The outstanding pathological changes observed in all forms of the disease are the pathognomic, greatly enlarged cells, particularly epithelial cells such as those lining the small bile ducts (Clark et al 1979). The diagnosis of CMV infection is established by the isolation of the virus from urine, secretions or tissues or by the presence of IgM antibody to CMV or persistent complement-fixing antibody (McDonald & Tobin 1978). There are a number of difficulties, since antibody tests may crossreact with other cell-associated herpes viruses and antibody concentrations may fluctuate wildly in normal individuals. Prolonged virus excretion may occur after infection. Some caution is necessary therefore in assuming an aetiological relationship between clinical features and the recovery of the virus or antibody changes.

There is no satisfactory treatment for CMV infections. The infection is so ubiquitous and its manifestation so protean that prevention is difficult. A vaccine is being developed.

Herpes simplex hepatitis

Herpes hepatitis occurs in some infants with generalized herpetic disease (Templeton 1970) and in adults who are immunosuppressed, including patients who have received liver transplantation. Fatal hepatitis has occurred in adults who were previously considered to be well.

Hepatic features

Hepatomegaly with tenderness, raised serum transaminases, and a prolonged prothrombin time are features of reported cases. On liver biopsy, small punctate areas of haemorrhagic necrosis are seen with a variable mononuclear reaction. Typical intranuclear inclusion bodies may be seen.

Diagnosis is established by virus isolation or identification using immunofluorescent or electronmicroscopic techniques.

Vaccines are currently being evaluated but are not yet available.

Immunosuppressed subjects should avoid contact with overt herpetic lesions. Infected infants should be isolated. Cytosine arabinoside (3–4 mg/kg/24 h) or acyclovir (10 mg/kg/24 h in 8 h boluses) should be used for patients with generalized infection (Oxford et al 1977).

Yellow fever hepatitis

Yellow fever is an acute infectious disease caused by a group B arbovirus. Infection is transmitted by the mosquito from man to man or from primate to man. The disease is endemic in parts of Africa and in South and Central America.

After an incubation period of 4–6 days, symptomatic infection is characterised by fever, prostration, headache and limb pain with jaundice appearing on the fourth day. The classical triad of symptoms, jaundice, haemorrhage and intense albuminuria is present only in severe infections. The fatality rate is still between 5 and 10% of symptomatic patients. Asymptomatic infection can occur (Francis et al 1972).

Hepatic involvement is characterized by necrosis in the mid-zone of the liver lobule with little inflammatory reaction (Kerr 1973). There is little connective tissue reaction and no permanent liver damage if the patient recovers.

The diagnosis is confirmed by antibody tests or by intracellular innoculation of mice or monkeys. Leptospirosis is the main differential diagnosis. There is no specific treatment.

The disease may be prevented by vaccination which provides protection for at least ten years. In towns, anti-mosquito measures help to control the spread of infection.

Other viruses affecting the liver

Involvement of the liver may occur in a wide range of other viral infections, including Coxsackie, adenovirus, varicella, measles and mumps. In most instances infection is asymptomatic and detected only by a rise in serum transaminases. In the presence of underlying liver disease jaundice may develop. Rare instances of fulminant hepatitis have been recorded with the majority of these viruses.

The liver appears to be a primary target for the relatively recently identified Lassa, Marburg and Ebola viruses. There are no specific treatments for these common or exotic viruses (Zuckerman & Simpson 1979)

PARASITIC INFECTIONS

Toxoplasmosis

Toxoplasmosis is a world-wide infection in man and animals caused by *Toxoplasma gondii*. 30% of adults in the UK have antibodies to the parasite.

Infection may occur in utero. Acquired infection is frequently asymptomatic. There may be mild fever with local or generalized lymph gland enlargement. Features may suggest infectious mononucleosis.

Hepatic involvement is evidenced by hepatomegaly with or without splenomegaly, elevation of serum transaminases and rarely mild jaundice (Tivari et al 1982).

The diagnosis is established by toxoplasma IgM antibody detection. Acquired toxoplasmosis is often so mild that treatment is unnecessary. If the disease is severe, combined pyrimethamine (1 mg/kg/24 h) for three weeks, and sulphadiazine 100 mg/kg/24 h may be given. A twice-weekly blood count is necessary while using pyrimethamine. A less toxic alternative is spiramycin in a dose of 100 mg/kg/24 h given for six weeks (Remington & Desments 1976).

Leishmaniasis

Leishmaniasis is an infectious disease caused by protozoa of the genus *Leishmania*, the intracellular form of which affects man and other mammals (Manson-Bahr 1983). Various species of sand-fly transmit the infection from host to host. *L. donovani* affects the entire reticuloendothelial system causing kala-azar. The domestic dog or wild canine and small rodents are the usual sources of infection. The incubation period is usually 4–6 months but may be up to ten years. A protracted febrile illness with much malaise, lymph gland enlargement, splenomegaly and hepatomegaly are the main clinical features. Jaundice develops in 10% of patients. Histological features vary from mild focal necrosis to extensive areas of haemorrhagic necrosis with extensive granulomatous nodules. Kupfer cells may contain Leishman-Donovani bodies. Scarring without cirrhosis occurs on healing (Verees et al 1974). The majority of infections are not apparent. Children of less than 5 years of age are the main victims.

The diagnosis is established by specific antibody tests or by the identification of Leishman-Donovani bodies in bone marrow, spleen or liver aspirates.

Intravenous or intramuscular sodium stibogluconate in a dose of 15 mg/kg/24 h for 30 days is effective in the vast majority of cases. Persistent cases are probably best treated with amphotericin B.

The disorder may be prevented by treatment of the disease in humans, the elimination of diseased dogs and rodents and the use of insecticide sprays directed against the sand-fly.

Toxocara and visceral larva migrans (see Ch. 10)

Hydatid disease (see Ch. 10)

The most frequent mode of presentation is the feeling of an epigastric mass. Less frequently, there may be abdominal pain, jaundice or very rarely, an anaphylactic reaction when a cyst has ruptured into the peritoneal cavity. Rupture into the bile ducts may lead to a cure, cholestatic jaundice or recurrent cholangitis. Calcification may occur. The finding of a typical cystic lesion on ultrasound or computerized tomography (CT) scanning supports the diagnosis which is confirmed serologically by indirect agglutination and complement fixation tests which are positive in 85% of cases.

The risks of rupture and secondary infection are such that the cysts should be removed surgically. It is important that they be removed completely without contaminating the peritoneum. Mebendazole in a dose of 10–15 mg/kg for 4–13 months should be tried in patients with ruptured cysts or *Echinococcus multilocularis* but is of no value in uncomplicated disease. It frequently does lead to a reduction in the size of the cysts but may not kill the *Echinococcus*. Side-effects are significant, but the drug is worth considering in patients who are too ill for surgery (Davidson 1984).

Amoebiasis

Amoebic dysentery and amoebic 'liver abscess' is caused by *Entamoeba histolytica*, a protozoan for which man is the only host (see also Ch. 10).

In acute amoebic dysentery tender hepatic enlargement with nonspecific hepatic inflammatory changes is quite common. With treatment of the intestinal infection, the liver returns to normal. There is no pathological evidence of invasion of the liver. Liver damage occurs when the parasite reaches the liver via the portal-venous system, survives, multiplies and blocks the small intrahepatic portal vein branches causing focal necrosis and lysis of liver tissue. The necrotic areas are commonly solitary but in children there may be multiple lesions. The largest may contain thick, red/brown fluid. The immediately surrounding liver tissue shows moderate inflammatory cell response but the remaining liver tissue is normal. The lesions heal with minimal scar formation.

The main clinical features are high fever, rigors, sweating, upper abdominal pain which may become pleuritic or be referred to the right shoulder, and weight loss. On examination there may be diminished respiratory movements, hepatomegaly with tenderness on deep palpation or percussion. Jaundice is rare. The lesion may be delineated by ultrasonography, hepatic scintigraphy and computerized axial tomography. Sensitive serological tests are positive in over 95% of patients. Seropositivity however, does not distinguish current tissue invasion from past disease. *Entamoeba histolytica* may be found in the stool as cysts or vegetative forms.

Metronidazole in a dose of 50 mg/kg/24 h for 5–8 days or tinidazole in a dose of 60 mg/kg/24 h for 5 days is the treatment of choice.

Surgical drainage or aspiration under ultrasonographic control is indicated for lesions with secondary infection, when rupture into other organs has occurred or when the lesion continues to enlarge in spite of drug treatment. The disease may be prevented by good sewage disposal facilities, adequate filtration of the water supply, and simple hygienic measures (Katzenstein et al 1982).

Schistosomiasis (Bilharziasis) (See also Ch. 10)

The severity of disease is related as much to the intensity of the inflammatory response which is of a delayed hypersensitivity type, as to the parasite load. In the liver, granulomata form around and near the portal tracts. They heal with intense fibrosis. There is little or no upset to the hepatic parenchyma but intrahepatic portal venous obstruction with the development of portal hypertension and portosystemic collaterals results (Nash et al 1982).

The course is extremely variable with features of portal hypertension commonly developing in late childhood or early adult life. Hepatomegaly, splenomegaly and haematemesis without clinical or biochemical abnormalities associated with cirrhosis, are the main hepatic features. Definitive diagnosis is made by the finding of the schistosome eggs in the excreta or in biopsy (particularly rectal) specimens. Immunodiagnostic (ELISA) techniques of high specificity have now been developed (Mitchell et al 1983). For *Schistosoma mansoni* infections oxamniquine in a single oral dose appears to be effective in the Americas and Caribbean, but in Africa, hycanthone in a singular intramuscular dose of 1.5 mg/kg is most effective. For *Schistosoma japonicum* infections praziquantel in a dose of 20 mg/kg administered orally three times in one day is the treatment of choice. In nonendemic areas it has also been used in treating all three forms of infection. The disorder may be prevented by an attack on the man/water/snail cycle but this is very costly. Mass chemotherapy has also been used.

Liver fluke diseases

Three major groups of liver flukes affect children and result in significant disease. The first is the *Opisthorchis* group which have cats as their definitive host, the second is the *Clonorchis* group which have fish as a second intermediate host, the third is the *Fasciola* group which live in the biliary tract of domestic herbivores. In all three types snails are involved in the life-cycle (see Ch. 10) (Sullivan & Koep 1980, Reshef et al 1982).

Clinically the disease falls into two parts. A migratory phase which may be symptomless or associated with fever, malaise, myalgia, eosinophilia and sometimes epigastric discomfort and tender hepatomegaly.

Secondly an obstructive phase with features of bile duct obstruction with cholangitis. Bacterial cholangitis, abscess formation, biliary cirrhosis, and bile duct carcinoma are long-term complications with *Opisthorchis* and *Clonorchis*.

The diagnosis may be suspected on the basis of the dietary history and the place of residence. It is confirmed by the finding of ova in the stools or from duodenal aspirate. Other causes of bile duct obstruction, including *Ascaris* have to be considered.

Praziquantel in a dose of 20 mg/kg/day for two days is effective for opisthorchiasis and clonorchiasis but treatment of structural abnormalities and bacterial infection may be required. Fascioliasis is treated with bithionol in a dose of 40 mg/kg/24 h given on alternate days for ten doses.

BACTERIAL INFECTIONS

Pyogenic liver abscesses

Classically, liver abscesses develop following portal pylephlebitis or from septic emboli in the portal-venous system arising from pelvic or intra-abdominal sepsis. Umbilical vein sepsis may be the cause in neonates. Currently, important causes include primary or iatrogenic immunosuppression, suppurative cholangitis associated with abnormalities in the biliary system, direct liver injury causing intrahepatic haematoma with secondary infection, septicaemia and direct infection from adjacent organs. In a large percentage of cases there is no obvious predisposing cause. (Stenson et al 1983)

Most commonly the infecting organisms are gram-negative but a very wide range of organisms have been incriminated including anaerobes, *Candida albicans* and actinomycosis.

The abscesses may be large, single and well encapsulated with fibrous tissue, or multiple and surrounded by disintegrating hepatic structures. They are centred around the biliary tree if secondary to cholangitis. Those arising from intra-abdominal causes or from septicaemia are mainly in the right lobe of the liver. The clinical features are often nonspecific with features of a febrile illness. The diagnosis may be suspected on the basis of a predisposing cause. At least 25% of cases have no clinical or laboratory features that indicate hepatic involvement. Hepatomegaly with tenderness on deep palpation is the most useful sign. There may be mild jaundice and a decreased range of respiratory movements.

Standard biochemical tests of liver function are relatively unhelpful although in some instances the serum alkaline phosphatase and bilirubin may be raised with the albumin depressed. The most useful investigation is an ultrasound scan of the liver which will show a fluid-filled cyst. Technetium colloid scans show a filling defect.

If an intrahepatic abscess is localized it has to be drained. A percutaneous catheter drainage, ultrasonographically directed is frequently effective. Surgery is usually required if there are multiple abscesses or peritonitis. Appropriate antibiotic therapy dictated by the bacteriological findings is essential. In some instances, particularly with multiple streptococcal liver abscesses a satisfactory response may be obtained with long-term parenteral and oral antibiotic therapy.

Leptospirosis

Leptospirosis is an acute infectious disease of varying severity caused by one of many serological types of spirochaetes of the genus *Leptospira*. The clinical illness may vary from an asymptomatic infection through a severe influenza illness to a fatal illness because of cardiac, renal or hepatic involvement. Although the serotype icterohaemorrhagica is classically associated with the severe form termed 'Weil's disease' the course of the disease is not related to the leptospira serotype (Feigin & Anderson 1975).

Sources of infection are the rodent, a wide range of domestic animals or household pets and many wild animals, reptiles and birds. Many are persistent, healthy excretors of leptospirae. Spirochaetes can survive for long periods outside their animal vectors and thus infection can occur without direct contact. Children are frequently infected.

The characteristic pathological feature of leptospirosis is an extensive vasculitis affecting all major organs and the skin. Hepatic features are those of a mild, diffuse hepatitis with Kupffer cell hypoplasia and portal infiltration with focal centalobular necrosis. On electronmicroscopy there is mitochondrial destruction. Histochemically, mitochondrial enzymatic activity is decreased.

After an incubation period of 2–21 days, there is an abrupt onset of septicaemic features with fever, chills, myalgia, headache, abdominal pain, skin rash, conjunctival injection, proteinuria and haematuria. Pneumonitis, myocarditis and meningitis may be evident. From 4–30 days later the septicaemic features settle but there is increasing damage to organs such as myocardium, kidneys or liver during an immune phase in which leptospirae are not found in the tissues.

Laboratory tests reflect the degree of organ involvement with a high alkaline phosphatase, the most frequent abnormality indicating liver disease. Leptospirae may be recovered from blood or cerebrospinal fluid (CSF) in the first ten days and in the urine up to the 30th day. Serological tests for antibodies show a progressive rise. Penicillin, erythromycin and tetracycline are effective if given within seven days of onset. Supportive treatment is required for congestive cardiac failure or renal or hepatic failure.

REYE'S SYNDROME

This is an acute disorder characterized by self-limiting mitochondrial dysfunction with diffuse fatty infiltration of the liver and a noninflammatory encephalopathy with marked cerebral oedema. The metabolism of proteins, carbohydrates, lipids and purines is disturbed. There are usually no clinical signs of hepatic involvement. Reye's sydrome occurs in a small proportion of infants and children during the recovery phase of a clinically unremarkable viral illness, e.g. chicken-pox or other exanthemata, respiratory and gastrointestinal disease (Mowat 1983). Mortality for recognized cases is currently approximately 30% in the United States and 60% in the UK. Neurological and psychological sequaelae may occur in the survivors (Reye's Syndrome 1984).

Epidemiology

The aetiology is unknown. At least 19 different viruses have been implicated in the prodromal illness. Epidemiological studies seek to implicate toxins such as salicylates, pteridines, isopropyl, alcohol, hypoglycins, 4-pentenoic acid, aflatoxins and emulsifiers, however the case for these is unproven. A currently favoured hypothesis is that Reye's syndrome occurs in a subject with a genetic predisposition and is triggered by an infection in the presence of an environmental toxin. The mechanism of mitochondrial injury is not clear.

Clinical features

The clinical features which suggest the diagnosis are vomiting, which is persistent and profuse, in an infant or child during the recovery phase of a viral illness when associated with a deterioration in the level of consciousness. This may proceed to brain death over a period of 4–60 hours, or may stabilize and improve at any stage short of this. 30% of cases have convulsions. Infants typically have tachypnoea, hyperventilation and, more commonly, hypoglycaemia and apnoea. Hepatomegaly is frequently found in infants but rarely in older children.

Diagnosis is suspected clinically when supported by laboratory evidence of hepatic involvement, namely increased aspartate aminotransferase activity to more than twice normal, prolongation of the prothrombin time of more than three seconds and high blood ammonia (Heubi et al 1984). Hypoglycaemia may be found in infants of less than 2 years. The diagnosis is confirmed by liver biopsy findings of histological evidence of reduced enzymatic activity of mitochondrial enzymes such as succinic dehydrogenase, or swollen distorted mitochondria on electronmicroscopy. These changes are most evident in the first three days of the illness and thereafter clear. There is also progressive glycogen depletion in the first 24 hours associated with a panlobular microvesicular lipid accumulation seen in its early stages only on electronmicroscopy or with lipid dyes, and progressing in severe cases to marked lipid accumulation 2–5 days into the illness. This clears by 9 days. The differential diagnosis includes many acquired encephalopathies and genetic disorders associated with hepatic dysfunction, particularly those involving mitochondria.

Treatment

The principles of treatment are to correct the metabolic abnormalities and to prevent cerebral oedema and tissue hypoxia using all the resources available with modern intensive care. Cases responsive to verbal stimuli may respond to 10–15% glucose infusions which maintain a blood glucose level greater than 8 mmol/l with a fluid intake at 70% of normal maintenance. With deeper coma, much more active measures are required to prevent death or neurological sequelae. The serum osmolarity is maintained at 300–320 mmol/kg, artificial ventilation maintains the $PaCO_2$ at 25 mm/hg and PaO_2 at 150 mm/hg. The intracranial pressure is kept at less than 20 mm/hg with a cerebral perfusion pressure of at least 50 mm/hg. The latter requires phenobarbitone and morphine coma, nursing at an angle of 40 ° and sometimes hypothermia and bifrontal decompressive craniectomy. The place of dexamethasone is controversial. Mannitol has an effect which is only temporary but may be useful while other measures are instituted.

NON-MICROBIAL CAUSES OF HEPATIC INFLAMMATION

There are many nonmicrobial causes of hepatic inflammation. In patients presenting with sporadic or isolated acute hepatitis, particularly if specific serological diagnostic tests are not available or negative, it is essential to exclude remedial causes of liver injury which may present in a similar way. The most important of these are Wilson's Disease (Chapter 18 and 21) galactosaemia and fructosaemia (Chapter 18), autoimmune chronic active hepatitis (Chapter 21) and biliary disorders, particularly choledochal cysts (Chapter 19).

Drugs and poisons

A careful history of systemic or topical exposure to drugs or hepatotoxins is essential since an increasing range of products (Table 20.4) are reported to cause or be associated with liver injury. The incidence is difficult to estimate since the association is frequently based on a single case report without confirmation by rechallenge or by in vitro testing. Adverse drug effects fall into four main categories, (Stricker & Spoelstra 1985, Neuberger & Davis 1983, Davis 1984, Mowat 1984a):
1. Interference with a specific metabolic process
2. A direct hepatotoxic effect of the drug
3. A metabolite-related toxic effect
4. An immunological reaction to the drug or its products
The patient's age, state of nutrition, presence or absence of gastrointestinal or renal disease and other xenobiotics which may influence drug metabolism, may contribute to adverse hepatic effects. The sporadic nature of many drug toxic effects is unexplained. The identification of an increasing number of isoenzymes of cytochrome P-450 may offer a possible explanation for interindividual differences in susceptibility while the effect of viral infection on hepatic metabolism may explain some isolated occurrences.

The range of hepatic pathology associated with drug exposure ranges from an asymptomatic rise in the serum transaminase with minimal structural abnormality of the liver through various forms of hepatic dysfunction

Table 20.4 Drugs and toxins causing liver damage

Antimicrobials
Tetracycline
Erythromycin
Estolate
Nitrofurantoin
Ampicillin
Flucloxacillin
Carbenicillin
Sulphonamides
Sulphasalazine
Trimetoprim-sulphamethoxazole
Ketoconazole
Chloramphenicol
Hycanthone

Antituberculous drugs
PAS
Isoniazid
Rifampicin
Pyrazinamide
Ethionamide
Ethambutol

Cytotoxic and immunosuppressive drugs
Methotrexate
6-mercaptopurine
Azathioprine
6-thioguanine
Mitomycin
Carbazine
Chlorambucil
Cyclophosphamide
Cyclosporin-A

Anaesthetics
Halothane
Enflurane
Chloroform

Anticonvulsants
Sodium valproate
Carbamazepine
Diphenylhydantoin
Dantrolene

Analgesics and antiinflammatory agents
Phenylbutazone
Indomethacin
Paracetamol
Salicylates
Dextroproxyphene
Ibuprofen
Glafenine
D-Penicillamine
Salindaac
Feproazone
Propafenone

Psychopharmaceutical agents
Phenathiazine
Tricyclic antidepressants
(e.g. amitriptyline)
Monamine oxidase inhibitors
(e.g. Iproniazid)
Haloperidol
Diazepam

Antithyroid drugs
Methimazole
Carbimazole
Thiouracil

Oral hypoglycaemic agents
Chlorpropamide
Tolbutamide

Other Agents
Methyltestosterone
Anabolic steroids
Methyldopa
Oxyphenisatin
Intravenous nutrients
Clofibrate
Allopurinol
Oral contraceptives

Poisons
Aflatoxin
Senecio alkaloids
Hypoglycins (Ackee fruit)
Amanita mushrooms
Crotolaria
Lupinous
Heletropium
Carbon tetrachloride
Tetrachlorethane
Chlorophenithone (DDT)
Benzine derivatives
Trinitrotoluene
Tannic acid
Phosphorus
Iron
Beryllium
? Arsenic
Hypothermia
Burns
Irradiation

such as cholestasis, to focal hepatic necrosis, granuloma formation, fulminant hepatic failure, venoocclusive disease, Budd–Chiari syndrome, cirrhosis and tumour formation.

FULMINANT HEPATIC FAILURE

Fulminant hepatic failure is a complex syndrome in which severe impairment of hepatic function and encephalopathy develops within 8 weeks of the onset of liver disease. Only patients without evidence of previous liver disease are included in this definition. All organ systems are secondarily affected. Mortality in childhood is up to 70% (Psacharopoulos et al 1980).

Causes

The liver injury may be due to viral hepatitis type A, type B, non-A, non-B hepatitis, infectious mononucleosis, yellow fever, leptospirosis, mushroom poisoning, or hepatotoxicity from drugs. In the newborn period the disorder may arise from metabolic causes such as galactosaemia, fructosaemia, or tyrosinosis. Leukaemia and reticulosis may present in this fashion. The factors which determine the severity of the hepatic injury are not known.

The pathological changes in the liver are of widespread hepatocellular necrosis with little or no effective regeneration. The reticulin framework collapses giving an apparent preponderance of portal tracts. There is marked inflammatory cell infiltrate in the portal tracts and hepatic parenchyma. If the patient survives, the liver frequently returns to normal over the course of 1–2 years. There is no characteristic cerebral pathology except oedema. The mechanism of the encephalopathy is unknown but is presumed to be due to a combination of metabolic factors, including hypoglycaemia, raised blood ammonia, fatty acids, mercaptans, an increased ratio of straight chain to branch chain aminoacids and an increased insulin to glucagon ratio. Disturbances of neurotransmitter metabolism (Roberts 1984) may lead to abnormal sympathetic and parasympathetic outflows to the heart and vascular system. Neuroactive and vasoactive bacterial products absorbed from a leaky intestine and traversing a faulty liver are also likely to be involved in causing changes in cerebral bloodflow, total cerebral glucose and oxygen utilization.

Macrophages responding to exogenously derived peptidoglycans may also contribute. Many factors may aggravate or precipitate encephalopathy. These include sedatives, anaesthetics, potassium depletion, gastrointestinal haemorrhage, hypovolaemia, diuretics, infection, constipation, high protein intake, renal failure and hypoxia.

Clinical features

Rarely, hepatic encephalopathy may precede or coincide with the onset of jaundice. More commonly it develops in the patient with an established hepatitis. Increasing anorexia, vomiting, abdominal pain and a bleeding diathesis are important features of impending encephalopathy. The single most important sign is a decrease in liver size, the liver frequently becoming impalpable with a markedly reduced area of hepatic dullness on percussion. The respiratory rate may increase.

Encephalopathy frequently starts with lethargy, interspersed with periods of confused, uncontrollable, often competitive or fight behaviour. It may remain stable at this stage or progress to deeper neurological depression, decerebrate rigidity and brain death. Some patients may regress slowly, others pass to decerebrate rigidity and brain death within hours of the onset. Rarely, patients follow a subacute course, with persisting features of severe hepatic necrosis and encephalopathy lasting for months.

Laboratory investigations

The laboratory features which confirm a diagnosis of hepatic failure are a persistent prolongation of the prothrombin time, a raised blood ammonia and frequently hypoglycaemia. When the disorder has been present for some weeks the serum albumin falls. The blood urea and cholesterol are typically low. Standard biochemical tests of liver function are deranged but are usually within ten times the upper limit of normal.

Management

The basis of treatment is to maintain effective respiration, an adequate circulation and biochemical homeostasis while awaiting spontaneous hepatic regeneration and elemination of the cause of liver injury. Children with fulminant hepatic failure require intensive care, close monitoring of their cardiovascular, respiratory and central nervous system status, fluid and electrolyte balance and food intake. Temperature, pulse, blood pressure, central venous pressure, cardiac output and body weight must be monitored, together with frequent estimations of serum and urinary pH, osmolarity and electrolyte concentration. A regular full blood count and biochemical tests of liver function, particularly measurement of clotting factors, are essential. Direct measurement of intracranial pressure should allow more rational use of measures to decrease intracranial pressure, but unfortunately, problems with bleeding at the insertion site and unreliability of the monitoring system, limit its use. It is essential to consider, and if necessary exclude, other causes of coma, e.g. subdural haematomata. Sedatives must not be given.

The patients usually require intravenous fluids which should take the form of 5–15% dextrose at an initial rate of 60% of the normal requirement. Potassium requirements will be high, sodium requirements low. Cardiac, pulmonary and renal function is impaired so great care is required in trying to correct abnormalities of homeostasis, particularly acidosis, alkalosis, or electrolyte depletion. Infusion of fresh frozen plasma to provide clotting factors, complement, albumin, and fresh whole blood for anaemia are useful but must be given with close monitoring of the central venous pressure. Platelet transfusions may be required for severe thrombocytopoenia.

Intravenous cimetidine reduces the risk of alimentary bleeding. Absorption of 'toxins' from the gastrointestinal tract is minimized by the withdrawal of dietary protein, gastrointestinal cleansing with enemas and lactulose in a sufficient dose to produce loose stools. Neomycin given by nasogastric tube, may have an additional effect.

Control of intracranial pressures (See under Reyes syndrome). Peritoneal dialysis or haemodialysis may be necessary for renal failure.

A wide range of experimental procedures such as charcoal column haemoperfusion are currently being assessed in the management of this syndrome. It is advisable to contact a unit specializing in the care of fulminant hepatic failure as soon as the diagnosis is made for advice on general management and in particular, the indications for the use of such procedures.

REFERENCES

Allen U R, Bass B H 1963 Fatal hepatic necrosis in glandular fever. Journal of Clinical Pathology 16:337

Beasley R P, Hwang L H, Chin-Yun L G et al 1983 Prevention of perinatally transmitted Hepatitis B virus infection with Hepatitis B immunoglobulin & Hepatitis B vaccine, Lancet ii:1099

Bianchi L 1982 The immunopathology of Acute type B hepatitis. In: Thomas H C, Miescher P A, Mueller-Eberhard (eds) Immunological Aspects of Liver Disease. Springer Verlag, Berlin. p 141

Botha J F, Ritchie M J J, Dusheko J M et al 1984 Hepatitis B carrier state in black children in Ovamboland. Lancet ii:1210

Cadrobbi P, Bortolotti M, Zacchello Z et al 1985 Hepatics B virus replication in acute glomerulo-nephritis with chronic, aggressive hepatitis. Archives of Disease in Childhood 65:83

Capps R B, Bennett A M, Stokes J 1952 Epidemic hepatitis in Infants' Orphanage. Archives of Internal Medicine, 86:6

Christie A B 1980 Infectious mononucleosis, Infectious Diseases, 3rd Edition. Churchill Livingstone, Edinburgh. p 890

Clark J, Craig R M, Saffro R et al 1979 Cytomegalovirus in granulomatous hepatitis. American Journal of Medicine 66:264

Davidson R A 1984 Issues in Clinical Parasitology: The management of hydatid cyst. The American Journal of Gastroenterology 59:397

Davis M 1984 Drugs and hepatotoxicity. In: Williams R, Madre W C (eds) Gastroenterology 4 (Liver). Butterworths International Medical Reviews. Butterworth, London. p 133

Dienhardt F, Gust I D 1982 Viral hepatitis. Bulletin of the World Health Organization 60:661

Dienstag J L 1982 Immunopathogenesis of the extrahepatic manifestations of Hepatitis B virus infection. In: Thomas H C Miescher P A, Mueller-Eberhard H J (eds) Immunological Aspects of Liver Disease. Springer-Verlag, Berlin. p 181

Duermayer W, Van den Veen J 1978 Specific detection of IgM antibodies by ELISA, applied to Hepatitis A. Lancet ii:684

Feigin R D, Anderson D C 1975 Human Leptospirosis. Clinical Research Centre Reviews in Clinical and Laboratory Science 5:413

Francis T I, Moore E L, Addington G N, Smith J A 1972 Clinico-pathological study of human Yellow Fever. Bulletin of the World Health Organization 46:659

Gianotti 1973 Papular acrodermatitis of childhood. Archives of Disease in Childhood 48:794

Hadler S C, DeMonzon M, Ponzetto A et al 1984 Delta virus infection in severe hepatitis. Annals of Internal Medicine 100:339

Harries J T, Fergusson A W 1968 Fatal infectious mononucleosis with liver failure in two sisters. Archives of Disease in Childhood 43:480

Heubi J E, Daugherty C C, Partin J S et al 1984 Grade 1 Reye's Syndrome — Outcome and predictors of progression to deeper coma grades. New England Journal of Medicine 331:1539

Katzenstein D, Rickerson V, Braude A 1982 New concepts of amoebic liver abscess derived from hepatic imaging, sero-diagnosis and hepatic enzymes in 67 consecutive cases in San Diego. Medicine (Baltimore) 61:237

Kerr J A 1973 Liver pathology in Yellow Fever. Transactions of the Royal Society of Tropical Medicine & Hygiene 62:882

Kirkpatrick Z M 1966 Structural and functional abnormalities of the liver in infectious mononucleosis. Archives of Internal Medicine 117:47

Locasciulli A, Alberti A, Barbieri R et al 1983 Evidence of non-A, Non-B hepatitis in children with acute leukaemia and chronic liver disease. American Journal of Diseases of Children 137:354

McDonald H, Tobin J O H 1978 Congenital cytomegalovirus infection: A collaborative study on epidemiological, clinical and laboratory findings. Developmental Medicine & Child Neurology 20:471

Manson-Bahr B A C 1983 Leishmaniasis. In: Weatherall D J, Leddingham J A G, Warrell D A (eds) Oxford Textbook of Medicine. Oxford Medical Publications, Oxford. p 5412

Manzel J A, Schalm S W, Gast P et al 1984 Passive-active immunization in neonates of HBsAg positive carrier-mothers. British Medical Journal 288:513

Melnick J L 1982 Classification of Hepatitis A virus as Enterovirus Type 72 and Hepatitis B virus as Hepadenavirus Type 1. Intervirology 18:105

Mitchell G F. Premier R R, Garcia E G et al 1983 Hybridoma antibody-based competitive ELISA in *Schistosoma japonicum* infection. American Journal of Tropical Medicine & Hygiene 32:114

Mondelli M, Mieli-Vergani G, Albertti A et al 1982 Specificity of T lymphocyte cytotoxicity to autologous hepatocytes in chronic hepatitis B virus infection. Evidence that T cells are directed against HBV core antigen expressed on hepatocytes. Journal of Immunology 129:2773

Mowat A P 1983 Reye's Syndrome: 20 Years on. British Medical Journal 286:1999

Mowat A P 1984a Pediatric liver disease. Drugs and Poisons. In: Arias I M, Frankel M, Wilson J H P (eds) Liver Annual 4. Elsevier, Amsterdam. p 323

Mowat A P 1984b Hepatitis A, B, non-A, non-B and other forms of hepatitis. In: Arias I M, Frankel M, Wilson J H P (eds) Liver Annual 4. Elsevier, Amsterdam. p 330

Nash T E, Cheever A W, Ottesnen E A, Cook J A 1982 Schistosome infections in humans: Perspective in recent findings. Annals of Internal Medicine 97:740

Neuberger J, Davis M 1983 Immune mechanisms in drug-induced liver injury. In: Thomas H C, MacSween R N M (eds). Recent Advances in Hepatology, 1. Churchill Livingstone, Edinburgh. p. 89

Noble R C, Kay M A, Reeves S A et al 1984 Post-transfusion hepatitis A in a neonatal intensive care unit. Journal of the American Medical Association 252:2711

Oxford J S, Draser F A, Williams J D 1977 Chemotherapy of Herpes Simplex viral infection. Academic Press, New York.

Provost P J, Conti P A, Giesa P A et al 1983 Studies in Chimpanzees of liver attenuated hepatitis A vaccine candidates. Proceedings of Society of Experimental Biology & Medicine 172:357

Psacharopoulos H T, Mowat A P, Davis M et al 1980 Fulminant hepatic failure in childhood. An analysis of 31 cases. Archives of Disease in Childhood 55:252

Remington V, Desments G 1976 Toxoplasmosis. In: Remington J S, Klein J O (eds) Infectious Diseases of fetus and newborn infant. Saunders, Philadelphia.

Repsher L H, Freebern R B 1969 Effective exercise on recovery from infective hepatitis. New England Journal of Medicine 281:1393

Reshef R, Lok A S F, Sherlock S 1982 Cholestatic jaundice in Fascioliasis treated with Niclofolan. British Medical Journal 285:1243

Reye's Syndrome, United States 1984. Morbidity and mortality National Statistics Review (1985) 34:13

Rizzetto M, Canes M J, Arico S et al 1977 Immuno-fluorescent detection of a new antigen — antibody system associated to HBV in liver and serum of HBsAg carriers. Gut 18:997

Rizzetto M, Morello C, Mannucci, P M 1982 Delta infection and liver disease in haemophilic carriers of HBsAg. Journal of Infectious Diseases 145:18

Roberts E 1984 The gamma aminobutyric acid system and hepatic encephalopathy. Hepatology 4: 342

Schusterman H N, Frauenhoffer C, Kindy M D 1978 Fatal massive hepatic necrosis and cytomegalovirus mononucleosis. Annals of Internal Medicine 88:810

Shafritz E A, Schouval D, Sherman H I et al 1981 Integration of hepatitis B virus, DNA into genome of liver cells in chronic liver disease and hepatocellular carcinoma: Studies in percutaneous liver biopsies and post-mortem tissue specimens. New England Journal of Medicine 305:1067

Siegal G, Frosner J G 1978 Characterisation and classification of virus particles associated with Hepatitis A. Journal of Virology 26:40 (a) and 26:48(b)

Skellie J, Howard C R, Zuckerman A J 1981 Hepatitis B polypeptide vaccine preparation in micelle form. Nature (London) 290:51

Stenson W F, Eckert T, Avioli L A 1983 Pyogenic liver abscess. Archives of Internal Medicine 143:126

Stricker B H C H, Spoelstra P 1985 Drug-induced hepatic injury. Elsevier, Amsterdam.

Sullivan W G, Koep L J 1980 Common bile duct obstruction and cholangiohepatitis in Clonorchiasis. Journal of the American Medical Association 243:2060

Templeton A C 1970 Generalised Herpes simplex in mal-nourished children. Journal of Clinical Pathology 23:24

Tivari I, Roland C F, Popple A W 1982 Cholestatic jaundice due to toxoplasma hepatitis. Postgraduate Medical Journal 58:299

Verees E, Malik M O, Satir A E, El Hasson A M 1974 Morphological observation in Leishmaniasis. Journal of Tropical Medicine and Hygiene 73:63

Vergani D, Locasciulli A, Masera G et al 1982 Histological evidence of Hepatitis B virus infection with negative serology in children with acute leukaemia who develop chronic liver disease. Lancet i:361

Weller T H 1977 Cytomegaloviruses, ubiquitous agents with protein manifestations. New England Journal of Medicine 285: 203–267

Yoakum G H, Korba E B, Lechner J F et al 1983 High frequency transfection and cytopathology of Hepatitis B virus core antigen gene in human cells. Science 222:385

Yong V C W, Ipp H M V, Resnik H V et al 1984 Prevention of the Hepatitis B surface antigen carrier state in newborn infants of mothers who are chronic carriers of HBsAg and HBeAg by the administration of the Hepatitis B vaccine and Hepatitis B immunoglobulin. Lancet 8383:921

Zanetti A, Faroni P, Magliano E M et al 1982 Perinatal transmission of Hepatitis B virus of the HBV associated delta antigen from mothers to offspring in Northern Italy. Journal of Medical Virology 9:139

Zuckerman A J 1984 Viral Hepatitis. In: Arias I M, Wilson J H P (eds) Liver Annual, Vol. 4. Elsevier, Amsterdam.

Zuckerman A J, Simpson D I H 1979 Exotic virus infections of the liver. In: Popper H, Schaffner F (eds) Progress in Liver Diseases, Vol. 6. Grune & Stratton, New York. p. 45

Chronic liver disease

A variety of infectious, metabolic or immunological causes lead to chronic liver disease in children (Chandra 1979). Most chronic diseases of the liver manifest as either chronic hepatitis, or cirrhosis. Cirrhosis leads to portal hypertension. These general categories of disorders along with some important specific disorders will be considered in the following section.

CHRONIC HEPATITIS

Chronic hepatitis is defined as continuing liver inflammation beyond the expected period of recovery. Nonresolution of jaundice or relapsing jaundice occurring within 10–12 weeks of onset of an acute episode of hepatitis is cause for concern. All patients with chronic hepatitis do not have an identifiable preceding episode of acute hepatitis. Many patients may directly present with signs and symptoms of chronic liver inflammation. Chronic hepatitis is usually divided into two main categories: chronic persistent hepatitis and chronic active hepatitis.

Chronic persistent hepatitis

Chronic persistent hepatitis is a relatively benign condition with minimal or no signs and symptoms (Dietrichson 1975). Patients usually present with persistent elevation of liver transaminases following an acute episode of hepatitis. Others may present with nonspecific symptoms like fatigue, malaise, anorexia, and right upper quadrant discomfort. Abnormal liver enzymes found during screening laboratory studies may be the first clue in patients with vague symptoms. The liver is infrequently enlarged and jaundice or splenomegaly are rare.

Serum alanine transaminase (ALT) and aspartate transaminase (AST) levels are consistently raised up to 100–500 μM/l. An elevation of liver enzymes does not always coincide with symptomatic episodes. Serum bilirubin is normal or mildly elevated. Prothrombin time (PT), alkaline phosphatase, gamma glutamyltranspeptidase, total protein, albumin and globulin levels are usually within normal limits.

Diagnosis is made by percutaneous liver biopsy. Histology reveals a mononuclear infiltrate limited to the portal areas with no disruption of hepatic lobular architecture. Hepatocytes may vary in size but hepatic cords are well maintained. Cobblestone arrangements of hepatocytes may be seen from central to portal areas. Occasionally hepatocytes with ground-glass material in their cytoplasm are seen and this usually represents hepatitis B surface antigen (HBsAg).

If fibrosis is present it is minimal. It should be kept in mind that the above hepatic picture can be caused by different mechanisms including infection (e.g. hepatitis B virus (HBV)), metabolic abnormalities (e.g. Wilson's disease and alpha$_1$-antitrypsin deficiency), and drugs (e.g. isoniazid, oxyphenisatin). Some of these conditions may be distinguished from others by their characteristic biopsy appearance (e.g. periodic acid Schiff acid (PAS) positive cytoplasmic deposits in alpha$_1$-antitrypsin deficiency, and orcein-staining ground-glass cytoplasmic material in HBV infection). This biopsy appearance can also be seen in the quiescent phase of chronic active hepatitis. Lymphoreticular malignancies may also give a similar appearance.

In general, no treatment is required as the condition is self-limited and the prognosis is excellent (Becker et al 1970). Patients should be regularly followed up until liver function returns to normal. No restriction of activity or nutrition is recommended. Episodes of malaise or fatigue usually remit spontaneously.

Prognosis is less good in patients with persistent HBsAg in serum. Studies in adults have shown that these patients can progress to chronic active hepatitis and even cirrhosis but little information is available as yet in children. No effective treatment is available for patients with hepatitis B-induced chronic hepatitis. Steroids or immunosuppressive drugs are definitely contraindicated.

Chronic active hepatitis

Chronic active hepatitis is a serious disorder which often results in permanent liver damage and cirrhosis. Though seen in all age-groups, it occurs more commonly in adolescents and young adults (50% of patients being between 11–30 years of age) and is one of the commonest causes of chronic liver disease in children. Contrary to the situation in adults, where most cases of chronic active hepatitis are due to HBV, chronic active hepatitis in children is usually HBV negative. The pathophysiology, prognosis and treatment of HBV positive is very different from HBV negative chronic active hepatitis.

Different names have been used to describe HBV negative chronic active hepatitis, including lupoid hepatitis, plasma cell hepatitis, active juvenile cirrhosis, and subacute hepatic necrosis. The cause has not been clearly established and it seems likely that the same clinical syndrome can be produced by a number of different insults to the liver. The final common pathway of liver injury seems to be autoimmune damage to the liver. Presence of mutiple autoantibodies in the serum, autoimmune damage to other organ systems including thyroid, kidney, small intestine and colon, and an excellent response to glucocorticoids and immunosuppressive agents give credence to this hypothesis. Drugs, including oxyphenisatin, alpha methyldopa, and isoniazid, are well documented causes of chronic active hepatitis. Other rarer causes are inflammatory bowel disease, Wilson's disease and alpha$_1$-antitrypsin deficiency.

Various immunoregulatory abnormalities have been found in patients with chronic active hepatitis. A defect in 'suppressor' T-lymphocytes, which could presumably lead to formation of autoantibodies has been reported. Antibodies against membrane lipoproteins, other liver antigens and a variety of other autoantibodies (see below) have been found in serum of patients with chronic active hepatitis.

Symptoms vary from chronic malaise, anorexia and fatigue to full-blown episodes of acute hepatitis. Over half the children present with acute onset jaundice. It may be difficult, in these patients, to distinguish chronic active hepatitis from acute hepatitis on clinical and laboratory data alone. Persistent jaundice is a feature in a majority of patients. Teenagers may have hirsutism, acne, or obesity. Autoimmune inflammation of other organs can produce arthralgias, haemolytic anaemia, thyroiditis, glomerulonephritis, pleuritis, enteropathy and inflammatory bowel disease. A history of easy bruising, bleeding, haematuria and purpura may be obtained.

On examination, hepatosplenomegaly is seen in up to 80% of patients. Other findings include jaundice, palmar erythema, spider naevi and skin rash. A few patients may appear clinically well, while some may present with evidence of advanced liver dysfunction in the form of ascites and cachexia.

Elevated serum bilirubin (around 8–10 mg/dl) and increased serum transaminases (usually around 500 μ/l but up to 1500 μ/l are almost always present. The other striking finding is the presence of a multitude of autoimmune antibodies. Antinuclear antibody (ANA) is positive in 50–75%, and anti dsDNA (deoxyribonucleic acid) is present in 42%. Rheumatoid factor is often positive. Antibodies against smooth muscle, mitochondria, gastric mucosa, thyroid, kidney and intestine are often found. Coombs positive haemolytic anaemia and lupus erythematosus (LE) cell phenomenon is seen in about 15%. An antibody against hepatic and renal microsomes has been detected in some patients. Nonspecific findings include elevation of serum gamma globulin components (especially IgG), hypoalbuminaemia, elevated prothrombin time, and other clotting abnormalities. Normocytic normochromic anaemia, thrombocytopaenia and neutropaenia may be present secondary to hypersplenism. A few patients have elevated serum cortisol levels.

Liver biopsy is required for confirmation of the diagnosis. The biopsy should be adequate in length as the hepatic damage varies from lobule to lobule (Soloway et al 1971). Hepatocellular necrosis is patchy and necrotic areas may be present adjacent to relatively healthy ones. Hepatocytes with multiple nuclei and many mitotic figures may be seen and these represent regenerating liver cells. The most striking biopsy finding is the destruction of lobular architecture. Mononuclear cell infiltrate extends beyond the portal tracts, causing destruction of the limiting plate. Lymphocytes, plasma cells and macrophages constitute most of the infiltrate. 'Piecemeal necrosis' occurs due to extension of the inflammatory cells from the portal tracts into the hepatic parenchyma. Hepatocytes assume pseudoductular or pseudoacinar arrangement. Mononuclear cells may aggregate to form lymphoid follicles. Hepatic necrosis activates fibroblasts. Fibrous strands extend into the hepatic lobule causing disruption of the sinusoidal pattern and formation of intralobular septa. The degree of fibrosis depends on the rate of collagen deposition versus collagen catabolism. When necrosis is extensive, collapse of entire lobules may be seen. Inflammatory cells along with necrotic hepatocytes may then connect portal tracts with adjacent portal tracts or with centrilobular veins. 'Bridging necrosis' and multilobular involvement are considered to be harbingers of eventual cirrhosis. If nodular regeneration surrounded by fibrous septae is seen, cirrhosis is already present and a diagnosis of chronic active hepatitis cannot be made.

Every child with an acute episode of jaundice should be fully investigated for chronic active hepatitis. Baseline screening tests should include anti-nuclear antibody, alpha$_1$-antitrypsin levels, serum albumin and gamma globulin levels. Studies should also be done to rule out Wilson's disease. Persistence of jaundice for more than 4–6 weeks should alert the physician to the possibility of chronicity and a liver biopsy should be done to clarify diagnosis. Chronic active hepatitis should also be considered in patients with extrahepatic symptoms like arthralgias, recurrent erythema nodosum, secondary amenorrhoea and clotting abnormalities.

Steroid treatment should be initiated as soon as the diagnosis is confirmed. The dose given to induce remission is 2 mg/kg/24 h of predni-sone or prednisolone, up to a maximum of 60 mg/day. The starting dose of prednisone is continued until remission is obtained or until side effects develop (e.g. obesity, growth retardation, osteoporosis etc). Monthly trans-aminase levels are carried out and if liver enzymes return to normal a follow up liver biopsy should be obtained. The dose of prednisone is tapered off if histology returns to normal or shows chronic persistent hepatitis. Alternatively the prednisone dose is tapered as soon as evidence of a biochemical and clinical response is obtained and without waiting for normalization of liver histology. The dose is reduced by 10 mg every week till a maintenance dose of 20 mg is reached. If the patient stops improving, the dose is increased by 10 mg for the next two weeks. Alternate day steroids may be used once biochemical remission has been achieved (Arasu et al 1979). Azathioprine has been used along with prednisone in an attempt to improve response rates. It is generally added if no response to prednisone is obtained after three months of therapy. The question of maintenance therapy is controversial.

A recent study has emphasized the importance of prompt therapy in preventing permanent sequelae (Vegnente et al 1984). Patients who were started on steroids within a month of diagnosis, had a much lower incidence of subsequent cirrhosis as compared to those who received treatment after waiting for six months. If a liver biopsy is contraindicated because of abnormal clotting time, steroid treatment should be begun without waiting for the biopsy.

Almost all patients with HBV negative chronic active hepatitis respond to prednisone. A reappraisal of the diagnosis should be made in patients who fail to respond. Once therapy is stopped, up to half the patients have a clinical or biochemical relapse (Hegarty et al 1983) but most will again respond to steroid therapy. Stable remissions are likely in patients who can be taken off medication within a period of two years of starting therapy. Over 70% of patients achieved stable remissions on prednisone or prednisone plus azathioprine (Czaja et al 1981). The histological lesion may change from chronic active to chronic persistent hepatitis or return to normal in 18–20% of patients. There is definite prolongation of life in patients treated with corticosteroids with a five-year survival in treated patients of approximately 70%.

Persistence of jaundice and recurrences are commonly seen in untreated patients. Patients who fail to maintain sustained remission continue to have smouldering liver disease (Czaja 1981) which often progresses to cirrhosis. Hepatic necrosis or cirrhosis on initial liver biopsy suggest a poor outcome. Recurrences may be precipitated by intercurrent infections or may develop insidiously. Up to one third of all patients progress to cirrhosis with development of ascites, portal hypertension, oesophageal varices and bleeding. Ultimately hepatocellular failure develops with spider angiomata, telangiectasias and encephalopathy.

Chronic active hepatitis B

Chronic active hepatitis due to HBV is quite common in children from countries where hepatitis B is endemic. In countries like Taiwan, there is a very high rate of transmission of HBV from mothers to infants (Tong et al 1981). The transmission occurs by ingestion of amniotic fluid, vaginal secretions, and placental or maternal blood by the fetus. It was initially believed that acquisition of HBV by the neonate did not commonly cause chronic hepatitis but it has now been shown that severe chronic liver disease can occur fairly frequently in infants who are HBsAg positive (Maggiore et al 1983). Most infants who acquire chronic HBV infection in the perinatal period develop biochemical and histological characteristics of chronic persistent hepatitis. In time, some of them may progress to chronic active hepatitis, and develop hepatocellular insufficiency and cirrhosis. The progression to cirrhosis may occur rapidly, and cases in which cirrhosis occurred within a year of birth have been described (Estada & Espinosa 1980, Shinozaki et al 1981). Chronic active hepatitis has also been described in patients who were presumably infected with the non-A non-B hepatitis virus (Knodell et al 1977, Rakela & Reedeker 1979).

Patients may also present soon after an episode of acute viral hepatitis. Some give a history of viral hepatitis months to years before development of chronic hepatitis but in other patients no history of hepatitis can be obtained and it is presumed that, in these patients, the initial infection was subclinical. Symptoms are similar to those seen in HBV negative chronic active hepatitis with jaundice, anorexia, malaise or loss of weight being common presenting features. Extrahepatic syndromes which include arthritis and arthralgias, skin lesions, glomerulonephritis and cryoglobulinaemia can be seen with HBV positive chronic active hepatitis. A significant proportion of patients are asymptomatic and are discovered during routine screening. This is especially true for neonates, who acquire the virus soon after birth. Physical examination reveals jaundice, hepatomegaly, splenomegaly, ascites and other stigmata of liver failure.

Laboratory tests show hyperbilirubinaemia and elevated liver enzymes and HBsAg is positive in almost all cases. Autoimmune antibodies are not found in serum of these patients. Other laboratory findings include an elevated alpha-fetoprotein, polyclonal hypergammaglobulinaemia, and anaemia.

Histological findings are similar to those seen in HBV negative chronic active hepatitis. The cytoplasm may have a ground-glass appearance. This represents HBV and stains positively with orcein (Hadziyannis et al 1973). Liver biopsy may be the only way of making a diagnosis in infants, who may otherwise be asymptomatic.

Recent trials have confirmed that administration of hepatitis B vaccine and hepatitis B globulin to neonates immediately after birth significantly protect against the development of a persistent HBsAg carrier state (Wong et al 1984). Besides prophylaxis against infection, there is no treatment available for HBV-induced chronic active hepatitis. Steroids and immunosuppressive agents are definitely contraindicated as they cause biochemical deterioration and are assoicated with a worse outcome (Lam et al 1981). Immunosuppressive therapy inhibits formation of antibodies against viral antigens and in one study, patients receiving steroids did not synthesize anti-HBeAg as opposed to untreated patients (Trevisan et al 1982). Formation of anti-HBeAg has been associated with a more favourable outcome (Realdi et al 1980, Centers for Disease Control 1984).

WILSON'S DISEASE

Wilson's disease, an inherited defect of copper metabolism, should always be considered in any child with chronic liver disease or cirrhosis. It is especially important that this condition be suspected and looked for in children with compatible liver abnormalities, as an early diagnosis is useful not only in the treatment of the patients but also in detection and treatment of asymptomatic siblings. Wilson's disease is commonly diagnosed during childhood as more than half the patients have symptoms early in the course of their illness.

Wilson's disease is transmitted in an autosomal recessive fashion, with a disease incidence of 5–30 per million and a prevalence rate of carriers of around 1:200 to 1:500. The precise defect in copper metabolism has not been identified. There is an increased hepatic content of copper, which is mainly intralysosomal, with decreased copper excretion in bile (Gibbs & Walshe 1980). Hence a defect in hepatic transport of copper is postulated. There is an increase in hepatic copper content early in the disease but once liver stores are saturated, necrosis of hepatic tissue occurs with release of copper in the serum. Subsequently, deposition of copper occurs in the brain, kidney, bone, lens and endocrine glands, especially the parathyroid (Carpenter et al 1983), leading to malfunctioning of these organs.

In children, the disease manifests with nonspecific symptoms of chronic liver disease. It may occasionally present as acute hepatitis and may lead to fulminant hepatic necrosis. Haemolytic anaemia is frequently seen. Acute intravascular haemolysis, due to sudden release of copper, may occur in patients who develop acute liver failure (Roche-Sicot & Benhamou 1977). Renal tubular defects causing glycosuria, aminoaciduria, hypercalcuria and hypophosphaturia may be present, which may lead to osteomalacia and rickets. Older patients may initially be identified by neurological symptoms including tremor, deterioration of handwriting and clumsiness. There can be rapid neurological deterioration with spastic dystonia, chorea, difficulty in speech, ataxia and dysphagia. Psychiatric manifestations like bizarre behaviour, psychosis or hysteria can be prominent. The sensory system is usually unaffected.

Many patients are fortuitously diagnosed by the detection of a Kayser–Fleischer ring during a routine ophthalmological examination. This ring is a golden brown discoloration of Descemet's membrane in the limbic region of the cornea. Kayser–Fleischer rings are not present in all patients and their absence does not therefore rule out Wilson's disease. These rings can also be seen in chronic active hepatitis with cirrhosis, cryptogenic cirrhosis, and primary biliary cirrhosis (Frommer et al 1977). In most other patients, a strong index of suspicion is needed to identify the disease, as it cannot be diagnosed by routine laboratory tests which only show mild elevation of liver enzymes, and an abnormal bromosulphothalein excretion.

Specific tests include serum ceruloplasmin and copper, urinary copper excretion with and without penicillamine, radiolabelled copper tests and the hepatic copper content. Serum ceruloplasmin, is usually low or absent. This test may be less reliable in children where only 70% were reported to have low serum ceruloplasmin (<20 mg/dl) versus 95% of adult patients. Low ceruloplasmin levels can be seen in other liver diseases (e.g. chronic active hepatitis) or in conditions associated with low plasma proteins (e.g. nephrotic syndrome and kwashiorkor). Serum copper levels may be high, normal or low depending on the stage of the disease. There is an increase in the easily dissociable albumin-bound copper. Urinary copper excretion is increased to greater than 0.75 μmol/24 h with most patients having values greater than 1.5 μmol/24 h. In patients with normal urine copper excretion, administration of 500 mg D-penicillamine increases urine copper excretion to 9–11 μmol in the next 6 hours. Sometimes it may be difficult to differentiate Wilson's disease with normal serum ceruloplasmin from chronic active hepatitis with elevated hepatic copper content (LaRusso et al 1976) and a radiolabelled copper excretion test should be used in such patients (Sternlieb & Scheinberg 1979). After administration of an oral dose of copper in normal subjects there is an initial rise in plasma radioactivity which declines in one to two hours as the radioactive copper is cleared by the liver. There is, subsequently, a secondary rise in plasma radioactivity over the next 48 hours, as ceruloplasmin containing radiolabelled copper reappears in the blood. In patients with Wilson's disease, this secondary rise does not occur, as they are unable to incorporate the administered radiolabelled copper into ceruloplasmin for release into the blood stream. Measurement of copper content per gram of dry liver tissue is useful for confirming the diagnosis. Hepatic copper content is greater than 250 μg per gram liver tissue in most patients whereas a normal hepatic copper content in an untreated patient rules out Wilson's disease.

Early liver pathology shows slight pleomorphism of hepatocytes with glycogen accumulation in the nuclei of periportal hepatocytes (Stromeyer & Ishak 1980). Fatty metamorphosis, vacuolated nuclei and focal necrosis are seen. Mallory's hyaline, if present, indicates the acute form of Wilson's disease. Some specimens show a picture similar to chronic active hepatitis, with periportal inflammatory cell infiltrates and piecemeal necrosis. When cirrhosis develops, the pattern is either macronodular or mixed micro-macronodular. Most liver specimens can be shown, by copper stains, to contain excessive deposition of copper. Histochemical staining for copper and orcein staining of copper-associated protein may however be normal in some patients despite an increased hepatic copper content (Jain et al 1978).

The management of Wilson's disease is based on lowering tissue copper by administration of chelating agents. D-penicillamine is the drug of choice

(Deiss et al 1971). It chelates copper and markedly enhances excretion of copper in the urine. To prevent rapid mobilization of tissue copper stores, which can precipitate acute haemolysis, therapy is started at a dose of 250 mg/day and this is increased by 250 mg per week till a final dose of 1000–1500 mg is achieved. Side effects include proteinuria with nephrotic syndrome, bone marrow suppression, lupus-like syndrome, cheilosis, glossitis and skin rash. Pyridoxine supplements should be given to prevent neuropathy. On regular penicillamine therapy, tissue copper stores diminish, liver function tests return to normal, the Kayser–Fleischer rings disappear, and neurological status improves. Hepatic transplantation, if successful, is curative. With a new liver, the defect in copper metabolism disappears. There is increased excretion of copper in the urine and tissue copper levels fall to normal.

If untreated the disease is fatal. Prognosis is good for patients who are detected and treated before the onset of symptoms. For patients without extensive liver necrosis and cirrhosis, reversal of the hepatic damage can be expected on therapy. Once cirrhosis with ascites and portal hypertension develops, the outlook is poor with most patients dying within one to two years.

ALPHA$_1$-ANTITRYPSIN DEFICIENCY

Alpha$_1$-antitrypsin, as its name suggests, is an alpha$_1$ globulin present in serum, which inactivates serine proteases. It has two alleles which are inherited in a codominant fashion. A normal person has two M alleles, while two Z alleles lead to alpha$_1$-antitrypsin deficiency. Between 1:1700 to 1:5000 people in the general population have the ZZ phenotype and have alpha$_1$-antitrypsin deficiency.

The unpredictability of the clinical associations of the ZZ phenotype and paucity of follow-up data makes genetic counselling difficult at this time. The development of safe, intrauterine fetal blood sampling at 17–18 weeks gestation permits the identification of the protease inhibitor phenotype sufficiently early to allow termination of pregnancy (Kidd et al 1984). At the present time, analysis of the outcome of liver disease in 47 families with more than one affected child suggests that if the first born child has unresolved or fatal liver disease there is a 75% chance that a further affected child in that family will have similar liver disease (Psacharopoulos et al 1983). After careful counselling, termination of pregnancy must be carefully considered for such a family if it is shown the infant has the ZZ phenotype.

Liver disease in alpha$_1$-antitrypsin deficiency was first reported by Sharp et al (1969). Since then, it has been recognized that liver disease is a frequent result of this deficiency and between 5–25% of all paediatric liver disease may result from alpha$_1$-antitrypsin deficiency.

The earliest manifestation of liver disease is prolonged neonatal cholestasis. It may persist for as long as six months. Other nonspecific symptoms include irritability, lethargy and failure to thrive. In older children, cirrhosis may develop with signs of portal hypertension. On palpation, firm hepatomegaly with a smooth margin is felt. The spleen may be palpable. Laboratory tests at this stage show nonspecific changes of biliary obstruction including conjugated hyperbilirubinaemia, raised alkaline phosphatase and hypercholesterolaemia. In most patients, the jaundice resolves spontaneously. Persistent jaundice is difficult to distinguish on clinical grounds alone from that due to extrahepatic biliary atresia and many patients have been subjected to exploratory laparotomy to make the diagnosis.

Alpha$_1$-antitrypsin levels should be measured in all children with liver disease. Homozygotes have levels below 100 mg/dl and heterozygotes between 100–200 mg/dl (normal 200–300 mg/dl). A decreased alpha$_1$ globulin peak on serum electrophoresis should alert the physician about the possibility of alpha$_1$-antitrypsin deficiency. Protease-inhibitor typing can be done by special techniques.

On liver biopsy, eosinophilic cytoplasmic granules are seen in the hepatocytes which stain strongly with periodic acid Schiff (PAS) but are not hydrolysed by diastase. These have been shown to consist of aggregation of alpha$_1$-antitrypsin protein in smooth endoplasmic reticulum. There appears to be some abnormality of the alpha$_1$-antitrypsin molecule which prevents it from being secreted in the usual fashion. In neonates, disorganization of the hepatic cords with formation of giant cells, and pseudoacini may be seen. Intracellular cholestatsis is also commonly seen. Some portal inflammation may be present. Early portal fibrosis, neoductular proliferation, or a paucity of interlobular bile ducts are associated with a higher incidence of cirrhosis. In older children, features of postnecrotic cirrhosis may be seen.

There is no specific treatment. Portal hypertension can be treated by surgical shunts. Patients who have undergone orthotopic liver transplantation, have recovered normal serum alpha$_1$-antitrypsin levels with a normal phenotype.

Prognosis varies from individual to individual. In a recent study of 74 children under the age of 17 years with chronic liver disease due to alpha$_1$-antitrypsin deficiency, 20 had died, 20 had established cirrhosis, 19 had persistent liver disease and 15 had made a complete recovery (Psacharopoulous et al 1983).

INDIAN CHILDHOOD CIRRHOSIS

Indian childhood cirrhosis is a relentlessly progressive disease of the liver which is almost exclusively found in children from the Indian subcontinent and which leads to hepatic cirrhosis and death (Chandra 1982). A few cases have recently been reported in American children (Lefkowitch et al 1982). The aetiology is not known, though infectious, toxic, metabolic, and

nutritional causes have been proposed. In view of the strikingly high concentrations of hepatic copper in this condition, it is likely that an inheritable
defect in copper metabolism has some role to play in its pathogenesis. The
disease is familial with an increased incidence of parental consaguinity in
affected families but the inheritance has not been formally defined.

The disease typically affects children aged 8 months to 4 years, though
cases as old as ten years have been reported. Onset in a majority of the
children is insidious with abdominal distension and malaise, followed by
fever and jaundice (Bhave et al 1982). Some may give a history of an acute
episode of jaundice before the development of these symptoms. Less
commonly, young patients may present with acute onset of rapidly
progressive abdominal distension, fever and jaundice.

All children have firm hepatomegaly and almost all have an associated
splenomegaly. Ascites and jaundice are present on admission in over half the
patients. Laboratory investigations are not usually helpful in distinguishing
Indian childhood cirrhosis from other hepatic disorders. There is
hyperbilirubinaemia with mild to moderate elevation of liver enzymes,
hypoalbuminaemia and elevated prothrombin time and other nonspecific
indicators of hepatocellular dysfunction. Anaemia is frequently seen and is
associated with a poor prognosis. Greatly elevated levels of serum alpha-
fetoprotein are found and serum copper and ceruloplasmin levels are
elevated. Renal tubular defects causing aminoaciduria and glucosuria may
be found. Many nonspecific immunological abnormalities have been
described (Chandra 1979) including elevation of serum immunoglobulins,
circulating immune complexes, and low levels of complement C3.

Liver biopsy is diagnostic with a pattern of 'micro-micronodular
cirrhosis' (Nayak 1979). There is widespread ballooning and necrosis of
hepatocytes, which are surrounded by a fine creeping fibrosis. Mallory's
hyaline may be present. Ultrastructurally, this material is made up of a
tangled mass of fibrils and electron-dense particles. Fibrosis and oedema
of central veins is seen, but in contrast to Wilson's disease, no fatty infiltration occurs.

The hepatic copper concentration is very high (ranging from 0.7–6 mg/g
dry liver) in most children with Indian childhood cirrhosis. There are
deposits of orcein staining copper-binding protein in liver biopsy specimens
(Portmann et al 1978). Rhodamine staining reveals copper deposition in
hepatocytes. It has been proposed that in Indian childhood cirrhosis high
levels of intracytoplasmic copper damage microtubules, which leads to
accumulation of synthesized proteins in the cytoplasm, ballooning of hepatocytes and formation of Mallory's bodies.

Treatment is supportive. No special form of therapeutic intervention has
been shown to be of benefit. Attempts to treat the condition with D-
penicillamine have been unsuccessful. The disease is almost uniformly fatal
within a few weeks to a year after diagnosis (Nayak & Ramalingaswamy
1975).

LIVER INVOLVEMENT IN CYSTIC FIBROSIS

Involvement of the liver and the biliary tract is commonly seen in patients with cystic fibrosis. The incidence varies from 20–40%, though figures as high as 90% have been reported (Isenberg & L'Heureuse 1976). With the increase in life expectancy of children with cystic fibrosis, more patients are now being seen with hepatic complications. Viscid biliary secretions are inspissated in biliary canaliculi, ultimately leading to biliary cirrhosis. With the exception of prolonged jaundice in the perinatal period, there may be very few signs and symptoms of liver involvement. Later in life, cirrhosis with jaundice, portal hypertension and ascites develop.

In a large series of patients (Psacharopoulos et al 1981), cirrhosis was the commonest liver complication seen. A few children had neonatal hepatitis or chronic active hepatitis. Splenomegaly was common and occasionally led to hypersplenism. Splenic pain was a major problem in two patients. Variceal bleeding occurred in 6 out of 74 patients, and was controlled by injection sclerotherapy.

Liver function tests are usually normal during the asymptomatic stage of liver involvement. Elevation of alkaline phosphatase or gamma glutamyl transpeptidase in a patient with cystic fibrosis should alert the physician to the possibility of underlying liver disease. Thrombocytopaenia, leukopenia and anaemia are signs of hypersplenism.

Fatty infiltration is the commonest histological change seen in infants (Silverman & Roy 1983). In older children intrahepatic and canalicular cholestasis, along with neoductular proliferation and fibrosis, are present. Focal biliary cirrhosis, with fibrosis and nodular regeneration, appear later. Finding of excess biliary mucus in intralobular bile ducts, suggests cystic fibrosis as the cause of biliary cirrhosis. Abnormal collection of haemosiderin and ceroid pigment may be found in hepatocytes.

Management is supportive. If oesophageal varices and bleeding develop the prognosis becomes grave. Sclerotherapy should be used in the first instance to control bleeding. Splenorenal or mesocaval shunt with splenectomy can be undertaken in an effort to decompress the portal system, but the results are not gratifying (Stern et al 1976). Many of these patients develop deterioration of pulmonary function. Surgery itself is made difficult by the presence of retroperitoneal fibrosis and oedema. Elective shunting has been attempted in a few children with good liver function after the first episode of variceal bleeding. All these measures however just delay the inevitable fatal outcome of the disease.

CONGENITAL HEPATIC FIBROSIS

This is a rare disease characterized by the presence of fibrous tissue in the portal and periportal veins (Alvarez et al 1981). The aetiology is unknown, but biliary dysplasia is assumed to play some role in its pathogenesis

(Alagille & Odievre 1979a). It is inherited in an autosomal recessive fashion. Many renal anomalies are associated with this condition including the infantile form of polycystic kidney disease (Anand et al 1975).

Clinically, patients have firm hepatomegaly with a smooth surface. Splenomegaly is often seen and may cause hypersplenism, with anaemia and thrombocytopenia. Many patients develop portal hypertension and its associated symptoms. The exact cause for the development of portal hypertension is not clear, but the block to blood flow is perisinusoidal. There are no signs of liver insufficiency or jaundice. Other patients may have repeated cholangitis with fever and severe right upper quadrant pain. If the infection is severe, septicaemia with shock may occur.

Laboratory investigations show normal bilirubin and transaminase activities but bromsulphalein (BSP) excretion time is prolonged and alkaline phosphatase is elevated. Anaemia, thrombocytopenia and leukopenia are manifestations of hypersplenism. A decreased urine specific gravity may be the only sign of renal involvement. Raised blood urea and creatinine are sometimes seen.

Splenoportography reveals abnormalities in the intrahepatic portal system with duplication of many veins. Oral or intravenous cholecystography or ultrasound reveals abnormally dilated biliary ducts. An intravenous pyelogram shows enlarged kidneys with opacities in the medulla radiating to the cortex. Other signs of precalyceal tubular ectasia include stretched and distorted cavities, and elongation of the calices.

Liver biopsy confirms the diagnosis. Open liver biopsy is desirable as the disease is not uniform throughout the liver. Pathologically, there is diffuse portal fibrosis, but the hepatic lobule is not invaded. The limiting plate is intact and the hepatic lobular architecture is preserved. The individual hepatic lobules may be greatly compressed. Numerous ectatic or dilated bile ducts, lined by cuboidal or columnar epithelium, are present in the fibrotic areas. Their lumen is empty. There is no inflammatory response and there are no regenerative nodules.

A splenorenal or a mesocaval shunt is performed after the first episode of variceal haemorrhage. The prognosis is excellent and patients do not develop hepatic decompensation after surgery. Some have advocated prophylactic shunts in these patients, even before gastrointestinal bleeding is seen. Eventually renal failure from associated kidney disease may develop in up to one quarter of all patients.

CIRRHOSIS

Cirrhosis represents ongoing fibrosis of liver surrounding regenerating nodules of hepatocytes. It results in portosystemic shunting of blood and thus causes decreased perfusion of hepatocytes.

Chronic diseases of the liver in children usually progress on to cirrhosis which can be classified according to the underlying pathogenetic mechanism into biliary cirrhosis or postnecrotic cirrhosis. Biliary cirrhosis accounts for more than half of all cases of childhood cirrhosis, largely as a result of extrahepatic biliary atresia. Conditions frequently leading to postnecrotic cirrhosis include alpha₁-antitrypsin deficiency, Wilson's disease, and chronic active hepatitis. A more complete list of the causes of cirrhosis in childhood can be found in Table 21.1. In a significant proportion of

Table 21.1   Causes of cirrhosis in children

Biliary cirrhosis
    Extrahepatic biliary atresia
    Bile duct stenosis and strictures
    Dilation of bile ducts
        Choledocal cyst
        Dilatation of intrahepatic bile ducts
        Caroli's disease
    Paucity of intrahepatic bile ducts
        Alagille's syndrome
        Zellweger's syndrome
    Byler's disease
    Ascending cholangitis
    Ulcerative colitis
    Cystic fibrosis*
    Extrinsic compression by tumors, etc

Postnecrotic cirrhosis
    Viral Hepatitis
        Hepatitis B virus*
        Hepatitis A virus (rare)
        Non-A non-B virus
    Chronic active hepatitis*
    Neonatal hepatitis
    Drugs
        Phenytoin
        Chlordiazepoxide
        Imipramine
    Congestive
        Budd–Chiari syndrome*
        Constrictive pericarditis
        Ebstein's anomaly
    Metabolic
        Wilson's disease*
        Alpha₁-antitrypsin deficiency*
        Galactosaemia
        Glycogen storage disease type IV
        Gaucher's disease
        Niemann–Pick disease
        Osler–Weber–Rendu syndrome
        Haemachromatosis
        Wolman's disease
    Indian Childhood cirrhosis*
    Jamaican Veno-occlusive disease*
    Haemangioendothelioma
    Kwashiorkor
    Radiation

*Discussed in the text

patients, no cause may be discovered but attempts should be made in every case to find the cause, as prompt treatment of underlying disorders may prevent further liver damage.

The primary defect in biliary cirrhosis is an obstruction to the flow of bile, leading to biliary stasis. This results in neoductular proliferation which stimulates periportal and perilobular fibrosis. Initially there is no direct damage to hepatocytes, but distortion of hepatic architecture ultimately results in hepatocellular damage. Hepatocellular injury further activates collagen synthesis and fibrosis. In postnecrotic cirrhosis, on the other hand, injury to the hepatocyte, whether due to an infectious agent, a toxin or some metabolic abnormality, is the initial event. Hepatocellular damage causes stimulation of fibroblasts which lay down collagen, thus causing fibrosis. Fibrous septae form around regenerating hepatocytes, giving rise to characteristic cirrhotic nodules. In cirrhosis due to passive venous congestion, fibrous septae bridging central veins to portal veins may be seen. Alternative channels for blood flow develop in these fibrous septae, depriving hepatocytes of their normal blood supply and this leads to further hepatocellular damage and local hypoxia, resulting in additional fibrosis. The liver ultimately becomes hard and nodular. Distortion of hepatic architecture results in increased resistance to blood flow through the liver, causing portal hypertension and development of portosystemic collaterals.

Biliary cirrhosis

Jaundice is almost always present in biliary cirrhosis due to an extrahepatic biliary atresia, choledochal cyst or stricture of the bile duct. A history of pruritis, dark-coloured urine and light-coloured stools can be elicited. In biliary cirrhosis due to Byler's disease or paucity of intrahepatic bile ducts, jaundice may be minimal or absent. In cystic fibrosis, presence of jaundice indicates advanced cirrhosis. Excoriations and xanthomas may be seen on the skin. Digital clubbing is frequently seen and nail beds may be cyanosed.

If splenomegaly with hypersplenism is present, purpura, petechiae or ecchymoses may be present. The liver may be enlarged, normal in size or shrunken. If palpable, it is firm to hard in consistency with an irregular margin. Cirrhotic nodules can sometimes be palpated. The spleen is generally enlarged in patients with portal hypertension. Ascites occurs earlier in patients with biliary cirrhosis and the abdomen is usually distended, either because of hepatosplenomegaly or ascites.

Laboratory investigations reveal a conjugated or mixed hyperbilirubinaemia, increased alkaline phosphatase, elevated serum bile acids, hypercholesterolaemia and hyperlipaemia. Serum 5'-nucleotidase and gamma glutamyltranspeptidase activities are elevated. The BSP retention test is abnormal which is consistent with obstruction of bile flow. Hypoalbuminaemia can give rise to falsely low BSP retention times and correction should be made for low serum albumin when analysing BSP retention studies. Elevated serum bile acids have been linked to pruritis.

Radiological examination, can be of considerable benefit in determining the site of an anatomical abnormality. Ultrasonography can detect minimal amounts of ascitic fluid and is useful in detecting dilated intra or extrahepatic bile ducts and abnormalities of the portal vein. Computerized tomography not only provides similar information, but can also visualize hepatic nodules. Radionuclide scans, using HIDA or DISIDA may be useful in the evaluation of bile ducts even in patients with significant jaundice. Percutaneous transhepatic cholangiography can be performed in patients with dilated bile ducts.

Liver biopsy is required for the histological analysis of liver tissue. Tissue should be obtained from both the nodules and the intranodular areas. There is a 50% chance of sampling error with percutaneous liver biopsy. Biopsy under vision, either during laparoscopy or minilaparotomy obviates this problem. Laparoscopy or laparotomy should be performed if no clear aetiology of biliary cirrhosis can be found (see Ch. 19).

Postnecrotic cirrhosis

This is usually seen in older children, many of whom may have a history of antecedent acute viral hepatitis, chronic active hepatitis or metabolic liver disease. The commonest causes in older children are neonatal hepatitis and chronic active hepatitis. Wilson's disease and alpha$_1$-antitrypsin deficiency may be seen in children of all ages and must be kept in mind. HBV infection, though not common in the west, is by far the commonest cause of postnecrotic cirrhosis in children from endemic areas. In a significant percentage of cases, the cause remains unknown and is labelled as cryptogenic cirrhosis.

Clinical signs are variable. Some patients may be asymptomatic, others may present with nonspecific complaints of malaise, fatigue or anorexia. Decreased libido in adolescents, primary or secondary amenorrhoea in girls, and epistaxis may be the presenting features. Jaundice and pruritis are late manifestations. Physical findings include hepatosplenomegaly, ascites, spider naevi, palmar erythema and malar flush. Gynaecomastia and testicular atrophy can occur as a consequence of increased circulating oestrogens. Distended veins may be present on the abdomen with blood flow away from the umbilicus. A bounding pulse and flow murmurs are signs of a high cardiac output. Bruits may be heard over the lungs and have been attributed to bronchopulmonary shunts. Finger clubbing may be present.

Serum bilirubin may be normal with a mild to moderate elevation in alkaline phosphatase, 5'-nucleotidase and gamma glutamyltranspeptidase. Hepatocellular dysfunction leads to decreased serum albumin, and decreased clotting factors with an increase in total proteins. Hypergammaglobulinaemia is frequently seen. Hypersplenism may manifest as thrombocytopenia, anaemia, and leukopenia. A hypokalemic metabolic alkalosis may be present. Serum alpha$_1$-antitrypsin, serum ceruloplasmin, urinary copper excretion and sweat chloride levels should be estimated in all patients with postnecrotic cirrhosis.

Oesophageal varices can be demonstrated radiologically by a barium swallow or by fibre-optic endoscopy. A liver scan with technetium[99] shows a mottled uptake in the liver. A liver biopsy is necessary to confirm the diagnosis.

Complications

The management of a patient with cirrhosis generally involves treating the ensuing complications. The major complication in children, besides ascites, portal hypertension, hypersplenism and encephalopathy is nutritional insufficiency with failure to thrive.

Ascites

Ascites in cirrhosis results from multiple factors (Wyllie et al 1980). Accumulation of fluid in the peritoneal space is due to an increased hydrostatic pressure from portal hypertension trying to drive fluid out of the vascular space against a reduced plasma oncotic pressure from hypoalbuminaemia trying to hold it back. It has also been postulated that there is an imbalance in the formation of lymph and that the lymphatics of the peritoneum are unable to return all the transudate to the intravascular compartment. A decrease in effective intravascular volume activates the renin-angiotensin system, causing retention of salt and water by the kidneys.

Slowly accumulating ascites does not cause much discomfort to the patient and does not need to be aggressively treated. Rapid accumulation of ascitic fluid is usually precipitated by gastrointestinal bleeding, infections and dietary indiscretions. This can cause abdominal discomfort and respiratory distress. Basilar atelactasis occurs due to raising of the diaphragm. Significant hypoxia can develop as a consequence of diminished diaphragmatic excursion, basilar atelectasis, pleural effusions (which are frequently seen in patients with ascites) and pulmonary shunts. Spontaneous bacterial peritonitis is a frequent complication of ascites and can be fatal if untreated. Increased abdominal pressure may cause umbilical and inguinal hernias, and gastroesophageal reflux. There is an increased risk of variceal haemorrhage in the presence of tense ascites.

Treatment of ascites should be very conservative. Inappropriately aggressive management can potentially do considerable harm. If the ascites is not too large and does not bother the patient too much, dietary sodium restriction should be tried. Ideally, daily sodium intake should be limited to 1–2 mEq/kg/24 h. This generally leads to an adequate diuresis, but in practice it is very difficult to maintain a child on a diet without salt (see Ch. 23).

Fluid is not restricted unless the patient develops signs of fluid overload like hyponatraemia and increasing weight. If these signs appear, fluid can be restricted to 1000 ml per day. Diuretics should be tried before fluid restriction is instituted. Spironolactone is used as the initial diuretic in a dose of 3 mg/kg/24 h. It takes 4–5 days to exert maximal action. If adequate diuresis does not result the dose can be safely doubled. Frusemide, in a dose of 1–3 mg/kg/24 h can be added to the above regimen, if necessary. In patients with peripheral oedema along with ascites, up to 500 ml of fluid can be diuresed safely every day. Patients with ascites without peripheral oedema should be diuresed more cautiously (200 ml/24 h) as they are prone to develop intravascular volume depletion. Another common side effect of diuretic therapy is hypokalaemia. Hypokalaemic alkalosis can precipitate hepatic encephalopathy by converting ammonium ions into ammonia. Potassium chloride supplements should be used in all patients on prolonged diuretic therapy. Hypochloraemia can occur and should be treated with lysine monochloride. Misuse of diuretics is one of the commonest causes of the hepatorenal syndrome, with oliguria and renal failure. Paracentesis should be done in patients having acute respiratory distress. Not more than 1000–2000 ml fluid should be removed in 24 hours, as hypotension may develop due to rapid reaccumulation of ascitic fluid. When ascites is resistant to medical management other forms of treatment should be considered. Paracentesis should be avoided as it only removes proteins that the patient can ill afford to lose. Apparatus is available by which the ascites can be ultrafiltered in order to remove water and electrolytes, the colloids being returned intravenously. The procedure allows the rapid removal of ascites and produces a good diuresis. A peritoneojugular shunt with a one-way pressure sensitive valve (Leveen shunt) has been used to treat patients with resistant ascites (Epstein et al 1980). This procedure has a number of complications including shunt-blockage, infection, consumption coagulopathy and hypokalaemia.

Gastrointestinal bleeding

This is a consequence of portal hypertension and will be discussed in that section (pp. 482–490).

Hepatic encephalopathy

This is a sign of advanced liver disease. It may present as increasing drowsiness, hyper-reflexia, incoordination and flapping tremor. The flapping tremor is due to the inability of the basal ganglia to maintain postural tone. Other findings include dysarthria, amnesia and ultimately coma. The aetiology of the neurological signs is not clear. Among the different substances incriminated are ammonia, false neurotransmitters (e.g.

octopamine), mercaptans, and free fatty acids. Encephalopathy can be precipitated by gastrointestinal bleeding, dietary indiscretions, diuretics, hypokalaemia, sedatives, and infection, all of which should be treated promptly.

The gastrointestinal tract is cleared of all blood and nitrogenous material by administering cathartics and enemas. Neomycin is used orally to sterilize the intestinal flora and decrease the breakdown of nitrogenous material into ammonia. Lactulose, a nonabsorbable disaccharide, is administered to reduce the intestinal pH and inhibit conversion of ammonium ion to ammonia. Dietary protein intake should be reduced to a minimum (0.5–1 g/kg/24 h). The prognosis is poor, and most patients succumb to their illness.

Malnutrition

Malabsorption with failure to thrive is a serious problem in children with biliary cirrhosis (Linscheer 1970). Because of decreased bile salt concentrations in the intestinal lumen there is inadequate solubilization of lipids and the fat soluble vitamins. An increased prothrombin time develops due to lack of vitamin K. It is correctable by administration of either a water soluble vitamin K preparation or intramuscular vitamin K. Defects in vitamin D absorption lead to rickets or osteomalacia. Large doses of oral vitamin D (up to 375 μg/day), 25 hydroxy cholecalciferol or 1,25 dihydroxycholecalciferol should be used. Prolonged steatorrhoea can cause a deficiency of vitamin E, which may lead to difficulty in walking, opthalmoplegia and areflexia. In general patients will not absorb oral preparations of vitamin E and typically intramuscular injections (of the order of 10 mg/week) must be given to correct serum vitamin E concentrations to normal. Medium chain triglycerides may be helpful in providing additional calories but are not a source of essential fatty acids. Enough protein, calories and vitamins should be given to fulfill the nutritional requirements of the child (see Ch. 23).

Haematological abnormalities

Bleeding disorders are frequent in cirrhosis. Malabsorption results in a decreased concentration of vitamin K which causes a prolongation of the prothrombin time and may lead to petechiae, ecchymoses, epistaxis and bleeding from other areas. Splenomegaly leads to thrombocytopenia due to sequestration and destruction of platelets in the spleen. Liver disease results in a reduced production of clotting factors. Anaemia is seen in almost all patients with advanced liver disease. This can be due to red cell destruction in the spleen, loss of blood in the gastrointestinal tract, or inadequate bone marrow production.

Portal hypertension

Portal hypertension is said to exist when the pressure in the portal veins becomes more than 10–12 mm of mercury or 17–20 cm of water. It may or may not be a consequence of liver disease, and is due to pre-, intra- or posthepatic portal vein destruction (Alagille & Odievre 1979b). The commoner causes are shown in Table 21.2.

Pathophysiology

Elevation in portal pressure leads to development of alternate channels which shunt venous blood from splanchnic to systemic circulation. Porto-systemic shunts are listed in Table 21.3. Of these, the gastroesophageal

Table 21.2   Causes of portal hypertension in children

Prehepatic causes
    Congenital hypoplasia of portal vein
    Umbilical vein catherization
    Omphalitis
    Phlebitis of the portal vein
    Extrinsic compression
        Pancreatitis
        Malignancy
        Portal lymphadenopathy
    Increased blood flow
        Atriovenous fistula
        Tropical splenomegaly
    Idiopathic

Hepatic causes
    Cirrhosis
    Congenital hepatic fibrosis
    Schistosomiasis
    Hereditary telangiectasia
    Infiltrative liver disease
        Gaucher's disease
        Hodgkins disease
        Haemangiomata
    Noncirrhotic portal fibrosis
    Nodular noncirrhotic regenerative hyperplasia
    Felty's syndrome

Posthepatic causes
    Budd–Chiari syndrome
    Inferior vena cava obstruction
        Bands
        Webs
        Strictures
    Veno-occlusive disease
    Cardiac causes
        Constrictive pericarditis
        Ebstein's anomaly
        Right atrial myxoma

Table 21.3 Portosystemic collaterals in portal hypertension. (Adapted from Alagille D & Odievre M 1979b)

Gastro-oesophageal shunts
    Left gastric vein to oesophageal vein to azygous and hemiazygous veins
    Short gastric vein and gastroepiploic vein to superior hemiazygous vein
    Gastro-oesophageal plexus to diaphragmatic veins

Left renal vein shunts
    Gastro-phreno-capsulo-renal shunts
    Spontaneous spleno-renal shunts

Rectal shunts
    Inferior and middle rectal vein to superior rectal vein
    Inferior rectal vein to right renal vein

Perisplenic shunts to
    Lumbar veins
    Perirenal veins
    Thoracic and abdominal walls

Porto-umbilico-caval shunts

Parieto-peritoneal collaterals

---

shunts are the most important. Here, portal blood reaches azygos or superior hemiazygous veins (i.e. the systemic circulation) via gastro-oesophageal anastomoses. Dilation of oesophageal veins occurs due to the large amount of blood flowing through them and this leads to oesophageal varices which may rupture and cause massive GI bleeding. Anastomoses between superior and inferior rectal veins may cause haemorrhoids; the umbilicoportocaval anastomosis can cause dilated venous channels on the abdomen; portopulmonary anastomoses may lead to pulmonary hypertension (Levine et al 1973).

Splenomegaly, is almost invariably present in patients with portal hypertension. The spleen is moderately enlarged and may secondarily lead to anaemia, leukopenia, and thrombocytopenia. Other causes of splenomegaly should be looked for and ruled out. These include haemolytic anaemias, haematologic malignancies, infections and storage disorders.

Gastrointestinal bleeding, as manifested by haematemesis or melaena is the presenting feature of portal hypertension in many patients. Haematemesis is usually followed by melaena. Melaena may occur in absence of haematemesis if the bleeding is not massive in amount and occurs over a period of time. As mentioned above, almost all bleeding is due to rupture of oesophageal varices, and these must be looked for in any patient with upper gastrointestinal bleeding. Presence of splenomegaly along with gastrointestinal bleeding, is very suggestive of portal hypertension. Fibreoptic endoscopy is the most accurate way of detecting oesophageal varices. The varices appear as irregular elevations on the mucosa of the oesophagous which do not subside on air insufflation, which distinguishes them from oesophageal folds. Accuracy is not however 100% and varices, especially if located in the fundus of the stomach, may be missed. Barium swallow is a noninvasive way of visualizing varices and is usually quite adequate in most patients. Very young patients may not be able to cooperate. Other causes of gastrointestinal bleeding should also be considered.

Ascites is most commonly seen in portal hypertension due to cirrhosis. It is almost always present in patients with portal hypertension due to posthepatic causes and is much less common in prehepatic portal hypertension, where it may be temporally related to occurrence of gastrointestinal bleeding. In these patients, ascites is painless and may spontaneously regress. Ascites is easily detected clinically if large amounts of fluid are present. Abdominal ultrasound is a very sensitive technique for demonstrating free fluid in the abdominal cavity.

Hepatic encephalopathy is a late complication, seen only in patients with severe liver disease. It is a consequence of collateral channels which bypass a significant portion of blood from portal to systemic circulation. Shunting of blood is not sufficient to cause hepatic encephalopathy, and patients with extrahepatic portal hypertension with normal liver function almost never develop encephalopathy.

Investigations are necessary to confirm the diagnosis and find the cause of portal hypertension, study any underlying liver disease, and acquire information needed to make accurate surgical decisions. A complete blood count, including a platelet count, is performed and a platelet count of less than $20 \times 10^9/l$ is a contraindication for any invasive technique. A liver-spleen scan gives some idea of liver morphology and function. Studies needed to determine the cause of underlying liver disease include hepatitis B antigen and antibody, hepatitis A antibody, liver enzymes, bilirubin, prothrombin time, BSP retention, serum ceruloplasmin, serum alpha$_1$-antitrypsin, sweat electrolytes, and urine for reducing sugars and organic acids. Liver biopsy forms an integral part of the work-up of a child with portal hypertension. The obvious contraindications are coagulation abnormalities, thrombocytopenia and impending liver failure. Other contraindications include ascites, and posthepatic portal hypertension.

To determine the exact site of the venous block and collateral circulation, and to measure portal pressure, requires invasive vascular studies. Table 21.4 lists the vascular studies which may be helpful in portal hypertension. Splenoportography is the procedure of choice in children with portal hypertension (Melhem & Rizk 1970). Not only is it technically easy and fast, it gives a lot of anatomical and haemodynamic information and can be done in very young children. The splenic pulp pressure, which accurately reflects portal pressure, can be measured. The precise location of venous block, presence of collaterals and patency of splenic and portal veins can be determined. Contraindications to splenoportography include defects in coagulation, ascites, and a percutaneous liver biopsy in the past 24 hours. Ascites impairs local haemostasis. A liver biopsy done shortly before splenoportography can confuse the clinical picture in cases where abdominal

Table 21.4 Vascular studies and their uses in management of portal hypertension

Splenoportography
　　Measurement of splenic pulp pressure
　　Patency and size of splenic vein
　　Patency and size of portal vein
　　Identification of major collaterals
　　Indication of intrahepatic disease

Superior mesentric angiography
　　Patency of superior mesenteric vein
　　Excellent visualization of portal vein
　　Visualization of gastro-oesophageal collaterals
　　Anatomy and vascular supply of kidney

Coeliac arteriography
　　Number and localization of hepatic arteries
　　Ruling out arteriovenous fistula
　　Hepatography, to look for intrahepatic disease
　　Anatomy and vascular supply of kidney

Hepatic vein catheterization
　　Measurement of free and wedged hepatic pressure
　　Visualization of hepatic veins

Saphenous venography
　　Visualization of inferior vena cava

Inferior vena cava catheterization
　　Presence and patency of inferior vena cava
　　Rule out external compression

Percutaneous transhepatic portography
　　Visualization of portal and hepatic veins
　　Treatment of bleeding varices by selective embolization of coronary veins

Operative umbilical portography
　　Excellent film quality due to injection of contrast under pressure.

bleeding develops. Complications of splenoportography include a subcapsular haematoma, haemoperitoneum and capsular adhesions.

Superior mesenteric angiography visualizes the portal system well. It also visualizes portosystemic shunts not seen during splenoportography, including those draining into the renal vein. Splenoportography visualizes best the left collaterals while superior mesenteric angiography visualizes the right collaterals. Renal anatomy and vascular supply can also be determined, which can be useful when considering surgery. The major risk is spasm of the femoral artery with subsequent thrombosis and limb ischaemia. In patients with biliary atresia, the inferior vena cava should always be studied, as it may be abnormal or absent (Odievre et al 1977).

Measurement of free and wedged hepatic vein pressures is done by retrograde catheterization of the hepatic vein via the femoral or the cephalic vein. This is helpful in determining the location of the block. Normal free and wedged hepatic vein pressures are seen in presinusoidal blocks. They may also be normal in certain hepatic disorders like Wilson's disease, congenital hepatic fibrosis and hepatic schistosomiasis. In intrahepatic conditions, there is normal free hepatic vein pressure, with an elevated wedged hepatic vein pressure. In posthepatic blocks, on the other hand, both free and wedged hepatic pressures are elevated.

Prehepatic portal hypertension

Prehepatic portal hypertension results from an obstruction to bloodflow before it reaches the hilum of the liver. A significant proportion of children with this problem have a history of umbilical vein catheterization during the neonatal period. The risk of portal vein thrombosis is directly related to the duration of catheterization, and the trauma produced by the catheter. If the catheter is placed by mistake in the left or right portal vein, the risk of portal vein thrombosis is greatly increased. Catheterization after the first 48 hours of birth has been associated with an increased risk of thrombosis. Portal webs, fibrosis and congenital anomalies account for another large group of patients. Obstruction of the portal vein leads to the formation of portal cavernomas, a name given to dilated, tortuous venous channels which develop in place of the obstructed portal vein. The cause of obstruction remains unknown in 30–50% of patients. Many of them have other congenital anomalies including heart defects, and anomalies of the inferior vena cava.

Extrahepatic portal hypertension usually presents before 5–7 years of age. Those with a history of umbilical vein catheterization present earlier, with most developing portal hypertension before two years of age. Gastrointestinal bleeding is the presenting feature in the majority of patients and may present as haematemesis, malaena or both. Transient ascites may be seen after an episode of major bleeding. Some cases are discovered during the work-up of an isolated splenomegaly. The liver is not enlarged and liver function tests and liver biopsy are usually normal. BSP retention time is abnormal in most patients.

Intrahepatic portal hypertension

Most chronic liver diseases ultimately lead to the development of portal hypertension and once cirrhosis is established it is almost invariably accompanied by portal hypertension. Non cirrhotic portal fibrosis, infiltrative liver diseases, Felty's syndrome, and congenital hepatic fibrosis are some other causes of intrahepatic portal hypertension. As a rule, patients with cirrhosis do worse than patients with non-cirrhotic liver disease. Presentation is usually due to upper GI bleeding or abdominal distension. Ascites and splenomegaly are commonly seen. Patients with cirrhosis may present with stigmata of hepatocellular insufficiency like spider angiomas and jaundice.

Invasive vascular studies reveal an elevated wedged hepatic pressure with a free hepatic vein pressure. The hepatic artery is enlarged to compensate for the decreased amount of blood flowing from the portal vein. The intra-hepatic vascular pattern is distorted by the regenerating nodules.

Management should be tailored around prevention and treatment of complications. If any specific therapy is available, as in Wilson's disease, it should be promptly instituted. Most patients do not tolerate gastrointes-tinal bleeding well and there is a risk of the development of hepatic encephalopathy. Portocaval shunting is useful in patients with adequate liver function and quiescent disease. The ultimate prognosis depends on the underlying liver disease.

Posthepatic portal hypertension

This is infrequently seen in children. Occlusion of the hepatic venous outflow leads to posthepatic portal hypertension. Conditions causing outflow obstruction include Budd–Chiari syndrome, veno-occlusive disease, hepatic vein thrombosis, strictures, bands or membranes in the inferior vena cava (Cabrera et al 1980), constrictive pericarditis, and right atrial myxoma.

Budd–Chiari Syndrome. This is an extremely rare syndrome caused by the occlusion of hepatic venous outflow. The causes are listed in Table 21.5. Patients present with rapidly accumulating, painful, tense, ascites. Periph-eral oedema and pleural effusions may be present. The liver is enlarged and tender. Splenomegaly and jaundice are other features. Haematemesis is unlikely as oesophageal varices do not commonly develop.

Splenoportography reveals a patent splenic and portal venous system. There is abnormal delay in clearance of the dye from the liver due to the

Table 21.5 Causes of Budd–Chiari syndrome

Idiopathic (70%)

Hepatic vein thrombosis
   Leukaemia
   Sickle cell disease
   Paroxysmal nocturnal haemoglobinuria
   Polycythaemia
   Inflammatory bowel disease
   Allergic vasculitis
   Visceral thrombophlebitis migrans

Extrinsic compression of hepatic vein
   Tumours
   Enlarged caudate lobe of liver
   Amoebic liver abscess

Bands or webs in the vena cava

Hepatic vein agenesis

posthepatic block. Free and wedged hepatic vein pressures should be measured as both are elevated. An inferior vena cavogram is needed to rule out a block (Takeuchi et al 1971, Taneja et al 1979). Posthepatic phlebography will demonstrate any block in the hepatic veins.

Histologically, abnormalities in the hepatic veins are seen. Thrombi, both fresh and organized may be present. There is some endophlebitis with proliferation of connective tissue. The liver shows stasis of blood in the central veins with pericentral hepatic necrosis. Later, there is fibrosis with destruction of hepatic architecture. Percutaneous liver biopsy is contraindicated because of a high incidence of bleeding and an open liver biopsy should be performed. If there is any precipitating cause, efforts should be made to eliminate it. A portocaval shunt is the procedure of choice if the inferior vena cava is patent. Webs or membranes in the inferior vena cava can be removed by transcardiac membranotomy. Surgical bypass, using Dacron grafts, can be attempted in cases where the vena cava is obliterated.

Veno-occlusive disease of the liver. This is a disease, associated with ingestion of certain alkaloids in 'bush tea', which causes occlusion of the smaller veins of the liver. It has been most commonly seen in Jamaica, though cases from Egypt, South America (Lyrord et al 1976), Middle East (Al-Hasany & Mohamed 1970), South Africa and India have also been reported. The alkaloids which are implicated belong to the pyrolizidine group which are converted by the liver into toxic pyrole derivatives (Stillman et al 1977). These cause endophlebitis in the smaller hepatic veins, ultimately leading to their occlusion.

Children between the ages of 2 and 6 are usually affected. Initially, there is hepatomegaly, abdominal pain and ascites; jaundice may or may not be present. Later the disease enters a chronic stage with centrilobular necrosis and fibrosis. Once portal hypertension occurs, splenomegaly and collateral circulation develop.

On histological examination, small hepatic veins are occluded with sparing of the larger veins. Central veins are congested and sinusoids are dilated. There is minimal or no thrombosis. Centrilobular hepatocytes become necrotic and fibrosis may appear in later stages.

Over half the children improve on supportive therapy and about one-third go on to develop cirrhosis.

Management of gastrointestinal bleeding

Parents of children with portal hypertension should be properly educated about the risk of bleeding. Under no circumstance should patients with portal hypertension consume preparations containing aspirin (acetylsalicylic acid).

GI haemorrhage is a medical emergency and treatment should be administered in a rapid and systematic way. Transfusion of blood, and irrigation of the stomach with ice-cold saline should be started immediately. Over-transfusion should be avoided as this causes distension of oeosphageal varices and leads to further bleeding. In case there are clotting abnormalities, fresh frozen plasma should be administered. Platelets are transfused if the patient has thrombocytopenia. Many patients will stop bleeding by these conservative steps alone. If bleeding continues despite the above measures, intravenous infusion of vasopressin at 0.2 to 0.4 μg/min has been found to be helpful (Johnson et al 1977). Hypertension, arrythmias and bradycardia may occur with this approach. Hence intravenous vasopressin cannot be administered for a long time. Administration of vasopressin selectively through the superior mesenteric artery can be continued for much longer periods. More recently the beta adrenoreceptor blocker propranalol has been used successfully for variceal haemorrhage (Lebrec et al 1980).

A triple-lumen Sengstaken–Blakemore tube is inserted if bleeding persists (Teres et al 1978). The tube is inserted into the stomach, the gastric balloon is inflated and pulled up against the cardia and the oesophageal balloon is then inflated to 30–40 mmHg. Continuous gastric drainage is maintained, and frequent oropharygeal suction is done to prevent aspiration. The balloon should be decompressed every 12 hours to prevent necrosis of the oesophageal mucosa. The Sengstaken–Blakemore tube is effective in stopping bleeding in 70–85% of patients.

Direct sclerosis of the bleeding varices by injection of a sclerosing agent can be performed instead of oesophageal tamponade (Lilly 1981) and it can also be used in patients who have failed to stop bleeding despite oesophageal tamponade. Experimental approaches include embolization of the coronary-gastro-oesophageal system using Gelfoam® pellets. As a last resort direct surgical ligation of the varices or an emergency shunt procedure can be done. These have a very high operative and postoperative mortality.

Surgical management

Definitive treatment of portal hypertension is the surgical creation of a shunt to transfer portal blood to the systemic circulation. Patients with extrahepatic portal hypertension and good liver function and those with congenital hepatic fibrosis do quite well after a portosystemic shunting procedure. Patients with cirrhosis and liver disease should be carefully screened before subjecting them to surgery. Operative and postoperative mortality is very high in improperly selected patients. Criteria, such as the presence of ascites, hepatic encephalopathy, nutritional status, serum albumin and bilirubin, are used to screen patients. A prolonged prothrombin time is a definite contraindication to surgery. The aetiology of portal hypertension is also important. Patients with Wilson's disease or hereditary tyrosinaemia and any active ongoing hepatic inflammation should not be subjected to a shunt.

Various shunt procedures are available. The three most popular ones are splenorenal, portocaval and mesocaval shunts. In extrahepatic portal hypertension, only mesocaval or splenorenal shunts can be done. Splenorenal shunts were thought to be better as they did not divert all the portal blood away from the liver. It now appears however that once the shunt is in place, almost all portal blood starts flowing through it. Selective decompression of oesophageal varices by a distal splenorenal shunt (Warren's shunt) or a coronarocaval shunt (Inokuchi's shunt) are other possible shunt procedures. For intrahepatic portal hypertension, a splenorenal shunt or a portocaval shunt can be done.

The patency of the shunt depends on the surgical expertise. With the advent of operating microscopes and microsurgery, vascular anastomoses can be done between the minute vessels present in children. Shunt patency is determined by intraoperative angiography and postoperative oesophagoscopy. In case oesophageal varices are still present, angiography should be repeated six months after surgery. Protein restriction should be enforced for several months to prevent the development of portosystemic encephalopathy. There may be some decrease in intellectual efficiency as a minor manifestation of portocaval encephalopathy.

REFERENCES

Alagille D, Odievre M 1979a Congenital hepatic fibrosis. In: Liver and Biliary Tract Disease in Children. Wiley-Falmmarion, Paris. pp 253–261
Alagille D, Odievre M 1979b Portal Hypertension. In: Liver and Biliary Tract Disease in Children. Wiley-Falmmarion, Paris. pp 262–297
Al-Hasany M, Mohamed A S 1970 Veno-occlusive disease of the liver in Iraq. Nine cases occurring in three Bedouin families. Archives of Disease in Childhood 45: 722–723
Alvarez F, Bernard O, Brunelle F, Hadchouel M, Leblanc A, Odievre M, Alagille D 1981 Congenital hepatic fibrosis in children. Journal of Pediatrics 99: 370–375
Anand S K, Chan J C, Lieberman E 1975 Polycystic disease and hepatic fibrosis in children. American Journal of Diseases of Children 129: 810–813
Arasu T S, Wyllie R, Hatch T F, Fitzgerald J F 1979 Management of chronic aggressive hepatitis in children and adolescents. Journal of Pediatrics 95: 514–522
Becker M D, Baptista A, Scheuer P J, Sherlock S 1970 Prognosis of chronic persistent hepatitis. Lancet i:53–57
Bhave S A, Pandit A N, Pradhan A M 1982 Liver disease in India. Archives of Disease in Childhood 57: 922–928
Cabrera J, Brugera M, Navarro F, Caralps J M, Pare C, Rodes J 1980 Budd–Chiari syndrome due to membranous obstruction of the inferior vena cava. Journal of Pediatrics 96: 435–437
Carpenter T O, Carnes D L, Anast C S 1983 Hypoparathyroidism in Wilson's disease. New England Journal of Medicine 309: 873–877
Chandra R K 1979 The Liver and Biliary System in Infants and Children. Churchill Livingstone, Edinburgh. pp 174–195, 242–328
Chandra R K 1982 Indian childhood cirrhosis. In: Rudolph A M, Hoffman J I E (eds) Pediatrics, 17th edn. Appleton-Century-Croft, Norwalk, Connecticut. pp 1028–1029
Czaja A J 1981 Current problems in the management of chronic active hepatitis. Mayo Clinical Proceedings 56: 311–323
Centers for Disease Control 1984 Post exposure prophylaxis of hepatitis B. Annals of Internal Medicine 101: 351–354

Czaja A J, Ludwig J, Baggenstoss A H, Wolf A 1981 Corticosteroid-treated chronic active hepatitis in remission. New England Journal of Medicine 305: 5–9

Deiss A, Lynch R E, Lee G R, Cartwright G E 1971 Long-term therapy of Wilson's disease. Annals of Internal Medicine 75: 57–65

Dietrichson O 1975 Chronic persistent hepatitis. A clinical, serologic and prognostic study. Scandinavian Journal of Gastroenterology 10: 249–255

Epstein M, Calia F M, Gabuzda G J 1980 The Leveen shunt for ascites and hepatorenal syndrome. New England Journal of Medicine 302: 598–607

Estrada A, Espinosa L 1980 Active chronic viral hepatitis type B in a 10-month-old child. Helvetica Paediatrica Acta 35: 165–168

Frommer D, Morris J, Sherlock S 1977 Kayser–Fleischer-like rings in patients without Wilson's disease. Gastroenterology 72: 1331–1335

Gibbs K, Walshe J M 1980 Biliary excretion of copper in Wilson's disease. Lancet ii: 538–539

Hadziyannis S, Geber M A, Vissoulis C, Popper H 1973 Cytoplasmic hepatitis B antigen in ground-glass hepatocytes of carriers. Archives of Pathology 96: 327–330

Hegarty J L, Nouri Aria K T, Portmann B S, Eddleston A L W F, Williams R 1983 Relapse following treatment withdrawal in patients with autoimmune chronic active hepatitis. Hepatology 3: 685–689

Isenberg J N, L'Heureuse D R 1976 Clinical observations on the biliary system in cystic fibrosis. American Journal of Gastroenterology 65: 134–139

Jain S, Scheuer P J, Archer B, Newman S P, Sherlock S 1978 Histological determination of copper and copper-associated protein in chronic liver diseases. Journal of Clinical Pathology 31: 784–790

Johnson W C, Widrich W C, Ansell J E et al 1977 Control of bleeding varices by vasopressin: a prospective randomized study. American Journal of Surgery 186: 369–376

Kidd V J, Golbus M S, Wallis R B, Itakura K, Woo S L C 1984 Prenatal diagnosis of alpha-1 antitrypsin deficiency by direct analysis of the mutation site in the gene. New England Journal of Medicine 310: 639–642

Knodell R G, Conrad M E, Ishak K G, 1977 Development of chronic liver disease after acute non-A non-B post-transfusion hepatitis. Gastroenterology 72: 902–909

Lam K C, Lai C L, Ng R P, Trepo C, Wu P C 1981 Deleterious effect of prednisone in HBsAg-positive chronic active hepatitis. New England Journal of Medicine 304: 380–386

LaRusso N F, Summerskill W H J, McCall J T 1976 Abnormalities of chemical tests for copper metabolism in chronic active liver disease: differentiation from Wilson's disease. Gastroenterology 70: 653–655

Lebrec D, Nouel O, Corbic M, Benhamou J P 1980 Propranolol a medical treatment for portal hypertension. Lancet ii: 180–182

Lefkowitch J H, Honig C L, King M E, Hagstrom J W C 1982 Hepatic copper overload and features of Indian childhood cirrhosis in an American sibship. New England Journal of Medicine 307: 271–277

Levine O R, Harris R C, Blanc W A, Mellins R B 1973 Progressive pulmonary hypertension in children with portal hypertension. Journal of Pediatrics 83: 964–973

Lilly J R 1981 Endoscopic sclerosis of oesophageal varices. Surgery 152: 513–514

Linscheer W G 1970 Malabsorption in cirrhosis. American Journal of Nutrition 23: 488–492

Lyrord C L, Vergara G G, Moeller D D 1976 Hepatic veno-occlusive disease originating in Ecuador. Gastroenterology 70: 105–108

Maggiore G, Giacomo C D, Marzani D, Sessa F, Scotta M S 1983 Chronic viral hepatitis in infancy. Journal of Pediatrics 103: 749–752

Melhem R E, Rizk G K 1970 Splenoportographic evaluation of portal hypertension in children. Journal of Pediatric Surgery 5: 522–526

Nayak N C 1979 Indian childhood cirrhosis. In: MacSween R N M, Anthony P P, Scheuer P J (eds) Pathology of the liver. Churchill Livingstone, New York. pp 268–269

Nayak N C, Ramalingaswami V 1975 Indian childhood cirrhosis. Clinical Gastroenterology 4: 333–349

Odievre M, Pige G, Alagille D 1977 Congenital abnormalities associated with extrahepatic portal hypertension. Archives of Disease in Childhood 52: 383–385

Portmann B, Tanner M S, Mowat A P, Williams R 1978 Orcein positive liver deposits in Indian childhood cirrhosis. Lancet i: 1338–1340

Psacharopoulos H T, Howard E R, Portmann B, Mowat A P, Williams R 1981 Hepatic complications of cystic fibrosis. Lancet ii: 78–80

Psacharopoulos H T, Mowat A P, Cook P J L, Carlile P A, Portmann B, Rodeck C H 1983 Outcome of liver disease associated with alpha-1 antitrypsin deficiency (PiZ). Archives of Disease in Childhood 58: 882–887

Rakela J, Reedeker A G 1979 Chronic liver disease after acute non-A non-B viral hepatitis. Gastroenterology 77: 1200–1202

Realdi G, Alberti A, Rugge M, Bartolotti F, Rigoli A M, Tremolada F, Ruol A 1980 Seroconversion from hepatitis Be antigen to anti-HBe in chronic hepatitis B virus infection. Gastroenterology 79: 195–199

Roche-Sicot J, Benhamou J P 1977 Acute intravascular hemolysis and acute liver failure associated as a first manifestation of Wilson's disease. Annals of Internal Medicine 86: 301–303

Sharp H L, Bridges R A, Krivit W, Freier E R 1969 Cirrhosis associated with alpha-1 antitrypsin deficiency: a previously unrecognised inherited disorder. Journal of Laboratory and Clinical Medicine 73: 934–939

Shinoazaki T, Saito K, Shiraki K 1981 HBsAg-positive giant cell hepatitis with cirrhosis in a 10-month- old infant. Archives of Disease in Childhood 56: 64–66

Silverman A, Roy C C 1983 Pediatric Clinical Gastroenterology. CV Mosby, St Louis.

Soloway R D, Baggenstoss A H, Choenfield L J, Summerskill W H J 1971 Observer error and sampling variability tested in evaluation of hepatitis and cirrhosis by liver biopsy. American Journal of Digestive Diseases 16: 1082–1086

Stern R C, Stevens D P, Boot T F, Doershuk C F, Jzant R J, Matthews I W 1976 Symptomatic hepatic disease in cystic fibrosis: incidence, outcome and course of porto-systemic shunting. Gastroenterology: 645–649

Sternlieb I, Scheinberg I H 1979 The role of radiocopper in the diagnosis of Wilson's disease. Gastroenterology 77: 138–142

Stillman A E, Huxtable R, Consroe P, Kohnen P, Smith S 1977 Hepatic veno-occlusive disease due to pyrrolizidine (Senecio) poisoning in Arizona. Gastroenterology 73: 349–352

Stromeyer F W, Ishak K G 1980 Histology of the liver in Wilson's disease. American Journal of Clinical Pathology 73: 12–24

Takeuchi J, Takada A, Hasumura Y, Matsuda Y, Ikegami F 1971 Budd–Chiari syndrome associated with the obstruction of the inferior vena cava. American Journal of Medicine 51: 11–20

Taneja A, Mitra S K, Moghe P D, Rao P N, Samanta N, Kumar L 1979 Budd–Chiari syndrome in childhood secondary to inferior vena caval obstruction. Pediatrics 63: 808–812

Teres J, Cecilia A, Bordas J M, Rimola A, Bru C, Rodes J 1978 Esophageal tamponade for bleeding varices. Gastroenterology 75: 566–569

Tong M J, Thursby M W, Lin J-H et al 1981 Studies on the maternal-infant transmission of the hepatitis B virus and HBV infection within families. In: Melnick J L (ed) Hepatitis B Virus and Primary Liver Cancer. Progress in Medical Virology, Volume 27. S. Karger, Basel.

Trevisan A, Cadrobbi P, Crivellaro C, Bartolotti F, Rugge M, Realdi G 1982 Virologic features of chronic hepatitis B virus infection in childhood. Journal of Pediatrics 100: 366–372

Vegnente A, Larcher V F, Mowat A P, Portmann B, Williams R 1984 Duration of chronic active hepatitis and the development of cirrhosis. Archives of Disease in Childhood 59: 330–335

Wong V C W, I H M H, Reesnik H W, Lelie P N, Refrink-Brongers E E, Yeung C Y, Ma H K 1984 Prevention of the HBsAg carrier state in newborn infants of mothers who are chronic carriers of HBsAg and HBeAg by administration of hepatitis-B vaccine and hepatitis-B immunoglobulin. Lancet i: 921–926

Wyllie R, Arasu T S, Fitzgerald J F 1980 Ascites: pathophysiology and management. Journal of Pediatrics 97: 167–176

Tumours of the gut and liver

INTRODUCTION

Tumours of the gastrointestinal tract and liver are uncommon in children. There has been some progress in management, different histological subgroups are recognized and treatment is becoming more effective.

Currently available anticancer therapy is not target-specific and a cure is rarely achieved without measurable and sometimes lasting effects on other tissues and organs. Individual cytotoxic drugs and photon irradiation may result in gastrointestinal and hepatic dysfunction. Some, such as intestinal crypt cell hypoplasia caused by the action of cell-cycle specific agents are predictable, whilst others are difficult to anticipate. Rather than 'cure at any cost', the principal goal should be 'cure at least cost'.

Aggressive chemotherapy commonly results in malnutrition although severe nutritional imbalance may be related to catabolic effects of the disease itself, secondary anorexia and the adverse psychological effects of prolonged hospitalization. Although some degree of weight loss is almost inevitable around the time of diagnosis and during the early stages of treatment it is important that nutritional status is regularly assessed, particularly during the induction phase of treatment as cytotoxic dose tolerance and haematological recovery are both influenced by nutrition. Prophylactic parenteral nutrition has been advocated when prolonged intensive chemotherapy is instituted but its value is controversial (Koretz 1984). In some patients simple dietary advice, encouragement and caloric supplementation may be adequate, but where there is progressive weight loss more active measures are required. The relative merits of the enteral route and intravenous feeding depend upon the individual and the clinical circumstances.

Where there is evidence of severe mucosal injury it is unlikely that even a disaccharide-free, oligoantigenic oral diet will be tolerated. When anorexia is the main problem or it is necessary to improve nutrition rapidly prior to intensive chemotherapy, continuous or intermittent nasogastric feeding may be very effective. When prolonged intravenous feeding is required, an indwelling venous catheter of the Hickman or Broviac type is best; a long Silastic® line may be inserted into the right atrium via a peripheral vein. Scrupulous attention to aseptic precautions are essential in handling such lines especially during episodes of neutropenia (see Ch. 24).

GASTROINTESTINAL TUMOURS

Benign tumours and tumour-like conditions

Haemangioma

Haemangioma of the bowel is a well recognized source of painless gastrointestinal bleeding. The lesions may be sessile or polypoid. They may involve only the mucosa and submucosa or extend through the muscle coats to involve serosa or adjacent mesentery. Intestinal haemangiomas are frequently multiple. Some patients have similar lesions in other organs, most frequently in the skin. Although angiomas occur most frequently in the small bowel they are also described in the oral cavity, stomach, duodenum and colon and comprise the commonest salivary gland 'tumour' in children. Because the lesions are small they are difficult to visualize radiologically. Fibreoptic endoscopy is the diagnostic method of choice and also allows therapy of those lesions which are accessible in the colon, stomach and duodenum. Laparotomy is only required for small intestinal and very large angiomas.

Other hamartomata

A variety of hamartomata (lipoma, leiomyoma, fibroma, lymphangioma and ganglioneuroma) though rare, have all been described in children from the new born period onwards. Most patients present with intestinal obstruction.

Fibromatosis

Localized fibromatosis (infantile fibrosarcoma) is occasionally seen in neonates. All those recorded have presented with symptoms of intestinal obstruction. Histologically the lesions are composed of sheets of interdigitating bands of elongated cells with plump cigar-shaped nuclei, and mitoses are often common. These tumours are not malignant by the usual criteria and when they occur in the intestine complete resection is possible without recurrence of the tumour.

Teratoma

The sacrococcygeal region is the commonest site for teratomata in child-hood. The majority are congenital and of benign behaviour. Intrapelvic extension may give rise to rectal obstruction, and associated malformations of the lower gastrointestinal and urinary tract have been described (Berry et al 1970).

Gastrointestinal teratomas are rare, and the commonest of these are gastric, with most presenting within the first months of life and nearly one half seen in the neonatal period. There is a striking male predominance, only 2 of 59 recorded cases occurring in girls.

The tumours are all histologically mature. Calcified structures may be identified radiographically within the tumour. Treatment is surgical although tumour size may necessitate extensive resection with regular vitamin B_{12} supplementation.

Occasionally retroperitoneal teratomas are seen which present as an abdominal mass. Obstructive symptoms may occur if the colon is stretched over such a tumour.

Histiocytosis X

The aetiology of this condition is still unknown although its fluctuant natural history suggests a reactive rather than a neoplastic disorder (Broadbent & Pritchard 1985). The skin, reticuloendothelial system, lungs, bones and pituitary gland are regularly involved. The oral cavity is involved in up to 50% of cases and is the most frequent site for gastrointestinal involvement.

Clinical manifestations include granularity of the mucosa (particularly over the palate) gingival hypertrophy and premature eruption or loosening of teeth. A palatal fistula may be produced very rarely.

There have been no systematic studies to determine the frequency of gastrointestinal involvement by histiocytosis X. Recent studies have shown that the incidence of bone marrow and lung involvement, when studied by trephine biopsy and lung function studies respectively, is considerably higher than is thought when only blood counts or chest X-rays are performed. It is likely that gastrointestinal involvement is also under-diagnosed. Specific lower intestinal symptoms are unusual. Although diarrhoea and malabsorption occur, they rarely dominate the clinical picture (Keeling & Harries 1973).

Radiological investigation of the small bowel may show evidence of malabsorption but intestinal biopsy is required for diagnosis. Histiocytosis X can be distinguished from other 'reactive' histiocytic conditions by light microscopy, cytochemical methods (particularly demonstration of α-mannosidase) and electron microscopy when the presence of the tennis racket-shaped Birbeck granule is diagnostic.

Children with histiocytosis X are now managed as conservatively as possible. Patients can be left untreated and observed regularly unless symptoms are troublesome. Gastrointestinal symptoms, particularly severe orodental involvement or significant malabsorption, are indications for systemic therapy. 40–50% of patients respond to a short course of prednisolone (2 mg/kg/24 h for four weeks, tailing off thereafter). Vincristine and VP16 are the best 'second line' agents.

Mortality is not as high as many authors suggest. Even patients with the Letterer–Siwe syndrome occasionally recover completely without treatment. About half of survivors have chronic symptoms which may continue for many years before finally remitting.

Polyps

Lymphoid polyps. Local nodular lymphoid hyperplasia is an exuberant response to intestinal infection. In view of the disposition of gut-associated lymphoid tissue it is not surprising that this condition commonly affects the terminal ileum although colon and rectum may also be involved. The prominent lymphoid nodules eventually become polypoid as a result of peristalsis and the passage of intestinal contents. Intestinal obstruction may result from intussusception. Colonic and rectal lesions present with haemorrhage. Histological differentiation from lymphomata is straightforward.

Juvenile (hamartomatous) polyps. These polyps may be single or multiple and whilst they are most commonly seen in the rectum they have been described in the stomach, small intestine and colon.

Multiple (hamartomatous/juvenile) polyposis may be seen as part of a syndrome in association with cardiac defects, hydrocephalus and incomplete intestinal rotation; this syndrome is not familial. Multiple (hamartomatous/juvenile) polyposis may occur without other manifestations when it appears to be inherited as an autosomal recessive condition (Bussey et al 1978). Juvenile polyps do not undergo malignant change.

The polyps are rounded with a slender stalk. Mucus-filled cysts are apparent on the cut surface. Histological examination shows tubules, often dilated by mucus and lined by normal mucus-secreting epithelium, embedded in a loose connective tissue stroma. Inflammation of the superficial parts of the lesion is usual.

Peutz–Jegher polyps. Hamartomatous polyps with a different histological appearance occur in children as part of the Peutz–Jegher syndrome. Affected individuals are most easily identified by the presence of small pigmented lesions in the oral mucosa, peri-oral skin, digits and anus. Multiple intestinal polyps occur usually in the jejunum but ileal and colonic polyps are also seen. The polyps produce anaemia because of haemorrhage into the gut lumen or intestinal obstruction because of intussusception. The syndrome is inherited as an autosomal dominant condition. There is a small increased risk of gastric and duodenal cancer in this syndrome but neoplastic change of polypi is not thought to occur (Dozois et al 1969). Regular radiological and endoscopic surveillance of these patients is carried out to look for new polyps in order to reduce the likelihood of obstructive bowel episodes.

Peutz–Jegher polyps are frequently sessile with a coarsely lobulated or fissured surface. Histological examination shows the polyps are composed of arborizing strands of smooth muscle covered by normal columnar epithelium.

Familial (adenomatous) polyposis syndromes. Familial polyposis coli (p. coli) is inherited in an autosomal dominant fashion and is characterized by the development of multiple (thousands) adenomatous polyps in the colon and rectum. The polyps do not usually occur in the first decade. The appearance of the polyps is identical with the adenomatous polyp of the adult, i.e. it is a benign epithelial tumour, which left alone, will undergo malignant change.

Similar adenomatous polyps occur in the colon and also in the stomach and small intestine as a manifestation of Gardner's syndrome (Gardner 1951). This syndrome also has an autosomal dominant inheritance. Other manifestations are multiple osteomas, epidermoid cysts and desmoid tumour. Some authors (Bussey et al 1978) regard familial p. coli as an incomplete manifestation of Gardner's syndrome. The risk of malignant change in polyps is extremely high, approaching 100% with time. After the age of 10 years, follow-up of affected individuals must be meticulous and is best done in a specialized unit. The decision about colectomy which is usually carried out in the second decade will be affected by the number and size of adenomas as well as the wishes of the individual and family. The rectum is usually retained and regular endoscopic examination undertaken.

There is firm evidence that there are families without evidence of colonic polyposis who are at increased risk (3–4 times) of developing colonic cancer compared with the rest of the population (Burt et al 1985).

Maligant tumours

Malignant tumours of the upper gastrointestinal tract are very rare in childhood and such children should be referred to specialist centres for confirmation of the diagnosis as well as for treatment. Tumours have been described in diverse sites and exhibit a variety of histological appearances (see Table 22.1). Clinical aspects are also discussed in Chapter 5.

Non-Hodgkin's lymphoma (NHL)

Intestinal lymphomas are invariably of B-cell type, presumably reflecting the predominance of 'B-dependent' lymphoid tissue associated with the intestine whilst T-cell tumours arise most commonly in the thymus and associated lymph nodes. The presenting features of abdominal NHL are

Table 22.1 Malignant tumours of the upper G. I. tract in children

	reference
Salivary gland	Krolls et al 1972
Rhabdomyosarcoma	
Non-Hodgkin's lymphoma	
Mucoepidermoid carcinoma	
Adenocarcinoma — actinic	
— cytochromic	
Tumours of the jaw	
Ewings sarcoma	
Osteogenic sarcoma	
Burkitt's lymphoma	
Odontogenic carcinoma	
Stomach	
Carcinoma	McNeer 1941
Pancreas	
Pancreatoblastoma (juvenile type carcinoma)	Horie et al 1977
Carcinoma	Taxy 1976

related to the site of origin. A few tumours, particularly those close to the ileocaecal junction, are unifocal and present with intestinal obstruction, and may result in intussusception (Berry & Keeling 1970). More frequently, the tumour is multifocal and many serosal tumour nodules are apparent at presentation; ascites is common. In advanced cases, the abdomen is 'frozen'. Pleural effusions, containing tumour cells, may be present in the absence of thoracic lymph node involvement. It is likely that unifocal and multifocal NHLs are part of a continuous spectrum of disease. A few ileo-caecal tumours have a follicular morphology rather than a diffuse pattern and have a better prognosis.

Diagnosis. Laparotomy should be avoided in children with multifocal intestinal lymphomas, as their general condition is usually poor. Examination of bone marrow aspirates, sometimes from several sites as involvement may be patchy, ascitic or pleural fluid and cerebrospinal fluid (CSF) for complete staging of disease is all that is necessary. Immunohistochemical staining of smears and cytospin preparations with monoclonal antibodies to identify lymphocyte subsets is sufficiently specific making tissue biopsy unnecessary in most cases.

Treatment. NHL spreads in a noncontiguous fashion and recurrence is usually at distant sites. Chemotherapy has, therefore, become the mainstay of treatment for all patients excepting the rare child with a follicular tumour. Local field radiation therapy is no longer indicated. A recent randomized controlled study has shown that radiation therapy to the original site of bulk disease offers no additional benefit (Mott et al 1984). Surgical excision of a single mass is indicated when the child presents with intestinal obstruction but there are conflicting views about the usefulness of 'debulking' surgery. It is likely that surgery like radiotherapy will be abandoned in the management of tumours with multifocal abdominal disease.

Chemotherapy regimes for NHL are based on high doses of cyclophosphamide with vincristine and methotrexate using folinic acid 'rescue' for adequate intrathecal therapy. Cytosine arabinoside, Adriamycin® and VM 26 and 6 mercaptopurine/6 thioguanine are also used. Because B-cell tumours are particularly sensitive to chemotherapy, patients are at risk of the tumour lysis syndrome (O'Regan 1977). Hyperuricaemia may occur despite prophylactic allopurinol together with hyperkalaemia and hyperphosphataemia during the first few days of chemotherapy. Despite awareness of these problems, some children die in the first weeks of chemotherapy from complications of this syndrome and some die from septicaemia during the period of myelosuppression. The majority (approximately 90%) will, however, survive and achieve complete remission.

Over 90% of children with stage II tumours and over half those with stage III will remain disease-free but those with very extensive stage III tumours and with stage IV disease usually relapse in the bone marrow or CSF. For these patients new 'aggressive' chemotherapy regimens usually incorporating high doses of cytosine arabinoside and methotrexate, and possibly bone marrow transplant procedures, are under study. Survival curves for patients with B-cell NHL show a 'plateau' after 12 months from the completion of therapy, and disease-free survival two years off treatment indicates almost certain cure. Current management is to treat for only six months, rather than for a longer period.

Other malignant lymphomas

It is extremely rare for Hodgkin's disease to involve the intestine in children. Whilst malignant histiocytosis is the commonest histological type of lymphoma to complicate coeliac disease in adults, no cases have been reported in children.

Carcinoma of colon

Carcinoma of the colon in children and young adults is much less common than in middle life and old age, and in children comprises between 0.3 and 1% of all colorectal cancers. When it does occur, it may arise de novo or be a complication of an inherited disorder such as multiple p. coli or Gardener's syndrome, or preexisting chronic inflammatory bowel disease (see ch. 6). The prognosis of colorectal cancer in children is poor with more than 95% of patients dying within five years, and most within 2 years of surgery because of metastatic disease (Anderson & Bergdahl 1978).

Carcinoid tumour

Only a very small proportion of carcinoid tumours occur in children. Over 90% of carcinoid tumours are clinically silent and the diagnosis is usually made following the discovery of a small mass in an appendicectomy specimen (Moertel 1983). Tumours are occasionally seen in other abdominal and nonabdominal sites but these are very rare in children. The size of the tumour is of major prognostic significance; those less than 1 cm in diameter being cured by excision whilst larger tumours are much more likely to recur. Carcinoid syndrome is usually seen in patients with large tumours and the full blown syndrome has not been reported in childhood although some systemic symptoms have been described.

HEPATIC TUMOURS

Benign tumours and tumour-like conditions

Benign space occupying lesions of the infant liver frequently present in the neonatal period and either die at that time or require no further treatment.

Hamartoma

A hamartoma is composed of tissue normally present in the site in which it arises, but they have an abnormal disposition and are in abnormal proportions. In the liver they probably represent the effect of fetal hypoxia or hypotension.

Liver hamartomata usually present in the first two years of life and many are found on routine examination of the infant either shortly after birth or during the ensuing months. There may be no symptoms other than a painless or slightly tender abdominal swelling. Occasionally large tumours may cause difficulties during delivery, or death from haemorrhage due to intrapartum trauma. Angiomatous hamartomata of the liver are a rare cause of neonatal jaundice (Claireaux 1960). A rapid increase in abdominal girth due to filling of cystic components with fluid or to haemorrhage into the tissue mass may occur and suggests a malignant tumour. In large angiomatous lesions arteriovenous shunting may cause high output cardiac failure (Bamford et al 1980). If the lesion is cystic, ultrasound appearances are distinctive and a malignancy can be confidently excluded; laparotomy may be necessary in order to distinguish between histologically benign lesions and hepatoblastoma. Serum alphafetoprotein levels are within the normal range.

Pathology. Two types of hamartoma are distinguished. The majority have a large vascular component and are variously called haemangioma and haemangioendothelioma, but careful examination shows that islands of hepatocytes and ductular structures often resembling portal triads are present (Fig. 22.1). Angiomas can be solitary or multiple and vary in size

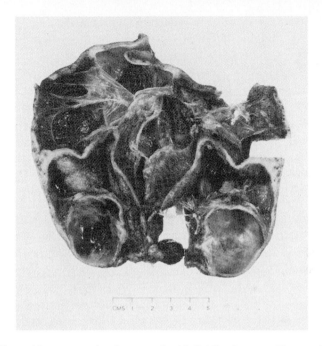

Fig. 22.1 Bisected hamartoma showing several epithelial-lined cysts and haemorrhages.

from 1 to greater than 15 cm. Small lesions are sometimes found incidentally at necropsy. The lesions may be encapsulated or they may merge
imperceptibly with normal liver at their periphery. A minority of hamartomata are composed of fluid-filled, epithelial-lined cysts (Fig. 22.1) whose
walls are composed of fibrous tissue containing bile ducts and islands of
liver cells (Srouji et al 1978).

Treatment. Surgery can be technically difficult but is curative if complete
excision is achieved. Treatment of large vascular lesions is particularly
difficult. Conservative management with digitalis and diuretics is usually
ineffective. Corticosteroids, radiation therapy (4–20 Gy) and hepatic artery
ligation or embolization have all been used successfully but the overall
mortality of the condition is high.

Adenoma

The adenoma is the only true benign tumour of the liver. It is uncommon,
but Type I glycogen storage disease and androgen therapy are recognized
predisposing causes. Angiographically, adenomas can seem vascular,
mimicking haemangioma or even malignancy.

The lesion may be single or multiple and range from 1–10 cm in diameter. Surgical excision of a solitary lesion results in cure. Histologically they
are composed of sheets of hepatocytes, often with adjacent areas of cells

with light and dark cytoplasm reflecting glycogen content. There are no portal triads within the nodules. Compression of surrounding liver, best seen with silver impregnation techniques for reticulin, may eventually produce a pseudocapsule. Adenomata may be difficult to distinguish from well differentiated hepatocellular carcinomas and probably account for the relatively good prognosis of that condition in some published series.

Focal nodular hyperplasia

Focal nodular hyperplasia (Stocker & Ishak 1981) affects girls more commonly than boys, and is usually asymptomatic although a few develop right upper quadrant pain. Imaging invariably shows a solitary lesion and surgery is curative. Histologically the tumours are nodular and aggregates of hepatocytes are separated by a characteristic stellate scar of fibrous tissue.

Benign teratoma

A small number of hepatic teratomata have been recorded, most occurring in infants less than 1 year of age (Witte et al 1983). Interpretation of serum α-fetoprotein results should take into account the child's age at the time of the sample. Surgery is curative.

Histiocytosis X

The exact incidence of liver involvement in this condition is difficult to determine but hepatomegaly is apparent at presentation in 10–20% of patients and develops later in another 10%. Histiocytes, admixed with lymphocytes and eosinophils infiltrate portal tracts. Jaundice is an uncommon but ominous sign, especially when it is accompanied by hypo-albuminaemia and a prolonged prothrombin time indicating early hepatic failure. Prognosis and management are discussed on pp. 495–496.

A histopathologically distinctive form of cirrhosis has been described in association with histiocytosis X (Leblanc et al 1981). It can evolve during or after the phase of active disease and should be suspected when the liver is clinically disproportionately large and hard. Portal hypertension compli-cated by varices and bleeding, commonly develops (Grosfeld et al 1976).

Maligant tumours

Primary liver malignancies account for less than 1% of all childhood cancer with an absolute incidence of only 10–15 per year in the UK, six times less common than Wilm's tumour. The majority are of hepatocellular origin (hepatoblastoma and hepatocellular carcinoma) but malignant tumours of the connective tissue (mesenchymal sarcoma) and biliary tree (rhabdomyosarcoma) and occasional malignant germ cell tumours, as well as rare predominantly hepatic manifestations of NHL, are also seen.

Hepatoblastoma

Hepatoblastoma is by far the commonest of the primary liver tumours in childhood and usually presents before the age of 3 years, although exceptionally it may occur in the older child (Ishak & Glunz 1967, Exelby et al 1975). Some tumours are undoubtedly congenital being recognized at birth or in the neonatal period. No generalized liver disorder has been reported in infants with hepatoblastoma nor has malignant change been found in a preexisting hamartomatous malformation. Children with Wiedemann–Beckwith syndrome are at increased risk of developing hepatoblastoma and there is 100-fold increase of dominantly inherited p. coli in families of children with hepatoblastoma (Kingston et al 1983). Hepatoblastoma has been described in several sibships.

The presenting symptoms include abdominal distension, vomiting and anorexia. Signs of precocious puberty may be present and both in vivo and in vitro production of chorionic gonadotrophin by hepatoblastoma has been demonstrated. A straight abdominal X-ray confirms hepatic enlargement and may show tumour calcification. An intravenous pyelogram should be performed to exclude Wilms' tumour. Liver scintillation scanning, inferior venacavography or hepatic arteriography will help to locate the tumour within the liver and distinguish between a solitary and a multifocal tumour. Arteriography may be of considerable assistance to the surgeon in anticipating possible planes of resection and may help to avoid extensive infarction of the liver which can be fatal following apparently complete resection of the tumour. α-fetoprotein estimation may be useful since elevated levels occur in hepatoblastoma as well as in hepatocellular carcinoma, whereas levels are normal in tumours metastasizing to the liver. Production of this protein by hepatoblastoma in tissue culture has also been demonstrated.

Biopsy is the only sure method of diagnosis. Open biopsy is preferred to needle biopsy since tumour samples may be confidently obtained and because of the danger from haemorrhage with such vascular tumours. As well as chorionic gonadotrophin and α-fetoprotein production, hepatoblastomas may secrete adenocorticotrophic hormone (ACTH) and insulin. Some tumours produce a megakaryocyte-stimulating factor and thrombocythaemia has been observed. Occasionally these tumours are accompanied by severe osteoporosis leading to fractures and suspicion of nonaccidental injury.

Pathology. Hepatoblastoma is an embryonic tumour of the infant liver comparable with nephroblastoma in its wide range of histological appearance. The tumour is a firm encapsulated brownish-tan mass and fibrous bands can be seen running across the cut surface. It occurs five times more commonly in the right lobe of the liver than in the left (Keeling 1971). The

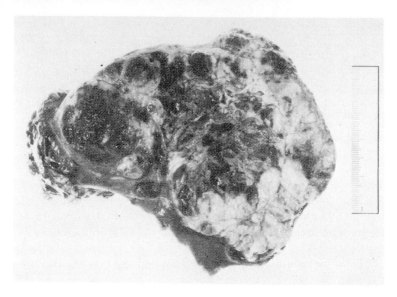

Fig. 22.2 Massive lobulated hepatoblastoma with multiple areas of haemorrhage (Keeling, 1971, by courtesy of the Editor of the *Journal of Pathology*).

tumour itself is a yellowish-tan and areas of haemorrhage several centimetres in diameter and of cystic degeneration are commonly seen (Fig. 22.2).

The histological types of hepatoblastoma are recognized which have prognostic and therapeutic connotation; a 'fetal' type where prognosis is relatively good (Fig. 22.3) and an 'embryonal' or mixed histological appearance where response to therapy is poor (Weinberg & Finegold 1983). The fetal pattern is as its name implies a pure epithelial tumour composed of relatively large cells which resemble fetal hepatocytes but are smaller than mature hepatocytes and are arranged in slender cords or trabeculae. Juxtaposed light and dark areas reflect cytoplasmic glycogen content. Embryonal tumours contain a mixture of cell types with areas resembling fetal hepatocytes together with smaller embryonal hepatocytes and foci of small dark staining cells with inconspicuous cytoplasm within which ductular structures may be found. These small dark cells are also capable of metaplasia to squamous cells and keratin pearls may be found within some tumours. Islands of osteoid may also be seen arising from the metaplastic bile duct cells. Sometimes, mineralization of the osteoid to bone may occur and this may be demonstrated radiographically. Embryonic mesenchyme is found in all hepatoblastomas if careful search is made.

Treatment. Chemotherapy can shrink most primary tumours (Weinblatt et al 1982) and probably eradicate small secondary deposits in the lung. Cure is rarely achieved without surgical removal of the primary tumour, and a radical procedure requiring accurate preoperative assessment with CT

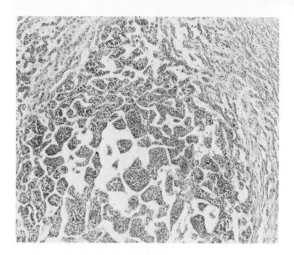

Fig. 22.3 Hepatoblastoma containing immature hepatocytes arranged in trabeculae (magnification × 31)

scanning and arteriography together with the services of an experienced paediatric surgeon are necessary. Multifocal tumours, especially when both lobes of the liver are affected, present problems for treatment. If the primary tumour can be controlled by chemotherapy and metastases do not appear, liver transplantation may be justified if the tumours remain inoperable. Because these tumours are so rare there are few reported studies of chemotherapy but vincristine, 5-fluorouracil, cyclophosphamide, Adriamycin® and cis-platinum are considered active agents. In a single-arm study, the United States Children's Cancer Study Group gave courses of vincristine, 5-FU, Adriamycin® and cyclophosphamide as adjuvant post-surgical therapy to patients with hepatoblastoma. Although the results for patients with stage III (macroscopic residual disease) and IV (metastases) tumours were disappointing with only 10–20% survival, the disease-free survival in stages I (complete removal) and II (microscopic residual disease) were 70–80%, which was a much better result than that achieved with single agent chemotherapy (Evans et al 1982). Recent case reports suggest that Adriamycin® and cis-platinum are currently the best adjuvants to surgery.

Hepatocellular carcinoma

Carcinoma of the liver, indistinguishable from the tumour found in adults, usually occurs in children over 6 years of age. Presenting symptoms include abdominal pain, vomiting, loss of weight and abdominal distension. Jaundice is uncommon in the early stages but often occurs terminally. Liver function tests are frequently normal but α-fetoprotein levels are usually elevated. Plain abdominal X-ray will confirm liver enlargement and other radiographic techniques can be used to localize the tumour. This tumour may arise in a previously apparently healthy liver or complicate other liver disease and metabolic disorders involving the liver. Carcinoma has been observed in livers with preexisting cirrhosis, extrahepatic biliary atresia and intrahepatic biliary atresia. It has been recorded in a child in whom giant cell hepatitis in infancy progressed to cirrhosis. Metabolic disorders which have been complicated by liver cell carcinoma include tyrosinosis, glycogen storage disease, Neimann–Pick disease, alpha$_1$-antitrypsin deficiency and hereditary tubular dysplasia (de Toni–Fanconi syndrome).

Complications of hepatocellular carcinoma in childhood include severe generalized osteoporosis and increased concentrations of serum lipids. The osteoporosis is thought to result from a protein-sparing mechanism and may be accompanied by growth retardation. A return to radiological normality has been observed following hemihepatectomy.

Pathology. Hepatocellular carcinoma may occur as a single mass occupying most of the liver lobe which is potentially suitable for resection, or as multiple tumour nodules present throughout the whole of the organ. The tumours are lobulated, encapsulated, and yellow in colour. Histologically the tumour is composed of large cells with lightly staining reticular nuclei with prominent nucleoli and large amounts of pale yellow eosinophilic cytoplasm resembling hepatocytes. Often there is little nuclear or cellular pleomorphism. Tumour cells are frequently arranged in irregular-sized trabeculae and bile ducts are absent. Intracellular bile is present imparting a yellow colour to the tumour. Hepatocellular carcinoma metastasize widely and early to local lymph nodes and to the lungs. The fibrolamellar variant of hepatocellular carcinoma occurs in noncirrhotic liver and has a better prognosis. Serum α-fetoprotein is normal, but serum transcobalamin I is useful for diagnosis and follow-up.

Treatment. Treatment, which is less successful than that of hepatoblastoma, consists of hemihepatectomy and Adriamycin®. It may prolong survival by months when compared with the natural course of the disease but long-term survival is poor. Liver transplantation may become part of management, especially when carcinoma complicates metabolic disease (Starzl et al 1985).

Rhabdomyosarcoma

Less than 1% of all rhabdomyosarcoma occur in the biliary tree (Hays & Snyder 1965), and usually in children over the age of 6 years. Differentiation from other causes of obstructive jaundice, choledochal cyst, stricture and gall stones, can usually be made by cholangiography and abdominal ultrasound. Chest X-ray and sometimes CT scans of lung, bone scan and bone marrow examination should be performed to exclude metastases.

Pathology. The tumours are cream-coloured and firm in texture. Yellowish areas of cystic degeneration are frequently found but no liver-like tissue is present within the tumour. Translucent botryoid nodules of tumour may protrude singly or in groups into dilated bile ducts resembling the appearance of rhabdomyosarcoma in the urogenital tract. The tumour may be solitary but frequently multiple tumours are found which may be widely separated with apparently healthy bile ducts between them.

Histologically, these tumours are composed of large, elongated, mesenchymal cells having large nuclei with spectacular pleomorphism; the cytoplasm is often foamy. Tubules lined by cuboidal cells are scattered through the tumour and are frequently surrounded by a halo of mesenchymal cells. Cytoplasmic striations can be demonstrated by phosphotungstic acid-haematoxylin staining in strap-like and 'tadpole' cells, but are not as frequently seen as in rhabdomyosarcoma of the urogenital sinus.

Treatment. Interdisciplinary management with chemotherapy, radiotherapy and surgery has transformed the outlook for patients with rhabdomyosarcoma at other sites. Although biliary tumours metastasize rarely and the primary tumour is usually small, they have a poor prognosis related to difficulty in resection and a tendency to spread within the biliary tree. The proximity of the liver, a relatively radiosensitive organ, precludes the administration of radiation doses higher than 25–30 Gy. Combination chemotherapy with either vincristine, actinomycin D and cyclophosphamide, or ifosfamide, vincristine and actinomycin D, is given for 6–12 months. Rhabdomyosarcoma is notorious for late recurrence but most 5 year disease-free survivors are probably cured.

Mesenchymal sarcoma

An occasional primary hepatic tumour arising from mesenchyme rather than hepatocytes has been described. Presenting features are similar to those of hepatoblastoma although the mean age is rather older. The serum α-fetoprotein level is normal. Management is similar to that for rhabdomyosarcoma.

Metastatic tumours in the liver

Metastatic tumours of the liver in children are much commoner than primary tumours. They are often asymptomatic and usually detected during routine staging investigations. although occasionally they cause marked hepatic enlargement in the presence of an unobtrusive primary tumour.

Factors which influence the site of tumour metastases are ill understood, but neuroblastoma frequently metastasizes to the liver whilst it is much less common for nephroblastoma and sarcomas to do so.

Neuroblastoma

Two patterns of metastatic involvement of the liver are recognized in

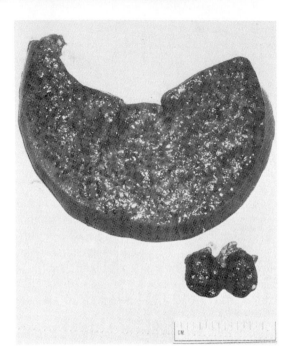

Fig. 22.4 Hepatomegaly results from diffuse involvement of the liver by metastatic tumour. The adrenal primary tumour is small.

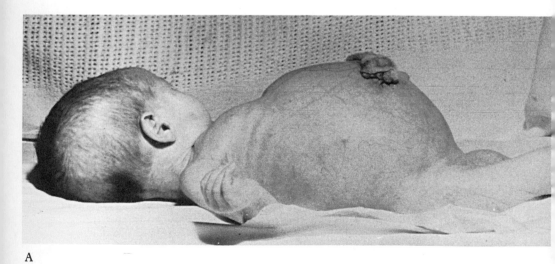

A

Fig. 22.5 Child with Stage IVs neuroblastoma. The primary adrenal tumour was small but there is massive liver infiltration (Fig. 22.5a). Respiratory distress was relieved by creation of an abdominal hernia, using Silastic® patch (Fig. 22.5b). The baby made a complete recovery.

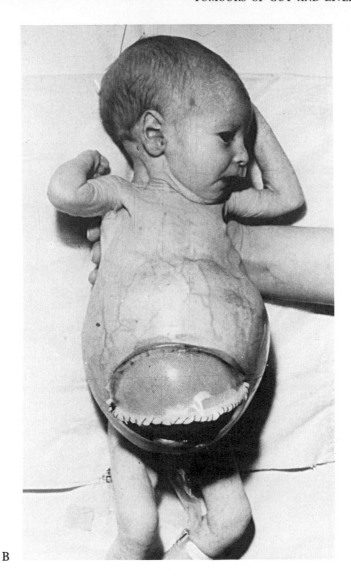

B

neuroblastoma. Focal deposits seen in stage IV disease commonest in children age 3–4 years, and diffuse infiltration (Fig. 22.4) stage IVs (s = special) (D'Angio et al 1971) which is virtually restricted to the first year of life. The extent of tumour infiltration is variable. In some cases the liver is only marginally enlarged while in others massive involvement may cause life-threatening respiratory embarrassment, (Fig. 22.5a and b) and filtration is so extensive that it is hard to identify normal hepatocytes on biopsy yet jaundice and other evidence of liver dysfunction is exceptional.

Some argue that all infants with stage IVs neuroblastoma should receive chemotherapy because a) The distinction between stage IV and IVs disease is not always clear cut b) Some infants die of respiratory or renal embarrassment and c) a number of children, whose IVs disease has previously undergone spontaneous remission, have relapsed at a later date with true stage IV disease. Most series, however, confirm that 60–80% of these babies undergo remission without any therapy or only low dose hepatic irradiation (Evans et al 1980). It therefore seems reasonable to adopt a policy of conservative management in asymptomatic children. Regression of hepatomegaly may take 3–12 months but liver function remains normal. The primary tumour is usually resected later. There is little information available about progressive changes in the liver; return to normality is usual, but cirrhosis has been described. It is not clear whether the cirrhosis is due to the tumour, or the treatment (especially postradiotherapy).

Leukaemia and lymphoma

Whilst there is no precise information about liver involvement based on liver biopsy appearances, most children with acute lymphoblastic leukaemia have liver enlargement and are presumed to have diffuse liver involvement at diagnosis. Perhaps because it indicates a large tumour load, the presence of hepatosplenomegaly is an adverse prognostic feature, independent of presenting blast cell count (Palmer et al 1980). Evidence of liver dysfunction is exceptional. Liver involvement in NHL is much less common (only 10–20% of our cases), and disease can be diffuse or multifocal. A patient presenting with hepatomegaly rarely proves to have NHL involving the liver alone (Miller et al 1983). The diagnosis should be suspected in a systemically unwell 5–10 year old boy where there is diffuse lymph node enlargement, especially if ascites is present. Response to chemotherapy is usually good and overall survival is over 50%. Two years disease-free survival following treatment usually equates with a permanent cure.

The liver is almost always involved in malignant histiocytosis and hepatomegaly with jaundice is seen in some patients. Response to combination chemotherapy and long-term survival is now being achieved.

Hepatic involvement in Hodgkin's disease in children is extremely uncommon and although hepatomegaly may be present involvement is focal.

Other tumours

Other tumours sometimes spread to the liver in children. Only 3–4% of patients with Wilms' tumour have liver secondaries at diagnosis and there is no association with a particular histological subtype. Single metastatic deposits may be surgically resectable but multiple metastases usually respond poorly to treatment.

ENTEROTOXICITY

Pathophysiology

Radiation therapy and chemotherapy inhibit cell division and therefore affect normal tissues with rapid cell turnover rates, such as bone marrow and oral and intestinal mucosa. The recent introduction of more aggressive treatment for child cancers — including 'massive therapy' with or without total body irradiation (TBI) — has inevitably led to an increased incidence of damage to both large and small bowel. Although irradiation can affect enterocytes at all stages of maturation, the primary target for most drugs is the enteroblast (Shaw et al 1971). Toxicity is both dose- and time-related. Sustained enteroblast mitotic inhibition prevents normal cell turnover. As a result, hypoplastic villus atrophy and even mucosal sloughing occur. Retarded drug elimination, because of renal failure for example, may enhance toxicity. This potential complication of high dose methotrexate (MTX) can be avoided by careful monitoring of plasma drug levels and the use of folinic acid rescue. Local intestinal toxicity may also be a problem, and there is evidence that enterohepatic recycling of MTX may produce a topical effect (Pinkerton et al 1985).

Prior treatment with radiosensitizing drugs such as Adriamycin® may increase the enterotoxicity of abdominal irradiation (Schenken et al 1979). Paradoxically, low dose cyclophosphamide given a few days before high dose melphalan reduces enterotoxicity in the experimental animal (Millar et al 1978). The mechanism of this 'priming' effect is unknown and, although used in clinical practice, its value is uncertain.

Acute enterocolitis

Severe toxicity may occur soon after high dose treatment with a number of single agents, e.g. melphalan, cyclophosphamide or with combinations of drugs such as cytosine arabinoside, daunorubicin and thioguanine. Its onset is related to the development of mucosal hypoplasia, usually around 5–7 days after treatment. Presenting features range from transient abdominal pain with or without loose stools to florid enterocolitis with severe colic and high volume, secretory diarrhoea. Stools may contain mucus or blood and in severe cases complete mucosal casts may be passed. Pain is a prominent feature and may be so severe that opiates are required. Vomiting is uncommon. The duration of the symptoms is dependent on both the drugs used and the length of time they are used for. Recovery only occurs when enteroblasts turn over once again. Once mucosal regeneration has occurred symptoms remit rapidly. The major causes of morbidity and mortality are secondary: septicaemia, fluid and electrolyte disturbances, intestinal perforation and haemorrhage. At necropsy, deep, haemorrhagic ulcers are seen in both large and small intestine (Fig. 22.6).

Anticipation of specific problems associated with particular intensive

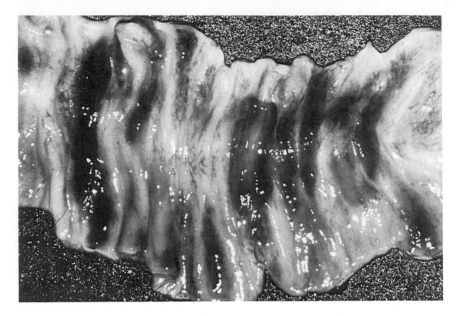

Fig. 22.6 Necropsy specimen of colon from a 12-year-old girl who developed severe haemorrhagic diarrhoea and septicaemia after intensive chemotherapy for acute myeloid leukaemia (daunorubicin, cytosine arabinoside, thioguanine). Multiple deep ulcers and areas of mucosal denudation were found, in addition to the generalized inflammation and haemorrhage.

treatment regimes, recognition of early symptoms and prompt intervention may be life-saving. Trivial symptoms may accompany rapidly progressive disease; secretion of fluid into the bowel lumen can cause profound hypovolaemia even in the absence of overt diarrhoea. The fluid and electrolyte disturbances are similar to those seen in any acute enteritis, although renal dysfunction following hypovolaemia, sepsis or antibiotics, especially amphotericin and aminoglycosides, may cause additional problems. Fluid replacement should be parenteral and monitoring of central venous pressure may be the only effective way to assess fluid balance. Symptomatic relief by loperamide has been reported in radiation-induced diarrhoea, but in high dose (greater than 1 mg/kg body weight) an ileus may occur. Opiates should be prescribed cautiously for severe pain. Patients are often in precarious nutritional balance and full parenteral nutrition is necessary when diarrhoea persists for more than a few days.

The 'acute abdomen'

The management of the 'acute abdomen' in a child who has received intensive chemotherapy requires a delicate balance between conservative supportive care and surgical intervention. Early examination and frequent reassessment by an experienced paediatric surgeon is essential. It is important to rule out common paediatric surgical emergencies. Localized tenderness or peritonism is unusual in uncomplicated cases and if the timing of symptoms is atypical, another aetiology should be sought. In cytotoxic drug-related enteritis early laparotomy may reveal an extensively inflamed and friable gut and do more harm than good. On the other hand, repair of localized perforation or resection of infarcted or necrotic bowel may be life-saving. Operative mortality in the immunosuppressed child has decreased substantially and encouraged early intervention (Schaller & Schaller 1983). Once the neutrophil count returns to normal, the patient's condition improves dramatically. Late complications such as adhesions or fistulae may lead to recurrent abdominal pain or obstruction and require surgical relief.

The damaged bowel offers easy access to bacteria, and septicaemia due to enteric organisms including *Escherichia coli*, *Pseudomonas*, *Klebsiella* and enterococci is common. The value of gut sterilization with oral colistin, neomycin, gentamicin and co-trimoxazole is controversial (Jacoby 1982) and in children its use is limited by oral drug tolerance, the development of resistant strains, the emergence of unusual pathogens and unwanted effects of the antibiotics on the intestine itself. An alternative strategy is careful surveillance of the gut flora with regular stool cultures to isolate all organisms and determine their sensitivities. Organisms which are normally regarded as nonpathogens must be included in such a screen. In this way it may be possible, in the absence of positive blood cultures, to prescribe rationally rather than empirically. Moreover regular stool screening may lead to identification of resistant strains. When diarrhoea is bloody, in the absence of thrombocytopenia, *Clostridium difficile* should be sought by both culture and toxin assay. Early treatment with oral vancomycin is indicated if a toxin-secreting organism is found. Intravenous metronidazole should be given in addition to broadspectrum antibiotics when there is fever with diarrhoea, as the risk of anaerobic septicaemia is high. Antibiotics should only be used in the face of infection or proven bacterial overgrowth.

The development of mouth ulcers is a common problem after chemotherapy and scrupulous attention to oral hygiene, with regular mouthwashes, is essential. Secondary infection with herpes simplex is usually responsive to acyclovir. Oral candidiasis is treated with topical Fungizone® or miconazole.

In the neutropenic patient, dysphagia and retrosternal pain suggest fungal oesophagitis. Barium swallow shows irregularity and narrowing of the oesophagus. Unless early systemic treatment is instituted with amphoteracin, systemic candidiasis may develop. In cases where the diagnosis is in doubt oesophagoscopy may be useful, and may help distinguish herpetic oesophagitis. Intestinal candidiasis can also occur and may cause ulceration and haemorrhage.

Malabsorption and diarrhoea

Morphological abnormalities of the intestinal mucosa are present in many patients on cytotoxic therapy, but only a minority are clinically relevant. Diarrhoea is the dominant symptom. It may occur at any stage and is unrelated to the cumulative drug dose. Symptoms usually disappear within days of stopping treatment but in some diarrhoea may be prolonged and require specific treatment. Protracted diarrhoea may occur after infective enteritis when continuing therapy prevents mucosal repair (Pinkerton et al 1983). Either overt steatorrhoea or loose watery stools may be present. Failure to thrive with progressive weight loss over several months in the absence of diarrhoea has been described. A jejunal biopsy may show partial villus atrophy or may appear completely normal. It has been suggested that the enteropathy may be due to folate deficiency following the use of folate antagonists.

The histological changes associated with chemoradiotherapy are well documented (e.g. Trier 1962, Pinkerton et al 1982) but the clinical picture is so characteristic that jejunal biopsy is rarely required. Jejunal intubation is, however, useful for the demonstration of pathogens such as *Giardia* which might be amenable to treatment. Stool examination and culture for common and unusual pathogens including viruses is essential. *Cryptosporidium* has been implicated as a causal factor in acute and protracted diarrhoea in immunocompromized patients (Miller et al 1984). Abnormalities of xylose transport and of small intestinal permeability have been demonstrated (Craft et al 1977, Pearson et al 1984) and may be useful in detecting subclinical malabsorption and for monitoring recovery, although simple parameters such as weight gain and stool frequency are usually adequate.

When significant malabsorption occurs, withdrawal of chemotherapy is usually a prerequisite for mucosal recovery but rarely for more than two weeks. When severe, parenteral nutrition may be used but when diarrhoea is not marked, oral or nasogastric feeding may be more appropriate. Exclusion of lactose, cow's milk, egg protein and reduced fibre is advisable, even though the hypothesis that transport of macromolecules across the damaged mucosa in chemotherapy enteropathy may lead to subsequent food intolerance (Donaldson 1977) remains unproven. Simple lactose intolerance is however a common concomitant of the enteropathy.

HEPATOTOXICITY

Liver dysfunction may be extra or intrahepatic (Table 22.2), the latter being commonly due to drugs or infection. Systemically administered drugs reach the liver via the hepatic artery whilst oral agents arrive in portal venous blood. The activity and toxicity of many drugs is affected by hepatic metabolism.

Table 22.2   Jaundice in children on cancer therapy

Extrahepatic origin:	Congestive cardiac failure Pancreatitis Intra-abdominal sepsis
Hepatic origin:	Metastatic disease Viral hepatitis A or B, Cytomegalovirus, Epstein-Barr virus Drug-induced abnormalities Veno-occlusive disease Graft-versus-host disease

Drug-related liver damage

The pattern of liver damage by a variety of cytotoxic drugs used in children is shown in Table 22.3. Many agents are cell-cycle specific and would not be expected to be hepatotoxic. Retention and concentration of toxic metabolites and interaction with cytoplasmic proteins may however be responsible.

Direct toxicity usually results in fatty degeneration and portal fibrosis, and occasionally progresses to cirrhosis. It may occur with long-term MTX treatment (Topley et al 1979) and the cumulative dose appears to be the critical factor. Whilst elevated serum transaminase and alkaline phosphatase (AP) activities may be difficult to interpret in the growing patient they are of little clinical significance in the absence of hepatomegaly, jaundice or splenomegaly. High dose MTX therapy is often followed by transient, marked elevation of transaminase levels, but these usually fall quickly to normal.

Transient elevation of liver enzymes have been described after vincristine

Table 22.3   Predominant patterns of drug-related hepatotoxicity

	Hepatocellullar	Cholestatic	Veno-occlusive
Irradiation	★		★
Methotrexate	★		
6MP and thioguanine	★	★	
M Amsacrine	★	★	
Dimethyl triazeno imidazole carboxamide (DTIC)★	★		
Bis-chloronitrosourea/chloro-ethyl cyclohexyl nitrosourea (BCNN/CCNU)	★	★	
Chlorambucil	★	★	
Busulphan		★	★
Melphalan			★
Cytosine		★	★
Daunorubicin	★		
Asparaginase	★		
Vincristine	★		

therapy and a causal relationship clearly established (Saghir & Hawkins 1984). L-asparaginase may cause elevation of transaminases sometimes associated with hypoprothrombinaemia and abnormalities of liver-produced clotting factors. This may be drug hypersensitivity or its effect on protein synthesis. Dimethyltriazenoimidazole carboxamide (DTIC) may also cause a hypersensitivity reaction in the liver. Intrahepatic cholestasis may complicate treatment with 6-mercatopurine (6MP) or thioguanine and usually resolves on cessation of therapy.

The combined effect of drugs and hepatic radiation is of particular importance. This may be radiosensitization, e.g. actinomycin D, when a recall phenomenon is observed, or may be due to enhancement of toxicity when given in association with abnormal irradation, e.g. vincristine and Adriamycin®. Toxicity of drugs metabolized and excreted by the liver. e.g. vincristine, Adriamycin®, daunorubicin and VP16 may be increased when there is liver dysfunction. Dose modification may then be necessary (Perry 1984).

Hepatitis

The frequent use of blood and blood products such as fresh frozen plasma, platelets and granulocytes increases the risk of blood-born hepatitis. As a result of donor screening, hepatitis B infection is uncommon and cyto-megalovirus (CMV) transmission is of more concern in the profoundly immunosuppressed patient. In some centres CMV-negative blood is available but it is expensive and may be difficult to obtain.

Hepatic veno-occlusive disease (HVOD)

This syndrome has been described after several intensive therapy regimes including total body irradiation, melphalan, busulphan and combinations such as daunorubicin, cytosine arabinoside and thioguanine (McDonald et al 1984). Early symptoms are unexplained weight increase, fever, oliguria and a tender liver; hepatosplenomegaly, abdominal distension and ascites are apparent. Liver function tests are variable, though severe hypoprotein-aemia is common. Abdominal ultrasonography may show a 'bright' liver but venous occlusion is rarely visualized unless there is associated extra-hepatic venous thrombosis. After allogeneic bone marrow grafting, HVOD is usually distinguishable from graft-versus-host disease (GVHD) by its earlier onset, pattern of symptoms and absence of extrahepatic manifes-tations of acute GVHD. HVOD may persist for several weeks and is usually self-limiting, but may contribute to death following intensive chemoradio-therapy. Histologically, centrilobular haemorrhage is seen and subintimal vascular proliferation leads to obliteration of venules.

Therapy comprises parenteral nutritional and regular plasma infusion.

Spironolactone may be of value when there is secondary hyperaldosteronism being primarily vascular in origin, but the ascites is resistant to most measures. The role of prophylactic heparin in this condition is controversial (Cahn et al 1985) and has not been critically assessed.

Graft-versus-host disease

High dose chemotherapy and TBI with bone marrow transplantation are currently used in a number of patients with a high risk of disease relapse, such as those with acute myeloid leukaemia, 'high count' acute lymphoblastic leukaemia (ALL) and disseminated solid tumours. GVHD results from the transfer of mature donor T-lymphocytes in bone marrow which attack recipient organs, particularly the skin, liver and gut.

Abnormal liver function tests, of either obstructive or hepatocellular origin, may be the first indication of acute GVHD. A generalized erythematous rash, particularly prominent on the palms and soles with extensive desquamation may occur. Jaundice and severe liver dysfunction with coagulation abnormalities may arise later. These signs occur 10–20 days after treatment and must be distinguished from CMV and hepatitis B infection. Liver biopsy will show the characteristic histological features of GVHD which include periportal lymphocyte infiltration and cellular atypia of small bile ducts. Focal parenchymal necrosis may occur (Slavin & Santos 1973, Farthing et al 1982). Gastrointestinal symptoms vary from a few loose motions to florid enterocolitis. Intestinal GVHD is usually distinguishable from drug-induced damage by its timing: the enterotoxic effects of irradiation and chemotherapy occur within a few days of ablative treatment, whilst GVHD is usually maximal around the time of graft take (15–20 days). Patients who have received allograft bone marrow are at risk of infection and it is important to exclude viral and bacterial causes of gastrointestinal disease. Histological features of acute intestinal GVHD can be seen in rectal biopsies. Features include necrosis of crypt glandular epithelium with extensive lymphocytic infiltration of the lamina propria (Slavin & Santos 1973).

Treatment of acute GVHD with high dose intravenous methylprednisolone (1–2 g/m^2) given daily for up to 3 days is usually effective but may cause glycosuria and hypertension. Oral prednisolone (2 mg/kg) is therefore substituted as soon as possible.

Chronic GVHD developing 3–18 months after grafting either succeeds acute GVHD or develops de novo (Derg 1984). The skin is almost invariably involved with dryness, depigmentation and a variety of maculopapular lesions. After several months, progressive sclerosis occurs often with debilitating joint contractures. Lichen planus-type lesions may occur in the oral mucosa and oesophagitis occasionally leads to stricture formation. Weight loss occurs in up to 50% of patients with chronic GVHD and although an enteropathy has been described, it is often multifactorial and related to anorexia, general ill health and alterations of intestinal flora associated with immunological dysfunction.

Chronic GVHD usually responds to long term steroid therapy or oral azothioprine. In severe cases the disease is intractable and mortality is around 25%.

Vomiting

Most cytotoxic agents are emetic and, although electrolyte imbalance and nutritional impairment do occur, it is the effect on the quality of life during treatment and on the child's attitude to therapy which is important. Anticipatory vomiting is a manifestation of the input from higher nervous centres and can occur minutes or hours prior to therapy. Drug-induced vomiting may occur during administration or several hours afterwards and may last from a few minutes to 2–3 days. Some agents, such as cisplatinum, cyclophosphamide and the anthracyclines are almost invariably emetic whilst vinca alkaloids rarely even cause nausea. Nausea and vomiting with antimetabolites may be dose-dependent. Low-dose MTX and cytosine arabinoside are well tolerated but dose elevation to several g/m^2 will usually produce vomiting. Similarly massive therapy regimens with bone marrow transplant require heavy sedation and intensive antiemetic treatment.

Assessment of antiemetic agents is difficult, and particularly in children (Trounce 1983, Morrow 1984). Antihistamines and metaclopramide are the most widely-used agents. High-dose metaclopramide and high-dose dexamethasone are useful for in-patient management (e.g. *cis*-platinum) but the former may be complicated by extrapyramidal side effects and both are difficult to control in the out-patient setting. Domperidone is helpful in some, but may be cardiotoxic. Delta-9-tetrahydrocannabinol has also been used and appears to be effective in some patients but is not readily available (Perry 1984).

It is important to achieve adequate antiemetic control during the first course of chemotherapy, as initial experiences greatly influence subsequent tolerance. With some drugs, e.g. cyclophosphamide, prehydration of the patient may reduce the severity of nausea and vomiting. Where treatment is given as an in-patient, sedative cocktails may be useful. With out-patients, an initial parenteral dose of antiemetic followed by regular oral or rectal administration for up to 24 hours is often successful. Some children find the sedative and psychotropic effects of the antiemetics themselves most unpleasant. A significant proportion would prefer to 'vomit and be done with it'!

HORMONAL EFFECTS OF TUMOURS ON GASTROINTESTINAL TRACT

Carcinoid syndrome (see also Ch. 5)

Carcinoid tumour is rare in childhood and, as indicated earlier, metastasizing carcinoids have been reported only very occasionally. The 'carcinoid syndrome' is the result of the production of physiologically active metabolites by about 10% of tumours. Diarrhoea, a well known feature of the syndrome, is thought to be due to secretion of serotonin which also gives rise to hypertension, arthropathy and endomyocardial fibrosis. Bradykinin and prostaglandins cause flushing whilst histamine may produce bronchospasm. Measurement of 24-hour urinary 5-hydroxy indole acetic acid can assist tumour diagnosis and the monitoring of treatment.

Those experienced in management of the syndrome in adults stress the need for a conservative approach. Symptomatic treatment with codeine, Lomotil® or loperamide is often successful, at least temporarily. Only in exceptionally severe cases are trials of inhibitors of serotonin release (e.g. parachlorophenylalanine), specific serotonin antagonists (e.g. cyproheptadine and methysergide) or corticosteroids indicated. Antitumour therapy is sometimes indicated; streptozotocin and 5-fluorouracil are the most useful agents.

Vasoactive intestinal polypeptide (VIP) hypersecretion

Diarrhoea is a rare symptom in newly-presenting patients with neuroblastoma and probably only occurs with VIP-secreting tumours. It is not related to catecholamine secretion. VIP is a gastrointestinal hormone, secreted by cells of 'APUD' origin. Hypersecretion leads to watery diarrhoea, often so severe as to be cholera-like, as well as hypokalaemia and gastric achlorhydria. In adults 'VIPomas' most often arise in the pancreas but in children neurogenic tumours (Tiedemann et al 1981) are the commonest cause of elevated plasma VIP levels. Immunohistochemical studies, using peroxidase-linked anti-VIP antibodies, show that VIP production is limited to the more differentiated components of these tumours, particularly ganglion cells (Mendelsohn et al 1979). VIP hypersecretion is thus almost exclusively associated with localized differentiated neural crest tumours, in ganglioneuroma and ganglioneuroblastoma, and may be interpreted as a favourable prognostic feature in neural crest tumours. The surgical removal of the offending tumour is usually curative. Experience of medical management of symptomatic VIP secretion in children is very limited. Streptozotocin can be helpful in adult 'VIPomas' but is not effective in neuroblastoma. Other agents such as corticosteroids, somatostatin and analogues, indomethacin and interferon are worth using to control the diarrhoea when surgery or chemotherapy are unsuccessful.

Zollinger–Ellison syndrome (see also Ch. 5)

Gastrin overproduction by a nonislet cell adenoma or carcinoma leads to gastric hypersecretion with hyperchlorhydria and thereby to severe peptic ulceration. Diarrhoea may also be a major feature, possibly resulting from the associated VIP hypersecretion. Though very rare, the syndrome has been seen in children in whom the identification of the primary tumour can be as difficult as in adults, especially as tumours can be small and are often multiple (Rosenlund 1967). If a single lesion can be identified, radical excision is the treatment of choice. In cases where the primary tumour(s) either cannot be found or are multiple, H_2 blocking agents (ranitidine or cimetidine) should be tried prior to removal of the target tissue.

REFERENCES

Anderson A, Bergdahl L 1978 Carcinoma of the colon in children: a report of six new cases and a review of the literature. Journal of Pediatric Surgery 11: 967–971
Bamford M F M, de Bono D, Pickering D, Keeling J W 1980 An arteriovenous malformation of the liver giving rise to persistent transitional (fetal) circulation. Archives of Disease in childhood 55:244
Berry C L, Keeling J W 1970 Gastrointestinal lymphoma in childhood. Journal of Clinical Pathology 23: 459–463
Berry C L, Keeling J, Hilton C 1970 Coincidence of congenital malformation and embryonic tumours of childhood. Archives of Disease in Childhood 45: 229–231
Broadbent V, Pritchard J 1985 Histiocytosis X — current controversies. Archives of Disease in Childhood 60: 605–607
Burt R W, Bishop T, Cannon L A, Dowdle M A, Lee R G, Skolnick M H 1985 Dominant inheritance of adenomatous colonic polyps and colorectal cancer. New England Journal of Medicine 312: 1540–1544
Bussey H J R, Veale A M O, Morson B C 1978 Genetics of gastrointestinal polyposis Gastroenterology 74: 1325–1330
Cahn J Y, Flesch M, Plouvier E, Fréquence des maladies veino-occlusives du foie après greffe de moelle osseuse. La Presse Medicale 14:1520
Claireaux A E 1960 Neonatal hyper-bilirubinaemia. British Medical Journal 1: 1528–1534
Craft A W, Kay H E M, Lawson D N, McElwain T J 1977 Methotrexate induced malabsorption in children with acute lymphoblastic leukaemia. British Medical Journal 2: 1511–1512
D'Angio G J, Evans A E, Koop C E 1971 Special pattern of widespread neuroblastoma with a favourable prognosis Lancet i: 1046–1049
Derg H J 1984 Bone marrow transplantation: A review of delayed complications. British Journal of Haematology 57: 185–208
Donaldson S S 1977 Nutritional consequences of radiotherapy. Cancer Research 37: 2407–2413
Dozois R R, Judd E S, Dahlin D C, Bartholomew L G 1969 The Peutz–Jeghers Syndrome. Is there a predisposition to the development of intestinal malignancy? Archives of Surgery 98: 509–517
Evans A E, Chatten J, D'Angio G J, Gerson J M, Robinson J, Schnaufer L 1980 A review of 17 IV-S neuroblastoma patients at the Children's Hospital of Philadelphia. Cancer 45: 833–839
Evans, A E, Land V J, Newton W A, Randolph J G, Sather H N, Tefft M 1982 Combination chemotherapy (Vincristine, Adriamycin®, Cyclophosphamide, and 5-Fluorouracil) in the treatment of children with malignant hepatoma. Cancer 50: 821–826
Exelby P R, Filler R M, Grosfeld J L 1975 Liver tumors in children in the particular reference to hepatoblastoma and hepatocellular carcinoma: American Academy of Pediatrics Surgical Section Survey — 1974. Journal of Pediatric Surgery 10: 329–337
Farthing M J G, Clark M L, Sloane J P, Powles R L, McElwain T J 1982 Liver disease after bone marrow transplantation. Gut 23: 465–474
Gardner E J 1951 A genetic and clinical study of intestinal polyposis: predisposing factor for carcinoma of colon and rectum. American Journal of Human Genetics 3: 167–176
Grosfeld J L, Fitzgerald J F, Wagner V M, Newton W A, Baehner R L 1976 Portal hypertension in infants and children with Histiocytosis X. American Journal of Surgery 131: 108–113
Hays D M, Snyder W H Jr. 1965 Botryoid sarcoma (rhabdomyosarcoma) of the bile ducts. American Journal of Diseases of Children 110:595

Horie A, Yano Y, Kotoo Y, Miwa A 1977 Morphogenesis of pancreatoblastoma, infantile carcinoma of the pancreas. Report of two cases. Cancer 39: 247–254

Ishak K G, Glunz P R 1967 Hepatoblastoma and hepatocarcinoma in infancy and childhood. Report of 47 cases. Cancer 20: 396–422

Jacoby G A 1982 Perils of prophylaxis. New England Journal of Medicine 306: 43–44

Keeling J W 1971 Liver tumours in infancy and childhood. Journal of Pathology 103: 69–85

Keeling J W, Harries J T 1973 Intestinal malabsorption in infants with histiocytosis X. Archives of Disease in Childhood 48: 350–354

Kingston J E, Herbert A, Draper G J, Mann J R 1983 Association between hepatoblastoma and polyposis coli. Archives of Disease in Childhood 58: 959–962

Koretz R L 1984 Parenteral nutrition: Is it oncologically logical? Journal of Clinical Oncology 2: 534–541

Krolls S O, Trodahl J N, Boyers R C 1972 Salivary gland lesions in children: a survey of 430 cases. Cancer 30: 459–469

Leblanc A, Hadchouel M, Jehan P, Odievre M, Alagille D 1981 Obstructive jaundice in children with histiocytosis X. Gastroenterology 80: 134–139

McDonald G B, Sharma P, Matthews D E, Shulman H M, Thomas E D 1984 Venocclusive disease of the liver and bone marrow transplantation; diagnosis, incidence and predisposing factors. Hepatology 4: 116–122

McNeer G 1941 Cancer of the stomach in the young. American Journal of Roentgenology, Radium Therapy and Nuclear Medicine 45: 527–555

Mendelsohn G, Eggleston J C, Olson J L, Said S I, Baylin S B 1979 Vasoactive intestinal peptide and its relationship to ganglion cell differentiation in neuroblastic tumours. Laboratory Investigation 41: 144–149

Millar J L, Phelps T A, Carter R L, McElwain T J 1978 Cyclophosphamide pre-treatment reduces the toxic effect of high dose melphalan on intestinal epithelium in sheep. European Journal of Cancer 11: 1283–1285

Miller R A, Holmberg R E Jr, Clausen C R 1984 Life-threatening diarrhea caused by Cryptosporidium in a child undergoing therapy for acute lymphocytic leukemia. Journal of Pediatrics 103: 256–259

Miller S T, Wollner N, Meyers P A, Exelby P, Jereb B, Miller D R 1983 Primary hepatic or hepatosplenic non-Hodgkin's lymphoma in children. Cancer 52: 2285–2288

Moertel C G 1983 Treatment of the carcinoid tumor and the malignant carcinoid syndrome. Journal of Clinical Oncology 1: 727–740

Morrow G R 1984 The assessment of nausea and vomiting. Past problems, current issues, and suggestions for future research. Cancer 53: Supplement, 2267–2280

Mott M G, Eden O B, Palmer M K 1984 Adjuvant low dose radiation in childhood non-Hodgkin's lymphoma (Report from the United Kingdom Children's Cancer Study Group — UKCCSG). British Journal of Cancer 50: 463–469

O'Regan S, Carson S, Chesney R W, Drummond K N 1977 Electrolyte and acid-base disturbances in the management of leukemia. Blood 49: 345–353

Palmer M K, Hann I, Jones P M et al 1980 A score at diagnosis for predicting length of remission in childhood acute lymphoblastic leukaemia. British Journal of Cancer 42:841

Pearson A D J, Craft A W, Pledger J V, Eastham E J, Laker M R, Pearson G L 1984 Small bowel function in acute lymphoblastic leukaemia. Archives of Disease in Childhood 59:460

Perry M C 1984 Hepatotoxicity of chemotherapeutic agents In: M C Perry, J W Yarbro (eds) Toxicity of Chemotherapy. Grune & Stratton, Orlando pp. 297–315

Pinkerton C R, Cameron C H S, Sloan J M, Glasgow J F T, Gwevava N J T 1982 Jejunal crypt cell abnormalities associated with methotrexate treatment in children with acute lymphoblastic leukaemia. Journal of Clinical Pathology 35: 1272–1277

Pinkerton C R, Glasgow J F T, Dempsey S I 1983 Intractable diarrhoea associated with continuation of cytotoxic chemotherapy during acute infective enteritis. European Journal of Pediatrics 140: 68–70

Pinkerton C R, Booth I W, Milla P J 1985 Topical methotrexate alters solute and water transport in the rat jejunum in vivo and rabbit ileum in vitro. Gut 26: 704–709

Rosenluid M L 1976 The Zollinger–Ellison syndrome in children: a review. American Journal of Medical Science 254:284

Saghir N S, Hawkins K A 1984 Hepatotoxicity following Vincristine therapy. Cancer 54: 2006–2008

Schaller R T Jr, Schaller J F 1983 The acute abdomen in the immunologically compromised child. Journal of Pediatric Surgery 18: 937–943

Schenken L L, Burholt D R, Kovacs C J 1979 Adriamycin-radiation combinations: drugs induced delayed gastrointestinal radiosensitivity. International Journal of Radiation Oncology, Biology, Physics 5: 1265–1269

Shaw M T, Spector M H, Ladman A J 1971 Effects of cancer, radiotherapy and cytotoxic drugs on intestinal structure and function. Cancer Treatment Reviews 6: 141–151

Slavin R E, Santos G W 1973 The graft versus host reaction in man after bone marrow transplantation: pathology, pathogenesis, clinical features and implication. Clinical Immunology and Immunopathology 1: 472–498

Srouji M N, Chatten J, Schulman W W, Ziegler M M, Koop C E 1978 Mesenchymal hamartoma of the liver in infants. Cancer 42: 2483–2489

Starzl T E, Zitelli B J, Shaw B W Jr et al 1985 Changing concepts: Liver replacement for hereditary tyrosinemia and hepatoma. Journal of Pediatrics 106: 604–606

Stocker J T, Ishak K G 1981 Focal nodular hyperplasia of the liver: A study of 21 pediatric cases. Cancer 48: 336–345

Taxy J B 1976 Adenocarcinoma of the pancreas in childhood. Report of a case and a review of the English language literature. Cancer 37: 1508–1518

Tiedemann K, Pritchard J, Long R, Bloom S R 1981 Intractable diarrhoea in a patient with vasoactive intestinal peptide-secreting neuroblastoma. Attempted control by somatostatin. European Journal of Pediatrics 137: 217–219

Topley J M, Benson J, Squier M V, Chessells J M 1979 Hepatotoxicity in the treatment of acute lymphoblastic leukaemia. Medical Pediatric Oncology 7: 393–399

Trier J S 1962 Morphological alterations induced by methotrexate in the mucosa of human proximal small intestine. 11. Electron microscopic observations. Gastroenterology 43: 407–424

Trounce J R 1983 Antiemetics and cytotoxic drugs. British Medical Journal 286: 327–328

Weinberg A G, Finegold M J 1983 Primary hepatic tumors of childhood. Human Pathology 14: 512–537

Weinblatt M E, Siegel S E, Siegel M M, Stanley P, Weitzman J J 1982 Preoperative chemotherapy for unresectable primary hepatic malignancies in children. Cancer 50: 1061–1064

Witte D P, Kissane J M, Askin F B 1983 Hepatic teratomas in children. Pediatric Pathology 1: 81–92

Dorothy E. M. Francis

Oral nutrition

Children differ from adults because their nutritional intake must provide not only for the replacement of tissues but also for growth (Falkner & Tanner 1979, McLaren & Burman 1982, Forfar & Arneil 1984). The nutritional adequacy of any diet is determined by the clinical state, growth and development of the child. Nutritional problems are, therefore, most likely during periods of rapid growth, and are frequently related to infections and other catabolic states. The sick child during infancy or adolescence is therefore at greatest risk of growth failure and nutritional disorders.

NUTRITIONAL REQUIREMENTS

The recommended nutrient intakes for populations of healthy people are given by a number of organisations (WHO 1974, NRC 1980, Aggett & Davies 1983, DHSS 1985). The recommendation for any one nutrient presupposes adequacy of all other nutrients, including the trace minerals and vitamins for which recommended intakes are not listed. Changes occur with the alteration in the composition and nature of the diet. Allowance is made for the needs of normal growth in children. The first year of life is the most critical for growth and development and the need for all nutrients are at a maximum at this time. The largest proportion of energy and protein intake is needed for growth in early infancy (Fig. 23.1) but rapidly decreases to only 1% of energy intake needed for growth at $2\frac{1}{2}$ years of age (Renate & Bergmann 1979). Energy requirements for activity increase, however, though the latter is very variable in any one individual (Burman 1982). The optimal intake for an individual is that which satisfies need and

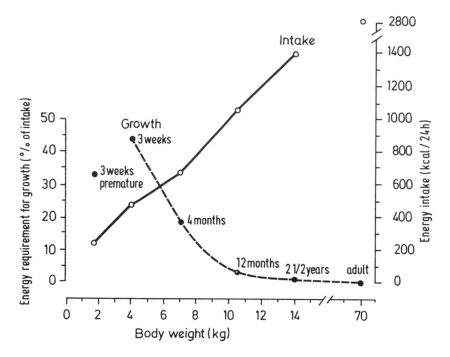

Fig. 23.1 Energy intake and percentage of energy required for growth, in relation to body weight. From Renate & Bergmann 1979.

allows for normal growth and activity. In some instances, excess is of little importance but in a few instances it may be harmful, e.g. excess vitamin D can cause hypercalcaemia.

Breast-feeding is strongly recommended during the first 6 months of life (DHSS 1983 Revision) as it not only provides adequate nutrition for growth (Ahn & MacLean 1980), but also protection against infection (Narayanan et al 1982, Holmes et al 1983) and may possibly protect against food intolerance (Soothill 1976). Weaning solids are normally introduced from about 4–6 months.

The recommended intakes do not cover additional needs arising from disease, for catch-up growth, malabsorption or metabolic abnormalities. Catabolism particularly increases the requirement of nutrients (p. 532). Restricted and synthetic diets require particular attention to be paid to all nutrients and supplements.

Protein

Protein is a source not only of energy but of nitrogen which is an essential part of all tissues, cells and enzymes. Protein requirements must be considered in conjunction with energy needs because unless fully met, protein will be used as an energy source rather than being available for essential functions and growth. Growth failure is frequently a consequence of protein energy malnutrition.

The amino group (NH_2) and the eight essential amino acids plus histidine in children cannot be synthesized by man, and must be provided in the diet (FAO/WHO 1973a and 1975). Several additional amino acids including cystine, tyrosine, arginine and possibly taurine, proline and glycine are considered semi-essential in young infants in whom enzyme systems are immature. Recently taurine has been considered essential at least in patients on long-term parenteral nutrition (Cooper et al 1984). Provided adequate nitrogen is available the nonessential amino acids can be synthesized in the body.

The optimal pattern of the essential amino acids for human protein synthesis is known as reference protein (FAO/WHO 1973a). A food protein whose amino acids pattern closely resembles this can be completely used for protein synthesis. Egg albumin and human milk closely resemble the reference protein pattern. Cereals, vegetable proteins, casein and some synthetic amino acid mixtures are limited in one or more essential amino acids and may only have a net protein utilization (NPU) score of 50–70, and therefore larger quantities of protein must be supplied in the diet to meet the needs for protein synthesis and growth. Better utilization of amino acids can be made for protein synthesis if complementary amino acids from different protein sources are given together.

The young infant has immature degradative enzymes in liver and kidney and as a result high protein intakes can lead to a raised blood urea, a high renal solute load and the risk of hypernatraemic dehydration or raised plasma amino acids (Smith & Francis 1982, DHSS 1983 Rev). Infants receiving human milk can maintain growth on approximately 1.8 g protein/kg per day in the first months of life and less by 6 months of age. Adults maintain nitrogen equilibrium on 0.35 to 0.45 g milk protein/kg per day providing energy and all other nutrient intakes are adequate.

Infants and patients fed enterally require a protein intake of high biological value. Infant feeds should mimic the amino acid profile of human milk or reference protein. The whey-based modified milk formulae have a higher biological value of protein compared to cow's milk because of their reduced methionine and phenylalanine, and increased cystine and arginine content. Many soya formulae contain little or no sulphur amino acids, thus methionine is often added to those formulae used for infant feeding to improve the protein quality, and some feeds are now also supplemented with taurine and/or carnitine. The amino acid formula Vivonex® does not however contain cystine or taurine, has a high osmolality and carbohydrate content and thus does not meet the nutritional need of young children. Casein-based formulae such as Portagen®, the older formula of Galactomin® MCT1® and Nutramigen® are high in protein but low in cystine and taurine and similarly are not recommended for young infants, whereas the hydrolysed casein formula Pregestimil® is supplemented with cystine, tyrosine and tryptophan and is one of the recommended formulae suitable for the young infant. Galactomin®, MCT (1)® and Nutramigen® are being reformulated in 1987. Hydrolysis and heat treatment of proteins reduces their sensitizing capacity and are preferable for patients at risk of allergy, if breast-feeding is not possible (McLaughlin et al 1981).

Energy

Utilization of protein for growth cannot occur unless adequate energy is provided. Likewise as the concentration of protein increases in the diet, the proportion used for body-building decreases; the remainder being used for energy. Diets should normally provide at least 10% of the energy as protein except in infants fed solely on human milk. Artificial feeds for the young infant should closely mimic the recommendations for breast milk substitutes (DHSS 1980).

The intake for each individual must supply the need for energy expenditure and growth and will depend on age, sex, physical activity and clinical condition and may vary widely from group recommendations (Heird et al 1972, Whitehead et al 1981, Grant & Todd 1982, McKillop & Durnin 1982).

For the majority of children a self-selected energy intake is appropriate and achieves satisfactory growth. Many young children benefit from 5 to 6 meals and snacks per day to ensure adequate opportunity to eat an appropriate intake. Modification by education on food priorities and high nutrient dense foods to encourage a better overall intake may be necessary (Francis 1986). Force feeding and concentrated energy supplements are not normally recommended. The nutrient content of dietary intakes can be calculated. This is particularly important for infants and young children on therapeutic regimes and for those with failure to thrive, in order to assess the adequacy of the nutrient intake for the individual.

Vitamins

The nutritional role of vitamins, the consequence of deficiency and excess intake are dealt with in many texts (Davidson et al 1979, McLaren & Burman 1982). Vitamins must be provided in an absorbable form. In some situations antivitamins compete with or inhibit the metabolic reaction in which the vitamin is involved or may be toxic themselves, e.g. avidin in uncooked egg white is an antivitamin to biotin. Drugs may also compete with or neutralize vitamins and also increase requirements. Vitamin K, niacin, riboflavin, B_{12} and folic acid are synthesized by the bacterial flora of the intestine but they are relatively poorly absorbed. Bacteria in the small intestine however also use dietary vitamins and make requirements difficult to determine. Synthetic diets alter the gut flora, and a change in dietary fibre intake, antibiotic therapy and infections can also alter bacterial flora and therefore the availability of vitamins. Catabolism increases requirements particularly of the water-soluble vitamins.

Therapeutic and synthetic diets, enteral and elemental diets must provide an adequate intake of all vitamins (Bunker & Clayton 1983, Francis 1986). Some diseases increase the need for supplements of a specific vitamin, e.g. folate in untreated coeliac disease; vitamin E in cystic fibrosis, vitamin A, E and K in hepatic failure.

In a few rare conditions a deficiency of a vitamin may result from an inherited deficit of absorption or metabolism, e.g. B_{12} and folate (Chanarin 1982), and vitamin E in abetalipoproteinaemia (Muller et al 1977, 1983).

Vitamin deficiency

Vitamin deficiencies are usually the result of insufficient vitamin intake or malabsorption. Rarely is a single vitamin deficient (except for vitamin D) and where a recognizable deficiency is identified, a severe lack of the vitamin can be assumed and may be associated with other vitamin deficiencies which are subclinical. Rashes and failure to thrive may result from deficiency of the lesser known vitamins (Mann et al 1965, Bunker & Clayton 1983, Francis 1986). Treatment with a comprehensive vitamin supplement is appropriate in order to prevent precipitation of other deficiencies, when the specific deficiency is corrected.

Vitamins in therapeutic diets

The artificial nature of many therapeutic diets will inevitably mean that certain essential vitamins will not be available from food and must therefore be provided as supplements. Comprehensive vitamin supplements such as Ketovite® tablets plus liquid or Cow & Gate vitamin-mineral supplementary tablets® are particularly useful. The complementary Ketovite® preparations are in a water miscible form free of carbohydrate, sorbitol and colouring agents, and are therefore suitable for most patients with various food intolerances. The Cow & Gate vitamin-mineral supplement tablets® need to be used in conjunction with a vitamin A and D preparation. They contain some trace minerals, and 70 mg sucrose per tablet as filler and are suitable except when traces of carbohydrates are significant, e.g. in patients with hereditary fructosaemia.

Minerals

The biological function of different minerals is well documented (FAO/WHO 1973b, Underwood 1977, Davidson et al 1979, McLaren & Burman 1982, Aggett & Davies 1983). A number of minerals including those required in so-called trace quantities are considered essential for man and include calcium, chlorine, chromium, cobalt, copper, iodine, iron, magnesium, manganese, molybdenum, phosphorus, potassium, selenium, sodium, sulphur, zinc. Others such as nickel, fluorine, tin, vanadium, silicon and arsenic have been reported essential in other mammals but direct evidence of a nutritional requirement in man is awaited (Davies 1981, Aggett & Davies 1983). Virtually every inorganic mineral is found in human tissue including the heavy metals, lead, mercury, cadmium and strontium.

Recommended allowances and estimated safe and adequate intakes have been suggested (NRC 1980, Aggett & Davies 1983, DHSS 1985) but no allowances for increased needs during illness are made, nor for the increased efficiency of absorption which may occur with low intakes. Any mineral in excess quantity may be toxic (Underwood 1977) but this is especially true of the heavy metals, e.g. cadmium, lead and mercury.

Factors influencing utilization and interactions of the trace minerals in nutrition have been recently reviewed (Aggett & Davies 1983, Chandra 1985, Francis 1986). For example, phytate which occurs naturally in many foods derived from plants has been recognized as a nutrient, because it contains phosphorus. It is however also toxic because it binds various essential minerals such as iron, calcium and zinc, and reduces their availability for absorption from the diet and reabsorption after their secretion in digestive juices (Wise 1983). The importance of identifying phytate as a major cause of mineral malabsorption lies in the widespread use of unprocessed bran and high fibre diets, especially in the treatment of constipation. To avoid the dangers of mineral imbalance, unprocessed bran should be avoided. A better source of fibre is wholemeal bread where the action of phytase in yeast considerably reduces the mineral-binding capacity of the phytate during fermentation. Alternatively, fruit, vegetables and unrefined cereals should be encouraged in high fibre diets. Dephytinized bran products are now becoming available and could be used if necessary (Andersson et al 1983). The increasing use in infancy of soya (isolate) formulae which contain phytate, necessitates their evaluation for trace mineral bioavailability.

Zinc and some other trace minerals are bound to proteins (Harzer & Kauer 1982) and may be removed during the manufacture of formulae. Organic supplements are often less well absorbed than their inorganic counterparts and therefore trace mineral deficiencies may result from otherwise desirable modifications.

The many interactions between trace minerals should be considered when planning dietary supplementation and trace mineral therapy (Aggett & Davies 1983). There should be a critical and practical evaluation of the level of trace elements provided by different diets, formulae, and parenteral nutrition. An evaluation, by trace mineral balance, of an 'in house' trace element supplement used with a casein-based formula, Galactomin®, highlights the difficulties encountered in devising supplements on theoretical grounds alone (Aggett et al 1983). The reduced bioavailability of zinc found when using a mineral mixture previously used in conjunction with the Comminuted Chicken (Cow & Gate)® based feed (Thorn et al 1978) is now thought to be related to the iron supplementation the infants were receiving before or during the balance studies (Aggett & Davies 1983).

Mineral deficiency

The risk of developing a deficiency depends on body reserves (Fell et al 1973). In the preterm infant such reserves have not accumulated, and this together with a high growth rate and inefficient absorption of trace minerals predisposes these infants to deficiency (Mendelson et al 1983).

Although it is relatively easy to confirm deficiencies associated with severe malnutrition marginal deficiencies are more difficult to detect and evaluation by calculated dietary intakes are inadequate due to the varying bio-availability and interaction of the minerals; clinical and laboratory criteria provide some indication but may only be confirmed in retrospect after correction of a defect following supplementation.

A number of situations predispose to a potential or actual deficiency of trace minerals. The most vulnerable infants are those with protein-energy malnutrition, with increased metabolic demands due to growth; malabsorption; catabolic states; and those on synthetic diets and or parenteral nutrition (Aggett & Davies 1983, Editorial Lancet 1983, Francis 1986).

Mineral supplements in therapeutic diets

The restriction of conventional foods and their replacement with synthetic substitutes as required in many therapeutic diets results in a reduction in mineral intake, and supplements may be needed. A single mineral supplement such as calcium in older children on a milk-free diet may suffice. For module and very restricted diets, either a comprehensive mixture is necessary or a combined vitamin-mineral supplement is required. Examples are given below:

(a) A comprehensive mineral mixture:
Aminogran Mineral Mixture® (Allen & Hanbury) and Metabolic Mineral Mixture® (Scientific Hospital Supplies) contain a range of macro and trace minerals but no chromium, selenium or nickel. They are contraindicated when an imbalance of minerals would occur because of the contribution of minerals from other sources. Care must be taken when they are used in infants so as to avoid a high renal solute load and hyperosmolar feed because of their sodium and potassium content.

(b) A combined vitamin-mineral supplement:
The new range of Seravit products combine vitamin and minerals including chromium and have recently become available from Scientific Hospital Supplies. They are currently being evaluated and may prove useful. They contain malto-dextrin as a carbohydrate base which must be included in calculations of the dietary regimen devised. Infant Seravit® (RD 222) contains selenium.

Essential fatty acids — EFA

Dietary fat and particularly vegetable oils provide an important source of EFA as well as energy in the diet. Linoleic acid, and possibly linolenic acid, are essential as they cannot be synthesized by man and must be provided in the diet. Deficiency leads to growth failure, skin changes with hair loses and an increase in metabolic rate (Hansen et al 1962). Steatorrhoea and low fat diets predispose to EFA deficiency. Although medium chain triglycerides (MCT) can be used as an energy supplement in the diet, they do not contain nor can they be metabolized to EFA, and thus a separate source of EFA must be included in the diet (see p. 548).

ACUTE INFECTION

Even minor intercurrent infections cause loss of appetite and in young children are often accompanied by diarrhoea and vomiting. It is important to prevent or correct dehydration with an oral rehydration solution (Booth et al 1984) (see Ch. 15). A temporary reduction in nutrient intake, apart from fluid and electrolytes, is insignificant in the majority of well nourished children but after the infection, losses must be made up to allow for catch-up growth. Usually the child's appetite is the best guide, provided ample opportunity is given to eat.

The parents of chronically ill children need guidance about an appropriate intake, replacements, and a list of priorities regarding different foods to offer, in order to prevent growth failure. This is particularly important if the child is on a therapeutic diet.

CATABOLIC STATES AND THE SEVERELY ILL CHILD

Children and particularly infants have far less body reserves of all nutrients including energy than adults (Heird et al 1972). Starvation is thus much more critical in infants and young children, than in adults

Table 23.1 Energy reserves during starvation in children of different ages compared to adults (data from Heird et al 1972)

| | Energy Reserve[1] | | Estimated No. days for total depletion of energy reserves | |
	kJ/kg	kCal/kg	Starvation	Partial starvation[2]
Small preterm infant	840	200	5	10
Large preterm infant	2500	600	12	32
Term infant	6700	1600	32	75
1 year-old child	9200	2200	42	110
Adult	7950	1900	90	400

[1] Non-protein energy + ¼ protein energy
[2] Partial starvation as represented by 10% dextrose supplying fluid requirement

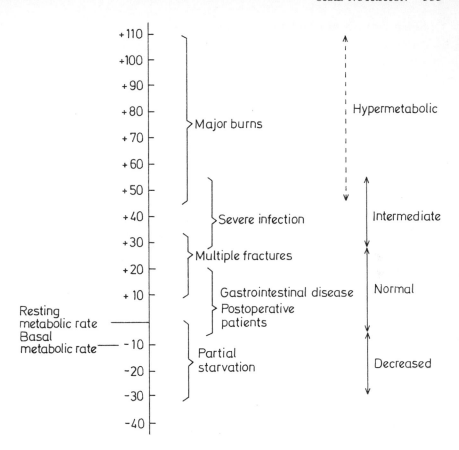

Fig. 23.2 Percentage change in resting metabolic rate in different clinical conditions in adults (modified from Elwyn 1980 cited in Enteral Parenteral Nutrition, Grant & Todd 1982).

(Table 23.1) (see Ch. 24). During starvation, glycogen stores are initially used, then fat and later protein to provide essential energy for basal metabolism (Grant & Todd 1982). The energy required by different organs of the body and the proportion needed by each varies with the weight of the patient. Brain metabolism requires approximately 65% of the basal metabolic energy in a 5 kg child and about 42% in a 20 kg child, compared to only about 25% in the adult (Heird et al 1972).

A summary of the changes in adult resting metabolic rates in different clinical situations is given in Figure 23.2 (Elwyn 1980). New protein synthesis is depressed and the rate of protein breakdown is increased (James 1981), with increased urinary nitrogen losses proportional to the severity of the illness (Cuthbertson 1980). Severe injury causes negative nitrogen balance and weight loss which cannot be prevented at the time of stress (Richards 1977). Protein depletion, sodium metabolic changes and potassium loss occur.

Severe catabolism with large nutrient losses result in poor wound healing, lethargy, anorexia, and impaired immune function with an increased risk of infections. Burman (1982), gives a guide to estimate the extent of protein catabolism:

If blood urea is constant;

g/24 hours urinary urea × 3.6

If the blood urea is rising;

g/24 hours urinary urea × 3.6 plus (rise in blood urea [g/litre] × 1.8 × kg body weight).

The primary aim of nutritional treatment is to provide fluid, maintain electrolyte homeostasis and give essential energy for basal metabolism, secondly to stop catabolism and correct nutritional deficiencies and thirdly to reverse catabolism to anabolism. In the anabolic phase, nutrient requirements are much higher than normal. Illness and tissue repair thus impose additional demands on the supply of nutrients and secondary nutritional deficiencies such as anaemia, vitamin deficiency and trace mineral depletion can subsequently result.

Nitrogen balance in seriously ill hypermetabolic patients can be improved by administering glucose, with exogenous insulin to maintain normoglycaemia (Woolfson et al 1979).

Nutrient requirements in the severely ill child

Nutritional requirements in the anabolic phase of illness are elevated, but estimates of intake can only be approximate. The child's daily weight, and clinical and biochemical state, with adjustment of intake appropriate for the severity of injury, should be used to ensure that the individuals requirements are met. Both energy and protein adjustments may be needed to maintain a positive nitrogen balance. Care must be taken to monitor the intake carefully in infants who have a low margin of tolerance both for excess as well as inadequate intake (Table 23.2).

Adequate intakes of fluid and electrolytes are essential and losses through urine, faeces and or skin must be corrected. Feeding actually increases water requirement because more urine is produced to excrete waste products and the total volume of feed is not the total fluid available, e.g. 100 ml milk provides only 87 ml free fluid.

Carbohydrate and fat can both be used to supply energy. Fat alone is ineffective at inhibiting protein breakdown for gluconeogenesis, but with some glucose it appears as effective at maintaining a positive nitrogen balance as glucose alone. To prevent ketosis, it is recommended that carbohydrate intake should always exceed that of fat and roughly an equal quantity of energy from both is recommended in enteral feeds (Elwyn 1980) unless either steatorrhoea or carbohydrate intolerance is present.

The osmolality of oral and enteral feeds should be as near that of plasma (approximately 300 mmol/kg) as possible and should not exceed

Table 23.2 A guide to nutrient intake for malnourished and catabolic infants.

Protein		0–6 months	3–4 g (maximum 6[1]) ⎫
		6–12 months	3–6 g (maximum 10[1]) ⎬ per kg actual weight per day.
Energy	high	0–6 months	540–630 kJ 130–150 kCal
	very high	6–12 months	630–900 kJ 150–220 kCal
Sodium	high ⎱	2.5 mmol ⎱ or as indicated biochemically	
Potassium	very high ⎰	3.0 mmol ⎰ and to meet faecal losses.	
Fluid (oral without IV)		200 (maximum 300) ml	
Calcium		At least 1.25–1.8 mmol/kg per day to 15 mmol per day 0.75–3 mmol/100 ml feed	
Phosphorus		0.5–1.9 mmol/100 ml feed	
Calcium : Phosphorus ratio		1.2:1 and not more than 2.2:1	
Magnesium		0.12–0.5 mmol/100 ml feed	
Iron[2]		0.18 mmol/day	
Zinc[2]		0–6 months 46 µmol/day	
		6–12 months 76 µmol/day	
Copper[2]		0–6 months 7.9–11 µmol/day ⎱ minimum	
		6–12 months 11–15.7 µmol/day ⎰ per day	
Vitamins at least normal requirement including:			
Thiamine		0.3 mg	
Riboflavin		0.4 mg	
Nicotinic acid equiv.		5.0 mg	
Total folate		50.0 µg	
Vitamin A retinol equiv.		450.0 µg	
Ascorbic acid		20.0 mg	
Vitamin D cholecalciferol		7.5 µg	

[1] Such high protein intakes will be partially used for energy and elevated blood urea or blood amino acids can occur; biochemical monitoring and adjustment of the intake is essential.

[2] Full details of trace mineral requirements and interactions are given by Aggett & Davies (1983). Higher intakes may be needed to compensate losses in malabsorption. Requirement of other minerals must also be provided with a full range of all essential nutrients (vitamins and EFA).

500 mmol/kg. High concentrations of carbohydrate (>15% mass/vol) increase the osmolality of the feed to unacceptable levels, and may precipitate an osmotic diarrhoea by exceeding the digestive and absorptive capacity of the intestine. In patients with impaired absorption and deficient proteolytic activity, and in those undergoing jejunal feeding, there may be advantages in providing protein as di- and tri-peptides from hydrolysed proteins of high biological value, as dipeptides are more rapidly absorbed than amino acids (Matthews 1975).

Choice of feeding the sick child

A patient who will not spontaneously take adequate nutrition from conventional meals should be encouraged to increase intake from extra appropriate snacks and drinks. Praise and reward should be used to encourage the child to eat, but reprimands are inappropriate. The dietary intake should be reviewed frequently. Supplements can be prescribed to make up deficits of energy, protein, vitamins and minerals, if the intake is still inadequate. Fortified drinks are particularly useful. A high protein intake without adequate total energy will result in the protein being used as an expensive source of energy, and the blood urea will rise. Energy intake without adequate protein will not totally prevent nitrogen losses, and growth and nutritional repletion will only occur if all nutrient needs are met. Protein depletion and an inadequate intake of nutrients are particularly common in the child with gastrointestinal disorders.

Fluid diets, enteral feeds and supplements

Infants and young children require individual assessment of their nutritional needs. An extra volume of an appropriate modified infant formula may be all that is necessary. However, in patients with increased nutritional needs due to malabsorption or catabolism, one of the following may be appropriate:

(i) selection of a higher protein modified milk or the 'follow-on' formula Progress® (John Wyeth Lab) after the first months of life. These can provide the basis of an enteral feed in older infants and toddlers.

(ii) selection of a 'preterm' formula which has a high nutrient density, e.g. Prematalac® (Cow & Gate). Osterprem® (Farley) may be inappropriate in these circumstances due to its very high vitamin D content.

(iii) a cautious increase in feed concentration, e.g. 15% dilution instead of the normal 13% reconstitution of Gold Cap SMA® (John Wyeth Lab) contains 1.8 g protein, 320 kJ (77 kCal)/100 ml.

(iv) a supplement of 3 g glucose polymer or 3 ml of a 50% fat emulsion (Calogen® or Liquigen®), can be added to each 100 ml of human milk or most infant formulae to increase the energy content to approximately 320 kJ

(77 kCal)/100 ml. It is essential to ensure an adequate volume of feed is taken to meet the protein and other nutrient requirements.

(v) Human milk can be fortified with up to 5 g Pregestimil® to each 100 ml to increase the protein to 1.9 g, energy to 385 kJ (92 kCal) and other nutrients proportionally.

(vi) An adult enteral feed can be used from the age of >2 years with appropriate supplements e.g. Isoclinifeed®.

The child who cannot eat, and in whom semisolids and supplements still do not provide adequate intake, requires a fluid diet or enteral feed. The psychological effect of a fluid diet or enteral feeding in a child must be considered, and unless contraindicated, snack foods are encouraged in addition. Enteral feeds should preferably be given as small frequent cyclical feeds orally, or by nasogastric or nasojejunal feeding tube. This is more physiological than continuous feeding and the feed is better absorbed than large bolus feeds. This also allows the child more freedom for play and social activities than continuous enteral feeds or parenteral nutrition. Small volume bolus feeds given frequently are also safer in that fluid overload is less likely to occur provided the feed is calculated appropriately for the child's age and weight, and there is less fear of the tube becoming displaced with subsequent feed inhalation. However, continuous feeds, often for only 20 hours per day, can be useful in patients requiring a large volume of feed, high nutrient intakes or in those in whom the feed is poorly tolerated or absorbed. It is essential that the position of the nasogastric feeding tube is checked (by aspirate or air) before each bolus feed and 4-hourly with continuous enteral feeding. This will also determine whether gastric emptying is occurring. Accurate monitoring of the feed volume by syringe pump in infants or paediatric enteral pump in children with a burette type giving set, is recommended. The 'Piggy-back' battery-operated portable pumps (Viomedex) give ambulatory patients more freedom of movement. The Comminuted Chicken (Cow & Gate) based module feed (p. 538) is a suspension of meat and cannot be given as a continuous feeding regime. A gastrostomy may be preferred or is occasionally necessary, for example in patients with oesophageal atresia or stricture. As the feeding tube used is much wider than the fine bore nasogastric type, more viscous feeds can be given. Jejunostomy or nasojejunal feeding are less desirable as a bolus regime, as both the dumping syndrome, specially with high osmolar feeds, and steatorrhoea can occur due to inadequate mixing of the feed with bile and pancreatic juice. An appropriate hydrolysed protein, elemental diet and/or MCT-containing feed (Table 23.3) can be used to overcome the problem and should be administered as a continuous feeding regime.

A variety of commercially available chemically defined enteral feeds designed for adult nutrition can be adapted for use in older children or a simple feed made from homogenized full fat milk and supplements (Francis 1986). These are not suitable for infants or as the sole source of nutrition in the young child under about 5 years. Most of the enteral feeds are based

Table 23.3   Lactose free formulae[1]

	Product	Company
Soya:	Prosobee®	Mead Johnson
	S. Formula®	Cow & Gate
	Wysoy®	John Wyeth Lab.
Hydrolysed protein:	Alfaré®	Nestlè[2 4 5]
semi-elemental paediatric	Pepdite 0–2®	Scientific Hospital
formulae		Supplies (SHS)[4]
	MCT Pepdite 0–2®	SHS[4]
	Pregestimil®	Mead Johnson[4]
	Nutramigen®	Mead Johnson[2 6]
	Pepdite 2+®	SHS[34]
	MCT Pepdite 2+®	SHS[34]
Casein based	Galactomin No 17®	Cow & Gate[5 6 7]
formulae:[7]	MCT (i)®	Cow & Gate[5 6 7]
	Portagen®	Mead Johnson[3 4 7]
	Triosorbin®	Merck[3457]
	Fructose-Formula-Galactomin No 19®	Cow & Gate[567]
Modular formulae	*Protein*:	
ingredients:	Comminuted Chicken®	Cow & Gate
	Albumaid complete® — beef serum	SHS[2]
	hydrolysate	
	Maxipro HBV® — whey protein	SHS[7]
	Casilan®; casein protein	Farley[2 7]
	Carbohydrate:	
	Glucose polymer	various
	Glucose	
	Fructose	
	Fat (oil emulsion):	
	Calogen®	SHS
	Liquigen MCT®	SHS[4]
	Minerals:	
	Aminogran mineral mixture®	Allen & Hanbury
	Metabolic mineral mixture®	SHS
	Vitamins:	
	Ketovite® tablets and liquid	Paines & Byrne
	Vitamins and Minerals:	
	Seravit® (various formula)	SHS
Elemental diet adult		
formula:[3]		
Hydrolysates:	Flexical®	Mead Johnson[3 4]
	Nutranel®	Roussel[3 4 5]
	Peptisorbon®	Merck[3 4]
Amino acids:	Elemental 028A® (unflavoured)	SHS[3]
	Elemental 028® (orange)	SHS[3]
	Vivonex®	Eaton Lab[3]
	Vivonex HN®	Eaton Lab[3]

Table 23.3 (*contd*)

	Product	Company
Elemental diet adult formula[3]:	Clinifeed® various	Roussel[3 7]
	Ensure®	Abbott[3 7]
	Ensure Plus®	Abbott[3 7]
	Isocal®	Mead Johnson[3 4 7]
	Nutrauxil®	Kabivitrum[3 4 7]
	Fortison Standard®	Cow & Gate[3 7]
	Fortison Soya®	Cow & Gate[3]
	Enteral 400®	SHS[3 4 7]

[1] The latest compositional data should be obtained from the manufacturer
[2] Not recommended for infants ≤ 3 months
[3] Not recommended for infants or as the sole source of nutrition in young children
[4] Contains MCT
[5] Contains trace lactose
[6] To be reformulated in 1987 as 'complete' formula suitable for infants
[7] Contains whole protein (casein/whey); unsuitable for cow's milk protein-free diets.

on cow's milk protein. Lactose-free formulae are available for patients with clinical lactose intolerance. MCT formulae are not necessary for routine use and should be reserved for patients who require low fat formulae. Feeds based on protein hydrolysates or amino acids are useful for those patients who are either intolerant to cow's milk protein, have a jejunostomy or compromised absorption. They are unpalatable, expensive and tend to have a high osmolality. They are frequently referred to as elemental diets.

Feed introduction in the severely ill child

Gastric emptying must be established before a fine bore tube can be used or a continuous feeding regime instigated. It is difficult to aspirate fluid through a fine bore tube and therefore, at least initially, a wider feeding tube is preferable. The feed is introduced gradually over several hours or days as clinically appropriate. A slow increase of volume and concentration of feed is important when introducing feeds to a rested gut, when absorption is compromised or the feed has a high osmolality. However, for the majority, a full strength feed can be given immediately and has nutritional advantages (Keohane et al 1984). The technique of tube feeding is described by Grant & Todd (1982).

Fluid diets must be prepared freshly and aseptically, pasteurized terminally, refrigerated and stored with care as they are easily contaminated and are a good media for microbial growth. The feed reservoir for continuous feeds should be changed every 4 hours in hospital and 6 to 8 hourly in the home. The giving sets should be changed daily to reduce the risk of microbial contamination from the patient infecting the feed and vice versa.

Diarrhoea in patients on enteral feeds should be investigated and the following considered:

(i) Intercurrent infection in the patient.

(ii) Antibiotic therapy.

(iii) Microbial contamination of feeds and/or equipment.

(iv) High osmolality of the feed or incorrect dilution of ingredients.

(v) Delivery time of the feed; a slower delivery enhances feed tolerance. Small frequent feeding regime, e.g. 2 hourly × 12 or continuous feeding may overcome diarrhoea.

(vi) Clinical intolerance to a dietary constituent, e.g. lactose, milk protein, soya.

Constipation is not usually a problem with fluid diets but when it does occur may be corrected by administering continuous feeds for only 20 hours per day. Brown sugar in place of part of the added carbohydrate in the feed, the provision of natural orange juice once or twice daily, or in the older child, cautious use of prune juice, can also be helpful. Methyl cellulose as Colagel® can be added to the feed or given medicinally.

INDICATIONS FOR SPECIAL DIETS IN CHILDREN

A number of clinical situations require therapeutic dietary regimes. The regimen so devised, must provide adequate nutrients to promote growth in the individual and yet eliminate all items which are clinically contraindicated, e.g. gluten in coeliac disease (see Francis 1987).

Carbohydrate intolerance

Carbohydrates are an important constituent of diets throughout the world and after intestinal hydrolysis and absorption, provide a critical source of metabolic energy. The major carbohydrates ingested by man are starch, lactose and sucrose. Defects in hydrolysis and absorption (Ch. 9) result in retention of osmotically active solutes within the intestinal tract and gastrointestinal symptoms result, i.e. carbohydrate intolerance (McNeish & Harran 1980). This is a common clinical problem and may have serious consequences particularly when it occurs in young children (Harries 1982a).

Both primary and secondary disorders of carbohydrate absorption occur and treatment is by the elimination of the carbohydrate(s) which are related to the symptoms. Details of the common major carbohydrates present in foods are given by Southgate et al (1978).

In the primary sugar intolerances, the diet must be continued indefinitely although symptoms are less severe after infancy and some relaxation of the diet is usually possible. The length of time when dietary treatment is required in the secondary conditions depends on clinical responses and on the primary underlying condition, and recovery usually correlates with the recovery of the small intestinal mucosa. Intolerance can be very transient as seen in protein energy malnutrition and kwashiorkor (Hansen et al 1982), and in most patients with secondary intolerance, reintroduction can be attempted within 2 to 3 months for lactose, and sooner for glucose (and starch) and even within days if sucrose exclusion is required at all. Symptomatic relapse after reintroduction of a specific carbohydrate on several occasions, in a clinically well child, suggests the possibility of a primary carbohydrate intolerance, which should be appropriately investigated.

Lactose

Lactose is by far the commonest and most important carbohydrate intolerance, as lactose is the carbohydrate present in all mammalian milks (human, cow, goat, ewe) ingested by man, and is present in the majority of infant formulae and some enteral feeds. Milk is an important source of nutrients in the diet of infants and young children. A nutritionally adequate replacement (see Table 23.3) is essential when milk is excluded from the diet to ensure a sufficiency of nutrients for normal growth and development. Older children requiring a lactose-free diet may only need a calcium supplement (400 mg elemental calcium per day) provided adequate protein, energy, vitamins and minerals are taken in the diet from a variety of conventional foods.

A lactose-free diet must exclude all lactose and milk products: whey, casein, caseinate, milk hydrolysate, and manufactured foods to which these are added, e.g. infant cereals and weaning foods. Lactose is frequently the filler in retail monosodium glutamate, some sugar substitutes and medicines in tablet form.

Frequently, both milk protein and lactose have to be excluded, either because a differential diagnosis (see Ch. 8) is not possible initially or because milk protein intolerance is the primary cause of the lactose intolerance. Although there are minor differences between a minimum lactose and milk protein-free diet, they are mostly unimportant, at least in the first instance. An appropriate milk substitute should be selected. Later, items such as butter and hard cheeses containing only traces of lactose but containing milk protein can be introduced if tolerated. Older patients with genetic hypolactasia or secondary lactose intolerance may have adequate lactase activity to tolerate a nearly normal diet with only the avoidance of visible milk.

Sucrose

Secondary sucrose intolerance occurs very rarely and is usually transient and of little importance as a clinical entity. When it occurs a low sucrose diet is required.

In the treatment of primary sucrase-isomaltase deficiency, a low sucrose diet is frequently all that is needed though some starch restriction may also be required in the young infant.

Sucrose is used extensively in the normal diet, mostly as added sugar and in manufactured foods. Fruit and many vegetables also contain natural sucrose (Southgate et al 1978). Initially these should be excluded from the diet, but subsequently many patients can tolerate them. The diet should include a suitable source of sucrose-free vitamin C, e.g. tomatoes or ascorbic acid tablets.

Starch

Some difficulty in digesting starch is found in patients with cystic fibrosis and Shwachman's syndrome due to pancreatic amylase deficiency, but this is treated with pancreatic enzyme replacement therapy. In sucrase-isomaltase deficiency, even though dietary sucrose needs to be eliminated or restricted, exclusion of starch is only required in small infants, because of the small percentage of α 1–6 linkages needing isomaltase for the digestion of the amylopectin in starch (Walker-Smith 1979).

Glucose-galactose

Glucose, galactose and the poly- and disaccharides from which they are derived by enzymatic action, are widely distributed in food and milk, necessitating their elimination from the diet in glucose-galactose intolerance (see Ch. 9). All dietary carbohydrate must be supplied as fructose (laevosan or laevulose), and the diet is extremely limiting. The only milk substitute formula which contains fructose as the sole carbohydrate is Fructose-Formula-Galactomin No 19® (Cow & Gate) (see Table 23.3). Alternatively a module-based feed must be devised, with fructose as the carbohydrate source. Some carbohydrate-free formulae are available internationally (Nestlé, Mead Johnson) to which fructose can be added. As this diet severely restricts conventional food intake, especially in infants and young children, the importance of all essential nutrients must be stressed, and carbohydrate-free supplements prescribed including the minor vitamins and trace minerals. Medicines should be carbohydrate and sorbitol-free.

Protracted diarrhoea

This is one of the most difficult problems in paediatric gastroenterology (see Ch. 16). The first step is to correct dehydration and any electrolyte-acid base balance with intravenous fluids. The temporary withdrawal of oral intake allows observation as to whether the diarrhoea persists without oral intake (Larcher et al 1977, Candy et al 1981). If this is the case, a period of parenteral nutrition (see Ch. 24) is almost invariably necessary and is life-saving.

Appropriate oral nutrition can be introduced gradually in conjunction with parenteral nutrition. Some food is always absorbed; long fasts are contraindicated. Even with parenteral nutrition it is our practice whenever possible, to offer small quantities of appropriate enteral nutrition, e.g. protein hydrolysate formula, or the Comminuted Chicken (Cow & Gate) based modular formula to maintain oral habits and avoid the atrophic changes associated with total parenteral nutrition.

Human milk, if tolerated, is the ideal feed for the young sick infant, and may have a therapeutic value in some instances (MacFarlene & Miller 1984). The recent demonstration of the presence of epidermal growth factor (Starkey & Orth 1977, Lucas 1984) which is trophic to intestinal epithelium may provide human milk with further advantages in this group of patients. It can be supplied by the infant's own mother or donated from human milk banks. Unpasteurized human milk has immunological advantages (Soothill 1976, Narayanan et al 1982), but must be monitored microbiologically (DHSS 1981), and the advantages must be counterbalanced with the risks associated with the use of unpasteurized donor milk. The heat-labile lipase in human milk enhances the absorption of the fat from unpasteurized human milk (Harries 1982b). Expressed human milk is higher in fat and energy than 'drip' human milk which constitutes much of the 'bank' human milk in this country. Careful administration of the feed is needed preferably by bottle or bolus nasogastric tube feeding to ensure the fat content is actually ingested (Narayanan et al 1984). Only on very rare occasions is human milk protein not tolerated and even the lactose when given as human milk may be tolerated. However, if lactose intolerance is a problem or human milk is not available, an alternative formula should be selected to suit the clinical situation (see Table 23.3).

A modular diet gives more scope to introduce nutrients singly and to tailor the feed to the individual's nutritional requirements. It can be used in conjunction with parenteral nutrition or as the sole source of nutrition. In our experience, the modular feed based on Comminuted Chicken (Cow & Gate) (see Table 23.3), is the most appropriate (Larcher et al 1977, Francis 1987) (see Ch. 16).

Monosaccharide intolerance

A few infants have a temporary intolerance to all carbohydrates, including glucose, galactose and fructose, usually due to acute gastroenteritis and occasionally gut resection or protracted diarrhoea. In these patients, parenteral nutrition is recommended or at least intravenous carbohydrate should be provided. In addition a carbohydrate-free modular feed can be used (Harries & Francis 1968). If intravenous carbohydrate is not given the infant must be kept under constant observation as hypothermia, hypoglycaemia and ketosis are serious risks (Lifshitz et al 1970). Frequent (4 hourly) blood sugar and electrolyte estimations should be made, and abnormalities immediately corrected whilst the infant is on such a regimen.

International products such as CF$_1$® or CHO-Free® can be used if available, instead of a modular feed but as they contain cow's milk protein they are less appropriate because of the risk of associated cow's milk protein intolerance. Adequate dietary energy intake is difficult to achieve whilst the feed is carbohydrate free, without exceeding the infant's limited capacity to excrete renal solute and degrade excess amino acids and fat. As soon as clinical improvement occurs, or if intravenous carbohydrate cannot be maintained, glucose, glucose polymer or fructose should be cautiously introduced. Later a simpler feed is often tolerated.

Protein intolerance and enteropathy

Continued diarrhoea and failure to gain weight following acute diarrhoea requires further investigation. An underlying primary cause such as coeliac disease, or cystic fibrosis must be excluded (See Chs. 8 and 16). Delayed recovery may be due to either carbohydrate intolerance (usually lactose), and/or a postenteritis enteropathy due to cow's milk protein, egg, soya, fish, chicken, rice or gluten. A postenteritis enteropathy mostly occurs in children under 2 years old with prolonged diarrhoea, and usually in those with the most severe illness. In these patients, whole milk protein (casein and whey) and other relevant proteins such as soya and/or gluten should be excluded from the diet for a temporary period of about 3 to 6 months, before re-introduction of a normal diet. Human milk may be tolerated otherwise the most appropriate milk-substitutes are those based on hydrolysed proteins (see Table 23.3).

The prophylactic use of an appropriate formula may prevent postenteritis enteropathy. Manuel & Walker-Smith (1981) have compared three infant formulae for the prevention of delayed recovery after infantile gastroenteritis and found advantages in using Pregestimil® in these patients. The length of time such a formula would need to be used and the cost of such recommendations must be considered. A highly heat-treated 'evaporated' milk formula with low sensitizing capacity (McLaughlin et al 1981) is a cheaper, practical alternative but no suitable formula is available for the young infant in the UK. Further controlled trials are needed to evaluate the benefit of such a regimen.

The gluten-free diet

Patients with coeliac disease require treatment with a gluten-free diet. Gluten is a large complex molecule that has been divided chemically into four heterogeneous proteins: gliadins, glutenins, albumins, and globulins. α-gliadin is the most toxic of these and is present in wheat protein except in a variant Chinese spring wheat (Kasarda et al 1978) which awaits full evaluation before it can be safely used by patients with coeliac disease. Rye is also toxic to coeliacs. However, controversy still exists over the need to exclude oats and barley (Anderson et al 1972). These cereals, particularly barley, are used less extensively in the national diet than wheat. Traditionally oats have been permitted in the gluten-free diet of our successfully treated children, though except for the five children quoted by Packer et al (1978), no scientific evidence of regular intake with biopsy results is available.

Other cereals are classified as gluten-free and are not implicated; these include rice, maize, millet, buckwheat, soya and other pulses. Conventional foods such as milk, meat, fish, egg, fruit, vegetables, butter, and margarine, cheese, pure fats and oils, are gluten-free, but manufactured foods must be carefully scrutinized for sources of gluten from ingredients such as flour, starch, farina, semolina and pasta. Many manufactured products do not list their ingredients in an easily recognizable way, but some companies now use the gluten-free symbol, $\left(\cancel{X}\right)$ to identify appropriate products. Some medicines contain gluten and are also contraindicated. The Coeliac Society regularly publish a list of gluten-free manufactured foods in the United Kingdom and their newsheets, Crossed Grain and Cefax, regularly give additions and corrections as they occur.

In the past, to obtain a successful gluten-free bread, wheat starch from which gluten had been removed was the only gluten-free flour and bread available. Controversy has arisen as to whether these products should be used in a gluten-free diet or indeed should be termed 'gluten-free'. Our patients, quoted by Packer et al (1978) treated with a gluten-free diet using wheat starch based bread and flour had normal prechallenge biopsies. Recently Ciclitera et al (1985) have suggested that intestinal mucosal damage can result from the use of a wheat starch product containing 0.64% protein by weight. This awaits confirmation from other units. Codex Alimentarius (WHO 1979) has given a proposed standard for the permitted residual protein of not more than 0.3% protein in dry matter in a wheat or gluten-containing cereal, starch based, gluten-free product. EEC proposed regulations require that the total nitrogen content of wheat, triticale, rye, barley or oats used in a gluten-free product should not exceed 0.05 g per 100 g of these grains on a dry matter basis and the nature of the source of the starch should be declared on the label. There is no evidence at present to suggest that products based on wheat starch which fulfills these WHO 1979 and EEC definitions of a gluten-free product are unsuitable for use in the treatment of patients with coeliac disease. However, new technology is making possible a range of naturally gluten-free (i.e. wheat-free) flours and breads which in time may totally replace those based on gluten-free wheat starches. In our experience, patients with wheat allergy frequently do *not* tolerate wheat starch based products (see Francis 1987).

Gluten challenge

Sequential biopsies before and after gluten challenge are essential to differentiate patients who have coeliac disease necessitating lifelong treatment.

Different age groups and different dietary patterns result in a widely varying intake of wheat protein, and therefore gluten, on a normal diet. The recent proposals to increase dietary fibre and cereal intake in the national diet will result in a higher wheat protein and gluten intake. An estimate of the wheat protein content expected in a normal diet ranges from

5–10 g/day in toddlers, 10–15 g/day in children and 15–30 g/day in children over 9 years of age. Wheat protein as the source of gluten has in our experience been found satisfactory for the gluten challenge and usually a diet containing approximately 10 g protein from wheat is advised, i.e. approximately 120 g of conventional bread or equivalent per day. Bread and cereals of wheat origin are more physiological than gluten powder (vital wheat protein) which is unpalatable and hard to incorporate into the diet, while its consistency makes it difficult to take as a medicine (Francis 1987).

Once a diagnosis of coeliac disease is confirmed, most children will return to a gluten-free diet without undue problem. More problems are, however, found in children under 8 years old at the time of the gluten challenge than older children who can understand the procedure more fully (Packer et al 1978). The optimal age for the gluten challenge is controversial though there is some advantage in confirming the need for a gluten-free diet before the child has to cope with social eating at school. The emotional stress of the biopsy and gluten challenge both to parents and child must be considered. Careful explanation of the procedure is essential, and the fear of so-called 'toxic' foods should not be overlooked whether using gluten powder or conventional foods. The optimal length of time for a gluten challenge has not been established (Packer et al 1978, Walker-Smith 1979) (see Ch. 8).

Inflammatory bowel disease (IBD); Crohn's disease and ulcerative colitis

The aim of treatment is to induce and maintain remission in both conditions. This is more easily achieved in ulcerative colitis than Crohn's disease. Nutritional measures, either enterally (Kirschner et al 1981) or if necessary parenterally (Kelts et al 1979) are extremely important in both diseases, but particularly in Crohn's disease where the associated growth failure frequently responds favourably to nutritional repletion (Kirschner et al 1981), and remission may be induced (O'Morain et al 1982) (see Ch. 6). Nutritional measures also play an important part in the restoration of specific nutritional deficits commonly seen in Crohn's disease (Booth & Harries 1984) (see Ch. 6).

Elemental diets have received a considerable amount of attention in the management of IBD (Navarro et al 1977) but most reported series are uncontrolled trials. Artificial supplementation is, however, not essential (Moriarty et al 1981). Kirschner and colleagues (1981) used an elemental diet for 12 months in 7 children, 6 of whom thereafter received only conventional foods. During a follow-up period of 4 years the energy intake was boosted from 56% to 91% of the recommended intake for height, and 5 of the children had improved growth such that their height came within 5% of their pre-illness height centile. We currently select a low antigen hydrolysate formula in preference to a whole protein milk or soya based feed because of the theoretical increased risk that these patients have, or acquire, intolerance or allergy (Jones et al 1985).

A nutritionally adequate formula is selected for the child's age and nutritional needs, e.g. Pregestimil® and or Flexical®; supplements are added as necessary. The newer hydrolysate and amino acid based formulae (see Table 23.3) may be equally appropriate and many are more palatable. The feed is usually administered by a continuous enteral feeding pump. Some patients however will take such formulae orally, either from an infant feeding bottle, teacher-beaker or with a straw and appropriate flavouring. It should be remembered that some flavourings will increase the osmolality of the feed to unacceptable levels, and others contain various antigens or additives which may be contraindicated in these patients, e.g. tartrazine.

After a period, usually 6 weeks to 2 months, of total enteral feeding, conventional foods (initially low antigen, e.g. milk and egg free) are gradually introduced and once oral intake is adequate to meet nutritional requirements the enteral feed is reduced to an overnight supplement. The regimen can be continued at home once the child is in remission and supplements are discontinued only once adequate conventional food is being taken to permit catch-up growth.

Allergic colitis in infants

In contrast to adults and older children, food allergy appears to play an important role in colitis in infancy and accounts for what previously appeared to be an increased incidence of ulcerative colitis in the first year of life (Jenkins et al 1982) (see Ch. 6). Prompt remission of symptoms occurs when a low antigen elimination diet is introduced. Cow's milk protein is the most common offending antigen. Differential diagnosis is important and provided the condition is recognized and appropriately treated with an exclusion diet and a suitable milk substitute (see Table 23.3), such as Pregestimil® or the new Pepdite® (SHS) range, the prognosis appears to be excellent.

Fat restriction

Steatorrhoea in association with biliary atresia and obstructive jaundice; pancreatic insufficiency (cystic fibrosis and Shwachman syndrome); loss of intestinal absorptive area following resection; lymphangiectasia and the rare condition abetalipoproteinaemia, necessitates a reduction of dietary fat intake with appropriate replacement of the dietary energy loss, and fat soluble vitamins.

The degree of fat restriction varies with the diagnosis and the age of the patient from the minimum fat intakes prescribed for lymphangiectasia and abetalipoproteinaemia of approximately 1 g per year of age to 10–15 g/day, whereas > 30% energy from dietary fat may be tolerated by patients with cystic fibrosis in whom pancreatic enzyme therapy is used to enhance absorption. As generous an intake of fat as can be tolerated should be prescribed at least in the young child.

Energy

Fat is the most calorie-dense food and a major source of energy in the diet of young children, e.g. human milk and infant formulae contain approximately 50% energy from fat (Francis 1986). In low fat diets the energy deficit must be replaced with sugars, starches, fruit and vegetables. Glucose polymers and/or MCT can be incorporated into the diet (Francis 1987), but the latter is not recommended in abetalipoproteinaemia (Muller et al 1977).

Essential fatty acids

Fat is an important source of essential fatty acids (EFA), particularly linoleic acid. Clinical evidence of EFA deficiency has rarely been reported even though blood levels of linoleic acid may be low in patients on low fat diets (Lloyd 1982). The role of EFA has, however, recently received attention in patients with cystic fibrosis (McCollum & Harries 1977, Silk 1984).

A small prescribed quantity of oils rich in polyunsaturated fatty acids (PUFA) such as safflower oil (2–5 ml/day) can be given in conjunction with low fat diets as a source of EFA, or a limited quantity of a margarine high in PUFA may be permitted in the diet. The fat content of chicken, turkey, fish, cereals and pulses are relatively rich in PUFA, and these foods can also provide an important contribution to the protein content of the low fat diet. Some milk substitutes and MCT 'filled' milks contain an EFA supplement.

Fat soluble vitamins

Dietary fat largely provides the fat soluble vitamins. Low fat diets should be generously supplemented with vitamins A, D, E and K, ideally in a water miscible form. A comprehensive range of all vitamins is advised, especially in patients with steatorrhoea or liver conditions e.g. Ketovite® tablets plus liquid. Vitamin E supplements are particularly important in patients with severe and chronic fat malabsorption such as abetalipoprotein-aemia and cholestatic liver disease (Muller et al 1983). Milk substitutes and MCT 'filled' milks are frequently supplemented with a range of vitamins.

Milk substitutes for use with low fat diets

The lipase in human milk and its fatty acid composition, enhances its fat absorption (Harries 1982b). Thus the majority of infants with cystic fibrosis can be breast-fed, though supplements of pancreatic enzymes may be needed.

Alternatively, a whey based modified milk can be used to devise a formula with 2% fat (mass/vol) which is high in PUFA (Table 23.4). Progress® (J Wyeth) may be suitable after the first months of life or a commercial MCT 'filled' milk can be selected such as MCT Pepdite 0–2® (SHS) or Pregestimil®. A minimum fat feed (Table 23.4) is occasionally required, for example in the treatment of chylothorax or lymphangiectasia, but such a feed is high in protein and renal solute and is not ideal nutritionally, especially in young infants. It should, therefore, be used with caution, supplemented with vitamins and EFA as appropriate. MCT1® (Cow & Gate) or Portagen® are suitable milk substitutes for the toddler and child or skimmed milk may suffice, provided adequate energy intake is ingested from other sources.

Enteral feeds or supplements of an appropriate formula either given orally or as a nasogastric/nasojejunal feed may be necessary to correct or avoid the growth failure commonly seen in patients with chronic steator-rhoea, e.g. patients with cystic fibrosis (Silk 1984).

Because of the high carbohydrate intake in patients on low fat diets, appropriate fluoride supplements and regular dental checks are important together with meticulous teeth cleaning to adequately remove dental plaque and thus reduce the risk of caries.

Protein restriction

Treatment of a number of conditions such as liver disease and the inborn errors of protein metabolism, the hereditary hyperammonaemias and organ-icacidaemias, require restriction of protein intake. Unabsorbed amino acids are decomposed by luminal bacteria producing ammonia, organic acids and amines which are absorbed and normally detoxicated by the liver. Increased amounts of these metabolites occur in blood when, for example, liver func-tion is impaired or production increased as in bacterial overgrowth of the small intestine, in transport defects or when specific liver enzymes for their degradation are deficient (Mowat 1979, Smith & Francis 1982, Francis 1987) (see Ch. 18).

Increased dietary protein above that required for growth and essential tissue synthesis, does not increase protein synthesis but increases the proportion of amino acids for degradation and hence ammonia and urea production. Any increase in gluconeogenesis caused by starvation, energy deficit, infection and catabolism also increases their production. Protein intake in diseases affecting protein degradation should be reduced and tailored to the individual's tolerance and growth needs. In addition use should be made of specific means to remove toxic metabolites, e.g. arginine in citrullinaemia to enhance the removal of ammonia (Brusilow 1985); sodium benzoate to detoxify ammonia by conjugation in the liver; lactulose to decrease ammonia absorption from the intestine (see Chs. 18 and 21) (Francis 1987).

550 HARRIES' PAEDIATRIC GASTROENTEROLOGY

Table 23.4 Feeds for infants requiring fat restriction (100 ml composition)[1]

	Protein g	CHO g	Fat g	Energy kJ	Energy kCal	Sodium mmol	Potassium mmol
(i) Human milk (mature) 100 ml	1.3	7.2	4.1[2]	289	69	0.6	1.5
(ii) Fortified human milk							
100 ml human milk (EBM)	1.3	7.2	4.1[2]	289	69	0.6	1.5
+ Pregestimil® powder (Mead Johnson)	0.6	3.1	0.9[3]	97	23	0.5	0.6
Total	1.9	10.3	5.0	386	92	1.1	2.1
(iii) Reduced fat formula[4]							
(a) 6.5 g Gold Cap SMA® (John Wyeth Lab)	0.8	3.6	1.8[2]	138	33	0.3	0.7
4.3 g Marvel® (Cadbury)	1.6	2.2	0.1	65	16	1.0	1.8
6.5 g Caloreen® (Roussel)	Nil	6.5	Nil	104	26	0.1	tr
Water to 100 ml							
Total	2.4	12.3	1.9[2]	307	75	1.4	2.5
(b) 6.2 g Premium® (Cow & Gate)	0.8	3.7	1.8[2]	138	33	0.4	0.9
4.6 g Marvel® (Cadbury)	1.7	2.4	0.1	69	16.5	1.1	1.9
6.5 g Polycal® (Cow & Gate)	Nil	6.5	Nil	104	26	0.1	tr
Water to 100 ml							
Total	2.5	12.6	1.9[2]	311	75.5	1.6	2.8
(c) Progress® 14.9% solution (John Wyeth Lab)	2.9	8.0	2.6	272	65	1.7	2.7

(iv) MCT® filled infant formula RD 231 (15% solution) (SHS)	2.1	10.5	1.4[3]	250	59.8	1.4	1.5
(v) Pregestimil® (15% solution) (Mead Johnson)	1.8	9.3	2.7[3]	291	69	1.5	1.8
(vi) Minimal fat temporary feed for infants[5]							
(a) 5 g Skimmed milk powder	1.8	2.2	trace	76	18	1.2	2.1
15 g Maxijul® LE (SHS)	Nil	15.0	Nil	240	60	trace	trace
Water to 100 ml							
Total	1.8	17.2	trace	316	78	1.2	2.1
(b) 2 g Maxipro® HBV (SHS)	1.8	trace	trace	30	7	0.2	0.2
15 g Maxijul® LE (SHS)	Nil	15.0	Nil	240	60	trace	trace
0.8 g Metabolic Mineral Mixture® (SHS)	Nil	Nil	Nil	Nil	Nil	1.4	1.7
Water to 100 ml							
Total	1.8	15.0	trace	270	67	1.6	1.9

[1] Vitamin supplements including A, D, E and K are essential, e.g. 3 Ketovite® tablets and 5 ml Ketovite® liquid
[2] Fat high in EFA and PUFA
[3] Fat high in PUFA and MCT
[4] Other brands of modified infant formula and glucose polymers can be calibrated to provide suitable formulae. Recipes (iii) (a) and (b) can be made using the scoop in the SMA® or Premium® packet for each ingredient as follows:
2 level scoops Gold Cap SMA® or Premium® powder
2 level scoops Marvel® granules
2 level scoops Caloreen® or Polycal® respectively } Total volume approximately 130 ml
120 ml/4 oz measured boiled water
[5] Essential fatty acid supplement may be required

During catabolic periods and in acute hepatic failure a temporary protein-free high-energy regimen to cover basal energy needs may be required, and can be provided orally by use of an appropriate volume of a 10–20% (mass/vol) solution of glucose polymer ±2.5–5% supplement of fat, e.g. Calogen® or Liquigen®, together with bicarbonate and potassium to correct acid base balance. This can be administered as 2-hourly drinks or given by nasogastric bolus feeds. The older child may prefer Lucozade®, fruit juice or coke, fortified with a glucose polymer, as a more palatable alternative. The liquid glucose polymer supplements e.g. Fortical®, Hycal®, Maxijul® liquid are, however, so concentrated that diarrhoea is almost inevitable in children unless they are diluted with at least an equal quantity of water. They are inappropriate for infants.

The minimum protein requirement for growth needs should be given immediately the child improves clinically or ultimately growth failure will occur. The diet must be monitored and adjusted on biochemical and clinical data.

Protein source

The source of protein should be of high biological value (Francis 1987) in order to meet the essential amino acid requirement for growth with a minimum of amines for degradation. Human milk and the whey based modified infant formulae have optimal amino acid profiles for infant nutrition. Milk, egg and meat are high biological sources of protein, and provided the protein prescription is sufficiently generous can be incorporated into the diet of the older child. Although pulses, bread and cereals have lower biological values than egg and meat proteins, they contribute a higher energy value for protein intake. In order to provide a variety in protein-restricted diets, protein intake is conveniently measured using an exchange system of foods (Francis 1987); the quantity of food containing 6 g protein for meat, milk, egg and 1 g protein for cereals, potato, bread, etc, or 50 mg of the amino acid(s) as appropriate in specific amino acid disorders. For practical purposes approximately 75% of the protein should come from the high biological sources. It is, however, important that the diet is eaten happily and therefore patient food preferences must be taken into account in the dietary prescription. The daily protein intake, together with energy sources should be distributed between the meals.

Replacement of part of the dietary protein intake with a supplement of essential amino acids, e.g. Dialamine® or Hepatamine® can reduce total nitrogen intake and improve the amino acid profile and their utilization for growth. Specific supplements of amino acids devoid of the amino acid(s) concerned in the particular inborn error of metabolism are used in tyrosinaemia, methylmalonicacidaemia, maple syrup urine disease, phenylketonuria, etc. (Francis 1987).

Energy source

Adequate energy intake is vitally important in all situations where protein intake is restricted. Endogenous protein catabolism contributes significantly to the raised ammonia or plasma amino acids and abnormal metabolites. Energy from carbohydrates and fats have a protein sparing action and should be provided in increased amounts in low protein diets. The energy requirement may be 25% higher than normal, and for catch-up growth and in hypercatabolic states even higher energy intakes may be temporarily necessary (pp. 532–536). Sugars, fats, selected vegetables, fruit and other foods of negligible protein content such as low protein breads, biscuits and pasta are permitted without measurement. Glucose polymers and fats in the form of vegetable oil emulsions such as Calogen® or margarine, butter and cream are concentrated sources of protein-free energy which can be added to the diet and incorporated into drinks. Supplements should be prescribed, where applicable, to ensure the regimen is nutritionally adequate in energy and other nutrients such as vitamins and minerals for growth and to correct any specific biochemical abnormalities associated with the diagnosed condition.

Complications

Gastroenterological symptoms may be related to increased gut ammonia produced by microorganisms. This is particularly important in young children, in poorly nourished patients and when fluid intake has to be restricted. Hyperosmolar solutions should be avoided or introduced gradually over several days and such solutions are better tolerated when given in small, frequent quantities. Anorexia and food refusal due to abdominal cramp and nausea can be caused by over-concentrated supplements. Excessive and unrealistic energy intakes are inappropriate as food refusal can result. Synthetic energy supplements in children with anorexia may simply replace food intake of better nutritional content without actually achieving an increased total energy intake (Francis 1987). As a result of the poor conventional food intake, the trace nutrients such as zinc, chromium, iron and vitamin content of the diet can be reduced resulting in chronic nutritional deficiencies. It is very important to review therapeutic diets frequently; in infants initially at 1–2 week intervals, and in older children at 1–2 month intervals. The diet must be modified in the light of clinical findings, growth, age and weight. This is essential where a minimum protein intake is used, since it could be outgrown and will then inhibit further growth.

Weaning solids should be encouraged at the appropriate age and are normally introduced from 3–4 months in order to establish good eating habits. The manufacturers of baby foods, will provide up-to-date lists of the composition of their products. Suitable foods should be carefully chosen according to the dietary prescription aad the quantity in an appropriate sized serving.

FOOD REFUSAL

Chronically ill children and especially those with gastrointestinal disorders such as Crohn's disease, Schwachman syndrome and disorders of protein metabolism are anorexic and notoriously poor eaters. The actual dietary intake should be assessed from time to time and compared with offered and recommended intakes. Advice should be given regarding the intake and manipulation needed to improve nutritional adequacy. Force feeding should be avoided. Snacks as well as meals should be encouraged in order to achieve a better total dietary intake in these children. Encouragement, praise, reward schemes and ingenuity are required to achieve optimal intake in the majority of these patients. Some patients may benefit from nasogastric tube feeding when growth failure is a major concern. A relaxed atmosphere at meal times encourages cooperation from mother and child so that food refusal is reduced to a minimum (see Francis 1986, 1987).

REFERENCES

Aggett P J, Davies N T 1983 Some nutritional aspects of trace metals. Journal of Inherited Metabolic Disease 6, Supplement 1: 22–30

Aggett P J, Moore J M, Thorn J M, Delves H T, Cornfield M, Clayton B E 1983 Evaluation of the trace metal supplement for a synthetic low lactose diet. Archives of Disease in Childhood 58: 433–437

Ahn C, MacLean W C 1980 Growth of the exclusively breast fed infant. American Journal of Clinical Nutrition 33: 183–192

Anderson C M, Gracey M, Burke V 1972 Coeliac disease: some still controversial aspects. Archives of Disease in Childhood 47: 292–298

Andersson H, Nävert B, Bingham S A, Englyst H N, Cummings J H 1983 The effect of breads containing similar amounts of phytate but different amounts of wheat bran on calcium, zinc and iron balance in man. British Journal of Nutrition 50: 503–510

Booth I W, Harries J T 1984 Inflammatory bowel disease in childhood — Progress report. Gut 25: 188–202

Booth I W, Levine M M, Harries J T 1984 Oral rehydration therapy in acute diarrhoea: medical progress. Journal of Pediatric Gastroenterology and Nutrition 3: 491–499

Bunker V W, Clayton B E 1983 Trace element content of commercial enteral feeds. Lancet ii: 426–428

Burman D 1982 Nutrition in early childhood. In: McLaren D S, Burman D (eds) Textbook of Paediatric Nutrition 2nd Edn. Churchill Livingstone Ch. 3 pp. 39–73

Brusilow S W 1985 Inborn errors of urea synthesis. In: Lloyd J, Scriver C (eds) Genetic and metabolic disease in paediatrics. International Medical Review. Butterworth, London. Ch. 7 pp 140–165

Candy D C A, Larcher V F, Cameron D J S, Norman A P, Tripp J H, Milla P J, Pincott J R, Harries J T 1981 Lethal familial protracted diarrhoea. Archives of Disease in Childhood 56: 15–26

Chanarin I 1982 Disorders of vitamin absorption. In: Harries J T (ed) Clinics in Gastroenterology: Familial inherited abnormalities Vol II No 1. Saunders, London pp 73–85

Chandra R K 1985 Trace elements in nutrition of children. Nestlé Nutrition Workshop Series, Vol. 8. Raven Press, New York

Ciclitera P J, Ellis H J, Evans D J, Lennox E S 1985 A radioimmunoassay for wheat gliadin to assess the suitability of gluten free foods for patients with coeliac disease. Clinical Experiment Immunology Vol 59 No 3: 703–708

Cooper A, Betts J M, Pereira G R, Ziegler M M 1984 Taurine deficiency in severe hepatic dysfunction complicating total parenteral nutrition. Journal of Pediatric Surgery 19: 462–465

Cuthbertson D P 1980 Alterations in metabolism following injury. Injury 2: 175–189, 286–303

Davidson S, Passmore R, Brock J F, Truswell A S 1979 Human Nutrition and Dietetics 7th Edn. Churchill Livingstone, London

Davies N T 1981 An appraisal of the newer trace elements. Philosophical Transactions of the Royal Society of Medicine, London. 294: 171–184

DHSS 1980 Artificial feeds for the young infant. Report No 18. HMSO, London

DHSS 1981 The Collection and storage of Human milk. Report No 22, HMSO London

DHSS 1983 (Revision) Present day practice in infant feeding. Report No 20, 1980 HMSO, London

DHSS 1985 (Revision) The recommended amounts of food energy and nutrients for groups of people in the United Kingdom. Report No 15, 1979, HMSO London

Elwyn D H 1980 Nutritional requirement of adult surgical patients. Critical Care Medicine 8: 9–20

Falkner F, Tanner J M (eds) 1979 Human growth 3. Neurobiology and Nutrition. Plenum Press, Bailliere Tindall, New York

FAO/WHO 1973a Energy and protein requirements. Report of a joint FAO/WHO ad-hoc expert committee (WHO technical report series No 522 and FAO Nutrition meetings report series No 52) Geneva

FAO/WHO 1973b. Trace elements in human nutrition. Technical report series No 532 Geneva

FAO/WHO 1975 Energy and protein requirements. Recommendations by a joint FAO/WHO informal gathering of experts. Food and Nutrition 1: 11–19

Fell G S, Cuthbertson D P, Morrison C, et al 1973 Urinary zinc levels as an indication of muscle catobolism. Lancet i: 280–282

Forfar J O, Arneil G C 1984 Textbook of Paediatrics 3rd Edn, Churchill Livingstone, Edinburgh

Francis D E M 1986 Nutrition for Children. Blackwell Scientific Publications, Oxford

Francis D E M 1987 Diets for Sick Children 4th Edn. Blackwell Scientific Publications, Oxford

Grant A, Todd E 1982 Enteral and Parenteral Nutrition. Blackwell Scientific Publications, Oxford

Hansen A E, Stewart R, Hughes G, Soderhjelm L 1962 The relation of linoleic acid to infant feeding. Acta Paediatrica Scandinavica Suppl. 137

Hansen J D L, Buchanan N, Pettifor J M 1982 Protein energy malnutrition PEM. In: McLaren D S, Burman D (eds) Textbook of Paediatric Nutrition 2nd Edn. Churchill Livingstone, Edinburgh. Ch. 7 pp 114–142

Harries J T 1982a Disorders of carbohydrate absorption. In: Harries J T (ed) Familial Inherited Abnormalities Vol II No 1. W B Saunders, London Ch. 2, pp 17–30

Harries J T 1982b Fat absorption in the newborn. Acta Paediatrica Scandinavica 299: 17–23

Harries J T, Francis D E M 1968 Temporary monosaccharide intolerance. Lancet i: 360

Harzer G, Kauer 1982 Binding of zinc to casein. American Journal of Clinical Nutrition 35: 981–987

Heird W C, Driscoll J M, Schullinger J N, Grabin B, Winters R W 1972 Intravenous alimentation in pediatric patients. Journal of Pediatrics 8: 351–372

Holmes G E, Hassanein K M, Miller H C 1983 Factors associated with infections among breast fed babies and babies fed proprietary milks. Pediatrics 72: 300–306

James W P T 1981 Protein and energy metabolism after trauma. Acta Chirurgica Scandinavica Supplement 507: 1–20

Jenkins H R, Milla P J, Pincott J R, Soothill J F, Harries J T 1982 Food allergy: the major cause of infantile colitis? Gut 23: A9

Jones V A, Workman E, Freeman A H, Dickinson R J, Wilson A J, Hunter J O 1985 Crohns Disease: maintenance of remission by diet. Lancet ii: 177–180

Kasarda D D, Qualsel C O, Mecham D K, Goodenberger D M, Strober W 1978 A test of toxicity of bread from wheat lacking alpha gliadins coded for 6A chromosone. In: McNickoll O B, McCarthy C F Fottrell P C (eds) Perspective in Coeliec Disease. M T P Press Lancaster. pp. 55–61

Kelts D G, Grand R J, Shen G, Watkins J B, Werlin S L, Boehme C 1979 Nutritional basis of growth failure in children and adolescents with Crohn's disease. Gastroenterology 76: 720–727

Keohane P P, Attrill H, Love M, Frost P, Silk D B A 1984 Relation between osmolarity of diet and gastrointestinal side effects in enteral nutrition. British Medical Journal 288: 678–680

Kirschner B S, Klich J R, Kalman S S, de Favoro M V, Rosenberg I H 1981 Reversal of growth retardation in Crohn's disease with therapy emphasising oral nutritional restitution. Gastroenterology 80: 10–15

Lancet Editorial 1983 Selenium perspective i: 685

Larcher V, Shephered R, Francis D E M, Harries J T 1977 Protracted diarrhoea in infancy. Analysis of 82 cases with particular reference to diagnosis and management. Archives of Disease in Childhood 52: 597–605

Lifshitz F, Coello-Ramirez P, Gutiẽrrez-Topete G 1970 Monosaccharide intolerance and hypoglycaemia in infancy with diarrhoea I + II. Journal of Paediatrics 77:(4) 595–603, 604–612

Lloyd J K 1982 Disorders of lipid metabolism. In: McLaran D S, Burman D (eds) Textbook of Paediatric Nutrition 2nd End. Churchill Livingstone, Edinburgh Ch 14. pp 285–294

Lucas A 1984 Hormones, nutrition and the gut. In: Tanner M S, Stocks R J (eds) Neonatal Gastroenterology: Contemporary Issues. Intercept, Newcastle-upon-Tyne

McCollum J P K, Harries J T 1977 Disorders of the pancreas. In: Harries J T (ed) Essentials of Paediatric Gastroenterology. Churchill Livingstone, Edinburgh. Ch 20, 335–353

MacFarlene P I, Miller V 1984 Human milk in the management of protracted diarrhoea in infancy. Archives of Disease in Childhood 59: 260–265

McKillop F M, Durnin J V G A 1982 The energy and nutritional intake of a random sample (305) of infants. Human Nutrition: Applied Nutrition 36A: 405–421

McLaren D S, Burman D (eds) 1982 Textbook of Paediatric Nutrition 2nd Edn. Churchill Livingstone, Edinburgh

McLaughlin P, Anderson K J, Widdowson E M, Coombs R R A 1981 Effect of heat on the anaphylactic sensitising capacity of cow's milk, goats milk and various infant formulae fed to guinea pigs. Archives of Disease in Childhood 56: 165–171

McNeish A S, Harran M J 1980 Clinical aspects of disordered carbohydrate absorption. In: Burman D, Holten J B, Pennock C A (eds) Inherited Disorders of Carbohydrate Metabolism. M T P Press, Lancaster Ch 3 pp. 39–57

Mann T P, Wilson K M, Clayton B E 1965 A deficiency state arising in infants on synthetic foods. Archives of Disease in Childhood 40: 364–375

Manuel P D, Walker-Smith J A 1981 A comparison of three infant feeding formulae for the prevention of delayed recovery after infantile gastroenteritis. Acta Paediatrica Belgica 34: 13–20

Matthews D M 1975 Intestinal absorption of peptides. Physiology Review 55:537

Mendelson R A, Bryan M H, Anderson G H 1983 Trace mineral balances in preterm infants fed their own mother's milk. Journal of Pediatric Gastroenterology and Nutrition 2: 256–261

Moriarty K J, Hegarty J E, Clarke M, Fairclough P D, Dawson A M 1981 A comparison of the relative nitrogen-sparing properties of whole protein, protein hydrolysate, and the equivalent amino acid mixtures in man. Gastroenterology 80:1234

Mowat A P (ed) 1979 Fulminant liver failure. In: Liver Disorders of Childhood. Butterworth, London, Ch 7 pp 228–230

Muller D P R, Lloyd J K, Bird A C 1977 Long term management of abetalipoproteinaemia. Possible role of vitamin E. Archives of Disease in Childhood 52: 209–214

Muller D P R, Lloyd J K, Wolff O H 1983 Vitamin E and neurological function. Lancet i: 225–228

Narayanan I, Praskash K, Prabhaker A K, Gujral V V 1982 A planned prospective evaluation of the anti-infective property of varying quantities of expressed human milk. Acta Paediatrica Scandinavica 71: 441–445

Narayanan I, Singh B, Harvey D 1984 Fat loss during feeding of human milk. Archives of Disease in Childhood 59: 475–477

Navarro J, Ricour C, Mougenot, Duhamel J F 1977 Constant rate enteral alimentation in Crohn's disease (at hospital and at home). Acta Paediatrica Belgica 30:195

NRC 1980 National research council recommended dietary allowances 9th Edn. National academy of Science, Washington

O'Morain C A, Segal A W, Levi A J 1982 Elemental diets in treatment of acute Crohn's disease. A controlled study. Gut 23: A 891

Packer S M, Charlton V, Keeling J W et al 1978 Gluten challenge in treated coeliac disease. Archives of Disease in Childhood 53: 449–455

Renate L, Bergmann K 1979 Nutrition and growth in infancy. In: Falkner F, Tanner J M (eds) Human Growth 3. Neurobiology and Nutrition. Plenum Press/Baillière Tindall, New York pp 331–360

Richards J R 1977 Metabolic response to injury, infection and starvation: an overview. In: Richards J R Kinney J M (eds) Nutritional aspects of care in the critically ill. Churchill Livingstone, Edinburgh p 273

Silk B D A 1984 Future directions in Supplemental Nutrition. In: Lawson D (ed) Cystic fibrosis: Horizons in Proceedings of the 9th International Cystic Fibrosis Congress, Brighton, June 9–15th 1984. John Wiley & Sons, Chichester pp 96–114

Smith I Francis D E M 1982 Disorders of amino acid metabolism In: McLaren D S, Burman D (eds) Textbook of Paediatric Nutrition 2nd Edn. Churchill Livingstone, Edinburgh Ch 15 pp 295–323

Soothill J F 1976 Breastfeeding: the immunological argument. British Medical Journal i: 1466

Southgate D A T, Paul A A, Dean A C, Christie A A 1978 Free sugars in food. Journal of Human Nutrition 32: 335–363

Starkey R H, Orth D N 1977 Radioimmunoassay of human epidermal growth factor (urogastrone). Journal of Clinical Endocrinology and Metabolism 45: 1144–1153

Thorn J M, Aggett P J, Delves H T, Clayton B E 1978 Mineral and trace metal supplement for use with synthetic diets on comminuted chicken. Archives of Disease in Childhood 53: 931–938

Underwood E J 1977 Trace Elements in Human and Animal Nutrition 4th Edn. Academic Press New York

Walker-Smith J A 1979 Disease of the Small Intestine in Childhood 2nd Edn. Pitman Medical Bath

Whitehead R G, Paul A A, Cole T J 1981 A critical analysis of measured food energy intake during infancy and early childhood in comparison with current international recommendations. Journal of Human Nutrition 35: 339–348

WHO 1974 Handbook on human nutritional requirements. Monograph series No 61. Geneva

WHO 1979 Codex alimentarius commission Alinorm 79/26 Appendix 2, pp 19–20

Wise A 1983 Dietary factors determining the biological activities of phytate. Nutrition abstracts and reviews in Clinical Nutrition Series A. Vol 53, No 9, pp. 791–806

Woolfson A M J, Ricketts C R, Hardy S M et al 1979 Prolonged nasogastric tube feeding in critically ill and surgical patients. Postgraduate Medical Journal 52: 678–682

Parenteral nutrition

The ability to provide enough nutrients parenterally to sustain growth in infants and children suffering from intestinal failure or severe functional intestinal immaturity, undoubtedly represents one of the most important therapeutic advances in paediatric gastroenterology of the last two decades. Many of the metabolic complications previously associated with parenteral nutrition are now avoidable by the use of more appropriate solutions and careful clinical and biochemical monitoring. However, the problems of catheter-related sepsis and cholestatic jaundice of uncertain aetiology remain largely unresolved, and should temper unqualified enthusiasm for the technique. Furthermore, parenteral nutrition is expensive, sometimes hazardous, and demands a high degree of nursing and medical expertise. As so commonly occurs with the availability of important life-saving technology, difficult ethical problems ensue and the decision to embark upon prolonged parenteral nutrition in patients with possibly irreversible intestinal failure is one which requires mature clinical judgment. However, in spite of these reservations, the number of children with severe gastrointestinal disease successfully treated with parenteral nutrition has increased greatly over the last 10 years, and this trend seems likely to continue.

INDICATIONS

In general, parenteral nutrition is indicated whenever insufficient nutrients can be provided enterally to prevent or correct malnutrition, or to sustain

Table 24.1 Indications for parenteral nutrition

Protracted diarrhoea in infancy
Major gastrointestinal surgery in the neonate
Very low birth weight neonates
Necrotizing enterocolitis
Crohn's disease (short gut, induction of remission and growth failure)
Short bowel syndrome
Cytotoxic therapy
Marrow and organ transplantation
Acute renal failure
Burns
Trauma

appropriate growth. It is not indicated in patients with adequate small intestinal function in whom nutrition may be maintained by oral, tube or gastrostomy feedings, possibly using a defined formula feed (see Ch. 23). The principal conditions in which parenteral nutrition is likely to be required are summarized in Table 24.1.

Prophylactic parenteral nutrition

When an extended period of gastrointestinal dysfunction seems likely, for example, following extensive intestinal surgery in the neonate, parenteral nutrition may be started prophylactically. In such circumstances, the timing of parenteral nutrition is largely determined by the expected duration of starvation and by the age and size of the patient.

Starvation and expected survival in paediatric patients

In small babies, parenteral nutrition should be started early. A small preterm baby weighing 1 kg contains only 1% fat and 8% protein, and has a nonprotein caloric reserve of only 460 kJ/kg. The nonprotein caloric reserve increases with body size and a one-year-old weighing 10.5 kg has a reserve of 9200 kJ. Thus, if it is assumed that all nonprotein and one-third of the protein content of the body is available for caloric needs at the rate of 210 kJ/kg/24 h in infants and children, and 84 kJ/kg/24 h in adults, estimates of the duration of survival during starvation and semistarvation may be made (Fig. 24.1). A small preterm baby has sufficient reserve to survive a mere four days starvation and a large preterm baby enough for only 12 days. Clearly, if severe malnutrition or death is to be avoided, early prophylactic parenteral nutrition is required in small infants when the enteral route is not available.

Parenteral nutrition in the management of malnutrition

Commonly patients are seen who have received an inadequate nutritional intake, perhaps over a prolonged period. In such patients the decision to

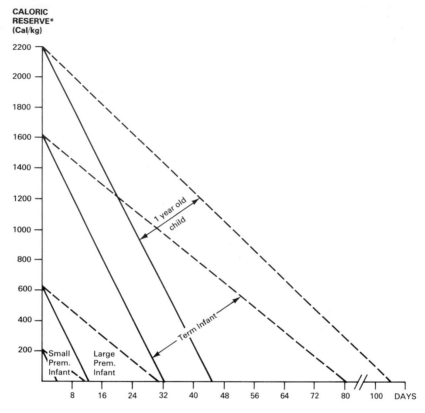

Fig. 24.1 Estimates of the duration of survival during starvation (solid line) and semistarvation (broken line); 10% glucose to supply fluid requirements. (Heird et al 1972).

begin parenteral nutrition is influenced not only by the likely duration of continuing nutritional depletion, but also by careful assessment of current nutritional status. This requires a full history and examination, dietary assessment and measurement of weight, height and plasma albumin in all patients. Only some patients will require a more complete assessment, and Merrit & Blackburn (1981) have proposed the following criteria:- >5% loss of body weight in past month (excluding dehydration), a diagnosis associated with possible protein-energy malnutrition; weight for height <5 percentile, or serum albumin <30 g/l. A convenient method for determining centiles for height, weight and weight for height at the bedside is by the use of a slide rule★ (Cole et al 1981), incorporating Tanner et al (1966) standards. On the basis of a complete assessment, patients may be

★Cole's slide rule, Castlemead Publications, Swains Mill, 4A Crane Mead, Ware, Hertfordshire, England

Table 24.2 Criteria for nutritional support and monitoring (after Merritt & Blackburn 1981)

Group 1: Repletion therapy required in the presence of any of the following:
Serum albumin less than 25 g/l
Transferrin less than 100 μg/100 ml
plus
Weight for height more than 2 SD below normal
Arm muscle area less than 5th percentile (Gurney & Jellife 1973, Frisancho 1981)

Group 2: Maintenance support and continued monitoring required in the presence of any of the following:
Weight for height more than 2 SD below normal
Arm muscle area less than 5th percentile
Serum albumin less than 30 g/l or transferrin less than 150 μg/100 ml

Group 3: No nutritional deficit
Nutritional support not required but continued asessment required in patients undergoing major surgery or nutritional stresses.

assigned to one of three groups for which appropriate treatment and monitoring is suggested (Merritt & Blackburn 1981). See Table 24.2.

Induction of remission or correction of growth failure in Crohn's disease

The rationale and indications for parenteral nutrition in Crohn's disease as a means of inducing remission or of reversing growth failure are discussed in Chapter 6.

SOURCES OF PARENTERAL MACRONUTRIENTS

Energy

Normal energy requirements and the requirements of other nutrients and minerals are given in Table 24.3 and in the Appendix. It is important to realise however that under certain circumstances caloric needs are increased over and above those shown in the table. Thus, each degree of fever above 37°C increases the caloric requirement by 12%, severe sepsis by 40–50%

Table 24.3 Daily intravenous nutritional requirements

Age (years)	Fluid (ml/kg)	Sodium (mmol/kg)	Potassium (mmol/kg)	Protein (g/kg)	Fat (g/kg)	Carbohydrate (g/kg)	Energy (kcal/kg)
0–1	150	2.5	2.5	3.0–3.5	4	13	100–120
1–3	100	2.5	2.5	2.6–3.0	4	10	90–110
3–6	90	2.0	2.0	2.0	4	8	90–100
7–12	70	1.5	1.5	2.0	4	8	80
Adults	35	1.0	1.0	1.2	2	2	35

Details of other mineral, trace element and vitamin requirements are given in Grotte et al (1982) and major surgery by 20–30%. When correcting long-term growth failure, for example in children with Crohn's disease, 40% more calories should be provided than those calculated on the basis of the child's height-age.

A simple method of estimating calorie requirements in children aged 6 months to 15 years (kcals/kg) is: 95 — (3 × age in years) (Wallace 1977).

Water

In order to achieve the desired caloric intake it may be necessary to cautiously increase the fluid intakes recommended in Table 24.3 (by 10 ml/kg/24 h in infants to a maximum of 200 ml/kg/24 h or by 10% of initial volume per day in patients over 10 kg to a maximum of 4000 ml/m^2/24 h, if *tolerated* (Kerner 1983).

A 12% increase in water is required for each 1°C rise in body temperature. Extra fluids are also required to replace ongoing losses resulting from diarrhoea, vomiting or hyperventilation.

Carbohydrate

Glucose is the carbohydrate of choice. It is used by all cells and prevents the hypoglycaemia in low birthweight neonates which results from impaired gluconeogenesis. Although fructose does not lead to hypoglycaemia or increased insulin secretion, it is rapidly metabolized to pyruvate and lactate and in large amounts results in a lactic acidosis. It is therefore unsuitable for use in parenteral nutrition.

There are a number of reasons why glucose should not be the sole caloric source. Fatty infiltration of the liver frequently occurs when glucose is used alone and this may be prevented by the concurrent use of lipid in a ratio of glucose 4:fat 1. Furthermore, glucose as a sole calorie source leads to greater water retention than when combined with lipids (MacFie et al 1981). Glucose oxidation also leads to a greater production of carbon dioxide than lipid and may therefore compromise respiratory function.

Nitrogen

Mixtures of crystalline l-amino acids are preferable to protein hydrolysates; nitrogen utilization is better as crystalline l-amino acid mixtures do not contain non-utilized short chain peptides and formulation is more precise. In addition to the 8 amino acids essential to older children and adults, histidine is essential to infants. Proline, tyrosine, cystine/cysteine and alanine cannot be synthesized in adequate amounts in infancy and should be regarded as 'semiessential.'

To promote efficient protein utilization, between 24 and 32 non-nitrogen calories should be given with each gram of protein used.

Fat

The use of lipid emulsions in parenteral nutrition regimens provides not only a concentrated energy source in a form which leads to less water retention than isocaloric amounts of glucose alone (MacFie et al 1981), but also prevents essential fatty acid deficiency (Friedman 1980). In order to prevent ketosis, lipid should comprise no more than 60% of the total caloric input.

The rate of elimination and metabolic fate of 0.5 μ particles of soya bean oil and egg yolk phospholipids (Intralipid®) is the same as naturally occurring chylomicrons. Thus, clearance from the plasma is dependent upon the activity of lipoprotein lipase on the capillary endothelium. Some intravenous fat emulsions are associated with a deposition of pigmented material in macrophages within the reticuloendothelial system (Passwell et al 1976). However, earlier reports that lipid emulsions impaired bacterial clearance and inhibited neutrophil chemotaxis have not been confirmed (Palmblad et al 1980, English et al 1981).

There is however an association between parenteral lipid-induced hyperlipaemia and diminished pulmonary function (Greene et al 1976). Furthermore, pulmonary fat accumulation has been described in preterm infants (Levine et al 1980). Lipid infusion may also be associated with a reduction in PaO_2 in preterm infants (Sun et al 1978, Pereira et al 1980), in whom its use is associated with increased lymphatic flow and pulmonary arterial pressure. Thus, in infants with increased pulmonary water or lymphatic flow secondary to chronic heart or lung disease, parenteral lipid emulsions, even at low rates of infusion should be used with caution.

Other potential problems related to the use of parenteral lipid emulsions are the displacement of bilirubin by free fatty acids following triglyceride hydrolysis in the neonate (Andrew et al 1976), interference with biochemical estimations on plasma samples, and hypocarnitinaemia (Schiff et al 1979).

Parenteral nutrition in the preterm neonate

Water requirements in preterm infants are extremely variable; insensible water losses are increased by such factors as radiant heaters and phototherapy, and decreased by heat shields and thermal blankets. Overhydration in the first few days of life is associated with an increased incidence of patent ductus arteriosus (Stevenson 1977) and subsequent bronchopulmonary dysplasia (Brown et al 1978); the need for fluid restriction may therefore limit the ability to use adequate calories. In general, an initial parenteral fluid intake of 40–60 ml/kg/24 h in low birthweight neonates is reasonable, increasing to 100 ml/kg/24 h by one week of age and to 130–140 ml/kg/24 h by the end of the second week. Fluid requirements are assessed on the basis of clinical examination, weight gain, urine output and osmolarity and measurement of plasma, urea and electrolytes.

Although a regimen providing between 70–90 kcal/kg/24 h will usually result in weight gain, the exact amount should be tailored to the requirements of the individual as judged by response. In very low birthweight infants, glucose intolerance may limit the calories administered and in some instances it may take 2–3 weeks before 70 kcal/kg may be tolerated. Infants weighing less than 1000 g rarely tolerate more than 6 mg glucose/kg/min and those between 1000–1500 g more than 8 mg/kg/min. The use of insulin to prevent hypoglycaemia is fraught with difficulties because of an extremely variable and unpredictable response and is not recommended.

Once the infant is able to tolerate 100 ml/kg/24 h of 10% glucose, amino acids may be commenced and increased up to a dose of 2.0–2.5 g protein/kg/24 h. Currently the composition of the available amino acid solutions may not be entirely appropriate for preterm infants. In particular, the concentrations of threonine and the aromatic amino acids may be too high and those of the branched chain amino acids, lysine and taurine too low (Rigo & Senterre 1983). Modified solutions are being evaluated.

Parenteral lipid emulsions appear safe to use in preterm babies and their use is associated with fewer apnoeic spells and less hyperbilirubinaemia (Cashore et al 1975). However, infants of less than 32 weeks gestation (Shennan et al 1977) and those who are small for gestational age (Gustafson et al 1974, Olegard et al 1975) have an impaired intolerance of parenteral lipid emulsions. Thus, in these infants lipid is introduced in a dose of 0.5 g/kg/24 h and increased to a maximum of 3 g/kg/24 h over 10 days. In full term, appropriate for gestational age infants, an initial dose of 1 g/kg/24 h is increased to a maximum of 4 g/kg/24 h over 6 days.

TECHNIQUES

Parenteral nutrition is ideally administered by a multidisciplinary nutrition support team (Suskind 1981, Poole & Kerner 1983), comprising physician, pharmacist, nutrition support nurse and dietitians. It seems likely that complications are fewer when protocols are administered by those familiar with the technique (Nehme 1980).

The administration of parenteral feeding solutions by the peripheral route is useful when the anticipated duration is likely to be about two weeks, and when calories appropriate to the patient's requirements may be delivered by a regimen using a 10% rather than a 20% dextrose solution. The use of central venous catheters in sick, malnourished infants carries an appreciable risk of sepsis which can be minimized by the use of peripheral veins. However, the infusion site should be changed frequently and by 2–3 weeks all suitable veins have often been used up. Moreover, the use of this route in the preterm infant requires extra handling which may in itself lead to apnoea and/or hypothermia. In these patients the peripheral, percutaneous insertion of central Silastic® catheters through a winged metal canula (butterfly), using a scalp or antecubital fossa vein may be extremely useful (Shaw 1973). In older, more mobile patients, the catheter inserted by this route often falls out within a week. When a more prolonged period of parenteral nutrition is anticipated, a central venous catheter is inserted surgically, usually under general anaesthesia. Recently two special Silastic® catheters have been introduced (Hickman & Broviac) which terminate in an integral Luer-Lok connector at the proximal end. This ensures secure connection with the giving set and enables the catheter to be heparin-locked* and used intermittently if this is desirable. Futhermore, a Dacron cuff is attached to the midpoint of both makes of catheter. This is positioned subcutaneously near the exit site and induces the formation of fibrous tissue which anchors the catheter in place after about two weeks. The catheters are removed by a steady pull; the Dacron cuff, which remains subcutaneously, undergoes spontaneous lysis or is removed surgically. A subcutaneous skin tunnel between the point of entry of the catheter into a central vein (e.g. internal jugular) and a distant exit site helps to stabilize the catheter and to reduce the risk of infection. Favoured exit sites are on the upper chest wall or over the deltoid muscle; both provide freedom of movement for the patient, while permitting the junction between catheter and giving set to be mounted on the chest wall or on a padded splint secured to the patient's upper arm.

The distal end of the catheter is ideally placed in the superior vena cava rather than the right atrium and its position should be checked radiologically before hypertonic solutions are infused. The injection of Conray 280 into the catheter before chest X-ray enables the catheter to be seen more easily.

Broviac and Hickman catheters are secured in position by cutaneous sutures, which may be removed after two weeks, when the Dacron cuff will have induced sufficient fibrosis to maintain the catheter in place. Smaller Silastic® catheters without Dacron cuffs may be anchored by spraying the entry site with Medical Adhesive Silicone Type A® (Dow Corning). This not only mobilizes the catheter but also produces a bacteria-proof barrier.

Infusion system

Figure 24.2 illustrates the arrangement of infusion pumps, giving sets and infusion bottles. Glucose, an amino acid solution (e.g. Vamin-glucose®), and a trace-element/mineral supplement (e.g. Ped-El® or Addamel®) are administered from a 3-litre bag, and a lipid emulsion (e.g. Intralipid®), fat and water soluble vitamins (e.g. Vitlipid Infant® and Solivito®) adminis-

---

*Injection of 2.5 ml heparin solution (100 units heparin per ml) through the injection cap every 12–24 hours.

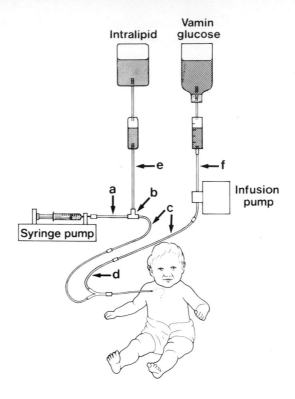

Fig. 24.2 Arrangement of infusion sets, pumps and infusates:
a) Braun LuerLok extension tube (425603/4)
b) 3-way tap
c) Avon Medicals 3 mm extension set (S 1028)
d) Avon Medicals Y-type extension set (A 64)
e) Braun Intrafix Air-P giving set (462710/8)
f) Abbott Soluset giving set (4965).

tered using a syringe pump (Booth & Harries 1982). Parenteral feeding
solutions and additives are made up under sterile conditions in a laminar
air-flow cabinet and delivered to the ward in sealed bags. Solutions and
giving sets are changed every 24 hours, using an aseptic technique for
disconnection and reconnection. The glucose-amino acid solution is infused
constantly over 24 hours, but the lipid emulsion is switched off for 4 hours
each day prior to blood sampling for biochemical and haematological
monitoring. When sterile conditions are not available for making up
parenteral feeding solutions, glucose and Vamin-glucose® are infused from
separate bottles, each with its own giving set. Ped-El® or Addamel® is
added to the Vamin-glucose® solution and additional potassium and phosphate to the glucose solution. Guidelines for the prescription of parenteral
nutrition fluids and a number of suggested regimens are given in the
Appendix.

Nursing care

Obsessional attention to detail pays dividends. An aseptic technique is essential when changing infusions and giving sets each day, and in the care of the catheter insertion site. The latter is best undertaken by a single nurse, as part of a nutritional support service. The optimal frequency and type of care given to the insertion site is not known. Daily inspection and dressing is probably unnecessary and meddlesome, and weekly nursing care is a reasonable alternative. The insertion site is inspected for sepsis, an alcoholic solution of providone-iodine applied, followed by a nonadherent dressing held in place by waterproof Elastoplast®.

Table 24.4 Monitoring parenteral nutrition

	First week	After first week
Body weight	Daily	Daily
Height	Weekly	Weekly
Sodium	Daily	2 ×/week
Potassium	Daily	2 ×/week
Calcium	2 ×/week	Weekly
Magnesium	2 ×/week	Weekly
Phosphate	2 ×/week	Weekly
Albumen	2 ×/week	Weekly
Alkaline phosphatase	2 ×/week	Weekly
Zinc	Weekly	Fortnightly
Copper	Weekly	Fortnightly
Glucose[1]	Daily	2 ×/week
Plasma turbidity[2]	Daily	2 ×/week
Bilirubin	2 ×/week	Weekly
Alanine aminotransferase	2 ×/week	Weekly
Haemoglobin	2 ×/week	Weekly
White cell count and differential	2 ×/week	Weekly
Platelet count	2 ×/week	Weekly

All variables should be measured before starting treatment
[1] Urinary glucose should be measured 2–6 ×/day during the first week and thence daily
[2] Checked visually, four hours after parenteral lipid discontinued

MONITORING TREATMENT

Many of the biochemical and haematological complications of parenteral nutrition may be avoided by regular and careful monitoring. Parenteral nutrition should not be performed unless all the investigations shown in Table 24.4 can be performed on capillary blood samples. The recommendations apply only to those patients who are free of large continuing losses, such as profuse diarrhoea, in whom more frequent biochemical monitoring is indicated.

Intravenous lipid emulsions may interfere with a wide variety of laboratory investigations and this infusion should therefore be discontinued for four hours prior to blood sampling (usually between 6.00 and 10.00). This period of time also enables lipid utilization to be assessed by examining the 10.00 am blood sample for lipaemia.

COMPLICATIONS

Catheter-related sepsis

Infection remains the most common complication of parenteral nutrition and the commonest reason for removing a central catheter. The strictest possible attention to aseptic technique when making up and changing solutions, a daily change of solutions and giving sets and obsessional attention to the nursing care of catheters are of the greatest importance in reducing the incidence of infection. Rates of sepsis do however remain higher in children than in adults. Silastic® catheters, giving sets and dressings are objects of great fascination to paediatric patients with enquiring minds.

Although a wide variety of organisms are implicated in catheter-related sepsis, the most frequently identified are those which are normally skin commensals: *Staphylococcus epidermidis and S. aureus. Candida albicans* is found less frequently but is particularly difficult to treat. Organisms may either colonize the internal surface of the catheter, a process which is enhanced by the formation of fibrin deposits at the catheter tip, or may track down the external surface of the catheter from the skin around the insertion site. The use of skin tunnels between the entry point in the skin and the point of entry into the circulation, may reduce the incidence of the latter phenomenon.

Table 24.5 Features of catheter-related sepsis in parenterally-fed children

Fever (or temperature instability)
Tachycardia, tachypnoea, and/or apnoea
Local signs of infection at entry site
Irritability/lethargy
Hepatosplenomegaly
Jaundice
Vomiting
Abdominal distension
Change in stool character or increase in volume
Rashes
Thrombocytopaenia

The symptoms and signs of sepsis are summarized in Table 24.5 and appropriate investigations are given in Table 24.6. No incontrovertible guidelines can be given about what to do when sepsis is suspected. Usually the most important question to be answered is whether the central line should be removed, and this decision is strongly influenced by the patient's clinical status. In general, catheters which are probably infected should be removed. However, in a severely malnourished patient with profuse diarrhoea and few alternative sites for insertion of central lines, attempts to treat the infection and leave the line in situ, may well be justified. The use of urokinase may be helpful in this respect (Glynn et al 1980). A suggested course of action when sepsis is suspected is given in Fig. 24.3.

Table 24.6 Investigation of suspected catheter-related sepsis

Full clinical examination, including fundoscopy for candida spots
Full blood count (including platelets)
Peripheral blood culture for anaerobic and aerobic bacteria and candida
Urine microscopy and culture
Gram stain of buffy coat (blood in heparinized tube)
Consider lumbar puncture
Swab for culture of male and female ends of connection between giving set and line

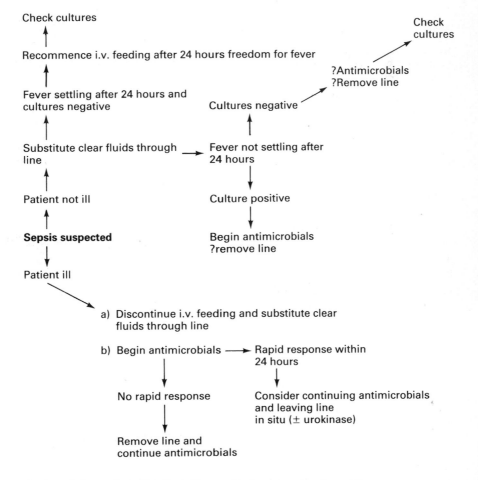

Check cultures

Recommence i.v. feeding after 24 hours freedom for fever

Fever settling after 24 hours and cultures negative

Substitute clear fluids through line

Patient not ill

Sepsis suspected

Patient ill

Cultures negative

Fever not settling after 24 hours

Culture positive

Begin antimicrobials
?remove line

?Antimicrobials
?Remove line

Check cultures

a) Discontinue i.v. feeding and substitute clear fluids through line

b) Begin antimicrobials ⟶ Rapid response within 24 hours

No rapid response

Consider continuing antimicrobials and leaving line in situ (± urokinase)

Remove line and continue antimicrobials

Aspirate infusate from line for culture, prior to removal and send tip in transport medium for culture.

Fig. 24.3 Suggested course of action in suspected catheter-related sepsis.

Metabolic complications

The metabolic complications of parenteral nutrition are summarized in Table 24.7. With the exception of hepatic dysfunction, they are largely avoidable by careful monitoring. Particular attention is drawn to hypophosphataemia which is a potentially serious complication, usually encountered in severely malnourished patients. It is associated with reduced cellular adenosine triphosphate (ATP) and red-cell 2,3-diphosphoglycerate, an encephalopathy, myocardial dysfunction and impaired neutrophil function. It may be avoided by introducing parenteral nutrition particularly slowly in severely malnourished patients and by extra-parenteral phosphate supplements.

Table 24.7 Metabolic complications of parenteral nutrition

Hyperglycaemia, glycosuria and osmotic diuresis
Rebound hypoglycaemia
Metabolic acidosis
Hypocalcaemia
Hypomagnesaemia
Hypophosphataemia
Hyperammonaemia
Amino acid toxicity
Hyperlipidaemia
Essential fatty acid deficiency (lipid-free infusions)
Trace metal deficiency
Hepatic dysfunction

A common and unexplained complication of parenteral nutrition is the development of liver disease; it may occur, for example in up to one-third of preterm infants (American Academy of Paediatrics 1983). Conjugated hyperbilirubinaemia with raised plasma alkaline phosphatase and transaminase activities are present, and the liver may be enlarged. Histologically there is a nonspecific hepatitis with bile duct proliferation, lymphocyte infiltration and variable fibrosis (Dahms & Halpin 1981). Cirrhosis may develop.

The aetiology of this serious complication remains unclear. In many patients there is intercurrent sepsis or recent abdominal surgery. It has been suggested that the constituents of the parenteral nutrition regimen, or bacterial endotoxins, may be responsible, but the evidence incriminating any individual component of the regimen is not good. It has also been suggested that cholestasis is the result of suppression of the release of those trophic hormones normally produced by the gut during enteral nutrition (Hughes et al 1983), but this remains speculative. The development of hepatobiliary dysfunction in adults is associated with the appearance of increased amounts of the secondary bile acid lithocholate in duodenal bile (Fouin-Fortunet et al 1982). Lithocholate is formed by bacterial 7-alpha-dehydroxylation of chenodeoxycholate, is hepatotoxic and produces a histological lesion in the liver similar to that seen in parenterally-fed patients. Thus, bacterial overgrowth of the small intestine may be the primary aetiological factor in the initiation of hepatic dysfunction in these patients. Metronidazole may therfore be useful in the management of this complication (Capron et al 1983).

ENTERAL NUTRITION

In the experimental animal the exclusion of luminal nutrients during total parenteral nutrition results in marked atrophic changes in the gut and pancreas with concurrent impairment of function (Hughes & Dowling 1980, Hughes et al 1980). Intraluminal nutrients are also important in adaptation of intestinal function following extensive gut resection (Feldman et al 1976), and possibly in the promotion of postnatal gut development and maturation. These trophic effects on the intestinal mucosa may be direct, and/or mediated by gastrointestinal hormones. It is therefore desirable to maintain a small oral nutritional intake during parenteral feeding whenever possible.

Following a period of parenteral nutrition the transition to enteral feeding should be made very gradually, as the abrupt interruption of parenteral nutrition may result in severe, rebound hypoglycaemia. The transitional period should not be less than one week and may extend to several weeks. Small volumes of dilute oral feedings are first introduced and then increased gradually to full strength. The volume of feeds may then be cautiously increased, while the volume of parenteral feeds is reduced pari passu. Many infants and children are reluctant to feed orally following prolonged parenteral nutrition for reasons which are not clear; patience is usually rewarded.

PSYCHOSOCIAL LIFE OF THE PARENTERALLY-FED INFANT

When infants are parenterally fed for prolonged periods of two months or more, they may become increasingly withdrawn and isolated and demonstrate impaired intellectual and emotional development, unless strenuous efforts are made to prevent this. These changes appear to be related not only to the physical constraints imposed by the apparatus used but also to parental separation and lack of stimulation.

The following measures should be adopted to minimize these sequelae:

a) Parents should be resident if possible. In many cases, owing to other family commitments or geographical separation, this is impractical and under these circumstances the parents should be encouraged to visit as frequently as possible.

b) Infants and children should be as active as possible and in most cases frequent excursions in pram or pushchair, using portable infusion pumps should be made.

c) When the mother is not resident, a permanent member of the ward staff should endeavour to form a close one-to-one relationship with the infant, with the object of providing a focus for emotional attachment. This member of staff should be excluded from direct involvement in painful procedures.

d) A clinical psychologist, with a special interest in the needs of infants and children who spend prolonged periods in hospital should be available to the parenteral nutrition team so that regular assessment and expert advice are readily available.

HOME PARENTERAL NUTRITION

The advent of suitable nutrients and well-tested methods of providing total parenteral nutrition has encouraged many groups to provide this form of nutritional support at home. Provided the logistical problems of monitoring, and supply of nutrients and hardware are solved many parents can be taught to care very effectively for the intravenous catheters. In the short-term such treatment by groups who have experience of managing patients at home seems successful. However, there is only scanty information regarding the outcome of long-term treatment and the experience of at least one group (Ralston et al 1984) suggests that it should be approached with caution.

ETHICS

The expertise is now available to keep infants with intestinal failure alive for very prolonged periods, i.e. for more than one year. However, in certain categories of infant such as those with lethal familial protracted diarrhoea following massive intestinal resection the chances of survival are small. The decision to feed such infants parenterally, with the resulting exposure of themselves, their parents and siblings to the unpleasant consequences of treatment which may extend for years, is often extremely difficult. Following carefully informed discussions with colleagues and parents, the withholding of parenteral nutrition may be practised in some instances.

APPENDIX

GUIDELINES FOR THE PRESCRIPTION OF PAEDIATRIC PARENTERAL NUTRITION

Feeding tables

Two basic solutions are usually prepared for paediatric use:
Solution 1 containing an amino acid solution, glucose solution, electrolytes and minerals.
Solution 2 containing a lipid solution plus fat and water-soluble vitamins.
A third solution may be needed to replace abnormal loses.

Tables 24.8–10 are intended as guidelines only, and the clinical condition of the child should be considered before prescribing intravenous nutrients. *Patients should be in fluid and electrolyte balance before TPN is commenced as it is difficult to correct gross imbalances using these solutions.* It is strongly recommended that the feeding regimens are introduced over 6 days, as illustrated in the feeding tables. During this time the amino acid and glucose concentrations are gradually increased to reach full amounts on day 6 of intravenous feeding. This ensures that glycosuria, hypophosphataemia and hyperglycaemia are avoided. The full requirements of both electrolytes and minerals may be introduced on day 1 of TPN, providing adequate renal function is present.

Rapid introduction of full TPN, particularly in the severely malnourished child almost invariably results in severe hypophosphataemia which may be life-threatening. Day 6 represents the full normal TPN regimens. The glucose concentration or fluid volumes may be *cautiously increased* beyond these values if this is necessary to maintain growth.

Additions to the basic solutions

Solution 1

This solution comprises Vamin-glucose®★, additional dextrose (either 10% or 15%) and added electrolyte trace element and mineral solutions as detailed in Tables 24.8–10. The amino acid solution (Vamin-Glucose®) and the trace element solutions (Addamel® and Ped-El®) contain some electrolytes and minerals, but many of these need to be supplemented to provide an adequate daily intravenous intake. Additions should be made after consulting the patient's current biochemical data and the reference intervals appropriate to the hospital's biochemical laboratory.

The paediatric daily intravenous requirements of electrolytes, minerals and vitamins are shown in Table 24.3. In addition to the amino acid and glucose solutions, the following ingredients may be added:

Ped-El®. This paediatric electrolyte solution is used to provide essential electrolytes and trace minerals to infants weighing less than 10 kg. Ped-El® contains a high sorbitol load (30%); it should therefore be used with caution in patients with fructose intolerance or impaired renal or liver functions. Usual dose: 5 ml/kg/24 h.

Addamel. This solution replaces Ped-El in those children weighing over 10 kilograms. Addamel® also contains 30% sorbitol, but since it is a more concentrated solution than Ped-El®, a smaller volume is used, resulting in a reduction in the amount of sorbitol administered in the older children. Addamel® is relatively low in some constituents compared with Ped-El® and these should be supplemented to provide an adequate daily intravenous intake. Usual dose: 0.2 ml/kg/24 h, maximum 10 ml/24 h.

★Vamin-glucose® Ped-El® Addamel® — Products of Kabi Vitrum Ltd

Table 24.8 Total parenteral nutrition for infants up to 10 kg — central line

	Prescription/kg/24 hour									Provision/kg/24 hours													
	Solution 1				Solution 2																		
Day of TPN	Vamin Glucose (V.G.)	Ped-el	Dextrose 10%	Dextrose 15%	Intra-lipid 20% (IL)	Vitlipid Infant (max 4 ml)	Solivito (max 10 ml)	Total fluid	Total Calories	Non-N Calories (in Kcals)	Fat (g)	Amino Acids (g)	Nitrogen (g)	CHO (g)	Na⁺	K⁺	Ca²⁺	Mg²⁺	P	Cl⁻	Fe²⁺	Zn²⁺	Cu²⁺
	mls	mls	mls	mls	mls	mls	mls	mls	K cals	Fat + Dextrose + Dextrose in V.G.	IL	V.G.	V.G.	V.G.+ Dex-trose	V.G.	V.G.	Ped-El® + V.G.	Ped-El®	Ped-El® Fat + V.G.	V.G. + V.G. Ped-El®	Ped-El®	Ped-El®	Ped-El®
															(mmol)	(mmol)	(mmol)	(mmol)	(mmol)	(mmol)	(μmol)	(μmol)	(μmol)
1	20	5	96	—	6	1	2	127	61	55.6	1.2	1.4	0.19	11.6	1	0.4	0.8	0.155	0.465	2.85	2.5	0.75	0.375
2–3	32	5	88	—	12	1	2	137	78	69.1	2.4	2.24	0.3	12	1.6	0.64	0.83	0.173	0.555	3.51	2.5	0.75	0.375
–	40	5	—	80	16	1	2	141	103	92.1	3.2	2.8	0.38	16	2	0.8	0.85	0.185	0.615	3.95	2.5	0.75	0.375
6⁺	48	5	—	80	20	1	2	153	116	103.1	4	3.36	0.45	16.8	2.4	0.96	0.87	0.197	0.675	4.39	2.5	0.75	0.375

Table 24.9 Total parenteral nutrition for infants up to 10 kg — peripheral line

Prescription/kg/24 hours					Provision/kg/24 hours*																
Solution 1			Solution 2																		
Vamin® Glucose (VG)	Ped-El® Dextrose 10%	Intralipid® 20% (1L)	Vitlipid® Infant (max 4 ml)	Solivito® (max 10 ml)	Total fluid	Total calories	Non-calories N (K cal)	Net energy per gram N (Kcal/g)	Fat (g)	Amino acids (g)	Nitrogen (g)	CHO (g)	Na⁺ (mmol)	K⁺ (mmol)	Ca²⁺ (mmol)	Mg²⁺ (mmol)	P (mmol)	Cl⁻ (mmol)	Fe²⁺ (μmol)	Zn²⁺ (μmol)	Cu²⁺ (μmol)
Day of TPN																					
ml	ml	ml	ml	ml	ml	Kcal			IL	V.G.	V.G.	V.G. + Dextrose	V.G.	V.G.	Ped-El® + V.G.	Ped-El®	Ped-El® Fat+ V.G.	Ped-El® + V.G.	Ped-El®	Ped-El®	Ped-El®
							Fat+ Dext.+ Dext. in V.G.														
1	20	5	6	1	2	127	61	55.6	321	1.2	1.4	0.19	11.6	1	0.4	0.8	0.155	0.465	2.85	2.5	0.75	0.375
2–3	32	5	12	1	2	137	78	69.1	260	2.4	2.24	0.3	12	1.6	0.64	0.83	0.173	0.555	3.51	2.5	0.75	0.375
4–5	40	5	16	1	2	143	88	77	234	3.2	2.8	0.38	12	2	0.8	0.85	0.185	0.615	3.95	2.5	0.75	0.375
6+	48	5	20	1	2	155	101	88	225	4	3.36	0.45	12.8	2.4	0.96	0.87	0.197	0.675	4.39	2.5	0.75	0.375

(i) The total fluid volume *does not* include the water and fat soluble vitamins (maximum 14 ml/24 hours).
(ii) The energy value of dextrose is calculated as 1 g = 3.76 Kcal.
(iii) Solivito® is dissolved in 5 ml of water and the appropriate volume removed, or in 4 ml of Vitlipid® infant if patient is > 5 kg
*The provision/kg/24 hours refers only to one quantity of electrolytes and trace elements present in the basic solutions; it may be necessary to add additional amounts to provide the daily intravenous requirements.

Table 24.10 Total parenteral nutrition for children weighing over 10 kg

Weight (kg)	Age (approx) (years)	Day of TPN	Vamin-Glucose amel® (VG) ml/kg/24hr	Add-amel® ml/kg/24hr	Dextrose 10% ml/kg/24hr	Dextrose 15% ml/kg/24hr	Intralipid® 20% (il) ml/kg/24hr	Vitlipid® Infant ml/kg/24hr Max 4 ml	Solivito® ml/kg/24hr Max 10 ml	Total Fluid ml/kg/24hr	Total Calories Kcal/24hr VG+IL+Dextrose	Kcal Non-N Kcal/24hr VG+IL+Dextrose	Fat (g) IL	Amino Acids (g) VG	Nitrogen (g) VG	CHO (g) VG+Dextrose	Na+ (mmol) VG	K+ (mmol) VG	Ca2+ (mmol) Addamel®+VG	Mg2+ (mmol) Addamel®+VG	P (mmol) Addamel® IL	Cl- (mmol) VG+Addamel®	Fe2+ (µmol) Addamel®	Zn2+ (µmol) Addamel®	Cu2+ (µmol) Addamel®
10–15	1–3	1	10	0.2	70	–	5	1	2	85.2	44.5	21	1	0.7	0.09	8	0.5	0.2	0.13	0.045	0.075	0.82	1.0	0.4	0.1
		2+3	20	0.2	60	–	10	1	2	90.2	57	34	2	1.4	0.19	8	1.0	0.4	0.15	0.065	0.155	1.37	1.0	0.4	0.1
		4+5	30	0.2	–	50	15	1	2	95.2	79.5	72	3	2.1	0.3	10.5	1.5	0.6	0.18	0.075	0.225	1.92	1.0	0.4	0.1
		6+	40	0.2	–	40	20	1	2	100.2	88.5	78	4	2.8	0.38	10	2.0	0.8	0.2	0.085	0.3	2.47	1.0	0.4	0.1
15–20	3–6	1	10	0.2	60	–	5	1	2	75.2	40.5	38	1	0.7	0.09	7	0.5	0.2	0.13	0.045	0.075	0.82	1.0	0.4	0.1
		2+3	15	0.2	55	–	5	1	2	80.2	51.8	48	2	1.05	0.14	7	0.75	0.3	0.14	0.055	0.155	1.12	1.0	0.4	0.1
		4+5	25	0.2	–	45	15	1	2	85.2	73.2	58	3	1.4	0.24	9.3	1.25	0.5	0.16	0.065	0.225	1.62	1.0	0.4	0.1
		6+	30	0.2	–	40	20	1	2	90.1	82	73.8	4	2.1	0.28	9	1.5	0.6	0.17	0.075	0.3	1.92	1.0	0.4	0.1
20–30	6–12	1	10	0.2	45	–	5	1	2	60.2	34.5	32	1	0.7	0.09	5.5	0.5	0.2	0.13	0.045	0.075	0.82	1.0	0.4	0.1
		2+3	15	0.2	40	–	10	1	2	65.2	45.8	42	2	1.05	0.14	5.5	0.75	0.3	0.14	0.055	0.155	1.12	1.0	0.4	0.1
		4+5	20	0.2	–	35	15	1	2	70.2	64	59	3	1.4	0.19	7.25	1.0	0.4	0.15	0.65	0.225	1.37	1.0	0.4	0.1
		6+	30	0.2	–	25	15	1	2	70.2	64.5	55.4	3	2.1	0.28	6.75	1.5	0.6	0.17	0.075	0.225	1.92	1.0	0.4	0.1
30+	12+	1	5	0.2	35	–	5	1	2	45.2	27.3	26	1	0.35	0.05	4	0.25	0.1	0.11	0.035	0.075	0.52	1.0	0.4	0.1
		2+3	10	0.2	30	–	10	1	2	50.2	38.5	36	2	0.7	0.09	4	0.5	0.2	0.13	0.045	0.155	0.82	1.0	0.4	0.1
		4+5	15	0.2	–	25	10	1	2	50.2	44.8	41	2	1.05	0.14	5.25	0.75	0.3	0.14	0.055	0.155	1.12	1.0	0.4	0.1
		6+	20	0.2	–	20	10	1	2	50.2	44.3	38.2	2	1.4	0.19	5	1.0	0.4	0.15	0.065	0.15	1.37	1.0	0.4	0.1

Table 24.11 Constituents of solutions used in preparation of TPN

Constituents of Solivito® (per ml)

Vitamin B1	0.24 mg
Vitamin B2	0.36 mg
Nicotinamide	2.0 mg
Vitamin B6	0.4 mg
Pantothenic Acid	2.0 mg
Biotin	0.06 mg
Folic Acid	0.04 mg
Vitamin B12	0.4 µg
Vitamin C	6.0 mg

Constituents of Infant Vitlipid® (per ml)

Vitamin A	100 µg (333 i.u.)
Vitamin D	2.5 µg (100 i.u.)
Vitamin K	50 µg

Although vitamin E is present in Intralipid® 20%, it is predominantly in the form of γ-tocopherol which has only 10% of the biological activity of α-tocopherol which in health is the major vitamin E species.

Constituents of Ped-El® (per 5 ml)

Calcium	0.75 mmol
Magnesium	125 µmol
Iron	2.5 µmol
Zinc	0.75 µmol
Manganese	1.25 µmol
Copper	0.375 µmol
Fluoride	3.75 µmol
Iodide	0.05 µmol
Phosphorus	375 µmol
Chloride	1.75 mmol
Sorbitol	1.5 g

Constituents of Addamel® (per 0.2 ml)

Calcium	0.1 mmol
Magnesium	30 µmol
Iron	1.0 µmol
Zinc	0.4 µmol
Manganese	0.8 µmol
Copper	0.1 µmol
Fluoride	1.0 µmol
Iodide	0.02 µmol
Chloride	0.27 mmol
Sorbitol	0.06 g

Vamin® — glucose (per 1000 ml)

Amino acids	70.2 g
Glucose (anhydrous)	100 g
Sodium	50 mmol
Potassium	20 mmol
Calcium	2.5 mmol
Magnesium	1.5 mmol
Chloride	55 mmol
Nitrogen per litre: 9.4 g	

Energy content per litre: 650 kcal of which 400 kcal are provided by glucose

Table 24.11   Constituents of solution used in preparation of TPN (*contd.*)

Intralipid® 20% (per 500 ml)
    Fractionated soya-bean oil   100 g
    Fractionated egg-phospholipids 6 g
    Glycerol   11 g
Water for injections to 500 ml

Energy content 2 kcal per ml of 20% Intralipid®

Electrolyte and mineral solutions used in TPN preparation

Ion	Solution	Commercial source	Ion (mmol/ml)
Na$^+$	Sodium chloride 30% (NaCl)	Macarthy	5.13
	Sodium phosphate 17.91% (Na$_2$HPO$_4$)	Macarthy	2.0
	Sodium bicarbonate 8.4% (NaHCO$_3$)	Macarthy	1.0
K$^+$	Potassium phosphate 17.42% (KH$_2$PO$_4$)	Macarthy	2.0
	Potassium chloride 15% (KCl)	Antigen	2.0
HPO+$^{2-}$	Potassium phosphate 17.42% (KH$_2$PO$_4$)	Macarthy	1.0
	Sodium phosphate 17.91% (Na$_2$HPO$_4$)	Macarthy	1.0
Zn^{++}	Zinc sulphate 50 mcmol/ml (ZnSO$_4$)	Macarthy	0.05
Mg^{++}	Magnesium sulphate 50% (MgSO$_4$ 7H$_2$O)	Evans	2.0
Ca^{++}	Calcium gluconate 10% (C$_{12}$H$_{22}$CaO$_{14}$.H$_2$O)	Antigen	0.22
	Calcium chloride (CaCl2)	Macarthy	1.0
Cu^{++}	Copper sulphate 0.4 mg/ml (CuSO$_4$.5H$_2$O)	Travenol	0.0016

Electrolytes. Patients receiving TPN, particularly those undergoing long term treatment, should be carefully monitored for deficiencies, special care being taken with the trace elements. Electrolyte requirements are requested on the prescription form as the *total amount* required *per kilogram per day.* This enables the pharmacist to deduct the amount present in the basic solutions and add any additional amounts required.

Sodium is usually added as sodium chloride injection 30% (containing 5.13 mmol Na$^+$ in 1 ml). If a different sodium salt is required, e.g. bicarbonate or phosphate, this should be indicated on the prescription form.

Potassium is usually added as potassium phosphate 17.42% (containing 2 mmol K$^+$ and 1 mmol phosphate in 1 ml). For infants weighing less than 10 kg, when more than 4 mmol/kg of potassium is requested, additional potassium should be added as potassium chloride 15% (containing 2 mmol K$^+$ in 1 ml) to prevent hyperphosphataemia developing. For children over 10 kg, extra potassium is usually added as potassium chloride 15%, although a small proportion may be added as potassium phosphate to provide the daily phosphate requirement. Patients receiving concomitant antibiotic therapy, particularly amphotericin, may have a higher than normal requirement for potassium during and immediately following the treatment period.

Phosphate is usually added as potassium phosphate 17.42%. It is present as Ped-El® and in small quantities in Intralipid®, where egg phospholipids are added as emulsion stabilizers, although it is not certain if the phosphate in this form is biologically available. If necessary, phosphate may be added as sodium phosphate 17.91% (containing 2 mmol Na^+ and 1 mmol phosphate in 1 ml of solution). This is of particular value if potassium is being restricted.

Infants weighing less than 10 kg receive their daily phosphate requirements from the Ped-El® and the additional potassium, as this is usually all added as potassium phosphate.

Patients weighing over 10 kg should receive at least 0.5 mmol phosphate/kg body weight/24 h. This may need to be increased in severely malnourished children or in those receiving high glucose concentrations.

Care should be taken when prescribing additional phosphate; it is always provided as the sodium or potassium salt and therefore its use may be limited by the concentrations of those ions requested.

Heparin is added to Solution 1 when a central line is in situ to help prevent thrombus formation at the catheter tip. Usually 1.0 unit/ml of solution is added, although care may need to be taken in the immediate post-op period.

Zinc. Both Ped-El® and Addamel® are relatively low in zinc. Therefore they need to be supplemented (as zinc sulphate 50 μmol in 1 ml) to provide a daily dosage of 2.0 μmol/kg/24 h. In patients with abnormally high fluid losses, e.g. chronic diarrhoea or fistulae, and in premature infants or severely malnourished children, stores of zinc may be depleted. In these patients it is necessary to provide additional zinc to supply the daily demand and to replete stores. In these cases doses in excess of 5.0 μmol/kg/24 h may be required.

Copper. Ped-El® contains sufficient copper to meet a basal requirement of 0.2 μmol Cu^{++}/kg/24 h. This may need to be increased in deficiency states or in patients with abnormal losses, to 0.5 μmol/kg/24 h. Addamel® is relatively low in copper and the basal requirements should be met using copper sulphate containing 1.6 μmol in 1 ml.

Calcium is present in adequate amounts in Ped-El®, but additional requirements can be met using calcium gluconate 10% (containing 0.223 mmol Ca^{++} in 1 ml). Addamel® has a relatively low calcium content. This should be supplemented to provide 0.5–1.0 mmol calcium/kg/24 h.

Calcium gluconate is more compatible with the phosphate present in Ped-El® and potassium phosphate, than is calcium chloride. However it is a very dilute solution and it may be more practical to use calcium chloride, particularly in the older children, if the additional chloride load can be tolerated. Calcium chloride 10% contains 1 mmol Ca^{++} and 2 mmol Cl^- in 1 ml.

Magnesium Ped-El® contains sufficient magnesium to meet basal requirements. Addamel® has a relatively low content, and therefore additional magnesium can be added as magnesium sulphate 50% (containing 2 mmol Mg^{++} in 1 ml) to provide 0.15 mmol/kg/24 h. Patients receiving amphotericin and some cytotoxics, particularly cisplatinum, may need additional magnesium supplements during and immediately following the treatment period.

Solution 2

Intralipid 20%* This lipid solution is used to provide essential fatty acids (EFA), and is also used as a calorie source. Patients on a fat-free intravenous diet, particularly if this continues for long periods, should be carefully monitored for EFA deficiency; this can be prevented by massaging 15 ml sunflower oil into the skin daily, or infusing 0.5–1 g/kg/24 h of fat as parenteral lipid emulsion.

Vitlipid Infant®* provides the fat-soluble vitamins A, D and K. Dose: 1.0 ml/kg/24 h, maximum 4 ml/24 h.

Solivito®* provides the water-soluble vitamins. *Solivito* is presented as a freeze-dried powder. This should be reconstituted immediately before use with either 5 ml water for injection (per vial of Solvito®) and added to solution 1, or with the required volume of Vitlipid Infant®, and added to Solution 2.

Dose: 2 ml/kg/24 h, maximum 10 ml/24 h (2 vials).

The water-soluble vitamins are degraded quickly by both natural light and amino acid solutions. The addition of Solivito® to Solution 2, if present, removes the amino acids and the whiteness of the lipid solution gives added protection to the light. The solution containing the water-soluble vitamins should always be protected from light using the red plastic bags provided; patients receiving these infusions should be moved away from windows to help protect the vitamins.

Solution 3

This solution is prepared to replace abnormal fluid losses, e.g. from ileostomies or gastric aspirate.

Single-bag system

This may be possible in some stable infants and children, but high losses and requirements often lead to incompatibility. High concentrations of divalent cations may lead to the formation of soaps with fat emulsions rendering both biologically unavailable.

Incompatibilities

TPN solutions are complicated mixtures and it may not always be possible to add all the ingredients requested. This is a special problem in patients of less than 10 kg receiving Ped-El® and potassium phosphate who need additional calcium, magnesium or bicarbonate. A precipitate of insoluble salts is favoured by high pH and by high concentrations of divalent cations in the solution.

Problems may also arise in patients who are fluid restricted, or where a peripheral line is in situ, since low glucose concentrations result in a solution with a relatively high pH allowing insoluble precipitates to form.

Other drugs may also cause precipitation of ingredients, or may themselves be precipitated or degraded by the TPN solutions. Due to the low pH of TPN solutions, it is not advisable to infuse some drugs at the same infusion site unless an adequate flushing procedure is adopted; penicillins are a particular example as they are rapidly degraded at low pH.

Storage of solutions

The compounded TPN solutions are stable for at least 96 hours, provided they are manufactured under strict aseptic conditions and are stored at 4°C in a refrigerator immediately prior to use. TPN solutions should *never* be warmed before infusion, but should be allowed to come slowly to room temperature.

*Intralipid, Vitlipid, Solivito — Products of Kabi Vitrum Ltd

REFERENCES

American Academy of Pediatrics: Committee on Nutrition 1983 Commentary on parenteral nutrition. Pediatrics 71: 547–552

Andrew G, Chan G, Schiff D 1976 Lipid metabolism in the neonate II. The effect of Intralipid on bilirubin binding in vitro and in vivo. Journal of Pediatrics 88: 279–284

Booth I W, Harries J T 1982 Parenteral nutrition in young children. British Journal of Parenteral Therapy 3: 31–40

Brown E R, Stark A, Sosenko I, Lawson E E, Avery M E 1978 Bronchopulmonary dysplasia: possible relationship to pulmonary oedema. Journal of Pediatrics 92: 982–984

Capron J P, Gineston J L, Herve M A, Braillon A 1983 Metronidazole in prevention of cholestasis associated with parenteral nutrition. Lancet i: 446–447

Cashore W J, Sedaghatian M R, Usher R H 1975 Nutritional supplements with intravenously administered lipid, protein hydrolysate and glucose in small premature infants. Pediatrics 56: 8–16

Cheek D 1968 Body composition, cell growth, energy and intelligence. In: Cheek D B (ed) Human Growth. Lea & Febiger, Philadelphia pp 353–371

Cole T J, Donnet M L, Stanfield J P 1981 Weight for height indices to assess nutritional status — a new index on a slide rule. American Journal of Clinical Nutrition 34: 1935–1943

Dahms B B, Halpin T C 1981 Serial liver biopsies in parenteral nutrition-associated cholestasis of early infancy. Gastroenterology 81: 136–144

English D, Roloff J S, Lukens J N, Parker P, Greene H L, Ghishen F K 1981 Intravenous lipid emulsions and human neutrophil function. Journal of Pediatrics 99: 913–916

Feldman E J, Dowling R H, McNaughton J, Peters T J 1976 Effects of oral versus intravenous nutrition on intestinal adaptation after small bowel resection in the dog. Gastroenterology 70: 712–719

Fouin-Fortunet H, Le Quernec L, Erlinger S, Lerebours E, Colin R 1982 Hepatic
alterations during total parenteral nutrition in patients with inflammatory bowel disease: a
possible consequence of lithocholate toxicity. Gastroenterology 82: 932–937

Friedman Z 1980 Essential fatty acids revisited. American Journal of Diseases of Children
134: 397–408

Frisancho A 1981 New norms of upper limb fat and muscle areas for assessment of
nutritional status. Amrican Journal of Clinical Nutrition 34: 2540–2545

Glynn M F X, Langer B, Jeejeebhoy K N 1980 Therapy for thrombotic occlusion of long-
term intravenous alimentation catheters. Journal of Parenteral and Enteral Nutrition
4: 387–390

Greene H L, Hazlett D, Demares R 1976 Relationship between Intralipid induced
hyperlipemia and pulmonary function. American Journal of Clinical Nutrition
29: 127–135

Grotte G, Meurling S, Wretlind A 1982 Parenteral Nutrition. In: McLaren D S, Burman D
(eds) Textbook of Paediatric Nutrition. Churchill Livingstone, Edinburgh. pp 228–258

Gurney J M, Jelliffe D B 1973 Arm anthropometry in nutritional assessment: normogram
for rapid calculation of muscle circumference and cross-sectional muscle and fat areas.
American Journal of Clinical Nutrition 26: 912–915

Gustafson A, Kjellmer I, Olegard R, Victorin L H 1974 Nutrition in low birth weight
infants II, Repeated intravenous injections of fat emulsion. Acta Paediatrica Scandinavica
63: 177–182

Hattner J A T, Kerner J A 1983 Indications for parenteral nutrition in pediatrics. In:
Kerner J A (ed) Manual of Pediatric Parenteral Nutrition. Wiley, New York pp 52–53

Heird W C, Driscoll J M, Schullinger J N, Grebin B, Winters R W 1972 Intravenous
alimentation in pediatric patients. Journal of Pediatrics 80: 351–372

Hughes C A, Dowling R H 1980 Speed of onset of adaptive mucosal hypoplasia and
hypofunction in the intestine of parenterally fed rats. Clinical Science 59: 317–27

Hughes C A, Prince A, Dowling R H 1980 Speed of change in pancreatic mass and in
intestinal bacteriology of parenterally fed rats. Clinical Science 59: 329–336

Hughes C A, Talbot I C, Ducker D A, Harran M K 1983 Total parenteral nutrition in
infancy: effect on the liver and suggested pathogenesis. Gut 24: 241–248

Kerner J A 1983 Fluid requirements. In: Kerner J A (ed) Manual of Pediatric Parenteral
Nutrition. Wiley, New York pp 69–73

Levine M J, Wigglesworth J S, Desai R 1980 Pulmonary fat accumulation after Intralipid
infusion in the pre-term infant. Lancet ii: 815–818

Macfie J, Smith R C, Hill G L 1981 Glucose or fat as a non-protein energy source? A
controlled clinical trial in gastroenterological patients requiring intravenous nutrition.
Gastroenterology 80: 103–107

Merritt R J, Blackburn G L 1981 Nutritional assessment and metabolic response to illness
of the hospitalised child. In: Suskind R M (ed) Textbook of Pediatric Nutrition. Raven
Press, New York. pp 285–307

National Center for Health Statistics Growth Charts 1976 Monthly Vital Statistics Report 25
(Suppl) No (HRA) 76–1120. Rockville, Md, Health Resources Administration

Nehme A L 1980 Nutritional supplement of the hospitalised patient: the team concept.
Journal of the American Medical Association 243: 1906–1908

Olegard R, Gustafson A, Kjellmer I, Victorin L 1975 Nutrition in low birth weight infants
III Lipolysis and free fatty acid elimination after intravenous administration of fat
emulsion. Acta Paediatrica Scandinavica 64: 745–751

Palmblad J, Bronstrom O, Uden A M, Venizelos N, Lahnborg G 1980 Intralipid and
reticuloendothelial blockade. Lancet ii: 1138–1139

Passwell J H, David R, Katznelson D, Cohen B E 1976 Pigment deposition in the
reticuloendothelial system after fat emulsion. Archives of Disease in Childhood
51: 366–368

Pereira G R, Fox W W, Stanley C A, Baker L, Schwartz J G 1980 Decreased oxygenation
and hyperlipemia during intravenous fat infusions in premature infants. Pediatrics
66: 26–30

Poole R L, Kerner J A 1983 The nutrition support team. In: Kerner J A (ed) Manual of
Pediatric Parenteral Nutrition. Wiley, New York pp. 281–4

Ralston C W, O'Connor M J, Ament M, Berquist W, Pannelee A M 1984 Somatic growth and developmental functioning in children receiving prolonged home total parenteral nutrition. Journal of Pediatrics 105: 842–846

Rigo J, Senterre J 1983 Parenteral nutrition in the very-low-birth-weight infant. In: Kretchmer N, Minkowski A (eds) Nutritional Adaptation of the Gastrointestinal Tract of the Newborn. Nestle, Vevey/Raven, New York pp 191–207

Schiff D, Chan G, Seccombe D 1979 Plasma carnitine levels during intravenous feeding of the neonate. Journal of Pediatrics 95: 1043–1048

Shaw J C L 1973 Parenteral nutrition in the management of sick low birth weight infants. Pediatric Clinics of North America 20: 333–358

Shennan A T, Bryan M H, Angel A 1977 The effect of gestational age on Intralipid tolerance in newborn infants. Journal of Pediatrics 91: 134–137

Stevenson J G 1977 Fluid administration in the association of patent ductus arteriosis complicating respiratory distress syndrome. Journal of Pediatrics 90: 257–261

Sun S C, Ventura C, Verasestakul S 1978 Effect of Intralipid-induced lipemia on the arterial oxygen tension in pre-term infants. Resuscitation 6: 265–270

Suskind R M 1981 The nutrition support service: an organised approach to the nutritional care of the hospitalised and ambulatory pediatric patient. In: Suskind R M (ed) Textbook of Pediatric Nutrition. Raven Press, New York pp 375–380

Tanner J M, Whitehouse R H. Takaishi M 1966 Standards from birth to maturity for height, weight, height velocity and weight velocity: British children 1965. Parts I and II. Archives of Disease in Childhood 41: 454–471, 613–635

Viteri T E, Alvarado J 1970 The creatinine height index, its use in the estimation of the degree of protein depletion and repletion in protein calorie malnourised children. Pediatrics 46: 696–706

Wallace W 1977 Fluid and electrolyte metabolism in infants and children: a unified approach. Ed: Weil W B, Balie M D Grune & Stratton, New York p 33

Index